I0044567

Diagnosis and Management of Chronic Liver Disease

Diagnosis and Management of Chronic Liver Disease

Editor: Heidi Hamlin

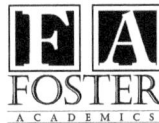

FA
FOSTER
ACADEMICS

www.fosteracademics.com

www.fosteracademics.com

FA
FOSTER
ACADEMICS

Cataloging-in-Publication Data

Diagnosis and management of chronic liver disease / edited by Heidi Hamlin.
     p. cm.
Includes bibliographical references and index.
ISBN 978-1-63242-680-2
1. Liver--Diseases. 2. Liver--Diseases--Diagnosis. 3. Liver--Diseases--Treatment. I. Hamlin, Heidi.
RC845 .D53 2019
616.362--dc23

© Foster Academics, 2019

Foster Academics,
118-35 Queens Blvd., Suite 400,
Forest Hills, NY 11375, USA

ISBN 978-1-63242-680-2 (Hardback)

This book contains information obtained from authentic and highly regarded sources. Copyright for all individual chapters remain with the respective authors as indicated. All chapters are published with permission under the Creative Commons Attribution License or equivalent. A wide variety of references are listed. Permission and sources are indicated; for detailed attributions, please refer to the permissions page and list of contributors. Reasonable efforts have been made to publish reliable data and information, but the authors, editors and publisher cannot assume any responsibility for the validity of all materials or the consequences of their use.

Trademark Notice: Registered trademark of products or corporate names are used only for explanation and identification without intent to infringe.

Contents

Preface   XI

Chapter 1

**Comparison of Efficacy and Safety of Tenofovir and Entecavir in Chronic Hepatitis B
Virus Infection**   1
Weixia Ke, Li Liu, Chi Zhang, Xiaohua Ye, Yanhui Gao, Shudong Zhou and Yi Yang

Chapter 2

Hepatitis B Surface Antigen Concentrations in Patients with HIV/HBV Co-Infection   9
*Jerzy Jaroszewicz, Thomas Reiberger, Dirk Meyer-Olson, Stefan Mauss, Martin Vogel, Patrick Ingiliz,
Berit Anna Payer, Matthias Stoll, Michael P. Manns, Reinhold E. Schmidt, Robert Flisiak,
Heiner Wedemeyer, Markus Peck-Radosavljevic, Jürgen Rockstroh and Markus Cornberg*

Chapter 3

**Impairment of the Organization of Locomotor and Exploratory Behaviors in Bile
Duct-Ligated Rats**   17
*Renata Leke, Diogo L. de Oliveira, Ben Hur M. Mussulini, Mery S. Pereira, Vanessa Kazlauckas,
Guilherme Mazzini, Carolina R. Hartmann, Themis R. Silveira, Mette Simonsen, Lasse K. Bak,
Helle S. Waagepetersen, Susanne Keiding, Arne Schousboe and Luis V. Portela*

Chapter 4

Hepatitis B Virus Gene Mutations in Liver Diseases   25
Abdul Malik, Deepak Kumar Singhal, Abdulmajeed Albanyan, Syed Akhtar Husain and P. Kar

Chapter 5

**A Genetic Validation Study Reveals a Role of Vitamin D Metabolism in the Response to
Interferon-Alfa-Based Therapy of Chronic Hepatitis C**   32
*Christian M. Lange, Stephanie Bibert, Zoltan Kutalik, Philippe Burgisser, Andreas Cerny,
Jean-Francois Dufour, Andreas Geier, Tilman J. Gerlach, Markus H. Heim, Raffaele Malinverni,
Francesco Negro, Stephan Regenass, Klaus Badenhoop, Jörg Bojunga, Christoph Sarrazin,
Stefan Zeuzem, Tobias Müller, Thomas Berg, Pierre-Yves Bochud and Darius Moradpour*

Chapter 6

**Serum Vitamin D Levels are not Predictive of the Progression of Chronic Liver Disease in
Hepatitis C Patients with Advanced Fibrosis**   40
*Kathleen E. Corey, Hui Zheng, Jorge Mendez-Navarro, Aymin Delgado-Borrego, Jules L. Dienstag and
Raymond T. Chung*

Chapter 7

Reproductive Status is Associated with the Severity of Fibrosis in Women with Hepatitis C   48
*Erica Villa, Ranka Vukotic, Calogero Cammà, Salvatore Petta, Alfredo Di Leo, Stefano Gitto,
Elena Turola, Aimilia Karampatou, Luisa Losi, Veronica Bernabucci, Annamaria Cenci,
Simonetta Tagliavini, Enrica Baraldi, Nicola De Maria, Roberta Gelmini, Elena Bertolini,
Maria Rendina and Antonio Francavilla*

Chapter 8

**Cancer-Associated Carbohydrate Antigens as Potential Biomarkers for
Hepatocellular Carcinoma**   57
*Chen-Shiou Wu, Chia-Jui Yen, Ruey-Hwang Chou, Shiou-Ting Li, Wei-Chien Huang,
Chien-Tai Ren, Chung-Yi Wu and Yung-Luen Yu*

Chapter 9

**Natural Killer Cells are Characterized by the Concomitantly Increased Interferon-c and
Cytotoxicity in Acute Resolved Hepatitis B Patients**   65
*Juanjuan Zhao, Yonggang Li, Lei Jin, Shuye Zhang, Rong Fan, Yanling Sun, Chunbao Zhou,
Qinghua Shang, Wengang Li, Zheng Zhang and Fu-Sheng Wang*

Chapter 10

**Clinical Usefulness of Measuring Red Blood Cell Distribution Width in Patients with
Hepatitis B**   76
YuFeng Lou, ManYi Wang and WeiLin Mao

Chapter 11

**The Treatment Cascade for Chronic Hepatitis C Virus Infection in
the United States**   82
Baligh R. Yehia, Asher J. Schranz, Craig A. Umscheid and Vincent Lo Re III

Chapter 12

**Dynamic Changes of Lipopolysaccharide Levels in Different Phases of Acute
on Chronic Hepatitis B Liver Failure**   89
*Calvin Pan, Yurong Gu, Wei Zhang, Yubao Zheng, Liang Peng, Hong Deng,
Youming Chen, Lubiao Chen, Sui Chen, Min Zhang and Zhiliang Gao*

Chapter 13

**The CXCR3(+)CD56Bright Phenotype Characterizes a Distinct NK Cell
Subset with Anti-Fibrotic Potential That Shows Dys-Regulated Activity in
Hepatitis C**   96
*Marianne Eisenhardt, Andreas Glässner, Benjamin Krämer, Christian Körner,
Bernhard Sibbing, Pavlos Kokordelis, Hans Dieter Nischalke, Tilman Sauerbruch,
Ulrich Spengler and Jacob Nattermann*

Chapter 14

**Discordance between Liver Biopsy and FibroScan in Assessing Liver
Fibrosis in Chronic Hepatitis B: Risk Factors and Influence of
Necroinflammation**   105
Seung Up Kim, Ja Kyung Kim, Young Nyun Park and Kwang-Hyub Han

Chapter 15

**High Hepatitis B Surface Antigen Levels Predict Insignificant Fibrosis in
Hepatitis B e Antigen Positive Chronic Hepatitis B**   113
*Wai-Kay Seto, Danny Ka-Ho Wong, James Fung, Philip P. C. Ip, John Chi-Hang Yuen,
Ivan Fan-Ngai Hung, Ching-Lung Lai and Man-Fung Yuen*

Chapter 16

Quantification of Hepatic Iron Concentration in Chronic Viral Hepatitis: Usefulness of T2-weighted Single-Shot Spin-Echo Echo-Planar MR Imaging   121
Tatsuyuki Tonan, Kiminori Fujimoto, Aliya Qayyum, Takumi Kawaguchi, Atsushi Kawaguchi, Osamu Nakashima, Koji Okuda, Naofumi Hayabuchi and Michio Sata

Chapter 17

Immunization with a Recombinant Vaccinia Virus that Encodes Nonstructural Proteins of the Hepatitis C Virus Suppresses Viral Protein Levels in Mouse Liver   128
Satoshi Sekiguchi, Kiminori Kimura, Tomoko Chiyo, Takahiro Ohtsuki, Yoshimi Tobita, Yuko Tokunaga, Fumihiko Yasui, Kyoko Tsukiyama-Kohara, Takaji Wakita, Toshiyuki Tanaka, Masayuki Miyasaka, Kyosuke Mizuno, Yukiko Hayashi, Tsunekazu Hishima, Kouji Matsushima and Michinori Kohara

Chapter 18

Psychological Stress Exerts Effects on Pathogenesis of Hepatitis B via Type-1/Type-2 Cytokines Shift toward Type-2 Cytokine Response   140
YingLi He, Heng Gao, XiaoMei Li and YingRen Zhao

Chapter 19

Predictability of Liver-Related Seromarkers for the Risk of Hepatocellular Carcinoma in Chronic Hepatitis B Patients   147
Yu-Ju Lin, Mei-Hsuan Lee, Hwai-I Yang, Chin-Lan Jen, San-Lin You, Li-Yu Wang, Sheng-Nan Lu, Jessica Liu and Chien-Jen Chen

Chapter 20

Decreased Peripheral Natural Killer Cells Activity in the Immune Activated Stage of Chronic Hepatitis B   157
Yuan Li, Jiu-Jun Wang, Shan Gao, Qian Liu, Jia Bai, Xue-Qi Zhao, You-Hua Hao, Hong-Hui Ding, Fan Zhu, Dong-Liang Yang and Xi-Ping Zhao

Chapter 21

Regulatory Phenotype, PD-1 and TLR3 Expression in T Cells and Monocytes from HCV Patients Undergoing Antiviral Therapy: A Randomized Clinical Trial   165
Shan-shan Su, Huan He, Ling-bo Kong, Yu-guo Zhang, Su-xian Zhao, Rong-qi Wang, Huan-wei Zheng, Dian-xing Sun, Yue-min Nan and Jun Yu

Chapter 22

Serum GP73, a Marker for Evaluating Progression in Patients with Chronic HBV Infections   175
Hongshan Wei, Boan Li, Renwen Zhang, Xiaohua Hao, Yubo Huang, Yong Qiao, Jun Hou, Xin Li and Xingwang Li

Chapter 23

Treatment of Naïve Patients with Chronic Hepatitis C Genotypes 2 and 3 with Pegylated Interferon Alpha and Ribavirin in a Real World Setting: Relevance for the New Era of DAA   183
Benjamin Heidrich, Steffen B. Wiegand, Peter Buggisch, Holger Hinrichsen, Ralph Link, Bernd Möller, Klaus H.W. Böker, Gerlinde Teuber, Hartwig Klinker, Elmar Zehnter, Uwe Naumann, Heiner W. Busch, Benjamin Maasoumy, Undine Baum, Svenja Hardtke, Michael P. Manns, Heiner Wedemeyer, Jörg Petersen and Markus Cornberg

Chapter 24

High Serum Levels of HDV RNA are Predictors of Cirrhosis and Liver Cancer in Patients with Chronic Hepatitis Delta   194
Raffaella Romeo, Barbara Foglieni, Giovanni Casazza, Marta Spreafico, Massimo Colombo and Daniele Prati

Chapter 25

The Association of HMGB1 Expression with Clinicopathological Significance and Prognosis in Hepatocellular Carcinoma   201
Lu Zhang, Jianjun Han, Huiyong Wu, Xiaohong Liang, Jianxin Zhang, Jian Li, Li Xie, Yinfa Xie, Xiugui Sheng and Jinming Yu

Chapter 26

Cys34-Cysteinylated Human Serum Albumin is a Sensitive Plasma Marker in Oxidative Stress-Related Chronic Diseases   209
Kohei Nagumo, Motohiko Tanaka, Victor Tuan Giam Chuang, Hiroko Setoyama, Hiroshi Watanabe, Naoyuki Yamada, Kazuyuki Kubota, Motoko Tanaka, Kazutaka Matsushita, Akira Yoshida, Hideaki Jinnouchi, Makoto Anraku, Daisuke Kadowaki, Yu Ishima, Yutaka Sasaki, Masaki Otagiri and Toru Maruyama

Chapter 27

Histological Changes in Kidney and Liver of Rats Due to Gold (III) Compound [Au(en)Cl$_2$]Cl   218
Ayesha Ahmed, Dalal M. Al Tamimi, Anvarhusein A. Isab, Abdulaziz M. Mansour Alkhawajah and Mohamed A. Shawarby

Chapter 28

A Serum MicroRNA Signature is Associated with the Immune Control of Chronic Hepatitis B Virus Infection   229
Maurizia Rossana Brunetto, Daniela Cavallone, Filippo Oliveri, Francesco Moriconi, Piero Colombatto, Barbara Coco, Pietro Ciccorossi, Carlotta Rastelli, Veronica Romagnoli, Beatrice Cherubini, Maria Wrang Teilum, Thorarinn Blondal and Ferruccio Bonino

Chapter 29

Genetic Association of Human Leukocyte Antigens with Chronicity or Resolution of Hepatitis B Infection in Thai Population   243
Nawarat Posuwan, Sunchai Payungporn, Pisit Tangkijvanich, Shintaro Ogawa, Shuko Murakami, Sayuki Iijima, Kentaro Matsuura, Noboru Shinkai, Tsunamasa Watanabe, Yong Poovorawan and Yasuhito Tanaka

Chapter 30

Effects of Nucleoside Analogue on Patients with Chronic Hepatitis B-Associated Liver Failure   249
Feng Xie, Long Yan, Jiongjiong Lu, Tao Zheng, Changying Shi, Jun Ying, Rongxi Shen and Jiamei Yang

Chapter 31

Anti-HDV IgM as a Marker of Disease Activity in Hepatitis Delta   257
Anika Wranke, Benjamin Heidrich, Stefanie Ernst, Beatriz Calle Serrano, Florin Alexandru Caruntu, Manuela Gabriela Curescu, Kendal Yalcin, Selim Gürel, Stefan Zeuzem, Andreas Erhardt, Stefan Lüth, George V. Papatheodoridis, Birgit Bremer, Judith Stift, Jan Grabowski, Janina Kirschner, Kerstin Port, Markus Cornberg, Christine S. Falk, Hans-Peter Dienes, Svenja Hardtke, Michael P. Manns, Cihan Yurdaydin and Heiner Wedemeyer

Chapter 32

**Genetic Variation in the Interleukin-28B Gene is Associated with Spontaneous
Clearance and Progression of Hepatitis C Virus in Moroccan Patients**   270
*Sayeh Ezzikouri, Rhimou Alaoui, Khadija Rebbani, Ikram Brahim, Fatima-Zohra Fakhir, Salwa Nadir,
Helmut Diepolder, Salim I. Khakoo, Mark Thursz and Soumaya Benjelloun*

Permissions

Contributors

Index

Preface

It is often said that books are a boon to mankind. They document every progress and pass on the knowledge from one generation to the other. They play a crucial role in our lives. Thus I was both excited and nervous while editing this book. I was pleased by the thought of being able to make a mark but I was also nervous to do it right because the future of students depends upon it. Hence, I took a few months to research further into the discipline, revise my knowledge and also explore some more aspects. Post this process, I begun with the editing of this book.

Chronic liver disease is a disease of the liver, which involves progressive destruction and regeneration of the liver parenchyma. This leads to fibrosis and cirrhosis. It encompasses a range of liver pathologies including chronic hepatitis, hepatocellular carcinoma and liver cirrhosis. The diagnosis of chronic liver disease is done through an examination of its symptoms which will vary according to the underlying cause such as nail clubbing, testicular atrophy, palmar erythema, leukonychia, asterixis, Dupuytren's contracture, parotid enlargement, cerebellar signs, etc. Some of the complications of chronic liver disease are synthetic dysfunction, portal hypertension, encephalopathy, hepatopulmonary syndrome, etc. Depending on the underlying cause, medications such as corticosteroids, antivirals, interferons, bile acids and other drugs may be prescribed. Supportive therapy including albumin, vitamin K, diuretics, antibiotics and nutritional therapy may help to prevent or manage complications of cirrhosis. This book aims to shed light on some of the unexplored aspects of chronic liver disease and the recent researches on this condition. It includes some of the vital pieces of work being conducted across the world, on the diagnosis and management of chronic liver disease. It is a vital tool for all researching or studying hepatology as it gives incredible insights into emerging trends and concepts.

I thank my publisher with all my heart for considering me worthy of this unparalleled opportunity and for showing unwavering faith in my skills. I would also like to thank the editorial team who worked closely with me at every step and contributed immensely towards the successful completion of this book. Last but not the least, I wish to thank my friends and colleagues for their support.

Editor

Comparison of Efficacy and Safety of Tenofovir and Entecavir in Chronic Hepatitis B Virus Infection: A Systematic Review and Meta-Analysis

Weixia Ke[9], Li Liu[9], Chi Zhang, Xiaohua Ye, Yanhui Gao, Shudong Zhou, Yi Yang*

Department of Epidemiology and Biostatistics and Guangdong Key Lab of Molecular Epidemiology, School of Public Health, Guangdong Pharmaceutical University, Guangzhou, Guangdong, China

Abstract

Objective: Tenofovir (TDF) and entecavir (ETV) are both potent antiviral agents for the treatment of chronic hepatitis B virus (HBV) infection. Multiple studies have compared efficacy and safety of these two agents, but yielded inconsistent results. Hence, we conducted a meta-analysis to discern comparative efficacy and safety.

Methods: Published data relevant to a comparison of TDF and ETV used in HBV were included. HBV DNA suppression rate, ALT normalization rate, and HBeAg seroconversion rate at 24 weeks and 48 weeks were reviewed. Drug safety profiles and resistance were also discussed.

Results: Seven articles met entry criteria. Four and six articles included data for 24 and 48-week HBV DNA suppression rates, respectively, and no significant differences for the rates between the two drugs were found in chronic HBV patients (TDF vs. ETV: relative risk [RR] = 1.10, 95% CI = 0.91–1.33 and RR = 1.07, 95% CI = 0.99–1.17 for 24 weeks and 48 weeks, respectively). For the ALT normalization rate (three studies for 24 weeks, four articles for 48 weeks) and HBeAg seroconversion rate (two and four studies for 24 weeks and 48 weeks, respectively), no difference was observed between TDF and ETV. Additionally, no significant distinction in short term safety was found for CHB patients.

Conclusions: TDF and ETV are similarly effective and safe in chronic HBV patients after 24 weeks and 48 weeks of anti-viral therapy. Nevertheless, the long-term efficacy and safety of TDF and ETV should be monitored in prolonged therapy.

Editor: Xiaoping Miao, MOE Key Laboratory of Environment and Health, School of Public Health, Tongji Medical College, Huazhong University of Science and Technology, China

Funding: This work was supported by Program for Guangdong Medical research Foundation (Grant No. B2012176), National Natural Science Foundation of China (NSFC-81302493) and Foundation for Distinguished Young Talents in Higher Education of Guangdong (Grant No. 2012LYM_0082). The funders had no role in study design, data collection and analysis, decision to publish, or preparation of the manuscript.

Competing Interests: The authors have declared that no competing interests exist.

* E-mail: yangyigz@163.com

[9] These authors contributed equally to this work.

Introduction

Chronic hepatitis B virus (HBV) infection remains a serious global health concern. Currently, approximately 2 billion people have been infected with HBV, and over 350 million are suffering from chronic hepatitis B (CHB) worldwide [1]. Cirrhosis, live failure, and/or hepatocellular carcinoma (HCC) are expected to develop in 15%–40% of patients with CHB without appropriate treatment [2], and approximately 1 million patients die annually of cirrhosis, liver failure, and HCC as a result of chronic HBV infection [3]. Therefore, the main goal of treatment of chronic infection is to effectively suppress viral replication, preventing liver disease, progression to cirrhosis, liver failure, and HCC [4–6]. Effective antiviral therapy via sustained HBV DNA suppression has become a priority research focus for chronic infection [4–6]. Available antiviral drugs include immunomodulatory drugs (interferon-alpha and pegylated interferon-alpha) and nucleotide analogue (NAs) polymerase inhibitors (lamivudine [LAM], adefo-

vir [ADV], entecavir [ETV], telbivudine [LdT], and tenofovir [TDF]). Since interferons are expensive, require parental administration, and cause side effects, oral nucleos(t)ide analogues are preferred [7]. Although LAM, ADV, and LdT are approved for the treatment of chronic HBV infection, high rate of resistance has plagued therapeutic use. At present, the two first line nucleoside/ nucleotides are ETV and TDF. ETV is a potent antiviral that effectively suppresses HBV DNA replication. It has a high genetic barrier for resistance in HBeAg-positive and HBeAg-negative patients [8–9] with a cumulative resistance probability of 1.2% after 5 years of treatment [10]. However, in lamivudine-refractory patients, the cumulative probability of genotypic ETV resistance developing over 5 years is 51% [11]. TDF is newer and considered a higher efficiency antiviral drug with a high genetic barrier. To date, no evidence exists to show development of resistance to TDF up to 144 weeks of therapy [12]. Moreover, TDF has been demonstrated to be effective in patients with both adefovir and lamivudine failure [13]. TDF is more effective than ETV to achieve rapid viral suppression in HBeAg-positive chronic HBV patients [14]. Additionally, the Bayesian meta-analysis by Woo *et al.* highlighted TDF as the more effective agent for HBeAg-negative patients during the first year of therapeutic intervention [15]. TDF is proposed to be superior to ETV for treating chronic HBV; however, a more promising result was shown by multiple studies claiming that both are similar in both efficacy and safety [16–21]. Due to the small sample sizes of past studies and subsequent limited data for comparing the two drugs, a more definitive conclusion is lacking. Herein, we conducted this meta-analysis by integrating published drug-based data to compare efficacy and safety of TDF and ETV and ultimately provide evidence for clinical decisions.

Materials and Methods

Literature search

Pubmed/Medline, Web of Science, EMBASE, The Wiley Online library, CNKI, WANFANG database, the Cochrane Central Register of Controlled Trials, and the Cochrane Database of Systematic Review databases were searched for relevant articles through June 30,2013 without language limitation. The search strategy was based on a combination of the key words "chronic hepatitis B virus or HBV or CHB", "entecavir or ETV", "tenofovir or TDF". Reference lists from retrieved documents were also scanned. Two reviewers independently screened citations and abstracts of each article (Wei-xia Ke and Chi Zhang).

Inclusion and exclusion criteria

The following inclusion criteria were used for this meta-analysis: (1) randomized and non-randomized control trials (included cohort or case-control studies), (2) study population consisting of patients with chronic HBV infection, and (3) intervention therapies of entecavir versus tenofovir monotherapy. The following types of studies were excluded: (1) studies of patients who were co-infected with HIV, HCV, or HDV, (2) studies of patients who adopted combination therapy or sequential therapy, (3) studies of individuals who used of immunomodulatory drugs or other nucleotide analogues within the preceding 6 months, (4) studies not reporting any efficacy measures or not conveying sufficient statistical information, and (5) studies not including either tenofovir or entecavir.

Efficacy measures

Efficacy was considered for patients 24 and 48 weeks post therapy by considering the following: HBV-DNA level (< 400 copies/ml), ALT normalization rate (<40 IU/ml), HBeAg seroconversion rate (HBeAg loss and the appearance of HBe antibody), and drug safety (adverse events, laboratory abnormalities, deaths, tolerability, etc).

Data extraction

Two authors extracted data independently and recorded the following for each publication: the first author's name, published year, country of study, time of study (start date and end date), number of patients, details of study design, patient characteristics (average age, gender, etc), treatment doses and duration, and outcome measures performed (described earlier). Where eligible, the authors of articles with insufficient data were contacted. If they did not provide data after contact, those articles were excluded from our meta-analysis.

Study quality

The two reviewers also assessed methodological quality based on following criteria: (1) Randomized controlled trials (RCTs) were assessed using the QUOROM guidelines and the Jadad scale [22]; (2) non-RCTs must have met the case matched by the patient's baseline data; (3) selected studies had defined inclusion and exclusion criteria for the study population and a clear definition of treatment responses. Reviewers resolved discrepancies through discussion.

Statistical analysis

Pooled rates for DNA suppression, ALT normalization, and HBeAg seroconversion were estimated using the inverse variance method. Relative risks (RRs) and 95% confidence intervals (CIs) as metrics of effect size were re-calculated for TDF versus ETV (as reference) in DNA suppression, ALT normalization, and HBeAg seroconversion rates. Inter-study heterogeneity was evaluated by the χ^2- based Cochran's Q statistic test and I^2 metric, with significance set at $P<0.10$ or $I^2>50\%$. In the absence of significant heterogeneity, the fixed-effect model,using Mantel-Haenszel method was applied to combine results [23]; In other cases, the random-effect method, using DerSimonian and Laird methods was applied [24]. Sensitivity analysis assessed whether a single study significantly affected overall estimates by sequentially removing studies. The Begg's rank correlation test and Egger's linear regression test were conducted for assessing publication biases. All statistical analyses were carried out in STATA V11.0, and all P values are two-tailed with a significant level at 0.05. This meta-analysis was conducted according to the Preferred Reporting Items for Systematic Reviews and Meta-analyses (PRISMA) statement (Checklist S1) [25].

Results

Search results and study characteristics

We identified 885 citations *via* electronic searches (Fig. 1). Seven were selected describing treatment of chronic HBV infection involving 844 patients (378 treated with TDF monotherapy and 466 treated with ETV monotherapy). Of these studies, two were RCTs [16–17], four were cohort studies [18–21], and one was a case-cohort study [14]. The detailed information of included studies is summarized in Table 1.

Study quality

Two manuscripts [16–17] were RCTs. One received Jadad scores of 5 and the other 3 (Table 2). For non-RCTs, all were well-matched based on baseline characteristics and clear definition of treatment response. With exceptions of Gao *et al.* [14] and Kurdas *et al.* [20] non-RCTs had defined inclusion and exclusion criteria for patients (Table 3).

HBV DNA suppression rate

For four studies evaluating patients post 24 weeks of therapy [14,17,20,21], the pooled HBV DNA suppression rates were 50% (95%CI = 25%–74%) and 46% (95%CI = 24%–68%) for TDF and ETV, respectively. No significant heterogeneity existed across studies (P for heterogeneity = 0.63; I^2 = 0%). In the fixed-effect model, no significantly difference was determined between TDF and ETV treatment groups in the HBV DNA suppression rate through 24 weeks of treatment (RR = 1.10, 95% CI = 0.91–1.33; Fig.2). Six studies compared HBV DNA suppression rates after 48 weeks of therapy (Fig.3), which were also similar for TDF (80%, 95%CI = 71%–90%) and ETV (76%, 95%CI 63%–88%). No significant heterogeneity was observed (P = 0.59, I^2 = 0%), and

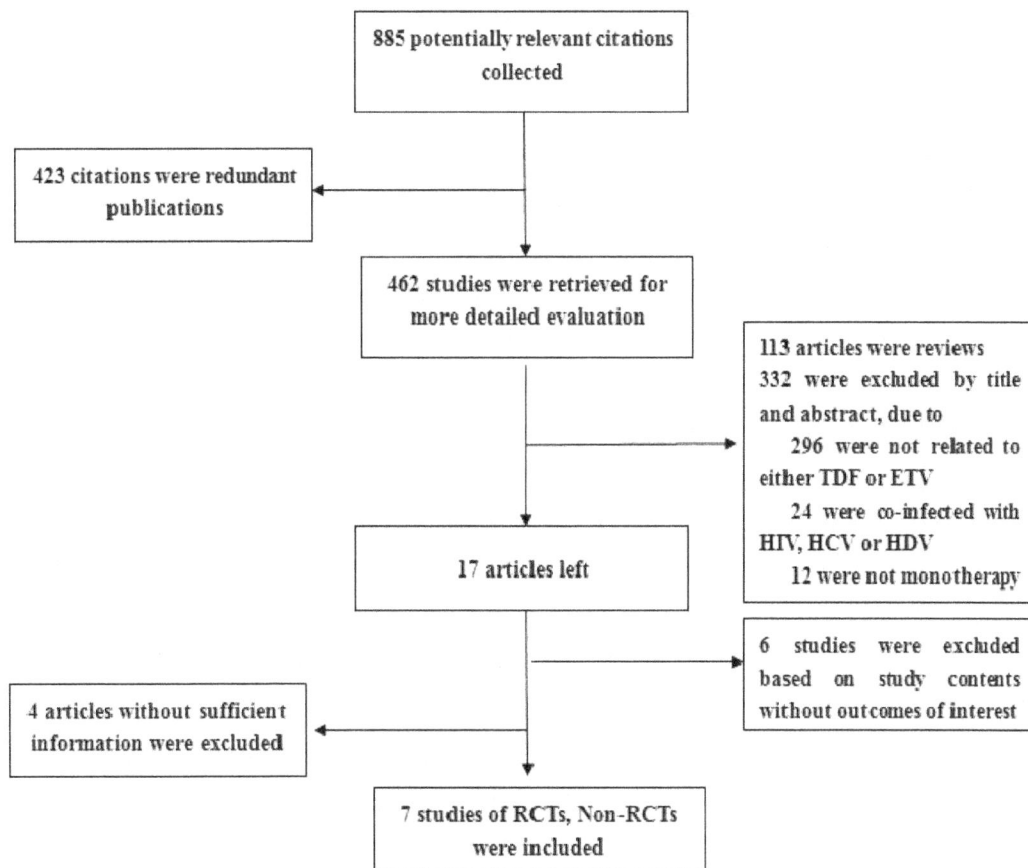

Figure 1. Flow diagram of selecting included studies.

no significant difference was also observed in that rate after 48 weeks treatment between the two treatment groups (RR = 1.07, 95%CI = 0.99–1.17). The statistic power for 24 and 48 weeks HBV DNA suppression rates were 92.08% and 85.03%, respectively.

ALT normalization rate

Pooled ALT normalization rates from three studies were 75% (95%CI = 59%–91%) and 76%(95%CI = 68%–83%) that included TDF and ETV groups 24 weeks post treatment, respectively. No significant heterogeneity was detected (P for heterogeneity = 0.19; I^2 = 40%). No significant difference between TDF and ETV for ALT normalization rate was calculated for 24 weeks post treatment (RR = 0.89, 95% CI = 0.77–1.04) (Fig.4). Four studies involved comparing ALT normalization rates after 48 weeks of therapy (Fig.5). The pooled rate for the TDF group (74%, 95%CI = 62%–86%) was similar to that of the ETV group (81.0%, 95%CI = 76%–86%). No significant difference was calculated after 48 weeks treatment between the two drugs (RR = 0.91, 95%CI = 0.83–1.01; P for heterogeneity = 0.26, I^2 = 26%).

HBeAg seroconversion rate

Two studies involved HBeAg seroconversion rates 24 weeks post treatment (Fig.6). Heterogeneity was found to be a concern (P for heterogeneity = 0.53; I^2 = 0%). The results of the two studies indicated that the pooled HBeAg seroconversion rate for the TDF group was 28% (95%CI = −10%–65%) and the ETV group

response rate was 29% (95%CI = −12%–59%). The pooled relative risk was 0.86 (95%CI = 0.45–1.66), suggesting no significant difference. Four studies were included to compare HBeAg seroconversion rates at 48 weeks post treatment (Fig.7). The pooled rates of 48 weeks post therapy were similar between TDF (16%, 95%CI = 0%–32%) and ETV (10%, 95%CI = 0%–20%). Heterogeneity was not found (P for heterogeneity = 0.39; I^2 = 1%), and a difference between the two groups was not significant (RR = 1.09, 95%CI = 0.57–2.11).

Tolerability and Safety of tenofovir and entecavir

Liaw et al. [16] found no significant differences between the TDF and ETV treatment groups for both co-primary safety endpoints (tolerability failures and confirmed changes in renal parameters) in decompensated CHB patients. Most adverse events (AEs) and laboratory abnormalities were consistent with decompensated cirrhosis, with few AEs related to these two agents. Sriprayoon et al. [17] reported no serious adverse events and no drop in renal function related to both agents. Additionally, for patients with HBV-related cirrhosis, Koklu et al. [18] concluded that TDF and ETV were similarly safe agents for long-term use. Furthermore, Dogan et al. reported that both drugs were well tolerated with minimal side effects. No significant increase in creatinine was detected. [19]

Virological breakthrough and resistance

Two studies referred to virological breakthrough or resistance. In the resistance surveillance by Liaw et al. [16], 13 patients (eight

Table 1. Main characteristics of included studies.

Study	Location	Ethnicity	Study design	Sample size TDF	Sample size ETV	Gender Male	Gender Female	Age(yrs) TDF vs. ETV	Baseline HBV DNA level	HBeAg (+)/(−) TDF	HBeAg (+)/(−) ETV	Status
Liaw [16]	Worldwide	Asian/White/Other	RCTs	45	22	54	13	Median (range): 52(48–57) vs. 54(47–58)	≥10³ copies/ml	14/31	7/15	Non-Naïve, Cirrhosis
Sriprayoon [17]	NA	NA	RCTs	100	100	NA	NA	Mean(SD): 42.4(11.5) vs. 40.8(11.0)	>2,000 IU/ml	52/48	54/46	Naïve, Cirrhosis
Koklu [18]	Turkey	NA	Cohort	72	77	114	35	Mean(SD): 54.2(10.5) vs. 52.4(11.2)	5.4±1.9log copies/ml	9/62	17/60	Non-Naïve, Cirrhosis
Dogan [19]	Turkey	NA	Cohort	65	29	58	36	NA	Detectable	29/36	10/19	Naïve, Cirrhosis
Kurdas [20]	Caucasus	Caucasian	Cohort	20	24	31	13	Mean (SD): 37.75(10.10) vs. 43.63(8.97)	≥6 log copies/ml	6/14	5/19	Naïve, Cirrhosis
Jayakumar [21]	India	NA	Cohort	19	20	35	4	Mean (SD): 34(9.60) vs. 42.15(17.11)	≥10⁴ copies/ml	10/9	15/5	Naïve, CHB
Gao [14]	U.S.	NA	Case Cohort	57	194	96	155	Mean: 41.6 vs. 43.2	>1,000,000 IU/ml	37/20	120/74	Naïve, CHB

Note: NA, not available; TDF, tenofovir; ETV, entecavir; SD, Standard Deviation; RCTs, randomized controlled trials; CHB, chronic hepatitis B.

Table 2. Methodical assessment of RCT studies.

Study	Adequate sequence genetation	Allocation concealment	Blinding	Incomplete outcome data addressed	Free of selective reporting	Free of other bias	Jadad
Liaw [16]	Yes	Yes	Yes	Yes	Yes	Yes	5
Sriprayoon [17]	Unclear	Unclear	Unclear	Unclear	Unclear	Unclear	3

Table 3. Methodical assessment of non-RCT studies.

Study	Case Matched	Well-defined inclusion and exclusion criteria	Clear definition of treatment responses
Dogan [19]	Yes	Yes	Yes
Jayakumar [21]	Yes	Yes	Yes
Koklu [18]	Yes	Yes	Yes
Kurdas [20]	Yes	Only inclusion criteria	Yes

TDF, two emtricitabine [FTC]/TDF, and three ETV) qualified for genotypic testing based on viremia through 48 weeks, and no patient developed resistance to any study drug throughout the 48 weeks. Two of three ETV patients with baseline lamividine resistance switched to open-label FTC/TDF due to insufficient viral suppression at week 24 (all three had HBV DNA < 400 copies/ml at week 48). Koklu *et al.* [18] reported that two of 77 patients switched from ETV to TDF at 24th and 40th month of treatment, respectively, because of virological breakthrough. No evidence for viral resistance to TDF was identified in these studies.

Sensitivity analysis

Sensitivity analysis was performed via the random-effect model only for the 48 weeks HBV DNA suppression rate (the rest of indicators confined to limited articles are not concerned). Pooled RRs were similar before and after removal of each study, and no single study significantly altered the pooled RRs, suggesting the robust stability of these results (Table 4).

Publication bias

Funnel plot shapes revealed no evidence of asymmetry for all efficacy measures. Begg's or Egger's test also showed no publication bias (all P values > 0.05).

Discussion

Entecavir (ETV) and tenofovir (TDF), two nucleotide analogs (NAs) are the most potent antiviral drugs for HBV infection [4–6]. Entacavir is a carboxylic analogue of guanosine that undergoes intracellular phosphorylation to its active 5' triphosphate metabolite. This form competes with the natural substrate deoxyguanosine triphosphate to inhibit HBV DNA polymerase, which is essential for viral replication [26]. Likewise, Tenofovir undergoes phosphorylation to mimic deoxyguanosine 5'-triphosphate. Once incorporated into the HBV DNA polymerase reaction, it functions as a chain terminator. ETV and TDF share a similar mechanism to suppress HBV DNA – they both compete with native substrates

for polymerase binding to terminate trascription [27]. Rates of HBV DNA suppression for TDF range from 68% to 90% and ETV from 61% to 92% after 48 weeks of therapy [28–32]. In our meta-analysis, results for pooled HBV DNA suppression rates for TDF and ETV were similar: 48 weeks post treatment were 80% and 76%, respectively, and 24 weeks post treatment were 50% and 46%, respectively. Furthermore, no significant differences in rates were seen between the TDF and ETV treatment groups (24 weeks: RR = 1.10 95% CI = 0.91–1.33; 48 weeks: RR = 1.07 95% CI – 0.99–1.17), suggesting similar efficacy for TDF and ETV in suppressing HBV DNA.

ALT level is a biomarker reflecting host immune response against virus-infected hepatocytes. ALT normalization usually follows a virological response and indicates cession of ongoing liver injury. In our meta-analysis, pooled ALT normalization rate for ETV was 76% and 75% for TDF. After 48 weeks of therapy, the pooled ALT normalization rate for ETV (81%) was similar to TDF (74%), indicating that both normalize ALT levels (24 weeks: RR = 0.89, 95% CI = 0.77–1.04; 48 weeks: RR = 0.91, 95%CI = 0.83–1.01).

Additionally, pooled HBeAg seroconversion for TDF was similar to the ETV group (24 weeks: 28% vs. 29%, RR = 0.86, 95% CI = 0.45–1.66; 48 weeks: 16% vs. 10%, RR = 1.09, 95% CI = 0.57–2.11). TDF and ETV do not greatly influence HBeAg seroconversion for HBV patients. Compared to pegylated interferon that enhances the host immune system to mount defense against HBV, oral NA therapy (including TDF and ETV) confers low HBeAg seroconversion rates at the end a year of treatment [33]. Furthermore, spontaneous seroconversion from HBeAg to anti-HBeAb during chronic hepatitis B is also immunologically mediated [3]. Therefore, it is plausible that TDF and ETV may have a marginal host immune system impact, yielding lower rates of seroconversion. This has yet to be supported.

Although oral nucleoside analogues, including ETV and TDF, are known to have relatively few side effects and are generally tolerated more than interferon, it is necessary to monitor long-

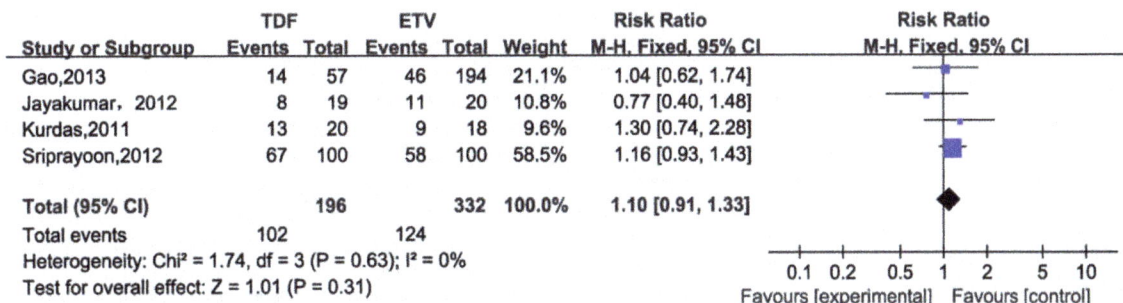

Study or Subgroup	TDF Events	Total	ETV Events	Total	Weight	Risk Ratio M-H, Fixed, 95% CI
Gao,2013	14	57	46	194	21.1%	1.04 [0.62, 1.74]
Jayakumar, 2012	8	19	11	20	10.8%	0.77 [0.40, 1.48]
Kurdas,2011	13	20	9	18	9.6%	1.30 [0.74, 2.28]
Sriprayoon,2012	67	100	58	100	58.5%	1.16 [0.93, 1.43]
Total (95% CI)		196		332	100.0%	1.10 [0.91, 1.33]
Total events	102		124			

Heterogeneity: Chi² = 1.74, df = 3 (P = 0.63); I² = 0%
Test for overall effect: Z = 1.01 (P = 0.31)

Figure 2. Forest plot for HBV DNA suppression rates 24 weeks post therapy.

Study or Subgroup	TDF Events	Total	ETV Events	Total	Weight	Risk Ratio M-H, Fixed, 95% CI
Dogan,2012	47	65	20	29	10.2%	1.05 [0.79, 1.40]
Gao,2013	39	57	120	194	20.1%	1.11 [0.90, 1.36]
Guzelbulut, 2012	19	20	21	24	7.0%	1.09 [0.91, 1.30]
Koklu, 2013	59	64	63	68	22.5%	1.00 [0.90, 1.10]
Kurdas,2011	19	20	21	24	7.0%	1.09 [0.91, 1.30]
Liaw,2011	31	44	16	22	7.8%	0.97 [0.70, 1.33]
Sriprayoon,2012	80	100	69	100	25.4%	1.16 [0.98, 1.37]
Total (95% CI)		370		461	100.0%	1.08 [1.00, 1.16]
Total events	294		330			

Heterogeneity: Chi² = 3.75, df = 6 (P = 0.71); I² = 0%
Test for overall effect: Z = 1.86 (P = 0.06)

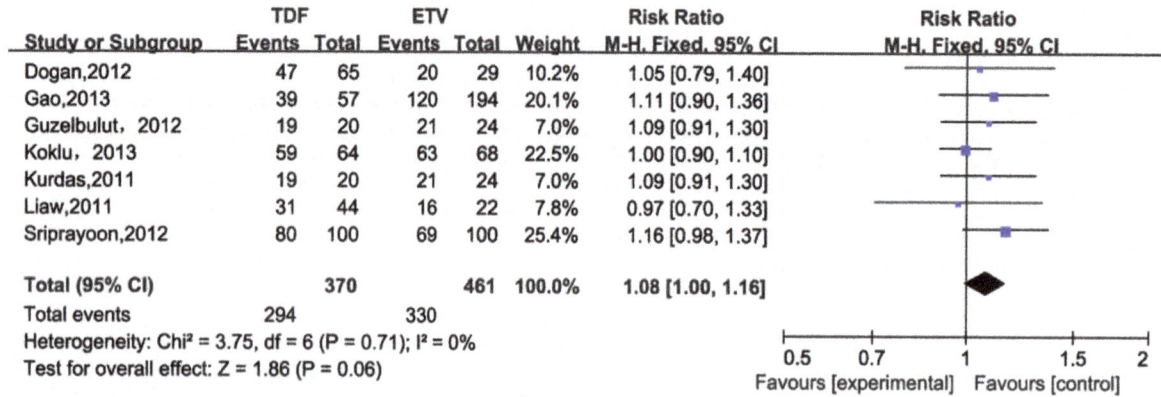

Figure 3. Forest plot for HBV DNA suppression rates 48 weeks post therapy.

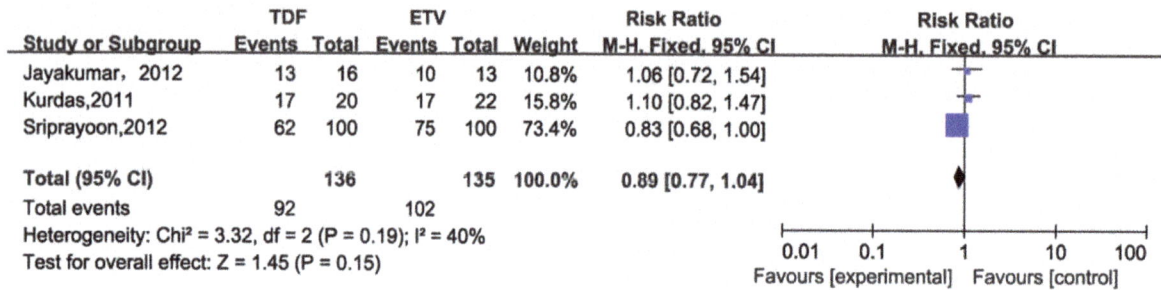

Study or Subgroup	TDF Events	Total	ETV Events	Total	Weight	Risk Ratio M-H, Fixed, 95% CI
Jayakumar, 2012	13	16	10	13	10.8%	1.06 [0.72, 1.54]
Kurdas,2011	17	20	17	22	15.8%	1.10 [0.82, 1.47]
Sriprayoon,2012	62	100	75	100	73.4%	0.83 [0.68, 1.00]
Total (95% CI)		136		135	100.0%	0.89 [0.77, 1.04]
Total events	92		102			

Heterogeneity: Chi² = 3.32, df = 2 (P = 0.19); I² = 40%
Test for overall effect: Z = 1.45 (P = 0.15)

Figure 4. Forest plot for ALT normalization rates 24 weeks post therapy.

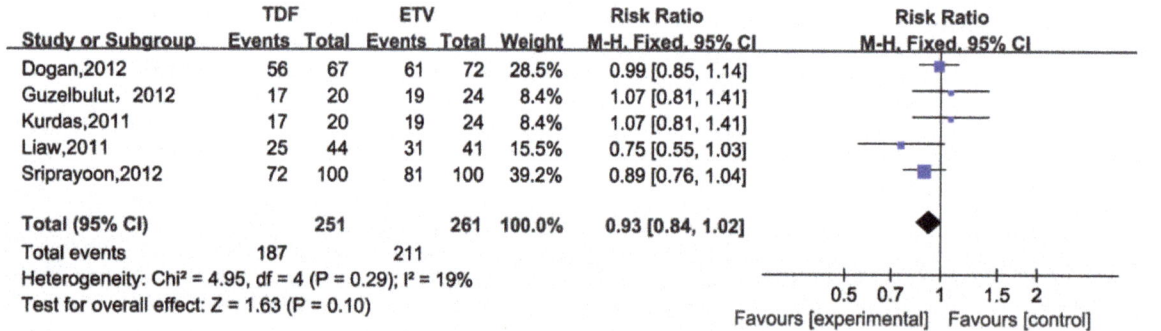

Study or Subgroup	TDF Events	Total	ETV Events	Total	Weight	Risk Ratio M-H, Fixed, 95% CI
Dogan,2012	56	67	61	72	28.5%	0.99 [0.85, 1.14]
Guzelbulut, 2012	17	20	19	24	8.4%	1.07 [0.81, 1.41]
Kurdas,2011	17	20	19	24	8.4%	1.07 [0.81, 1.41]
Liaw,2011	25	44	31	41	15.5%	0.75 [0.55, 1.03]
Sriprayoon,2012	72	100	81	100	39.2%	0.89 [0.76, 1.04]
Total (95% CI)		251		261	100.0%	0.93 [0.84, 1.02]
Total events	187		211			

Heterogeneity: Chi² = 4.95, df = 4 (P = 0.29); I² = 19%
Test for overall effect: Z = 1.63 (P = 0.10)

Figure 5. Forest plot for ALT normalization rates 48 weeks post therapy.

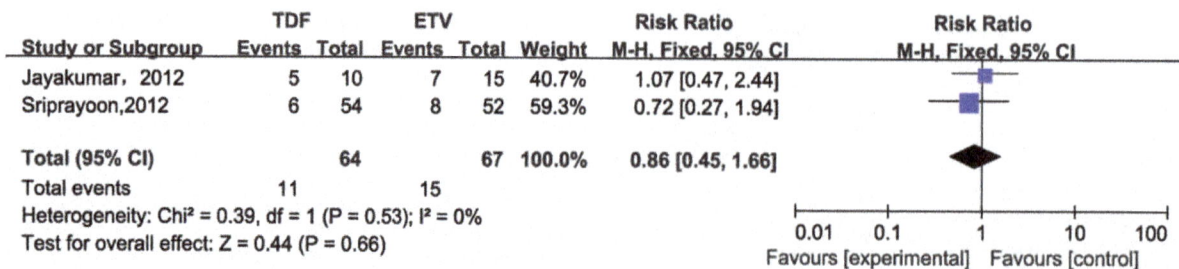

Study or Subgroup	TDF Events	Total	ETV Events	Total	Weight	Risk Ratio M-H, Fixed, 95% CI
Jayakumar, 2012	5	10	7	15	40.7%	1.07 [0.47, 2.44]
Sriprayoon,2012	6	54	8	52	59.3%	0.72 [0.27, 1.94]
Total (95% CI)		64		67	100.0%	0.86 [0.45, 1.66]
Total events	11		15			

Heterogeneity: Chi² = 0.39, df = 1 (P = 0.53); I² = 0%
Test for overall effect: Z = 0.44 (P = 0.66)

Figure 6. Forest plot for HBeAg seroconversion rates 24 weeks post therapy.

Study or Subgroup	TDF Events	Total	ETV Events	Total	Weight	Risk Ratio M-H, Fixed, 95% CI	Risk Ratio M-H, Fixed, 95% CI
Dogan,2012	0	65	1	29	14.7%	0.15 [0.01, 3.61]	
Kurdas,2011	3	6	1	5	7.8%	2.50 [0.36, 17.17]	
Liaw,2011	3	14	0	7	4.7%	3.73 [0.22, 63.66]	
Sriprayoon,2012	10	54	10	52	72.8%	0.96 [0.44, 2.12]	
Total (95% CI)		139		93	100.0%	1.09 [0.57, 2.11]	
Total events	16		12				

Heterogeneity: Chi² = 3.02, df = 3 (P = 0.39); I² = 1%
Test for overall effect: Z = 0.26 (P = 0.79)

0.005   0.1   1   10   200
Favours [experimental]   Favours [control]

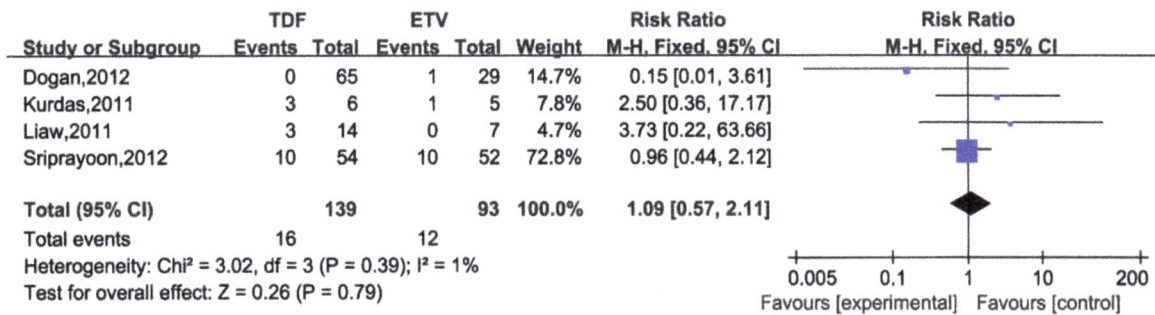

Figure 7. Forest plot for HBeAg seroconversion rates 48 weeks post therapy.

Table 4. Sensitivity analysis for the 48 weeks HBV DNA suppression rate.

Study omitted	RR	95% CI
Dogan, 2012	1.08	0.99–1.17
Gao, 2013	1.07	0.98–1.16
Koklu, 2013	1.10	0.99–1.22
Kurdas, 2011	1.07	0.98–1.17
Liaw, 2011	1.08	1.00–1.18
Sriprayoon, 2012	1.04	0.95–1.14
Combined	1.07	0.99–1.17

Note: RR, Relative Risk; CI, Confidence Interval.

term potential risks. ETV is classified as a category C drug and as it is associated with potential risk of fetal injury, it should be avoided during the first trimester of pregnancy [34]. TDF is eliminated mainly through nephrotoxicity [35], so all patients receiving TDF, creatinine clearance must be determined before and during therapy. Renal failure was not observed in Phase III clinical trials of TDF in patients with HBV monoinfection after up to 192 weeks of treatment [36–37]. Observation periods to date been too short, resulting in insufficient data to appraise whether difference exists for safety profiles of ETV and TDF.

To achieve long-term antiviral success, a high barrier to resistance is also critical for antiviral agents [38]. TDF and ETV both present low rates of resistance and have had success in patients failing to previous NA therapy [39–40]. Although resistance to ETV requires three mutations, pre-existing LAM resistance-associated mutations provide some foundation for ETV resistance [41–42] since resistance to ETV shares two common mutations (rtM204V and rtL180M) with LAM. In patients with LAM-resistant HBV, a high 6-year resistance rate of 57% has been suggested for ETV [10,43]. Undetectable HBV DNA is not always achieved and virological breakthrough has occurred with ETV [44]. Additionally, it has been reported that sequential monotherapy of ETV can further promote multidrug resistant mutations [45]. Therefore, ETV monotherapy no longer be considered an optimal first-line therapy against LAM-resistant HBV. Moreover, TDF is a beneficial alternative for LAM failure patients, despite an incomplete resistance profile [13,38,39].

Some limitations merit consideration. In our study, major included studies were non-RCTs (5 of 7 studies). It has been reported that some factors, geographic, ethnic or disease status

(CHB or cirrhosis) differences are possibly associated with agent efficacy. However, considering limited studies numbers for each factor, further analysis was restricted. Besides, due to the limited number of studies, analysis for some effect indicators might be underpowered (The power for 24 and 48 weeks HBV DNA suppression rates were 92.08% and 85.03%, respectively. The rest of indicators' powers are less than 80%). Although current related studies have shown TDF may be used as an alternative agent against HBV infection in drug safety and resistance, this study results still need more studies and reasonable statistic methods used to explore safety and tolerability of these drugs.

Our meta-analysis indicates that ETV and TDF are comparable in efficacy and safety to sustain HBV DNA suppression with limited side effects. However, in considering limited efficacy of ETV in patients with LAM resistance, TDF is an alternative agent against HBV infection. Nonetheless, long-term efficacy and safety of TDF and ETV should be monitored in prolonged therapy in well-designed prospective studies with large sample sizes.

Author Contributions

Conceived and designed the experiments: YY WXK. Performed the experiments: WXK CZ. Analyzed the data: WXK CZ. Contributed reagents/materials/analysis tools: XHY YHG SDZ YY. Wrote the paper: WXK LL.

References

1. Safioleas M, Lygidakis NJ, Manti C (2007) Hepatitis B today. Hepatogastroenterology 54: 545–8.
2. Lavanchy D (2004) Hepatitis B virus epidemiology, disease burden, treatment, and current and emerging prevention and control measures. J Viral Hepat 11: 97–107.
3. Ganem D, Prince AM (2004) Hepatitis B virus infection natural history and clinical consequences. N. Engl. J. Med 350: 1118–1129.
4. Liaw YF, Leung N, Kao JH (2008) For the chronic hepatitis B guideline workshop party of the Asian-Pacific Association For The Study Of The Liver. Asian-Pacific consensusstatement on the management of chronic hepatitis B: a 2008 update. Hepatol Int 2: 263–283.
5. Lok ASF, McMahon BJ (2009) Chronic hepatitis B: update 2009. Hepatology 50: 1–36.
6. European Association For The Study Of The Liver. (2009) Clinical practice guidelines: management of chronic hepatitis B. J Hepatol 50: 227–242.
7. Aggarwal R, Ghoshal UC, Naik SR (2002) Treatment of chronic hepatitis B with interferon-alpha: cost-effectiveness in developing countries. Natl. Med. J. India 15: 320–7.
8. Ayoub SB, Keefe EB (2008) Review article: current antiviral therapy of chronic hepatitis B. Aliment Pharmacol Ther 28: 167–77.
9. Leung N, Peng CY, Hann HW (2009) Early hepatitis B virus DNA reduction in hepatitis B e antigen-positive patients with chronic hepatitis B: A randomized international study of entecavir versus adefovir. Hepatology 49: 72–9.
10. Tenney DJ, Rose RE (2009) Long-term monitoring shows hepatitis B virus resistance to entecavir in nucleoside-naive patients is rare through 5 years of therapy. Hepatology 49:1503–14.
11. Tenny DJ, Pokornowsky KA, Rose RE (2008) Entecavir at five years show long term maintenance of high genetic barrier to hepatitis B virus resistance. Hepatol Int 2: A88–9.
12. Heathcote EJ, Marcellin P, Buti M (2011) Three-year efficacy and safety of tenofovir disoproxil fumarate treatment for chronic hepatitis B. Gastroenterology 140:132–43.
13. Patterson SJ, George J, Strasser SI (2011) Tenofovir disoproxil fumarate rescue therapy following failure of both lamivudine and adefovir dipivoxil in chronic hepatitis B. Gut 60: 247–54.
14. Gao L, Huy NT (2013) Tenofovir is more effective than Entecavir for achieving rapid viral suppression in HBeAg-Positive chronic hepatitis B patients with high HBV DNA levels. Gastroenterology 144: S–971.
15. Woo G, Tomlinson G, Nishikawa Y (2010) Tenofovir and entecavir are the most effective antiviral agents for chronic hepatitis B: a systematic review and Bayesian meta-analyses. Gastroenterology 139: 1218–29.
16. Liaw YF, Sheen IS, Lee CM (2011) Tenofovir disoproxil fumarate (TDF), emtricitabine/TDF, and entecavir in patients with decompensated chronic hepatitis B liver disease. Hepatology 53: 62–72.
17. Sriprayoon T, Lueangarum S, Suwanwela C (2012) Efficacy and safety of Entecavir versus Tenofovir treatment in chronic hepatitis B patients: A randomized controlled trial. Gastroenterology 1421: S695–S695.
18. Koklu S, Tuna Y, Taner M (2013) Long-term efficacy and safety of lamivudine, entecavir, and tenofovir for treatment of hepatitis B virus-related cirrhosis. Clin Gastroenterol Hepatol 11: 88–94.
19. Dogan UB, Kara B (2012) Comparison of the efficacy of tenofovir and entecavir for the treatment of nucleos(t)ide-naive patients with chronic hepatitis B. Turk J Gastroenterol 23: 247–52.
20. Kurdas O, Guzelbulut F (2011) Comparison of the efficacy of Entecavir and Tenofovir in chronic hepatitis B patients with high viral load and/or high fibrosis scores at week 48 of therapy. Gastroenterology 140: S930–931.
21. Jayakumar R, Joshi YK, Singh S (2012) Laboratory evaluation of three regimens of treatment of chronic hepatitis B: tenofovir, entecavir and combination of lamivudine and adefovir. J Lab physicians 4:10.
22. Jadad AR, Moore RA, Carroll D, Jenkinson C, Reynolds DJ, et al. (1996) Assessing the quality of reports of randomized clinical trials: is blinding necessary? Control Clin Trials 17: 1–12.
23. Mantel N, Haenszel W (1959) Statistical aspects of the analysis of data from retrospective studies of disease. J Natl Cancer Inst 22: 719–48.
24. DerSimonian R, Laird N (1986) Meta-analysis in clinical trials. Control Clin Trials 7: 177–88.
25. Moher D, Liberati A, Tetzlaff J, Altman DG, (2009) Preferred Reporting Items for Systematic Reviews and Meta-Analyses: The PRISMA Statement. PLoS Med 6(6): e1000097.
26. Langley DR, Walsh AW, Baldick CJ (2007) Inhibition of hepatitis B virus polymerase by entecavir. J Virol 81: 3992–4001.
27. Fung J, Lai CL, Seto WK (2011) Nucleoside/nucleotide analogues in the treatment of chronic hepatitis B. J Antimicrob Chemother 66: 2715–25.
28. Buti M, Morillas RM, Prieto M (2010) A viral load reduction > 3 log at 12 week of Entecavir treatment correlated with HBe seroconversion in HBeAg positive patients. Results from a real-life setting study. Hepatology 52: A409.
29. Lampertico P, Vigano M, Soffredini R (2011) Entecavir monotherapy for nuc-naïve chronic hepatitis B patients from field practice: high efficacy and favorable safety profile over 3 year. Hepatology 54: A1436.
30. Carey I, Nguyen HL, Joe D (2011) Denovo antiviral therapy with nucleos(t)ide analogues in 'real-life' patients with chronic hepatitis B infection: comparison of virological response between lamivudine + adefovir, entecavir vs. tenofovir therapy. Hepatology 54: A1396.
31. Ridruejo E, Adrover R, Cocozzella D (2011) Effectiveness of entecavir in chronic hepatitis B NUC-naive patients in routine clinical practice. Int J Clin Prac 65: 866–70.
32. Lampertico P, Sffredini R, Vigano M (2011) 2 year effectiveness and safety of tenofovir in 302 NUC-naïve patients with chronic hepatitis B: a multicenter European study in clinical practice. Hepatology 54: A1433.
33. Lin CL, Kao JH (2011) The clinical implications of hepatitis B virus genotype: Recent advances. J Gastroenterol Hepatol 26: 123–30.
34. Fontana RJ (2009) Side effects of long-term oral antiviral therapy for hepatitis B. Hepatology 49: S185–95.
35. Duarte-Rojo A, Heathcote EJ (2010) Efficacy and safety of tenofovir disoproxil fumarate in patients with chronic hepatitis B. Therap Adv Gastroenterol 3: 107–19.
36. Marcellin P, Buti M, Krastev Z (2010) Continued efficacy and safety through 4 years of tenofovir disoproxil fumarate treatment in HBeAg-negative patients with chronic hepatitis B (study 102): preliminary analysis. Hepatology 52:145A.
37. Heathcote EJ, Marcellin P, Buti M (2010) Three-year efficacy and safety of tenofovir disoproxil fumarate treatment for chronic hepatitis B. Gastroenterology 140: 132–143.
38. Zoulim F, Locarnini S (2009) Hepatitis B virus resistance to nucleos(t)ide analogues. Gastroenterology 137: 1593–608.
39. Van Bommel, de Man RA, Wedemeyer H (2010) Long-term efficacy of tenofovir monotherapy for hepatitis B virus-monoinfected patients after failure of nucleoside/nucleotide analogues. Hepatology 51: 73–80.
40. Reijnders JG, Deterding K, Petersen J (2010) Antiviral effect of entecavir in chronic hepatitis B: influence of prior exposure to nucleos(t)ide analogues. J Hepatol 52: 493–500.
41. Suzuki Y, Suzuki F, Kawamura Y (2009) Efficacy of entecavir treatment for lamivudine-resistant hepatitis B over 3 years: histological improvement or entecavir resistance? J Gastroenterol Hepatol 24: 429–35.
42. Karino Y, Toyota J, Kumada H (2010) Efficacy and resistance of entecavir following 3 years of treatment of Japanese patients with lamivudine-refractory chronic hepatitis B. Hepatol Int 4: 414–22.
43. Tenney DJ, Pokornoski KA, Rose RE (2009) Entecavir maintain a high genetic barrier to HBV resistance through 6 years in naïve patients. J. Hepatol 50: S10
44. Sheng YJ, Liu JY, Tong SW (2011) Lamivudine plus adefovir combination therapy versus entecavir monotherapy for lamivudine-resistant chronic hepatitis B: a systematic review and meta-analysis. Virol J 8: 393.
45. Petersen J, Buti M (2012) Considerations for the long-term treatment of chronic hepatitis B with nucleos(t)ide analogs. Expert Rev Gastroenterol Hepatol 6: 683–93.

Hepatitis B Surface Antigen Concentrations in Patients with HIV/HBV Co-Infection

Jerzy Jaroszewicz[1,7,8], Thomas Reiberger[2], Dirk Meyer-Olson[3,8], Stefan Mauss[4], Martin Vogel[5,8], Patrick Ingiliz[6], Berit Anna Payer[2], Matthias Stoll[3,8], Michael P. Manns[1,8], Reinhold E. Schmidt[3,8], Robert Flisiak[7], Heiner Wedemeyer[1,8], Markus Peck-Radosavljevic[2], Jürgen Rockstroh[5,8], Markus Cornberg[1,8]*

1 Department of Gastroenterology, Hepatology and Endocrinology, Hannover Medical School, Hannover, Germany, 2 Division of Gastroenterology and Hepatology, Department of Internal Medicine III, Medical University Vienna, Vienna, Austria, 3 Department of Clinical Immunology and Rheumatology, Hannover Medical School, Hannover, Germany, 4 Center for HIV and Hepatogastroenterology, Düsseldorf, Germany, 5 Department of Internal Medicine I, University of Bonn, Bonn, Germany, 6 Medical Center for Infectious Diseases (MIB), Berlin, Germany, 7 Department of Infectious Diseases and Hepatology, Medical University of Bialystok, Bialystok, Poland, 8 German Center for Infectious Disease Research (DZIF)

Abstract

HBsAg clearance is associated with clinical cure of chronic hepatitis B virus (HBV) infection. Quantification of HBsAg may help to predict HBsAg clearance during the natural course of HBV infection and during antiviral therapy. Most studies investigating quantitative HBsAg were performed in HBV mono-infected patients. However, the immune status is considered to be important for HBsAg decline and subsequent HBsAg loss. HIV co-infection unfavorably influences the course of chronic hepatitis B. In this cross-sectional study we investigated quantitative HBsAg in 173 HBV/HIV co-infected patients from 6 centers and evaluated the importance of immunodeficiency and antiretroviral therapy. We also compared 46 untreated HIV/HBV infected patients with 46 well-matched HBV mono-infected patients. HBsAg levels correlated with CD4 T-cell count and were higher in patients with more advanced HIV CDC stage. Patients on combination antiretroviral therapy (cART) including nucleos(t)ide analogues active against HBV demonstrated significant lower HBsAg levels compared to untreated patients. Importantly, HBsAg levels were significantly lower in patients who had a stronger increase between nadir CD4 and current CD4 T-cell count during cART. Untreated HIV/HBV patients demonstrated higher HBsAg levels than HBV mono-infected patients despite similar HBV DNA levels. In conclusion, HBsAg decline is dependent on an effective immune status. Restoration of CD4 T-cells during treatment with cART including nucleos(t)ide analogues seems to be important for HBsAg decrease and subsequent HBsAg loss.

Editor: James Fung, The University of Hong Kong, Hong Kong

Funding: This study was supported by the BMBF funded German Center for Infectious Disease Research (DZIF). The funders had no role in study design, data collection and analysis, decision to publish, or preparation of the manuscript.

Competing Interests: The authors have the following conflicts: Lamivudine, GlaxoSmithKline (GSK); Tenofovir and Emtricitabine Gilead; HBsAg test, Abbott, Roche, Siemens. Dr. Jaroszewicz received lecture fees or travel grants from Roche, Gilead and Abbott. Dr. Reiberger received support from Roche (travel grant, lecture fee, grant support), MSD (travel grant, lecture fee) and Gilead (travel grant, grant support). Dr. Meyer-Olson received lecture fees or travel grants from Abbott, Bristol Myers-Squibb, Boehringer Ingelheim, Chugai, Pfizer, Roche. Dr. Mauss received lecture fees Abbott, BMS, Gilead, Janssen, MSD, Roche, advisory board BMS, Gilead, Janssen, Roche. Dr. Vogel has been employed at Janssen-Cilag since June 2011. Dr. Ingiliz has received lecture fees/consultancy fees from Roche, MSD, Gilead, BMS, Abbott, Tibotec. Dr. Payer received support from Roche (grants, lecture fees), MSD (travel grants) and Janssen (travel grants). Dr. Stoll received lecture fees and/or consult fees by Abbott, BMS, Boehringer-Ingelheim, Glaxo-Smith-Kline, ViiV-Healthcare, Roche, Gilead, Janssen-Cilag, Tibotec, Pfizer, and Merck, Sharp & Dohme. Dr. Manns received grants, lectural fees and/or consult fees from GSK, Gilead, Novartis, BMS, and Abbott. Dr. Schmidt received grants lecture fees or consult fees from Gilead, Abbott and Roche. Dr. Flisiak received advisory Board fee from Gilead; Lecture fees from Gilead, Abbott and Roche. Dr. Wedemeyer received grants, lectural fees and/or consult fees from Gilead, Novartis, BMS, and Abbott. Dr. Peck-Radosavljevic received lecture fee/advisory board from Roche, BMS, Gilead, speaker fees/consulting fees from MSD and grant support from Roche and MSD. Dr. Rockstroh received lecture fees and consult fees from Abbott, BMS, Boehringer, Gilead, GSK, Janssen, Merck, Roche Tibotec, and ViiV. Dr. Cornberg received lecture fees and/or consult fees from GSK, Gilead, Novartis, BMS, Roche, MSD and grant support from Roche and MSD.

* E-mail: Cornberg.Markus@mh-hannover.de

Introduction

Chronic Hepatitis B virus (HBV) infection affects more than 350 million people worldwide. HBsAg clearance and anti-HBs seroconversion is associated with the best outcome in patients with HBV infection [1,2]. In the natural course of HBV infection and during antiviral therapy quantification of HBsAg is a useful tool to predict the chances for HBsAg clearance [3]. The decline of HBsAg concentrations may correlate with an effective immune response against HBV and is less dependent on direct viral suppression with HBV polymerase inhibitors. This statement is supported by data that interferon alpha induced stronger HBsAg decline compared to NA therapy [4,5]. Moreover, in a recent study HBsAg decline during NA therapy was correlated with high baseline interferon-inducible protein-10 (IP-10) levels [6], reflecting increased activity of the endogenous interferon pathway. Highest HBsAg levels are observed in immunotolerant HBeAg positive patients while lowest are detected in HBsAg carriers [7–9].

The link of the immune status and HBsAg concentrations may be of even greater clinical relevance in patients co-infected with the human immunodeficiency virus (HIV). The prevalence of chronic hepatitis B virus (HBV) infection in patients with HIV infection is 6–14% due to the shared routes of transmission [10]. The natural course of HBV infection can be more severe and progression of HBV related liver cirrhosis is faster in HIV positive patients [11]. Several nucleoside and nucleotide analogues (NA), inhibitors of the HIV reverse transcriptase, are also effective against HBV. One of the most frequently used NA as backbone of combined antiretroviral therapy (cART) against HIV is tenofovir, which is highly effective against HBV [12,13]. It has been documented that long-term therapy with tenofovir reduces the risk of liver cirrhosis in HIV/HBV co-infected patients [14]. Still, HBsAg clearance and subsequent seroconversion, which represents the ultimate goal of HBV treatment, is rare. A recent study in HIV/HBV co-infected patients documented a yearly HBsAg seroconversion rate of 2.6% [15]. Monitoring of HBsAg concentrations has so far mainly been studied in HBV mono-infected patients. Two recent studies have investigated HBsAg concentrations in HIV/HBV co-infected patients [16,17]. Both studies documented that HBsAg levels decreased only slowly despite complete suppression of HBV DNA replication during tenofovir treatment similar to reports in mono-infected patients [3]. The smaller study including 33 patients showed that HBsAg decline was not associated with HIV parameters such as HIV RNA or CD4 T-cell count. [16]. In contrast, the larger study from France including 143 patients demonstrated that HBsAg decline during TDF therapy was influenced by HIV induced immunodeficiency [17]. In HBeAg positive patients, HBsAg decline was significantly slower in patients with CD4 T-cell count <350/mm^3. This study suggests that the immune status is relevant for HBsAg decline but the body of evidence is limited.

Here we aimed to investigate the correlation of quantitative HBsAg and HIV parameters in 173 HIV/HBV co-infected patients in a cross-sectional study. Our data provide further evidence that the immune status is important for HBsAg decline.

Patients and Methods

Patients and Study Design

Two hundred and fifteen HIV/HBV co-infected patients were recruited in this multicenter, cross-sectional retrospective study in 6 centers in Germany, Austria and Poland between 2001–2011. In all subjects HIV infection (positive screening and confirmatory serological tests) and chronic hepatitis B virus infection (positive HBsAg for at least 6 months) have been documented. Participating centers included Vienna (n = 72), Hannover (n = 42), Duesseldorf (n = 36), Bonn (n = 26), Berlin (n = 21) and Bialystok (n = 8). Out of 215 patients, 42 had concomitant HCV and/or HDV infection. These patients were excluded from the analysis; the final cohort consisted of 173 HIV/HBV co-infected patients. There were 148 male (85%) patients with a median age of 40 (range 17–76 yrs), 123 (71%) were receiving combination antiretroviral therapy (cART) active against HBV for a median duration of 47 (7–95) months. Predominant route of infection was MSM (n = 93, 54%), followed by IVDU (n = 20, 12%) and heterosexual transmission (n = 14, 7%), while in 46 (n = 27%) the mode of infection was unclear or endemic. The detailed characteristics of the study cohort are given in Table 1. HIV/HBV co-infected patients not receiving cART (n = 46) were compared with HBV mono-infected subjects (n = 46) without history of anti-HBV therapy. Four untreated HIV/HBV co-infected patients could not be matched due to low HBV DNA and HBeAg positivity. The control group of

HBV mono-infected patients was selected from a well-defined cohort [7] and was matched for age, gender, HBeAg status and HBV DNA concentration (Table 2), which are the most relevant factors associated with HBsAg levels [3,7]. We analyzed HBsAg levels and HIV parameters at one time-point. In addition, nadir CD4 T-cell count was recorded.

This retrospective study was conducted in accordance with the guidelines of the Declaration of Helsinki, the principles of Good Clinical Practice and according to standards of the local ethics committees. The ethical committee of Hannover Medical School approved this research project and waived the need for written informed consent because routine diagnostic data have been analyzed anonymously.

Serum HBsAg Quantification

Serum HBsAg levels were retrospectively quantified from serum samples stored at −20°C. Serum HBsAg levels were quantified using the Abbott ARCHITECT® assay (Abbott Diagnostics, Abbott Park, IL). The test has a dynamic range of 0.05–250 IU/ml. Samples were diluted 1:100 in horse serum and if results were >250 IU/ml, samples were retested at a higher dilution. Samples with HBsAg levels <0.05 IU/ml were retested undiluted. Results are given in IU/ml. The inter- and intra-assay variability is approximately 10% (6.7–8.8%), according to the manufacturer datasheet. In addition, 26 HIV/HBV patient samples were also tested with the Roche Elecsys assay (Roche Diagnostics GmbH, Mannheim). The correlation of both assays was excellent (r = 0.99) (Figure S1).

HBV-DNA, HIV-RNA and T-cells Measurement

HBV-DNA was quantified with COBAS AmpliPrep/COBAS TaqMan (Roche Diagnostics, Mannheim, Germany) with a lower limit of detection (LLOD) of 12 IU/mL in Hannover, Vienna, Duesseldorf and Bialystok. In Bonn and Berlin HBV DNA was quantified with the Abbott RealTime assay which has a LLOD of 10 IU/ml. HIV RNA was measured COBAS TaqMan HIV-1 Test (Roche Diagnostics, Mannheim, Germany) with LLOD of 50 copies/mL (Hannover, Vienna, Duesseldorf, Bialystok) and by Abbott Real-time HIV-1 test with LLOD 40 copies/mL (Bonn and Berlin). CD4, CD8 and CD3 T-lymphocyte counts were evaluated by flow cytometer Navios in Hannover and Duesseldorf (Beckman Coulter, Krefeld, Germany), FACS Calibur in Vienna, Berlin and Bialystok (Becton Dickinson, Heidelberg, Germany or Schwechat, Austria).

Statistical Analyses

Serum HBsAg, HBV DNA and HIV RNA levels were logarithmically transformed. Data are presented as median (10–90% CI), unless indicated. Non-parametric (distribution-free) tests were applied. Mann–Whitney U and Kruskall–Wallis ANOVA tests were used for univariate and multivariate comparisons of independent continuous variables, Fisher's exact test for discrete variables comparison. Multivariate analyses were performed by a stepwise linear regression with HBsAg levels as dependent value. The significance level (α) was assumed for P-value <0.05 for a two-sided tests. Statistical analyses were performed with Statistica 9.0 (Statsoft, Tulsa, USA) and GraphPad Prism 5.0 (GraphPad Software, Inc, La Jolla, USA).

Results

HBsAg levels were quantified in 173 HIV/HBV co-infected patients (148 male, median age 40 yrs) recruited in 6 centers in Germany, Austria and Poland. In this large, multicenter, real-life

Table 1. Characteristics of HIV/HBV co-infected patients.

	Complete cohort (n = 173)	HBeAg(+) (n = 103)	HBeAg(−) (n = 70)
Age, years (median, 10–90% CI)	40 (27–53)	50 (25–54)	41 (28–52)
Gender, n (M/F)	148/25	93/10	55/15
cART (n, %)	123 (72)	72 (70)	51 (73)
cART duration, months (median, 10–90% CI)	47 (7–95)	49 (12–96)	46 (5–94)
Anti-HBV compound of cART:			
TDF+FTC (n,%)	71	44	27
LAM (n, %)	20	11	9
TDF+LAM (n, %)	18	10	8
TDF (n, %)	11	6	5
LAM+FTC (n, %)	3	1	2
CDC class:			
A (n,%)	60	29	31
B (n,%)	45	26	19
C (n, %)	49	36	13
Unknown (n, %)	19	12	7
HBeAg(+), n (%)	103 (59)	103 (100)	0 (0)
HBV DNA, $\log_{10}$ IU/mL (median, 10–90% CI)	1.30 (0.77–7.22)	1.94 (0.77–7.74)	1.30 (0.77–3.24)
HIV RNA, log10 copies/mL (median, 10–90% CI)	1.69 (1.60–4.49)	1.69 (1.60–5.12)	1.69 (1.60–4.87)
CD4 count, cells/μL (median, 10–90% CI)	373 (120–734)	355 (87–664)	417 (177–742)
Nadir CD4 count, cells/μL (median, 10–90% CI)	161 (16–409)	148 (11–393)	173 (23–420)
ΔCD4 count, cells/μL (median, 10–90% CI)	166 (0–501)	158 (0–431)	182 (0–518)
CD8 count, cells/μL (median, 10–90% CI)	845 (432–1691)	805 (406–1660)	915 (447–1811)
ALT, IU/mL (median, 10–90% CI)	33 (16–97)	34 (17–98)	30 (16–87)
AST, IU/mL (median, 10–90% CI)	34 (22–93)	37 (19–91)	32 (24–96)
INR (median, 10–90% CI)	1.00 (1.00–1.12)	1.05 (1.00–1.22)	1.00 (1.00–1.10)
Platelets, 10^3/L (median, 10–90% CI)	199 (117–291)	191 (111–289)	207 (117–315)

setting cohort more than half of patients were HBeAg positive (n = 103, 59%). One hundred twenty three patients (72%) received cART active against HBV for a median duration of 47 (7–95) months. The detailed characteristics of the study cohort are presented in Table 1.

Table 2. Characteristics of 46 HIV/HBV co-infected patients and 46 matched HBV-mono-infection patients not receiving anti-HBV therapy. Matched for age, sex and HBeAg status.

	HBV/HIV co-infection (n = 46)	HBV mono-infection (n = 46)	P-value
Age, years (median, 10–90% CI)	34 (23–51)	34 (22–54)	0.93
Gender, n (M/F)	40/6	40/6	1.00
HBV DNA, $\log_{10}$ IU/mL (median, 10–90% CI)	4.82 (1.07–8.04)	5.48 (2.27–8.06)	0.64
HBeAg(+), n (%)	26 (56)	26 (56)	1.00
ALT, IU/mL (median, 10–90% CI)	40 (23–228)	69 (18–207)	0.54
AST, IU/mL (median, 10–90% CI)	46 (30–131)	46 (24–149)	0.34
INR (median, 10–90% CI)	1.08 (0.90–1.50)	1.08 (0.95–1.45)	0.75
Platelets, 10^3/L (median, 10–90% CI)	175 (124–289)	213 (106–291)	0.22
HBsAg, $\log_{10}$ IU/mL (median, 10–90% CI)	4.29 (2.51–5.26)	3.94 (1.68–4.47)	0.02
HBsAg to HBV DNA ratio (median, 10–90% CI)	0.83 (0.54–2.56)	0.63 (0.46–1.32)	0.01

HBsAg Levels in the Entire HIV/HBV Co-infected Cohort

HBsAg levels showed a significant negative association with CD4 T-cell counts (R = −0.33, P<0.001, Fig. 1a). HBsAg levels did not correlate with CD8 T-cell counts (r = −0.08, P = 0.27). Thus, a negative association between CD4/CD8 T-cells ratio and HBsAg levels (r = −0.29, P<0.001) was analogous to the one observed between CD4 T-cell counts and HBsAg. Furthermore, the highest HBsAg levels were observed in patients with most advanced stage of HIV-infection (CDC C: 4.03, CDC B: 3.11, CDC A: 3.53 log10 IU/mL, ANOVA P = 0.01, Fig. 1b). HIV/ HBV co-infected patients with CD4 T-cell count below $200/mm^3$ had 1 $\log_{10}$ IU/mL higher HBsAg levels compared to patients with higher CD4 counts (4.30 vs 3.31 $\log_{10}$ IU/mL, P = 0.001, Fig. 1c). Nevertheless, HBV DNA remains the most important factor associated with HBsAg levels. Patients with undetectable HBV DNA had more than 1 $\log_{10}$ lower HBsAg level compared to patients with detectable HBV DNA (HBsAg 2.96 vs 4.33 $\log_{10}$ IU/ mL, P<0.0001, Fig 1d).

HBsAg Levels in HIV/HBV Co-infected Patients Treated with cART

123 HIV/HBV co-infected patients received cART active against HBV (Table 1). Median HBsAg levels in patients on therapy were lower by almost 1 $\log_{10}$ in comparison to untreated individuals (3.32 vs 4.23, P<0.001, Fig 2a). Comparing HBeAg positive and HBeAg negative patients, the difference in HBsAg levels between untreated and treated HIV/HBV co-infected patients was only significant in HBeAg positive patients (HBeAg positive 4.62 vs 3.71 IU/mL, P = 0.0003; HBeAg-negative 3.53 vs 3.02 IU/mL, P = 0.20). This suggests that anti-HBV therapy has more impact on HBsAg levels in HBeAg positive patients as also seen in HBV mono-infection [18].

HBsAg levels were higher in cART treated patients with HBeAg positive disease compared to HBeAg negative disease (4.62 vs 3.54, P = 0.002) and HBsAg was associated with HBV DNA (r = 0.56, P<0.001), while there was no correlation with ALT activity (r = 0.08, P = 0.34). Surprisingly, neither duration of anti-HBV therapy (r = −0.06, P = 0.51, Fig 2b) nor the anti-HBV regimen (ANOVA P = 0.59, Fig 2c) was associated with HBsAg levels. On the other hand, again the stage of HIV-infection was associated with HBsAg levels, with highest levels observed in CDC-C category (A: 3.31, B: 3.03 and C: 3.77, P = 0.01).

In this large cohort of patients receiving cART an inverse correlation between HBsAg levels and CD4 T-cell counts was observed (r = −0.34, P<0.001) (Table 3). Again, this association was much more pronounced in HBeAg positive patients (r = −0.38, P = 0.001) as compared to HBeAg negative HBV-infection (r = −0.31, P = 0.04). Of note, HBsAg levels were higher in patients with CD4 T-cells $<200/mm^3$ (4.03 vs, 3.22 $\log_{10}$ IU/mL, P = 0.003, Fig. 2d).

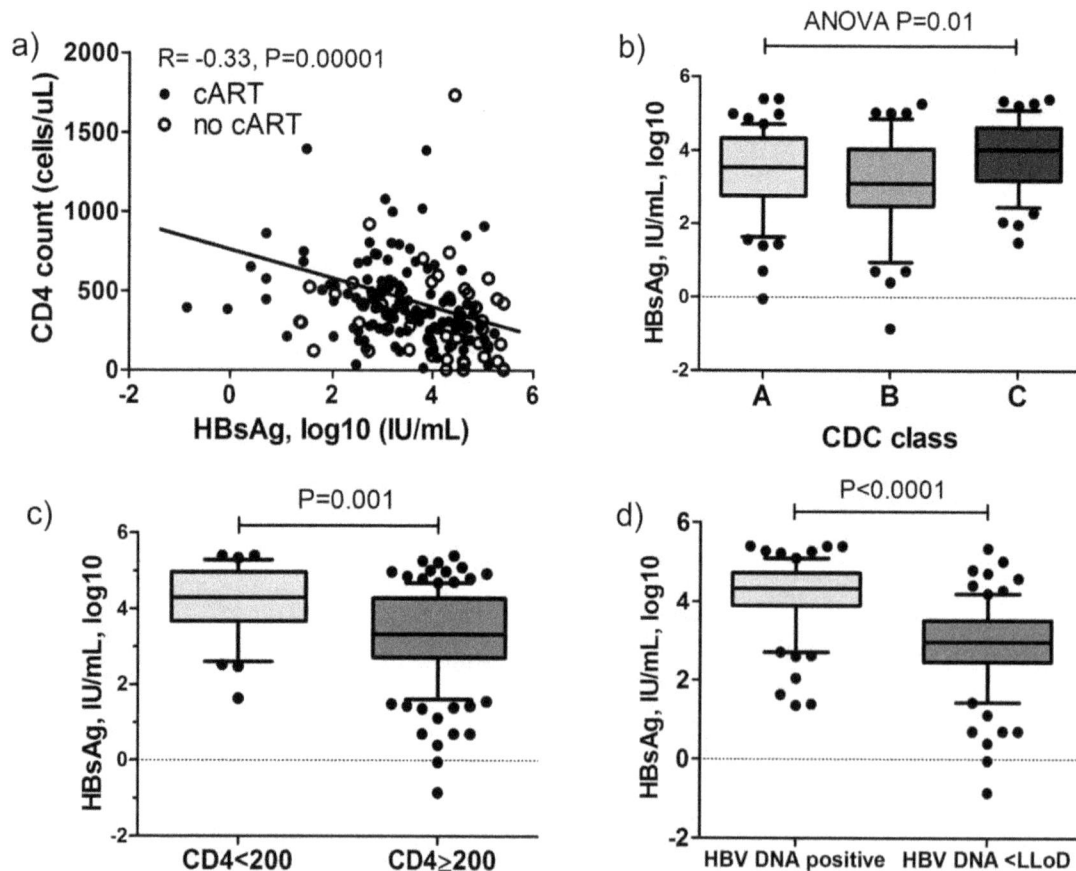

Figure 1. HBsAg levels in overall HIV/HBV cohort. a) Correlation of HBsAg levels with current CD4 T-cell count in all HIV/HBV co-infected patients. b) HBsAg levels in patients with different CDC stages. c) HBsAg levels in patients with CD4 T-cell counts <200 and $\geq 200/mm^3$ and d) in patients with undetectable HBV DNA (lower limit of quantification = LLOD) versus detectable HBV DNA. P-values obtained by Spearman correlation, U-Mann Whitney and Kruskall-Wallis ANOVA tests.

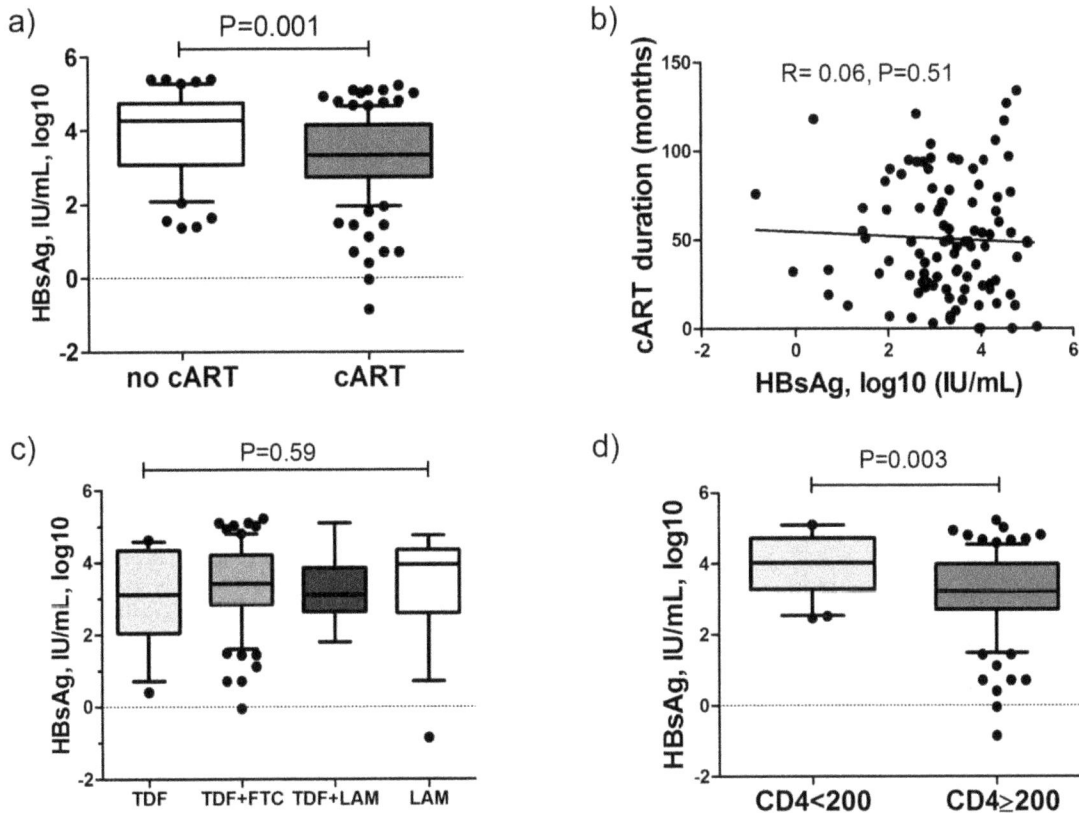

Figure 2. HBsAg levels in HIV/HBV patients receiving cART. a) Comparison of HBsAg levels in HIV/HBV co-infected patients receiving cART and not undergoing antiviral therapy. Lack of association between HBsAg levels and b) cART duration and c) cART regimen. d) HBsAg levels in patients receiving cART with current CD4 T-cell counts <200 and ≥200/mm³. P-values obtained by Spearman correlation, U-Mann Whitney and Kruskall-Wallis ANOVA tests.

In order to confirm these findings a multiple regression analysis with HBsAg levels as dependent value was performed in HIV/HBV co-infected patients receiving cART. HBsAg levels showed the strongest association with HBV DNA ($\beta = 0.51$, P<0.001). Among other factors with marginal significance CD4 T-cell count ($\beta = -0.21$, P = 0.06) and age ($\beta = -0.20$, P = 0.06) were noted

(Table 3). When we exclude HBV DNA from this analysis (because 77% of patients had undetectable HBV DNA), CD4 T-cell count was the only significant factor independently associated with HBsAg levels ($\beta = -0.30$, P = 0.006).

Finally, to explain an association between HIV related immunodeficiency and HBsAg levels in more detail we have

Table 3. Univarite correlations and linear stepwise multivariate regression analysis of HBsAg levels and clinical and laboratory parameters in HIV/HBV co-infected patients receiving cART.

Serum HBsAg (IU/mL) vs	Univariate correlations		Multivariate regression
	R-value	P-value	P-value
Age (years)	−0.17	0.06	0.06
Therapy duration (months)	−0.06	0.52	
HBV DNA (IU/mL)	0.45	<0.001	<0.001
HIV RNA (cps/mL)	0.24	0.02	0.15
CD4 count (cells/µL)	−0.34	<0.001	0.06
Nadir CD4 count (cells/µL)	−0.06	0.57	
ΔCD4 (cells/µL)	−0.25	0.01	
CD8 count (cells/µL)	0.02	0.98	
ALT (IU/mL)	0.09	0.34	
Platelets (10⁹/mL)	−0.13	0.17	

analyzed the effect of cART induced immune restoration, in this case a difference between current CD4 T-cell count and nadir CD4 T-cell count (ΔCD4). In patients receiving cART the median CD4 T-cell count increase was 166/mm^3 (16–409) and was not different between HBeAg positive and HBeAg negative patients (158 vs 182 cells/μL, P = 0.61). ΔCD4 showed a correlation with the duration of cART therapy (R = 0.25, P = 0.02) and also with HBsAg levels (R = -0.24, P = 0.02, Fig. 3a), suggesting a link between a restoration of immune functions and HBsAg levels. In patients receiving cART with ΔCD4>200/mm^3 HBsAg levels were significantly lower compared to patients with ΔCD4<200/mm^3 (3.31 vs 3.73 log10 IU/mL, P = 0.03, Fig. 3b). The distribution of HBeAg positive patients in the two groups was comparable (57% vs 62%, P = 0.59, respectively). The effect of immune reconstitution on HBsAg was more pronounced in HBeAg positive patients (Fig. 3c).

HBsAg Levels in Untreated Patients with HIV/HBV Co-infection

To assess a potential influence of HIV infection on HBsAg levels, we compared HBsAg levels in 46 HIV/HBV co-infected patients not receiving anti-HBV therapy with 46 HBV mono-infected untreated individuals matched for age, sex, HBeAg status and HBV DNA concentration, which are considered the most relevant factors associated with HBsAg concentrations [3,7]

(Table 2). HBsAg levels were higher in HIV/HBV co-infected patients vs. HBV mono-infected patients (4.29 vs 3.94 log10 IU/mL, P = 0.016) despite similar HBV DNA concentration (Fig. 4a). Thus, HBsAg productivity (HBsAg/HBV-DNA ratio) was significantly higher in patients with HIV/HBV co-infection (0.83 vs 0.63, P = 0.008, Fig. 4b).

Similar to previous reports in HBV mono-infected patients [7,8], HBsAg levels were significantly higher in HBeAg positive HIV/HBV patients compared with HBeAg negative HIV/HBV patients (4.62 vs 3.54 log10 IU/mL, P<0.001). Moreover, HBsAg levels showed a negative association with age (r = -0.28, P = 0.04) and a positive one with HBV-DNA (r = 0.37, P = 0.02). These correlations were less pronounced in HIV/HBV than in HBV mono-infected controls (r = -0.49, P<0.001 and r = 0.57, P<0.001, respectively). Not only HBV related factors influenced HBsAg concentrations. Also in untreated patients, HBsAg levels were higher in patients with more advanced stages of HIV-infection (CDC-A: 3.98, B: 4.46 and C: 4.63 log10 IU/mL, ANOVA P = 0.03, Fig. 4c). Secondly, in this limited number of patients we observed a trend towards a negative association between HBsAg levels and current CD4 T-cell counts (r = -0.24, P = 0.08). HBsAg levels tended to be higher in patients with CD4 T-cell counts below 200/mm^3 (4.61 vs 4.19 log10 IU/mL, P = 0.08, Fig 4d).

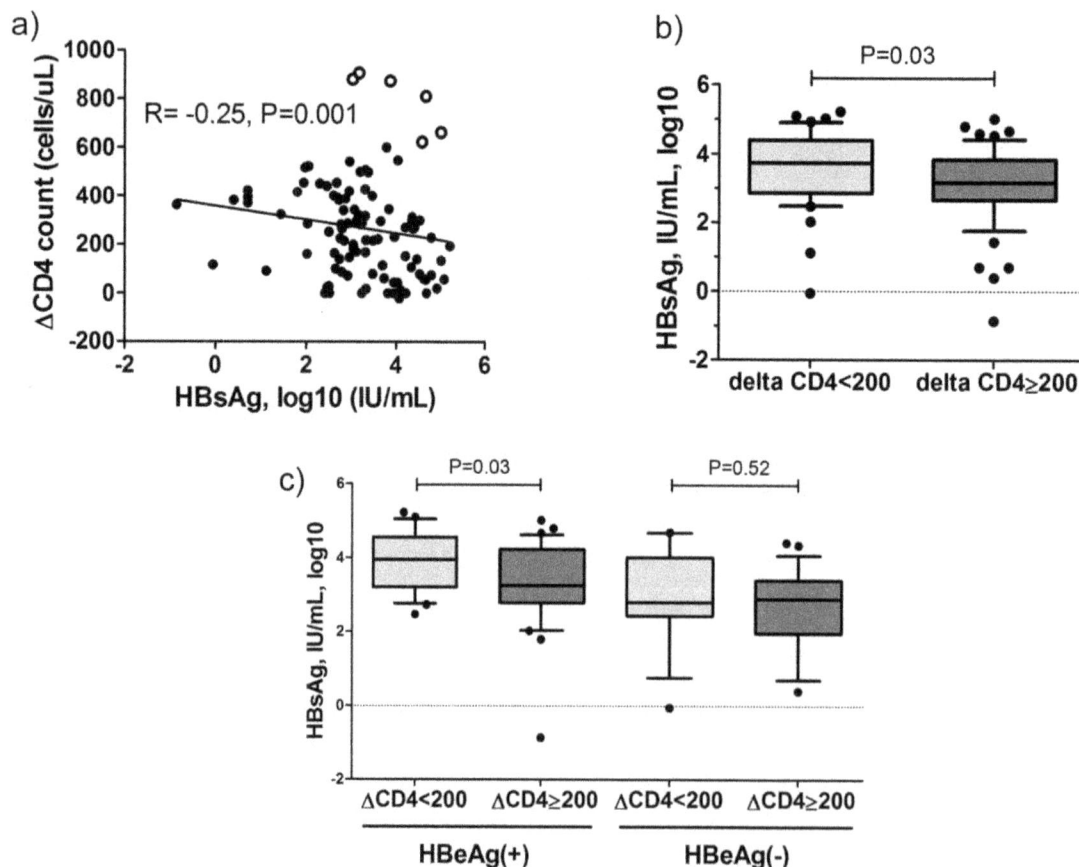

Figure 3. HBsAg levels and CD4 T-cell count dynamics. a) The correlation between CD4 T-cell count increase on cART (ΔCD4) and HBsAg levels (open circle denote outlier patients with delta CD4 T-cell >600/mm^3 but high HBsAg concentrations. 5/6 HBeAg positive, 3/6 (50%) had initially very low nadir CD4 T-cell count (9, 38 and 95 cells/μL). b) Differences in HBsAg levels in HIV/HBV co-infected patients with ΔCD4 T-cell counts <200 and $\geq$200/mm^3 in patients receiving cART and c) in HBeAg positive and HBeAg negative disease. P-values obtained by Spearman correlation and U-Mann Whitney tests.

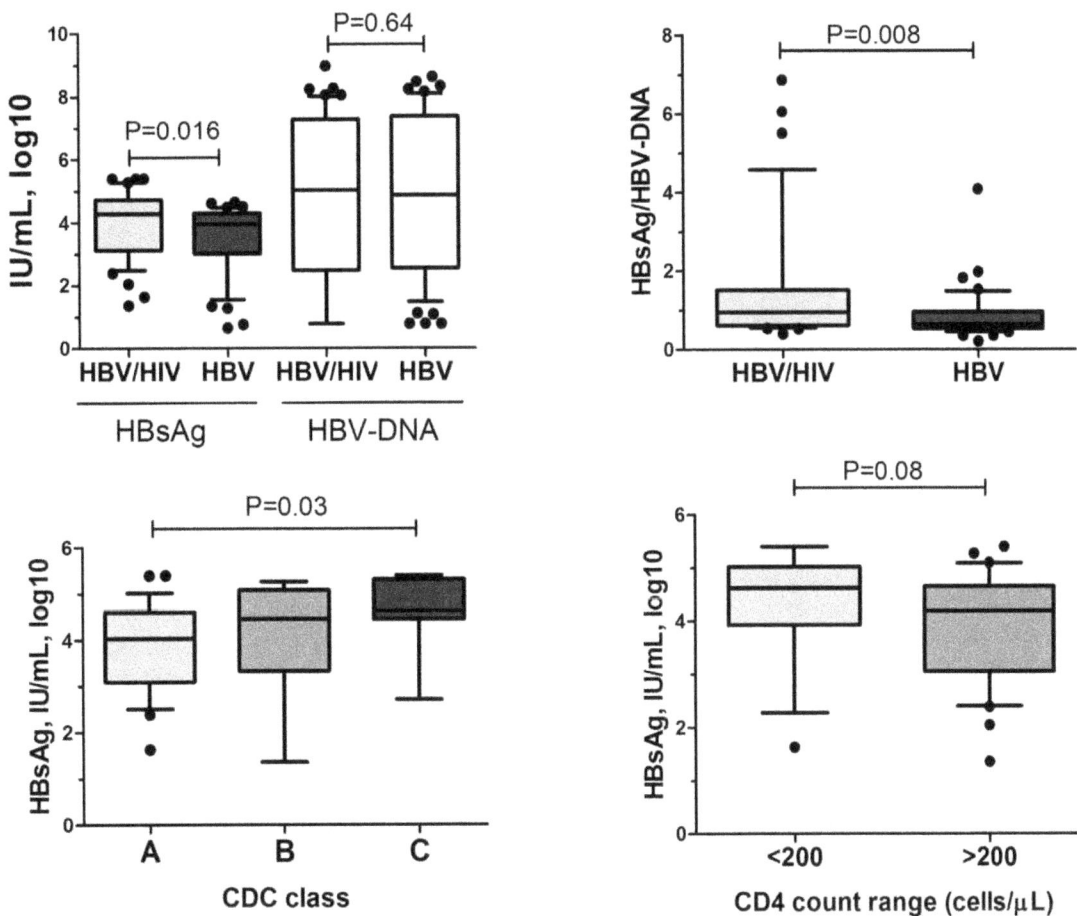

Figure 4. HBsAg levels in HIV/HBV patients not receiving cART. Comparison of HBsAg and HBV-DNA levels a) and HBsAg/HBVDNA b) in HIV/HBV co-infected patients not receiving cART with HBV mono-infected individuals without anti-HBV therapy matched for age, gender, HBeAg status and HBV DNA. HBsAg levels in HIV/HBV co-infected patients without cART in c) different CDC stages and d) in patients with CD4 T-cell counts <200 and ≥200/mm³. P-values obtained by U-Mann Whitney and Kruskall-Wallis ANOVA tests.

Discussion

In this retrospective multi-center study we provide data on HBsAg concentrations in a large cohort of HIV/HBV co-infected patients that further support the important role of the immune status for HBsAg decline.

In the overall cohort of 173 HIV/HBV patients we show a significant negative correlation between CD4 T-cell counts and HBsAg levels (Fig. 1a). We demonstrate that patients with less than $200/mm^3$ CD4 T-cells had significantly higher HBsAg levels compared to patients with higher CD4 T-cell counts (Fig. 1c) supporting the hypothesis that an intact immune status is important for inhibiting HBsAg production [6].

Combination antiretroviral therapy does not only restore CD4 T-cell counts but also inhibits HBV DNA, which both are relevant factors associated with HBsAg levels, especially in HBeAg positive disease [19] (Fig. 1d). Many studies have shown that HBV suppression by NA has only a limited effect on HBsAg decrease [5,6,18,20] with approximately $0.15–0.81 \log_{10}$ decline after 2 years during effective entecavir or tenofovir therapy [18]. The decline was documented to be higher in HBeAg positive patients than in HBeAg negative patients. In this study, patients on cART (median duration 3.9 years) had approximately $1 \log_{10}$ lower HBsAg levels compared to untreated HIV/HBV co-infected

patients (Fig. 2a). Considering that 60% of the HIV/HBV patients are HBeAg positive, the effect of NA therapy seems to be in the same range as in HBV mono-infected patients. We did not find a significant association between the NA regimen and HBsAg levels (Fig. 2c) and also HBV DNA (data not shown). This is in agreement with our data in HBV mono-infected patients where we did not observe a difference between potent NA (tenofovir, entecavir) and less potent NA (lamivudine, adefovir) in HBsAg decrease [6]. We also did not observe a correlation between treatment duration and HBsAg level. This could suggest that some patients may have experienced a stronger HBsAg decline and others not at all. In HBV mono-infected patients we have shown that approximately $1/5^{th}$ of patients experienced a pronounced HBsAg decline, while 28% had no decline at all during up to 9 years treatment [6]. The recent study by Thibault also confirmed that only 39% of HIV/HBV co-infected patients achieved any HBsAg decline during treatment containing tenofovir [16].

Most data suggest that direct targeting the HBV polymerase has limited impact on HBsAg levels. Nevertheless, HBV DNA suppression is important for HBsAg reduction. Also in HIV/HBV patients on cART, HBV DNA levels were the strongest factor associated with HBsAg concentrations (Table 3). After complete suppression of HBV DNA replication, some level of immune response is required to achieve further reduction of

HBsAg or even HBsAg loss. In HIV co-infected patients, cART including HBV polymerase inhibitors can restore CD4 immune responses that may explain the impact on HBsAg levels in HIV/HBV patients. Importantly, the difference of nadir CD4 T-cell count and CD4 T-cell count at the time of HBsAg quantification (ΔCD4) was significantly correlated with HBsAg concentrations in patients on treatment (Fig. 3a). For example, patients with a ΔCD4 count of $>200/mm^3$ had significant lower HBsAg levels than patients with ΔCD4$<200/mm^3$ (Fig. 4b). Our data suggest that the effect of ΔCD4 T-cell count on HBsAg levels may be stronger in HBeAg positive patients than in HBeAg negative patients (Fig. 3c). Patients with HBeAg positive wildtype HBV infection are in an earlier stage of infection. The immune status may have more impact during earlier stages of HBV infection compared to later stages of HBV infection where T cell responses against HBV might already be exhausted [21].

The most convincing data for the important influence of the immune status on HBsAg levels is given by our data in untreated HIV/HBV co-infected patients. Here we show for the first time that HBsAg levels and HBsAg production were significantly higher in untreated HIV/HBV co-infected patients compared to a well-matched control cohort of HBV mono-infected patients (Fig. 4). Importantly, both groups had similar levels of HBV DNA, which was the strongest factor associated with HBsAg (Table 3). Also in this cohort, the highest HBsAg concentrations were observed in patients with more advanced HIV disease (Fig. 1c). Older studies published before the era of potent antiretroviral/anti-HBV treatment showed that chronic hepatitis B in co-infected patients takes a more progressive disease compared to mono-infected patients [11]. The higher HBsAg concentrations in HIV/HBV co-infected patients may be one reason for this observation as high HBsAg levels have recently been associated with disease progression independent of HBV DNA levels [22]. However, a limitation of this study is that we cannot correlate HBsAg levels with the stage of liver disease, as liver biopsies have not been performed in the majority of patients.

In conclusion our data support the hypothesis that significant HBsAg decline requires both, HBV DNA suppression and an effective immune response. This study helps to explain why immunmodulatory therapies such as IFN are more effective in reducing HBsAg levels than NA alone [5] supporting the demand for new immunomodulatory treatment concepts to increase the rates of HBsAg clearance. Our results also support the recommendations to initiate cART early in HBV/HIV co-infected patients. Restoration of the immune response in an earlier phase of HBV infection may be important to achieve significant HBsAg decline during cART including HBV polymerase inhibitors. The study has limitations due to its cross-sectional approach. HBV mutations, adherence to therapy and HBV genotypes were not considered, which may have influenced HBsAg levels. Prospective longitudinal data are necessary to validate whether CD4 immune reconstitution has an impact on HBsAg decline and which specific immunologic pathways are involved.

Author Contributions

Conceived and designed the experiments: JJ MPM HW MC. Performed the experiments: JJ TR DMO SM MV PI BP MS. Analyzed the data: JJ HW MC. Contributed reagents/materials/analysis tools: JJ TR DMO SM MV PI BP MS MPM RES RF HW MPR JR MC. Wrote the paper: JJ HW MC. Drafting the article or critically revising it and final approval: JJ TR DMO SM MV PI BAP MS MPM RES RF HW MPR JR MC.

References

1. European Association for the Study of the Liver(2012) EASL Clinical Practice Guidelines: management of chronic hepatitis B. J Hepatol 57: 167–185.
2. Cornberg M, Jaroszewicz J, Manns MP, Wedemeyer H (2010) Treatment of chronic hepatitis B. Minerva Gastroenterol Dietol 56: 451–465.
3. Chan HL, Thompson A, Martinot-Peignoux M, Piratvisuth T, Cornberg M, et al. (2011) Hepatitis B surface antigen Quantification: Why and How to use it in 2011 - A Core Group Report. J Hepatol 55: 1121–31.
4. Brunetto MR, Moriconi F, Bonino F, Lau GK, Farci P, et al. (2009) Hepatitis B virus surface antigen levels: a guide to sustained response to peginterferon alfa-2a in HBeAg-negative chronic hepatitis B. Hepatology 49: 1141–1150.
5. Reijnders JG, Rijckborst V, Sonneveld MJ, Scherbeijn SM, Boucher CA, et al. (2010) Kinetics of hepatitis B surface antigen differ between treatment with peginterferon and entecavir. J Hepatol 54: 449–54.
6. Jaroszewicz J, Ho H, Markova A, Deterding K, Wursthorn K, et al. (2011) Hepatitis B surface antigen (HBsAg) decrease and serum interferon-inducible protein-10 levels as predictive markers for HBsAg loss during treatment with nucleoside/nucleotide analogues. Antivir Ther 16: 915–924.
7. Jaroszewicz J, Calle Serrano B, Wursthorn K, Deterding K, Schlue J, et al. (2010) Hepatitis B surface antigen (HBsAg) levels in the natural history of hepatitis B virus (HBV)-infection: a European perspective. J Hepatol 52: 514–522.
8. Nguyen T, Thompson AJ, Bowden S, Croagh C, Bell S, et al. (2010) Hepatitis B surface antigen levels during the natural history of chronic hepatitis B: a perspective on Asia. J Hepatol 52: 508–513.
9. Brunetto MR, Oliveri F, Colombatto P, Moriconi F, Ciccorossi P, et al. (2010) Hepatitis B surface antigen serum levels help to distinguish active from inactive hepatitis B virus genotype D carriers. Gastroenterology 139: 483–490.
10. Alter MJ (2006) Epidemiology of viral hepatitis and HIV co-infection. J Hepatol 44: S6–9.
11. Thio CL (2003) Hepatitis B in the human immunodeficiency virus-infected patient: epidemiology, natural history, and treatment. Semin Liver Dis 23: 125–136.
12. van Bommel F, Wunsche T, Schurmann D, Berg T (2002) Tenofovir treatment in patients with lamivudine-resistant hepatitis B mutants strongly affects viral replication. Hepatology 36(2): 507–508.
13. Heathcote EJ, Marcellin P, Buti M, Gane E, De Man RA, et al. (2011) Three-year efficacy and safety of tenofovir disoproxil fumarate treatment for chronic hepatitis B. Gastroenterology 140: 132–143.
14. Tuma P, Medrano J, Resino S, Vispo E, Madejon A, et al. (2010) Incidence of liver cirrhosis in HIV-infected patients with chronic hepatitis B or C in the era of highly active antiretroviral therapy. Antivir Ther 15: 881–886.
15. Martin-Carbonero L, Teixeira T, Poveda E, Plaza Z, Vispo E, et al. (2011) Clinical and virological outcomes in HIV-infected patients with chronic hepatitis B on long-term nucleos(t)ide analogues. AIDS 25: 73–79.
16. Thibault V, Stitou H, Desire N, Valantin MA, Tubiana R, et al. (2011) Six-year follow-up of hepatitis B surface antigen concentrations in tenofovir disoproxil fumarate treated HIV-HBV-coinfected patients. Antivir Ther 16: 199–205.
17. Maylin S, Boyd A, Lavocat F, Gozlan J, Lascoux-Combe C, et al. (2012) Kinetics of HBs and HBe antigen and prediction of treatment response to tenofovir in antiretroviral-experienced HIV-HBV infected patients. AIDS 26: 939–949.
18. Zoutendijk R, Hansen BE, van Vuuren AJ, Boucher CA, Janssen HL (2011) Serum HBsAg decline during long-term potent nucleos(t)ide analogue therapy for chronic hepatitis B and prediction of HBsAg loss. J Infect Dis 204: 415–418.
19. Thompson AJ, Nguyen T, Iser D, Ayres A, Jackson K, et al. (2010) Serum hepatitis B surface antigen and hepatitis B e antigen titers: disease phase influences correlation with viral load and intrahepatic hepatitis B virus markers. Hepatology 51: 1933–1944.
20. Wursthorn K, Jung M, Riva A, Goodman ZD, Lopez P, et al. (2010) Kinetics of hepatitis B surface antigen decline during 3 years of telbivudine treatment in hepatitis B e antigen-positive patients. Hepatology 52: 1611–1620.
21. Rehermann B (2007) Chronic infections with hepatotropic viruses: mechanisms of impairment of cellular immune responses. Semin Liver Dis 27: 152–160.
22. Chen CJ, Lee MH, Liu J, Batrla-Utermann R, Jen CL, et al. (2011) Quantitative serum levels of hepatitis B virus DNA and surface antigen are independent risk predictors of hepatocellular carcinoma. Hepatology 54: 881A–881A.

Impairment of the Organization of Locomotor and Exploratory Behaviors in Bile Duct-Ligated Rats

Renata Leke[1][*][¤], Diogo L. de Oliveira[1], Ben Hur M. Mussulini[1], Mery S. Pereira[1], Vanessa Kazlauckas[1], Guilherme Mazzini[1], Carolina R. Hartmann[2], Themis R. Silveira[3], Mette Simonsen[4], Lasse K. Bak[6], Helle S. Waagepetersen[6], Susanne Keiding[4,5], Arne Schousboe[6], Luis V. Portela[1]

1 Department of Biochemistry, ICBS, Federal University of Rio Grande do Sul, Porto Alegre, Rio Grande do Sol, Brazil, 2 Department of Pathology, Hospital de Clínicas de Porto Alegre, Porto Alegre, Rio Grande do Sol, Brazil, 3 Experimental Hepatology and Gastroenterology Laboratory, Research Center of Hospital de Clínicas de Porto Alegre, Post-Graduation in Child and Adolescents Health, Federal University of Rio Grande do Sul, Porto Alegre, Rio Grande do Sol, Brazil, 4 Positron Emission Tomography Centre, Aarhus University Hospital, Aarhus, Denmark, 5 Department of Medicine V, Hepatology and Gastroenterology, Aarhus University Hospital, Aarhus, Denmark, 6 Department of Drug Design and Pharmacology, Faculty of Health and Medical Sciences, University of Copenhagen, Copenhagen, Denmark

Abstract

Hepatic encephalopathy (HE) arises from acute or chronic liver diseases and leads to several problems, including motor impairment. Animal models of chronic liver disease have extensively investigated the mechanisms of this disease. Impairment of locomotor activity has been described in different rat models. However, these studies are controversial and the majority has primarily analyzed activity parameters. Therefore, the aim of the present study was to evaluate locomotor and exploratory behavior in bile duct-ligated (BDL) rats to explore the spatial and temporal structure of behavior. Adult female Wistar rats underwent common bile duct ligation (BDL rats) or the manipulation of common bile duct without ligation (control rats). Six weeks after surgery, control and BDL rats underwent open-field, plus-maze and foot-fault behavioral tasks. The BDL rats developed chronic liver failure and exhibited a decrease in total distance traveled, increased total immobility time, smaller number of rearings, longer periods in the home base area and decreased percentage of time in the center zone of the arena, when compared to the control rats. Moreover, the performance of the BDL rats was not different from the control rats for the elevated plus-maze and foot-fault tasks. Therefore, the BDL rats demonstrated disturbed spontaneous locomotor and exploratory activities as a consequence of altered spatio-temporal organization of behavior.

Editor: Judith Homberg, Radboud University, The Netherlands

Funding: This work has been supported by Brazilian funding agencies Coordenação de Aperfeiçoamento de Pessoal de Nível Superior (CAPES), Fundação de Amparo à Pesquisa do Estado do Rio Grande do Sul (FAPERGS), Conselho Nacional de Desenvolvimento Científico e Tecnológico (CNPQ), Instituto Nacional de Ciência e Tecnologia em Excitotoxicidade e Neuroproteção (INCT-EN). The funders had no role in study design, data collection and analysis, decision to publish, or preparation of the manuscript.

Competing Interests: The authors have declared that no competing interests exist.

* E-mail: renataleke@hotmail.com

¤ Current address: Experimental Hepatology and Gastroenterology Laboratory, Research Porto Alegre, RS, Brazil

Introduction

Hepatic encephalopathy (HE) is a neuropsychiatric complication that arises from acute or chronic liver diseases [1,2]. According to the etiology of liver injury, HE is classified as follows: type A, derived from acute liver failure; type B, associated with hepatic portal-systemic vascular shunting in patients without liver disease; and type C, associated with liver cirrhosis and portal-systemic vascular shunting due to portal hypertension [3]. The clinical manifestations of HE range from sleep disturbances and slight attention deficits to somnolence-sopor and coma [4]. Moreover, patients with HE experience altered motor function, such as hypokinesia, bradykinesia, ataxia and asterixis [4,5]. These psychomotor manifestations and the cognitive and emotional behavior dysfunctions impair the quality of life of HE patients [6,7].

Various models of chronic liver disease in rats leading to HE type B and C have been used to study changes in biochemical and psychomotor activities, such as bile duct-ligated (BDL) rats [8–11], porto-caval anastomosis (PCA) [12–14], portal vein-ligated (PVL) [15] and thioacetamide-induced liver damage [16]. Most studies report a decreased spontaneous locomotor activity in these animals [9,12,14], but some results are controversial, describing no differences in locomotor activity between PCA and control rats [17,18] and even increased locomotor activity in PCA rats compared to control rats [19]. This discrepancy might be due to the diversity of the animal models employed, the protocols and the analysis of the locomotor and exploratory behaviors. The majority of the psychomotor studies in rats analyzed the total distance traveled or the number of crossings in the arena as well as the total number of rearings, which primarily describe the quantity of activity. However, these studies did not explore the sequential (spatio-temporal) structure of behavior [20].

A frequently used animal model is the BDL rat, which according to the members of the ISHEN (International Society for Hepatic Encephalopathy and Nitrogen Metabolism) commission on experimental models of HE, reflects HE associated with cirrhosis and portal hypertension [21,22]. It is described that animals that are subjected to this surgical model of type C HE develops liver failure, jaundice, portal hypertension, bacterial translocation, immune system dysfunction, hyperammonemia and low-grade encephalopathy [21]. Using this animal model we have obtained evidence that the biosynthetic machinery for transmitter GABA is disturbed [23], which may be of interest since GABAergic neurotransmission has been related to aberrations in the behavioral parameters that are normally associated with HE [12,24].

On this basis, the present study was undertaken to investigate the structure of locomotor and exploratory behaviors in BDL rats in an open-field task. BDL rats exhibited an altered spatio-temporal organization of locomotor and exploratory behavior in the open-field behavioral task.

Methods

Animals

Adult female Wistar rats (n = 25, weight 182±2.5 g, 60 days old at the initiation of the surgical procedure) were obtained from the *animalarium* of the Biochemistry Department (Federal University of Rio Grande do Sul). The rats were housed three animals per cage and maintained in a controlled environment (room temperature 21±1°C, standard light/dark cycle of 12 h – lights on at 07:00 am) with standard food and water *ad libitum*. The handling and care of the animals were conducted according to the guidelines of the Guide for the Care and Use of Laboratory Animals (NIH-USA). The Ethics Committee of the Federal University of Rio Grande do Sul approved all procedures.

Bile duct ligation

The animals were randomly distributed into two groups: bile duct-ligated (BDL group, n = 10) and sham-operated (control group, n = 15) rats. The bile duct ligation procedure was conducted as described previously [22,25]. The rats were anaesthetized with ketamine (90 mg/kg) and xylazine (12 mg/kg) i.p. and placed in the supine position on an operating table. A thermal controlled mattress (37°C) was used to assure a constant body temperature during the surgical procedure. A middle abdominal incision was performed and the hepatic ligament was exposed. The common bile duct was ligated with two 4-0 non absorbent surgical sutures. The first suture was placed below the junction of the biliary hepatic ducts and the second suture was placed above the entrance of the pancreatic ducts. The common bile duct was resected between the two ligatures. The abdominal

incision was closed with 4-0 non absorbent suture in two layers. The rats were placed on another thermal mattress until consciousness was regained. The rats were then returned to their home-cages. The control rats consisted of sham-operated rats, i.e. rats that had the hepatic ligament exposed and manipulated, but the common bile duct was not ligated. All animals were maintained in the animal colony room for 6 weeks following surgery.

Sample collection

Rats were anesthetized as described previously and blood was withdrawn by cardiac puncture. The animals were decapitated and the liver and spleen were removed and stored in a 10% formaldehyde solution (10% formaldehyde in 0.1 mM phosphate buffer containing 21.6 mM Na2HPO4 and 81 mM NaH2PO4, pH 7.4). All organs were stored at 4°C until histological analysis. Blood samples were centrifuged for 5 minutes at 5000×g and 20°C and serum samples were stored at −20°C until analysis.

Histopathological examination

The livers and spleens of control and BDL rats were weighted and examined macroscopically. Subsequently, liver and spleen tissues were sampled for histological examination using Haematoxylin & Eosin (H&E) and Picrosirius (liver tissue) staining.

Biochemical parameters

Serum samples from the control and BDL groups were analyzed for aspartate aminotransferase (AST), alkaline phosphatases, bilirubin (total and direct) and albumin using an auto-analyzer (Cobas Integra 400, Roche Diagnostics Corporation®, USA).

Behavioral studies

The BDL and control rats were divided into two groups, 7 control and 5 BDL rats in the first group and 8 control and 5 BDL rats in the second group. The first group underwent open-field and plus-maze tasks, and the second group underwent foot-fault task. All experiments were conducted between the sixth and seventh week after surgical procedures. During the time between surgery and behavior tasks the rats were weekly manipulated to monitor weight gain and to avoid stress. Before each behavior task the rats were placed in the testing room (room size of 2 x 2.3 m, total area of 4.6 m^2) for one hour to allow habituation with the environment and researchers. Inter-task intervals were 2 days and all behavioral tasks were performed between 9:00–16:00 h. All behavioral parameters were recorded and analyzed using the appropriate video tracking system (Any-maze®, Stoelting CO, USA).

Open-field

Individual animals were placed in a 60-cm diameter circular black arena with 50-cm walls facing the wall. The animals were free to explore the arena for 15 min. The area was divided in two main sections, the center (0.1534 m^2) and periphery (0.1293 m^2) sections. Two halogen lamps (100 lx) pointed towards the room walls illuminated the room. After each trial, the apparatus was cleaned with 30% ethanol solution. The following parameters were quantified according to Eilam [20]: (1) activity (total distance traveled, time mobile/immobile, number of stops, inter stop distances, total numbers of rearing and grooming); (2) temporal organization of behavior (number of trips, trip lengths and the ratio between stops per trip); and (3) spatial distribution of activity (distance traveled within the center of the arena-calculated as a percentage of the total distance traveled, and time spent

Table 1 Biochemical parameters.

Parameters	Control	BDL	t	df	p
AST (U/L)	37.83±2.48	93.67±9.19*	7.721	16	<0.0001
Alkaline Phosphatases (U/L)	65.83±3.76	340.83±24.41*	15.66	16	<0.0001
Direct Bilirubin (mg/dL)	0.001±0.00	6.43±0.28*	32.96	16	<0.0001
Total Bilirubin (mg/dL)	0.06±0.01	10.54±0.32*	47.73	16	<0.0001
Albumin (g/dL)	4.45±0.09	2.08±0.16*	14.20	16	<0.0001

Biochemical parameters in serum of control (n = 12) and BDL rats (n = 6). Data are presented as means ± SEM. * = p<0.05 by Student's t test. df = degrees of freedom.

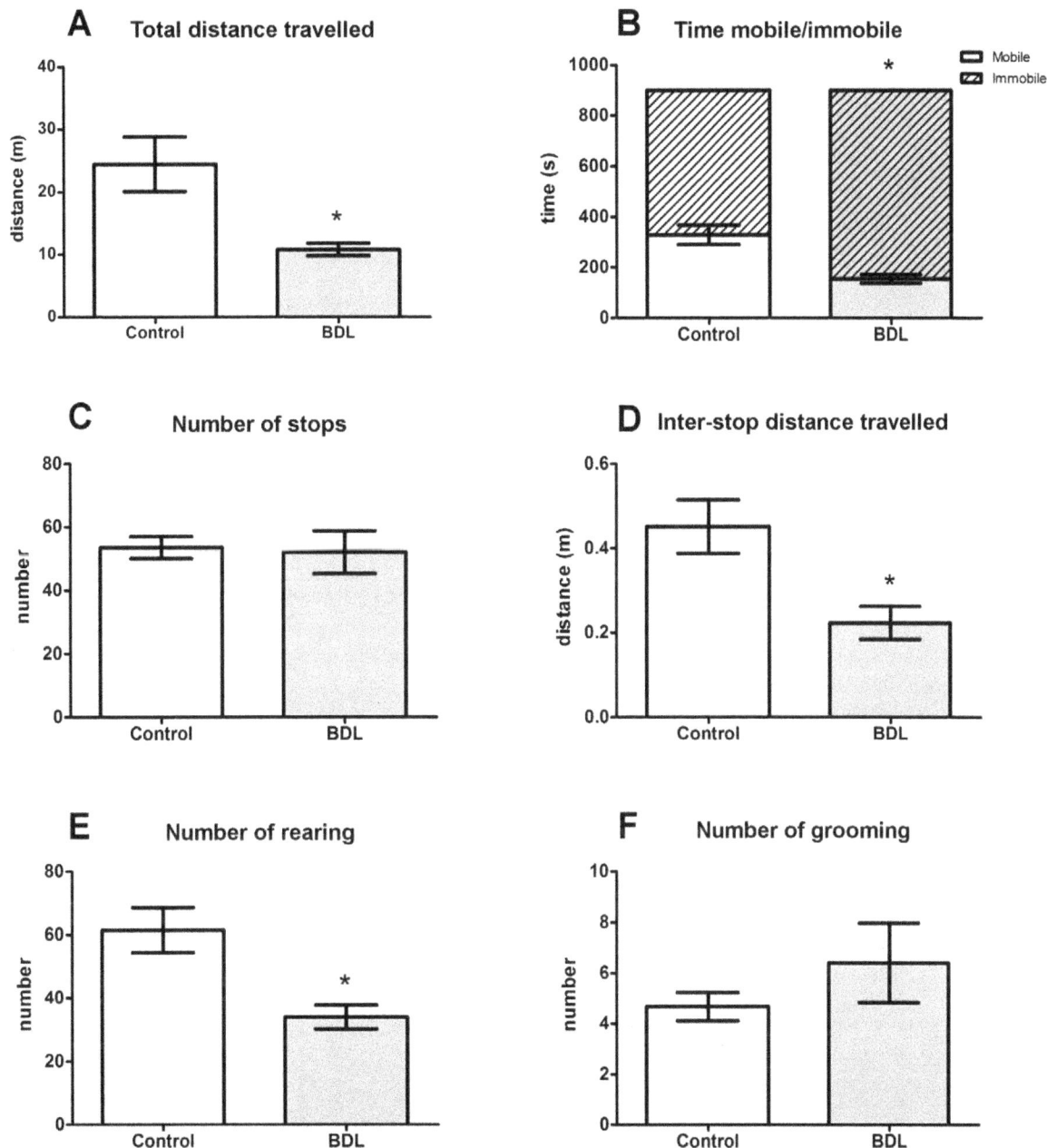

Figure 1. Locomotor and exploratory behavior. Control (n = 6) and BDL (n = 5) rats were evaluated for (A) total distance traveled, (B) time mobile/immobile, (C) number of stops, (D) inter-stops distance traveled, (F) number of rearings and (F) number of grooming. Data are presented as means ± SEM. * = $p<0.05$ by Student's t test.

locomoting in the center of the arena-calculated as a percentage of the total locomotion time).

Elevated plus-maze

Anxiety behavior was assessed in an elevated plus-maze according to Walf and Frye [26]. This task relies on the rodent's proclivity to dark enclosed spaces and an unconditioned fear of heights and open spaces. The apparatus consisted of four 50-cm long and 10-cm wide arms with two 40-cm high walls on two opposite arms. The apparatus was 50-cm above the floor and situated in the center of a red-lit room (60 lx). Red light was employed instead white light since it was demonstrated that the white light increases the open space avoidance [27]. The rats were

placed individually at the center of the apparatus facing the open arm and they were free to explore it for 5 min. After each trial, the apparatus was cleaned with 30% ethanol solution. The following parameters were quantified: (1) percentage of the number of entries in the closed arms by the total number of entries into the closed and open arms, and (2) percentage of time spent in the closed arms by the total time spent in both the closed and open arms.

Foot-fault

The rats were placed on a grid, and the number of failed attempts to accurately grasp the rungs was analyzed to examine coordinated fore- and hind-limb placement during spontaneous

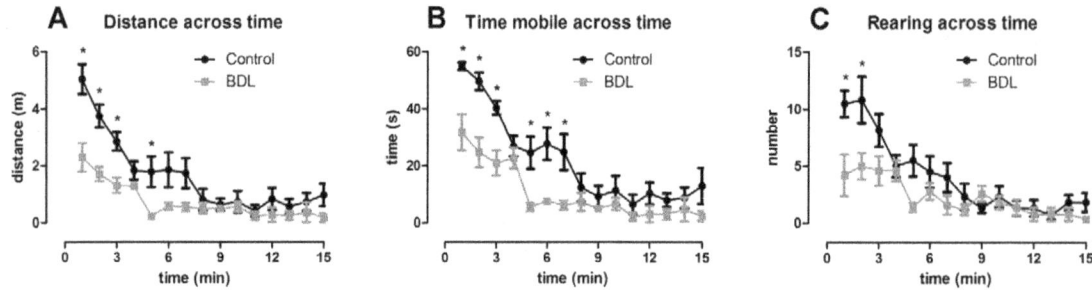

Figure 2. Locomotor and exploratory behavior across time. Control (n = 6) and BDL (n = 5) rats were evaluated for (A) distance traveled across time, (B) time mobile across time, (C) number of rearings across time. Data are presented as means $\pm$ SEM. * = $p < 0.05$ by two-way ANOVA followed by Bonferroni post-hoc test.

exploration. The apparatus was an elevated 80 cm$\times$60 cm wire grid platform with 3-cm^2 holes that was placed 76.5-cm above the floor. The animals freely explored the platform for 3 min. A foot-fault was scored when the rat misplaced its paw and the limb fell between the rungs. The total number of foot-faults was quantified.

Statistical analysis

Data are expressed as means $\pm$ standard error of the mean (SEM). The data were analyzed using Student's t-test for the open-field, elevated plus-maze and foot-fault tasks. Locomotor and exploratory parameters were analyzed across time using two-way ANOVA followed by the Bonferroni post-hoc test. A p value <0.05 was considered significant for all parameters. Data analysis was performed in Microsoft Excel 2007 and GraphPad Prism 5.0 softwares.

Results

Experimental cirrhosis

BDL rats exhibited yellowish fur and tails and enlarged abdomens. The body weights were not different between the control (225.5$\pm$5.0 g) and BDL (226.4$\pm$5.4 g) rats at the sixth week postsurgery. All BDL rats had ascites and their livers were tinged yellow with cystic bile duct remnants. Hepatomegaly and splenomegaly were observed in all BDL rats. One BDL rat in each group died prior to sample collection.

Histopathological and biochemical characterization

Histological analysis of the H&E- and picrosirius-stained liver tissue samples revealed that all BDL rats exhibited bile duct proliferation, disturbed cytoarchitecture, formation of septa

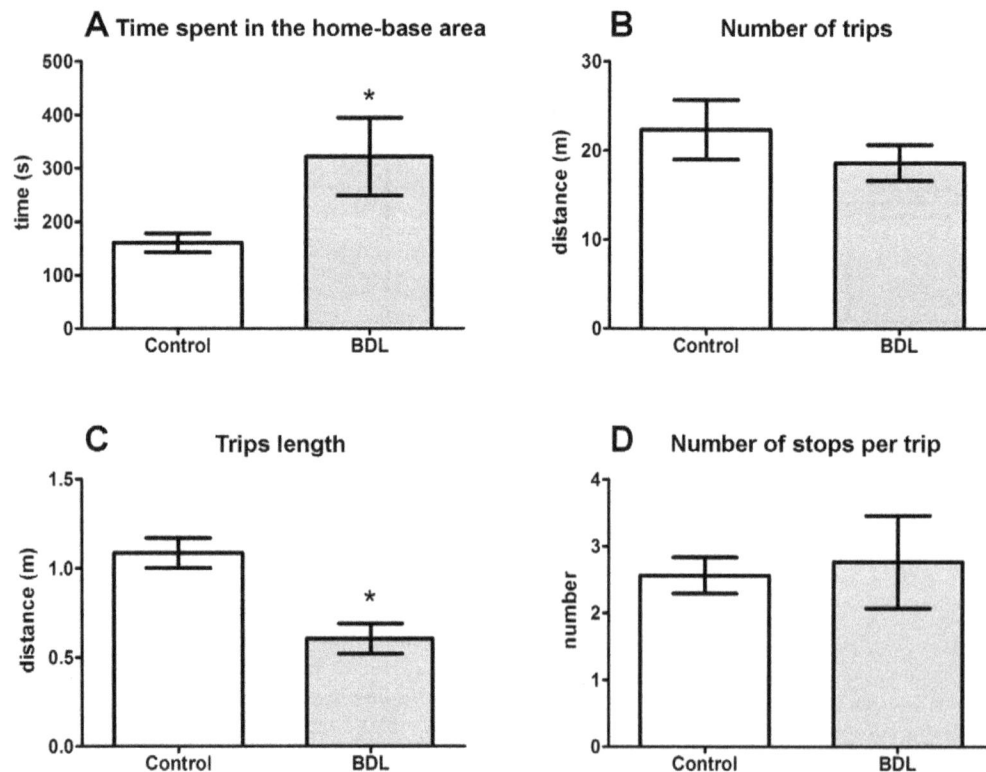

Figure 3. Temporal organization of behavior. Control (n = 6) and BDL (n = 5) rats were evaluated for (A) time spent in the home base area, (B) number of trips, (C) trips length and, (D) number of stops per trip. Data are presented as means $\pm$ SEM. * = $p < 0.05$ by Student's t test.

A Distance travelled in the center zone

B Time spent in the center zone

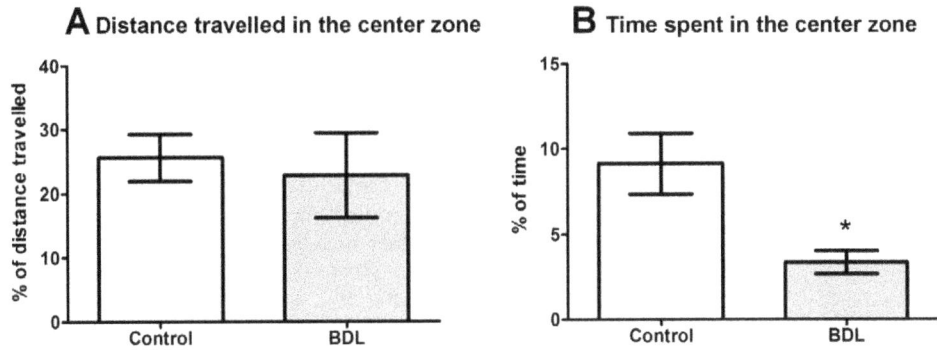

Figure 4. Spatial distribution of behavior. Control (n = 6) and BDL (n = 5) rats were evaluated for (A) percentage of total distance traveled in the center zone and (B) percentage of time spent in the center zone. Data are presented as means ± SEM. * = $p < 0.05$ by Student's t test.

between portal areas and a noticeable increase in collagen fibers. Control rats exhibited normal liver parenchyma. The spleen tissue samples of the BDL rats exhibited blood congestion, which is in agreement with portal hypertension. Serum AST, alkaline phosphatases and bilirubin (total and direct) were significantly increased in the BDL rats (Table 1). Albumin concentration was lower in the BDL rats compared to the control rats. These findings confirmed chronic cholestatic liver cirrhosis in the BDL rats.

Behavioral studies and Open-field task

Activity. BDL rats exhibited a significantly smaller total distance traveled in the open arena ($t = 2.788$, $df = 9$, $p = 0.0211$), a higher duration of immobile episodes ($t = 3.0801$, $df = 9$, $p = 0.0042$) and consequently, a smaller duration of mobile episodes, compared to the control rats (Figs. 1A,B). When analyzing the distance traveled across time it was observed that both groups presented the same pattern of behavior, i.e. both the control and BDL rats traveled larger distances during the first minutes and then decreased their locomotor activity over time. However, the BDL group exhibited a significantly smaller distance traveled in the first 6 minutes compared to the control rats (Fig. 2A, $F = 15.49$, $df = 14$, $p < 0.0001$ for variable time). The same pattern of behavior was observed in mobility across exploration time (Fig. 2B, $F = 19.46$, $df = 14$, $p < 0.0001$ for variable time). The total number of stops during the exploratory activity was not different between the BDL and control rats (Fig. 1C), albeit, the distance traveled between these stops was significantly smaller in the BDL group (Fig. 1D, $t = 2.919$, $df = 9$, $p = 0.0171$). The total number of rearings during this task was significantly decreased in

the BDL group (Fig. 1E, $t = 3.230$, $df = 9$, $p = 0.0103$), and the analysis across time revealed that this difference was only apparent during the first two minutes of the task (Fig. 2C, $F = 10.73$, $df = 14$, $p < 0.0001$ for variable time). Grooming behavior did not differ between groups (Fig. 1F).

Temporal organization of behavior. A significant increase was observed in the time that the BDL animals remained in the home-base area compared to the control rats (Fig. 3A, $t = 2.348$, $df = 9$, $p = 0.0434$). The number of trips during this task was not different between the groups (Fig. 3B), but the length of each trip was considerably shorter in the BDL group (Fig. 3C, $t = 3.983$, $df = 9$, $p = 0.0032$). The number of stops made in trips between two successive stops at the home-base (stops/trips) was not different between groups (Fig. 3D).

Spatial distribution of activity. The percentage of the distance traveled within the center zone was not different between the BDL and control rats (Fig. 4A). However, the percentage of time spent in the center of the arena was significantly smaller in the BDL rats compared to the control rats (Fig. 4B, $t = 2.824$, $df = 9$, $p = 0.0199$).

Elevated plus-maze

No difference in the percentage of the number of entries either in the percentage of time spent in the closed arms was observed between the BDL and control rats (Table 2).

Foot-fault

No difference in the total number of foot-faults was observed between the BDL and control rats (Table 2).

Table 2 Results of the plus-maze and foot-fault tasks.

Plus-maze					
Parameter	Control	BDL	t	Df	p
Number of entries (%)	55.84±5.60	49.75±3.06	1.117	9	0.2931
Time spent in the arm (%)	67.96±8.39	48.11±6.38	1.720	9	0.1196
Foot-fault					
Parameter	Control	BDL	t	Df	p
Number of faults	11.00±1.36	11.00±2.34	0.000	11	1.000

Control (N = 6) and BDL (N = 5) in the plus-maze and control (N = 8) and BDL (N = 5) in the foot-fault tasks. Data are presented as means ± SEM. Statistical analyses were performed using Student's t-test. df = degrees of freedom.

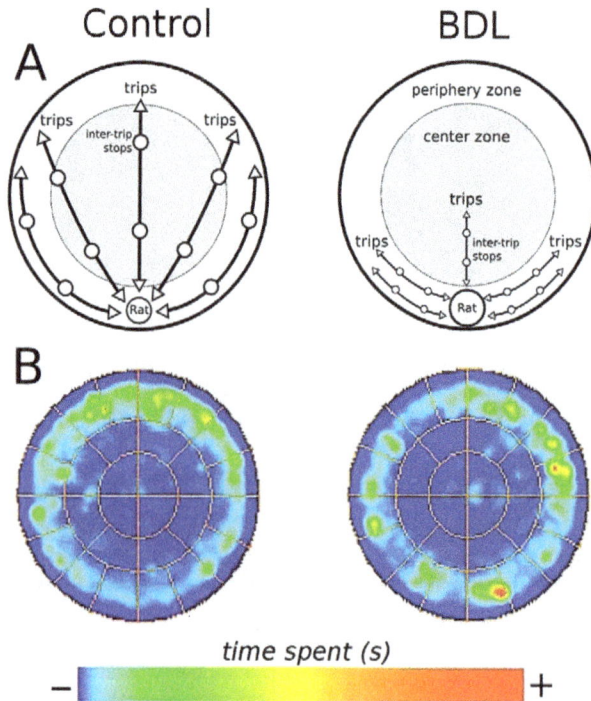

Figure 5. Schematic representation of behavior of control and BDL rats in the open-field task. (A) Representation of the spatio-temporal organization of locomotor and exploratory behavior in the control and BDL rats in the open-field task. (B) Occupancy plot of the open-field is presented as time (s) spent in the arena in the control and BDL groups. Control and BDL rats exhibited no differences in number of trips, number of stops and number of stops per trip during exploration of the arena; however, the length of the trips was shorter for BDL rats (A). BDL rats exhibited a decrease in the percentage of time spent in the center of the area and an increase in the time spent in the home base area (A and B).

Discussion

The BDL rat is an experimental model of secondary biliary cirrhosis that leads to chronic HE type C [21]. Studies described that rats with chronic liver failure developed by different models, exhibit impaired locomotor and exploratory behaviors [9,12,14]. In the present study the BDL rats, which exhibited chronic liver disease, had impaired locomotor and exploratory activities in the open-field task, characterized by a decrease in the total distance traveled and an increased immobility time. Furthermore, the BDL rats also traveled shorter distances between stops during the exploratory activity, but the total number of stops was not different from the control rats. Reinforcing the concept of altered locomotor and exploratory activities, the total number of rearings was smaller in the BDL rats. These results are in accordance with previous studies that demonstrated that different models of chronic liver disease exhibit locomotor dysfunction. Specifically, rats subjected to PCS have been shown to exhibit hypolocomotion in the open-field task [12,14,24] and BDL rats have been shown to exhibit a decreased locomotor activity when underwent the open-field behavioral task [8,9]. Contrary to these results, Méndez et al. [28] did not observe differences in locomotor behavior when studying the PCS rats and the thioacetamide-induced liver failure rat models. However, the majority of the locomotor and exploratory behavior studies have just focused only on parameters that depict animal activity in the apparatus. The present study

explored the open-field task in more detail, since the temporal and spatial structures of the behaviors were also investigated.

It is known that rats after being introduced to the open field establish a home base, which is the most visited location in the arena in which they spend an extended period of time and this is the place from which the rats will initiate trips [20]. Further analysis of the temporal (sequential) structure of the locomotor behavior of the BDL rats demonstrated that these animals remained in the home base area for longer periods of time than the control rats, but both groups performed the same number of exploratory trips. Therefore, the decreased in the total distance traveled by the BDL rats in the open-field is likely not related to the number of trips nor to the number of stops per trip performed by the animals. However, the distance traveled per trip was smaller in the BDL group, which consequently reduced the total distance traveled. With regard to the spatial distribution of locomotion, the BDL rats did not differ from the control rats in the percentage of distance traveled in the center zone of the arena. However, the time spent in this area was decreased in the BDL rats. This pattern of behavior could be interpreted as avoidance of the open area, which suggests an anxiety-like behavior. For this reason, the elevated plus-maze task was conducted to investigate anxiety; interestingly, it was found that the BDL rats did not exhibit greater anxiety behavior than the control rats. In agreement with this result, Sergeeva et al. [13] did not observe anxiety behavior in PCS rats, however, the animals moved less and more slowly in the open-field task compared to the control rats. In addition, it has been shown that rats with chronic liver failure induced by thioacetamide intoxication did not show anxiety behavior; it is notable, however, that they did not display locomotor and exploratory deficits either [28]. Furthermore, the diminished locomotor activity exhibited by the BDL rats in the present study was not a consequence of impaired motor coordination because the BDL rats were as coordinated as the control rats when performing the foot-fault task. In accordance with this result, Jover et al. [9] demonstrated that BDL rats exhibited mild coordination impairment in the the rotarod test whereas there was no statistical difference between the BDL and control rats in the beam walking test. Taken together, our results clearly demonstrate altered spatio-temporal organization of locomotor and exploratory activities in the BDL rats, but the hypolocomotion observed did not appear to be the result of anxiety or impairment of motor coordination (schematic representation in Fig. 5). It should be noted that we found no differences between the locomotor and exploratory behaviors of female and male BDL rats (data not shown).

Patients with HE exhibit impaired motor function and coordination and present the clinical manifestations such as asterixis, ataxia, dysarthria, rigor, tremor, hypomimia and hypokinesia [3,4,29]. It has been described that disturbances in motor function, such as hypokinesia and bradykinesia, are a consequence of altered basal ganglia function [6,29]. Amondio et al. [30], suggested that motor alterations were due to altered neuronal circuits between the basal ganglia and prefrontal cortex. The mechanisms underlying the HE-induced alterations in these cerebral areas are still unclear, although several studies have been undertaken to elucidate these mechanisms. Joebges et al. [5] showed in patients with minimal HE, i.e. a condition in patients with chronic liver disease and signs of HE that are not clinically manifested, that cortical brain areas such as the cingulate gyrus as well as the frontomesial and parietal cortex, which are related to movement initiation, exhibited decreased glucose uptake.

Studies in animals have further investigated the underlying mechanisms of induced motor alterations during HE. Oria et al.

[31] found that PCS and BDL rats did not exhibit alterations in motor-evoked potentials in conscious rats and suggested that the behavioral abnormalities that have been described might be a consequence of the dysfunction of other neuronal circuits. Another study using PCS rats demonstrated an increase in extracellular glutamate and metabotropic glutamate receptor mGluR1 activation in the substantia nigra reticulate, which may be related to the reduced motor activity observed in these animals [12]. It has been shown that the function of the neuronal pathway related to motor function, i.e. the circuits between the basal ganglia, thalamus and cortex was impaired in PCS rats [11]. In addition, increased levels of neurosteroids and consequently dysfunction in GABAergic neurotransmission might also participate in the altered locomotor activity observed in PCS rats [14]. In this context, it may be important to note that BDL rats have been shown to have impairments of the biosynthesis of neurotransmitter GABA [23].

Overall, different studies have described alteration in the function and neurochemistry of brain areas that are related to motor function, which have been related to the dysfunctions in the locomotor and exploratory activities. However, it is important to consider that other brain areas might be involved. According to that, it has been demonstrated that different rat models of chronic liver disease and HE type B and C exhibit deficits in tasks related to visual orientation [28]. Moreover, it has been described that patients with HE have impairments in visual perception, visual orientation and attention [32–34]. BDL rats, in the present study, exhibited an altered spatio-temporal organization of locomotor and exploratory behaviors. It should be considered that visual and spatial perception deficits might also interfere with locomotor and exploratory activities.

In conclusion, BDL rats with chronic liver disease and mild HE exhibited altered spatio-temporal organization of locomotor and exploratory activities compared to control rats. The mechanisms underlying these behavioral impairments are not completely understood, and further studies will be fundamental for the elucidation of which brain areas and neurochemical mechanisms that are involved.

Acknowledgments

The technical assistance of Ms Liz M.B.P. Brum from the Instituto de Cardiologia do Rio Grande do Sul from Porto Alegre was highly appreciated.

Author Contributions

Conceived and designed the experiments: RL DLdO VK MS SK. Performed the experiments: RL BHMM MSP GM. Analyzed the data: RL DLdO LKB. Contributed reagents/materials/analysis tools: TRS CRH LKB. Wrote the paper: RL AS DLdO TRS HSW SK LVP.

References

1. Hazell AS, Butterworth RF (1999) Hepatic encephalopathy: An update of pathophysiologic mechanisms. Proc Soc Exp Biol Med 222: 99–112.

2. Albrecht J, Jones EA (1999) Hepatic encephalopathy: molecular mechanisms underlying the clinical syndrome. J Neurol Sci. 170: 138–146.

3. Ferenci P, Lockwood A, Mullen K, Tarter R, Weissenborn K, et al. (2002) Hepatic encephalopathy-definition, nomenclature, diagnosis, and quantification: final report of the working party at the 11th World Congresses of Gastroenterology, Vienna, 1998. Hepatology 35: 716–721.

4. Weissenborn K, Bokemeyer M, Krause J, Ennen J, Ahl B (2005) Neurological and neuropsychiatric syndromes associated with liver disease. AIDS 19 Suppl 3: S93–98.

5. Joebges EM, Heidemann M, Schimke N, Hecker H, Ennen JC, et al. (2003) Bradykinesia in minimal hepatic encephalopathy is due to disturbances in movement initiation. J Hepatol. 38: 273–280.

6. Jover R, Compañy L, Gutiérrez A, Lorente M, Zapater P, et al. (2005) Clinical significance of extrapyramidal signs in patients with cirrhosis. J Hepatol. 42(5): 659–665.

7. Groeneweg M, Quero JC, De Bruijn I, Hartmann IJ, Essink-bot ML, et al. (1998) Subclinical hepatic encephalopathy impairs daily functioning. Hepatology 28: 45–49.

8. Chan CY, Huang SW, Wang TF, Lu RH, Lee FY, et al. (2004) Lack of detrimental effects of nitric oxide inhibition in bile duct-ligated rats with hepatic encephalopathy. Eur J Clin Invest. 34: 122–128.

9. Jover R, Rodrigo R, Felipo V, Insausti R, Sáez-Valero J, et al. (2006) Brain edema and inflammatory activation in bile duct ligated rats with diet-induced hyperammonemia: A model of hepatic encephalopathy in cirrhosis. Hepatology 43: 1257–1266.

10. García-Ayllón MS, Cauli O, Silveyra MX, Rodrigo R, Candela A, et al. (2008) Brain cholinergic impairment in liver failure. Brain.131: 2946–2956.

11. Rodrigo R, Cauli O, Gomez-Pinedo U, Agusti A, Hernandez-Rabaza V, et al. (2010) Hyperammonemia induces neuroinflammation that contributes to cognitive impairment in rats with hepatic encephalopathy. Gastroenterology 139: 675–684.

12. Cauli O, Llansola M, Erceg S, Felipo V (2006) Hypolocomotion in rats with chronic liver failure is due to increased glutamate and activation of metabotropic glutamate receptors in substantia nigra. J Hepatol. 45: 654–661.

13. Sergeeva OA, Schulz D, Doreulee N, Ponomarenko AA, Selbach O, et al. (2005) Deficits in cortico-striatal synaptic plasticity and behavioral habituation in rats with portacaval anastomosis. Neuroscience 134: 1091–1098.

14. Ahboucha S, Jiang W, Chatauret N, Mamer O, Baker GB, et al. (2008) Indomethacin improves locomotor deficit and reduces brain concentrations of neuroinhibitory steroids in rats following portacaval anastomosis. Neurogastroenterol Motil 20: 949–957.

15. Brück J, Görg B, Bidmon HJ, Zemtsova I, Qvartskhava N, et al. (2011) Locomotor impairment and cerebrocortical oxidative stress in portal vein ligated rats in vivo. J Hepatol. 54: 251–257.

16. Méndez M, Méndez-López M, López L, Aller MA, Arias J, et al. (2009) Associative learning deficit in two experimental models of hepatic encephalopathy. Behav Brain Res. 198: 346–351.

17. Martin JR, Dedek J, Driscoll P (1983) Portacaval anastomosis in rats: Effects on behavior and brain serotonin metabolism. Pharmacol Biochem Behav 18: 269–272.

18. Apelqvist G, Hindfelt B, Andersson G, Bengtsson F (1999) Altered adaptive behaviour expressed in an open-field paradigm in experimental hepatic encephalopathy. Behav Brain Res. 106: 165–173.

19. Campbell A, Jeppsson B, James JH, Ziparo V, Fischer JE (1984) Spontaneous motor activity increases after portacaval anastomosis in rats. Pharmacol Biochem Behav 20: 875–878.

20. Eilam D (2003) Open-field behavior withstands drastic changes in arena size. Behav Brain Res. 142: 53–62.

21. Butterworth RF, Norenberg MD, Felipo V, Ferenci P, Albrecht J, et al. (2009) Experimental models of hepatic encephalopathy: ISHEN guidelines. Liver Int. 29: 783–788.

22. Scott-Conner CEH, Grogan JB (1994) The pathophysiology of biliary obstruction and its effect on phagocytic and immune function. Journal of Surgical Research 57: 316–336.

23. Leke R, Bak LK, Iversen P, Sørensen M, Keiding S, et al. (2011) Synthesis of neurotransmitter GABA via the neuronal tricarboxylic acid cycle is elevated in rats with liver cirrhosis consistent with a high GABAergic tone in chronic. J Neurochem. 117: 824–32.

24. Cauli O, Mlili N, Llansola M, Felipo V (2007) Motor activity is modulated via different neuronal circuits in rats with chronic liver failure than in normal rats. Eur J Neurosci. 25: 2112–2122.

25. Kountouras J, Billing BH, Scheuer PJ (1984) Prolonged bile duct obstruction: a new experimental model for cirrhosis in the rat. Br J Exp Pathol. 65: 305–311.

26. Walf AA, Frye CA (2007) The use of the elevated plus maze as an assay of anxiety-related behavior in rodents. Nat Protoc. 2: 322–328.

27. Violle N, Balandras F, Le Roux Y, Desor D, Schroeder H (2009) Variations in illumination, closed wall transparency and/or extramaze space influence both baseline anxiety and response to diazepam in the rat elevated plus-maze. Behav Brain Res 203: 35–42.

28. Méndez M, Méndez-López M, López L, Aller MA, Arias J, et al. (2008) Spatial memory alterations in three models of hepatic encephalopathy. Behav Brain Res. 188: 32–40.

29. Giewekemeyer K, Berding G, Ahl B, Ennen JC, Weissenborn K (2007) Bradykinesia in cirrhotic patients with early hepatic encephalopathy is related to a decreased glucose uptake of frontomesial cortical areas relevant for movement initiation. J Hepatol. 46: 1034–1039.

30. Amodio P, Montagnese S, Gatta A, Morgan MY (2004) Characteristics of minimal hepatic encephalopathy. Metab Brain Dis. 19: 253–267.

31. Oria M, Chatauret N, Chavarria L, Romero-Giménez J, Palenzuela L, et al. (2010) Motor-evoked potentials in awake rats are a valid method of assessing hepatic encephalopathy and of studying its pathogenesis. Hepatology. 52: 2077–2085.

32. Tarter RE, Hegedus AM, Van Thiel DH, Schade RR, Gavaler JS, et al. (1984) Nonalcoholic cirrhosis associated with neuropsychological dysfunction in the absence of overt evidence of hepatic encephalopathy. Gastroenterology. 86: 1421–1427.

33. Weissenborn K, Heidenreich S, Giewekemeyer K, Rückert N, Hecker H (2003) Memory function in early hepatic encephalopathy. J Hepatol. 39: 320–325.

34. Amodio P, Schiff S, Del Piccolo F, Mapelli D, Gatta A, et al. (2005) Attention Dysfunction in Cirrhotic Patients: An Inquiry on the Role of Executive Control, Attention Orienting and Focusing. Metab Brain Dis. 20: 115–127.

4

Hepatitis B Virus Gene Mutations in Liver Diseases: A Report from New Delhi

Abdul Malik[1,2,3]*, Deepak Kumar Singhal[2], Abdulmajeed Albanyan[1], Syed Akhtar Husain[3], P. Kar[2]

1 Department of Clinical Laboratory Science, College of Applied Medical Sciences, King Saud University, Riyadh, Saudi Arabia, 2 Department of Medicine, Maulana Azad Medical College, University of Delhi, New Delhi, India, 3 Department of Biosciences, Jamia Millia Islamia, New Delhi, India

Abstract

Objectives: The study was designed to characterize the surface, core promoter, precore/core region sequences for the presence of mutations in hepatitis B virus (HBV) associated with different liver diseases.

Methods: 567 HBV associated patients with different liver diseases were enrolled in this study. All samples were analyzed for HBV surface, core promoter, precore/core region mutations and genotypes using PCR and direct sequencing.

Results: HBV genotype D (72.8%) was the predominant type followed by genotype A (27.2%). The serum viral load of HBV was highest in HBsAg carriers group and lowest in patients with hepatocellular carcinoma. 17.9% patients with cirrhosis and 24.6% hepatocellular carcinoma cases were ADV-resistant with rtA181T/V mutations in the S-gene. A1896T was found more frequently in fulminant hepatic failure compared to acute viral hepatitis patients (p = 0.038). T1753V mutation was significantly higher in patients with cirrhosis of liver (34.6%) than in chronic hepatitis (18.9%) and hepatocellular carcinoma patients (21.2%; p = 0.001). T1762/A1764 mutation was observed in all the groups. C1914G core gene mutation was associated with the hepatocellular carcinoma (32.2%) compared to other groups. HBV genotype D predominated in comparison to genotype A. An increased frequency of precore mutation and BCP double mutations amongst the population studied was also observed.

Conclusion: Mutations such as T1762/A1764, T1753V and C1914G were usually associated with advanced forms of liver disease and had an increased risk of HCC. The nucleotide variability in the basal core promoter and precore regions possibly plays a role in the progression of HBV disease. Prospective studies on the sequence variations of the preC/C region of the HBV genome and the molecular mechanisms in relation to progression of liver disease would aid in better understanding of the biological significance of HBV strains in India.

Editor: Anand S Mehta, Drexel University College of Medicine, United States of America

Funding: The authors are grateful to the Indian Council of Medical Research for providing assistance. The funding agency had no role in study design, data collection and analysis and it was purely an authors' decision to publish.

Competing Interests: The authors have declared that no competing interests exist.

* E-mail: abdul.ksu@gmail.com

Introduction

Hepatitis B virus (HBV) infection is one of the most important infectious diseases worldwide and is a major global health problem. Approximately one million people die annually because of acute and chronic HBV infection despite the availability of effective vaccines and effective antiviral medications [1]. HBV replicates *via* the reverse transcriptase enzyme system which lacks proofreading ability; therefore, new virions possess diverse genetic variability [2]. Different election pressures such as host immunity (endogenous pressure), and vaccine or antiviral agents (exogenous pressure) influence the production of HBV quasispecies in infected individuals. It has been demonstrated that mutations in the HBV genome not only impact the replication fitness of the virus (phenotypical effect) but can also influence the disease outcome, as well as the response to treatment (clinical effect) [3]. Mutations in the HBV surface (S), precore (PC) and basal core promoter (BCP) genes are observed frequently in HBV infected patients, and studies show that these mutations are associated with the clinical

outcomes of HBV disease [4], [5]. The most clinically relevant mutations in the S region arise in the immunologic "a determinant" domain and neutralizing antibodies (anti-HBs) are targeted against this epitope [6]. The basic core promoter (BCP, nt 1742–1849) and its adjacent precore (preC) region are crucial for replication of HBV. BCP binds various liver factors and preC forms ε structure in pregenomic RNA (pgRNA) as the encapsidation signal [7]. Changes in viral replication may influence the progression of liver diseases, particularly in fulminant hepatitis and acute exacerbation of chronic hepatitis [8], [9]. Mounting evidence has emerged to demonstrate that BCP and preC mutants are predisposed to severe and progressive liver diseases after HBV infection, causing an increased risk for hepatocellular carcinoma (HCC) [10], [11], [12]. For instance, mutations T1762/A1764 and A1899 have been reported to be independent risk factors for HCC [13], and T1653 and/or V1753 mutations are believed to promote the process of liver degradation [14]. However, the association of these mutations with severe symptoms is manifested in certain populations but not in others [15], [16], [17].

Studies have shown that G1896A is involved in HBeAg negativity by introducing a stop codon in the preC region [18]. Although the T1762/A1764 double mutation, commonly occurring in HBeAg-negative patients, was observed in vivo to suppress the production of preC mRNA independent of G1896A, recent in vitro research suggested other single site substitutions rather than these two which may be responsible for the reduction of HBeAg expression [9], [19].Unknown mutation in this core promoter may impede the seroconversion of HBeAg during antiviral treatment [20].

The prevalence of hepatitis B surface antigen (HBsAg) in India varies from 1–13%, with an average of 4.7% [21], [22]. Without any organized HBV prevention programme, and with 25 million live births each year, nearly 1 million HBV infections are added to the HBV pool yearly, contributing to its rapid expansion [23]. In this situation, HBV epidemiology is presumed to be an important determinant of the global HBV burden in the future. Molecular epidemiological data regarding HBV infection provides information about the emerging worldwide epidemiology of HBV, which is likely to shift its focus to South Asia in general, and India in particular, in the years to come, in view of the growing HBV burden therein and in the absence of interventions.

In a recent Indian study, a substantial proportion of anti-HBe positive chronically infected individuals continued to circulate preC wild-type HBV [24], and also documented an HBeAg positive CHB patient with a pre-C mutant. Further more a substantial proportion of anti-HBe positive subjects carry the precore wild-type strain, which suggests that predominance of pre-C mutants can never be solely responsible for the absence of HBeAg [25]. The HBV profile of Indian patients, a zone of intermediate prevalence, is believed to be an important determinant of the global HBV burden in the near future. The present study was designed to detect and characterize mutations in the precore/core and surface genes of the hepatitis B virus using direct sequencing, and its association with clinical outcome in HBV infected patients in different stages of liver disease.

Materials and Methods

Patients

Five hundred sixty seven HBsAg-positive patients comprising of 115 Acute Viral Hepatitis (AVH) patients, 40 patients of Fulminant Hepatic failure (FHF), 100 HBsAg carriers (ASC), 116 chronic hepatitis patients (CH), 78 patients with liver cirrhosis (LC) and 118 patients with hepatocellular carcinoma (HCC) and admitted in the wards of Lok Nayak hospital, New Delhi, were enrolled in the study from march 2003 till February 2006. All patients were interviewed and examined by gastroenterologists to evaluate the clinical findings and the results of the investigations (liver histology, ultrasonography, and laboratory tests such as serology, biochemical tests and virological markers) in order to determine the clinical status of the patient. AVH was diagnosed when patients exhibited overt jaundice and/or increased alanine aminotransferase levels (at least 3 times above the normal value) documented at least twice at a 1-week interval without any history of pre-existing liver disease [26]. FHF was considered to exist when, after a typically acute onset, the patient become deeply jaundiced and went into hepatic encephalopathy within 8 weeks of onset of the disease, with no past history of chronic hepatitis [27]. The patients with CH and liver cirrhosis were diagnosed by histopathological criteria laid down by International Study Group on Chronic Hepatitis [28]. The diagnosis of underlying cirrhosis was based on clinical, histological, endoscopic (presence of varices), and radiological documentation [ultrasound (US) and CT scan].

Histological evidence was used wherever available. All patients with HCC enrolled in the study were diagnosed, based on either pathological or cytological examination or an elevated ∝-fetoprotein level (≥400 ng/ml) combined with at least one positive image on angiography, sonography and/or computerized tomography. Cases were enrolled only if they met the EASL diagnostic criteria for HCC [29]. Written consent was obtained from each participant before inclusion in the study. Sera from patients with different liver diseases were obtained once the diagnosis was made. Serum samples were collected from all inpatients and outpatients with different stages of HBV-linked hepatic diseases and stored at −70°C until analysis. Ethical review board of Maulana Azad Medical College, New Delhi, had approved the study protocol.

Serological and Biochemical Parameters

All patients were tested for HBV serological markers (HBsAg, anti-HBs, IgM/IgG anti-HBc and HBeAg), hepatitis C virus (anti-HCV) and hepatitis A virus and hepatitis E virus using commercially available kits (DIA PRO Diagnostic Bioprobes, Srl., Italy). Patients with co-infections patients (HIV, HDV and HCV) were excluded from the study. Liver function tests such as serum albumin, total bilirubin, ALT, AST and ALP were measured by an auto-analyzer.

DNA Extraction from Serum

DNA was extracted from 200 µl of serum samples using QIAmp DNA mini-extraction kit (Qiagen K.K., Tokyo, Japan). The extracted DNA was dissolved in 50 µl of TE buffer.

Amplification of Precore/core Gene

For sequence analysis, nested PCR for amplification of Precore/core was performed. For the first stage PCR, 25 µl of reaction mixture containing 2 µl of the DNA sample, 1X PCR buffer (10 mM tris-HCl, pH 9.0, 50 mM KCl, 1.5 mM MgCl2, 0.01% gelatin and 0.1% triton X-100), 10 mM of each dNTP, 100 ng of each outer primer and 1U of Taq DNA polymerase was amplified in a thermal cycler (Perkin-Elmer Cetus, Norwalk, CT) for 35 cycles. Each cycle entailed denaturation at 95°C for 60s, primer annealing at 55°C for 30s and extension at 72°C for 60s with final extension step at 72°C for 10 min. After the first amplification, 1 µl of the PCR products was re-amplified for another 35 cycles with 100 ng of each inner primer.

For the Precore/core region, the outer sense primer was 5'-CTGGGAGGAGTTGGGGGA-3', nucleotide positions 1770–1787; the outer antisense primer was 5'-CAATGCTCAGGAGAC TCTAA-3', nucleotide positions 2476–2495; the inner sense primer was 5'-GGTCTTTG TACTCGGAGGCT-3', nucleotide positions 1788–1808; the inner antisense primer was 5'-GTCA-GAAGGCAAAAAAGA GA-3', nucleotide positions 2467–2486.

Amplification of Basal Core-promoter (BCP) and Surface Gene

For the first stage PCR, 25 µl of reaction mixture containing 2 µl of the DNA sample, 1X PCR buffer (10 mM tris-HCl, pH 9.0, 50 mM KCl, 1.5 mM MgCl2, 0.01% gelatin and 0.1% triton X-100), 10 mM of each dNTP, 100 ng of each outer primer and 1U of Taq DNA polymerase was amplified in a thermal cycler (Perkin-Elmer Cetus, Norwalk, CT) for 35 cycles. Each cycle entailed denaturation at 95°C for 60 s, primer annealing at 52°C for 30 s and extension at 72°C for 60 s with final extension step at 72°C for 10 min. After the first amplification, 1 µl of the PCR products was re-amplified for another 35 cycles with 100 ng of each inner primer. For the basal core-promoter, the outer sense primer was 5'-CTAGCCGCTTGTTTTGCTCG-3', nucleotide positions 1282–1301; the outer antisense primer was 5'-CACAGCTTGGAGGCTT GAAC-3', nucleotide positions 1881–1862; the inner sense primer was 5'-CTCATCTGCCGGA CCGTGTG-3', nucleotide positions 1342–1361; the inner antisense primer was 5'-TAGGACAT GAACAAGAGATG-3', nucleotide positions1840–1859. For the surface gene amplification, the outer sense primer was (HB1: 369–388) 5'-ATCGCTG-GATGTGTCTGCGG-3' and the outer anti-sense primer was (HB2:1136–1155) 5'-GGCAACGGGGTAAAGGTTCA-3'. The inner sense primer was (HB3: 822–842) 5'-TTAGGGTT-TAAATGTATACCC-3' and the inner anti-outer sense primer was (HB4: 427–448) 5'-CATCTTCTTGTTGGTTCTTTCTG-3', respectively.

Direct Nucleotide Sequencing

The PCR products were sequenced twice in forward and reverse directions using the inner primer pair of surface gene and precore/core genes. The nucleotide sequences of the amplified products were directly determined using fluorescence-labelled primers with a 3100 Automatic Sequencer (Applied Biosystems, Foster City, CA, USA). Sequencing conditions were specified in the protocol for the Taq DyeDeoxy Terminator Cycle Sequencing Kit (Applied Biosystems). (Representative samples submitted in the Genbank are as follows: EF158128-EF158294, DQ328773-DQ328791 and DQ184651-DQ184670.

Statistical Evaluation

Data were expressed as means ± standard deviations (SD). Statistical analyses were performed using a Chi square test and Fisher's exact test for categorical variables and Mann-Whitney's U test or one-way analysis of variance for continuous variables, as appropriate. Differences were considered significant for p values less than 0.05. The statistical analysis software used was SPSS software, version 12.0.

Results

Clinical and Demographic Data

Based on the clinical and laboratory findings the patients were divided into five categories which include 115 patients of AVH, 40 patients of FHF, 116 patients of CH, 78 patients with LC and 118 patients of HCC. Also 100 HBsAg carriers were inducted as controls. The clinical and laboratory findings (serologic, biochemical and virological profile) of AVH and CH are summarized in Table 1 and 2. Amino acid sequences of a portion of the S region of all 567 isolates of the study patients were compared with the amino acid sequences retrieved from the GenBank as reference genes. Only HBV genotype D and A were detected in all the study samples, which were respectively distributed in 72.8% and 27.2% of the total samples.

Characteristics of Nucleotide Substitution in the Surface Region of HBV related Different Liver Disease Patients

Amino acid mapping reveals that the S region was relatively conserved; however, an important substitution of P120T/S was observed in 7.8% (9/115) of AVH and 11.2% (13/116) in CH patients. Some substitutions such as P127T, V128A and D144N were observed in the immunologic domain of the "a determinant" region. No G145R substitution was identified in any of the isolates. In the S gene, an A184V mutation was found in 17.9% of the cirrhotic and 24.6% HCC patients included in this study, respectively. Among the patients of LC, SW172stop (6.4%) and SL173F (4.2%) mutations were also detected.

The Clinical, Biochemical and Virological Profile of HBV Related Acute and Fulminant Hepatitis Patients

Table 1, compares the clinical and virological characteristics between patients with AVH and FHF. The mean age of AVH patients was 32.09±15.73 yeas and that of FHF patients was 29.08±10.7, respectively. Male predominance was observed amongst AVH and FHF cases. Levels of AST, ALT, Total Bilirubin and alkaline phosphatase were significantly higher in patients with FHF compared to AVH. Distribution of HBV genotypes was no different between patients with FHF (genotype D accounted for 72.5% & genotype A- 27.5%) and AVH (genotype D accounted for 67.8% & genotype A- 32.2%), and the difference was statistically non-significant (p = 0.724). Mean HBV DNA levels were comparable in patients with AH and FHF (3.5±1.45 Vs. 3.7±1.28 log copies/ml; NS).

We compared our core promoter mutation data with previously reported HBV sequences [13]. Mutations at nt. 1762 and 1764 and 1766 and nt. 1753 were found when they were compared with each respective prototype sequence. The numbers of patients with T1762/A1764 are shown in Table 1. There was no difference in the frequency of these mutations between patients with FHF and those with AVH (32/115 (27.8%) v 15/40 (37.5%); NS). Double mutation T1764/G1766 was found only in 3/40 (7.5%) patients of FHF (Table 1). The numbers of patients with C/A/G 1753 mutation are higher in FHF group (7/40; 17.5%) compared to AVH group (6/115; 5.2%; p = 0.040). Mutation in the precore region, the number of AVH and FHF patients with A1896 is shown in Table 1. A1896 was found more frequently in patients with FHF compared to patients with AVH (p = 0.038). Other precore mutations were G1899A and C1914G which were comparable in AVH and FHF patients. A1993T and T2077C mutations were only found in FHF cases (Table 1).

The Clinical, Biochemical and Virological Profile of HBV Related Chronic Liver Diseases

The demographic, virological, and clinical characteristics of the patients with different stages of chronic HBV infection are summarized in Table 2. Male patients predominated in different stages of chronic HBV infection. The male-to-female ratio was lower in the asymptomatic carrier group than in the CH, Cirrhosis and HCC groups, respectively. The serum levels of ALT, AST and T. Bil were significantly higher in the Chronic hepatitis group than those in the other groups (p<0.05). Among all patients, the prevalence of HBeAg decreased gradually with clinical spectrum types from ASC (76.0%; 76/100), CHB (62.1%; 72/116), LC (37.2%; 29/78) and HCC (22.9%; 27/118). The highest serum viral load of HBV was observed in the ASC group, and a markedly lower viral load was found in the HCC group. The majority of patients belonged to genotype D (306/412; 74.3%), with 75.0% (75/100) in the ASC group, 69.8% (81/116) in the CH group, 73.1% (57/78) in the LC group, and 78.8% (93/118) in the HCC group. Although, genotype D was most common in each group, no statistically significant differences were found in the distribution of genotypes in various stages of chronic HBV infection. Genotype A was found in 25.7% (106/412) cases of various stages of CH infection (Table 2).

The HBV DNA sequences bearing the core promoter/precore/core regions were successfully amplified and following nucleotide substitutions were observed among studied strains (Table 3). Analysis of the nucleotide at position 1753 showed that a T-to-V (A/G/C) mutation was significantly higher in LC (34.6%) in comparison with CH (18.9%) and HCC (21.2%) (p = 0.001), suggesting that this mutation could be an indicator of liver

Table 1. The clinical, biochemical and virological profile of HBV related patients.

	Acute Viral Hepatitis (N = 115)	Fulminant Hepatitis (N = 40)	Chronic Hepatitis (N = 116)	Liver Cirrhosis (N = 30)	Hepatocellular Carcinoma (N = 30)
Age (Mean ±SD)	32.09±15.73	29.08±10.7	33.35±14.25	46.24±15.02	51.60±15.27
Sex (M/F)	1:1.1	0.8:1	1.9:1	6:1	9:1
ALT (IU/L)	280.61±568.58	1106.9±989.94	80.70±75.04	95.38±97.32	82.86±64.36
AST (IU/L)	219.39±415.154	1154.6±1245.70	76.25±71.84	76.08±60.73	64.20±45.96
ALP (IU/L)	88.30±123.63	267.70±193.68	39.50±61.53	89.55±135.33	202.60±196.01
T. Bil. (mg/dL)	2.78±1.38	5.68±2.67	0.96±0.24	1.2±0.49	1.6±0.82
HBsAg	115	40	116	30	30
Anti-HBc	115	40	116	30	30
HBeAg positive	43	19	37	10	12
HBV DNA (log copies/mL)	3.5±1.45	3.7±1.28	4.9±1.59	5.3±1.92	6.83±2.05

Abbreviations: ALT:Alanine Transaminases; AST:Aspartate Transaminases;
ALP:Alkaline Phosphatases; T. Bil.:Total Bilirubin.
HBsAg: Hepatitis B surface antigen; HBeAg: Hepatitis B e antigen.

cirrhosis. Mutations at positions 1762 and 1764, either as a double mutation or an independent mutation, were significantly higher in LC and HCC than CH and ASC (Table 2). Particularly, the double mutation (T1762/A1764) was found in 20.7%, 38.5% and 44.9% of CH, LC and HCC, respectively (p<0.001) and the difference was significant. The frequency of 1896 mutation was significantly high among CH, LC and HCC with respect to ASC (p<0.05).However, there was no difference in the percentage of patients with precore mutations between the HCC group (37.3%) compared with that of CH (24.1%) and LC (32.1%), respectively. The prevalence of the A1899 substitution was also higher in HCC (19.5%), LC (23.1%) and CH (14.7%) than in ASC (7.0%). Further, the C1914G core gene mutation was associated with the HCC cases (32.2%) compared to ASC (5.0%), CHB (7.8%) and LC (10.3%), respectively. No significant differences were observed in other mutations prevalent among the studied strains.

The clinical features of HBeAg-positive patients and anti-HBe-positive patients are shown in Table 3. Based on the HBeAg serology status, 205 patients were HBeAg positive and 362 patients were HBeAg-negative. There was no significant difference in age, ALT, AST, and bilirubin levels (biochemical parameters), and HBV viral load between HBeAg-positive and HBeAg-negative groups; however, a significant difference in the gender distribution

was observed (p = 0.001) (Table 3). Majority of chronic hepatitis B patients with HCC were HBeAg negative and were older than the other groups. The rate of precore 1896 mutant and core 1914 mutants were significantly higher (p = 0.001) in HBeAg-negative patients (43.4% and 23.4%) compared to HBeAg-positive patients (11.9% and 4.7%), respectively. There was no significant difference in the rate of BCP (T1762/A1764) double mutation between HBeAg-positive and HBeAg-negative patients (Table 3).

Discussion

Many studies have shown that virus mutations, including mutations of surface, BCP, and precore are linked to the severity and outcome of HBV infection. In the present study, amino acid mapping of the S gene showed a high rate of homology between the sequences. It has been shown that amino acid substitutions within the "a determinant" domain in the HBV S region may lead to conformational changes in the S protein. Some of these changes may create important medical and public health problems including vaccine escape, failure of hepatitis B immune globulin (HBIG) to protect liver transplant patients and babies born to HBV carrier mothers, and failure to detect HBV carriers with certain diagnostic tests [30]. In this study, the P120T/S was the most important substitution. This substitution was located at the

Table 2. Characteristics of patients with hepatitis B virus (HBV) infection according to hepatitis B e antigen (HBeAg) status.

Characteristics	HBeAg-positive (N = 121)	Anti-HBe-positive (N = 210)	P
Age (yr; mean ± SD)	35.06±12.8	38±12.2	NS
Sex : Male/Female	95 (78.5)/26 (21.5)	194 (92.4)/16 (7.6)	0.001
ALT (IU/L)	67.3±56.7	86.3±105.9	0.066
AST (IU/L)	64.8±89.2	81.5±92.8	0.110
T-Bil (mg/dL)	1.27±0.86	1.59±1.81	0.0684
Genotype A/D	32 (26.5)/89 (73.5)	43 (20.5)/167 (79.5)	0.211
HBV DNA (log copies/mL)	6.39±5.4	5.17±7.08	0.1019

Abbreviations: ALT:Alanine Transaminases; AST:Aspartate Transaminases;
ALP:Alkaline Phosphatases;T. Bil.:Total Bilirubin.

Table 3. Prevalence of Precore, Core and Surface region mutations in HBV isolated among different clinical groups.

Mutations	Acute Viral Hepatitis (N = 115)	Fulminant Hepatitis (N = 40)	Chronic Hepatitis (N = 116)	Liver Cirrhosis (N = 30)	Hepatocellular Carcinoma (N = 30)	Total %
T1753C/G	7 (7.1)	2 (5.0)	22 (18.9)	10 (33.3)	14 (46.7)	55 (16.6)
A1762T/G1764A	32 (27.8)	15 (37.5)	39 (33.6)	14 (46.7)	20 (66.7)	120 (36.3)
T1764/G1766	0 (0.0)	3 (7.5)	24 (20.7)	4 (13.3)	11 (36.7)	42 (12.7)
G1896A	20 (17.4)	18 (45.0)	38 (32.7)	12 (40.0)	17 (56.6)	105 (31.7)
G1899A	13 (12.2)	10 (25.0)	39 (33.6)	16 (53.3)	13 (43.3)	101 (30.5)
C1914G	2 (1.7)	6 (15.0)	12 (10.3)	7 (23.3)	19 (47.5)	46 (13.9)
A1993T	0 (0.0)	1 (2.5)	13 (11.2)	4 (13.3)	8 (26.7)	26 (7.8)
T2077C	0 (0.0)	3 (7.5)	23 (19.8)	8 (26.7)	7 (23.3)	41 (12.4)

outside of the "a determinant" immunologic domain. The P120T/S was detected in 7.8% of chronic hepatitis and 11.2% in patients with cirrhosis. As previously reported, the P120T/S substitution may cause problems with diagnostic assays, and may also cause vaccine escape and poor response to HBIG therapy [31]. Drug resistant mutations to ADV have been reported mainly in the HBV polymerase domain D rtN236T or the domain B rtA181V/T [32], [33], whereas a domain D rtN236T mutation does not overlap with the envelope gene, a mutation at rtA181T can result in a stop mutation in the envelope region of the S gene (SW172stop). In addition, an ADV-resistant mutation at rtA181V results in a concomitant change at SL- 173F. The S gene mutation, A184V, was detected in the ADV resistant rtA181T/V chronic hepatitis. This mutation site overlaps with the rt192 region in the polymerase gene. However, the A184V mutation did not result in amino acid changes in the polymerase region. There is one published report that the A184V mutation was related to reduced or negative HBsAg signal [34]. In our study, however, changes in HBsAg titer were not observed. The clinical implications of this remains to be determined. We detected sW172stop (6.4%) and sL173F (4.2%) mutations in LC patients with ADV-resistant rtA181T/V polymerase mutations. A large percentage of the cases with rtA181T mutations developed SW172stop mutations. In cases with ADV treated LMV-resistant mutations, the rtA181T mutation was reported at the ADV treatment baseline with low HBV DNA titers [35].

HBeAg negative patients with HBV DNA had significantly more severe liver disease than in other groups, suggesting that the accumulation of mutations due to host immune pressure in the due course of viral persistence could lead to the progression of liver damage. It is unlikely that the severity of illness is dependent solely on the prevailing precore/core sequence; it probably relates to such other factors like viral load, host immune response, etc. Some studies have also shown association of mutation in the preC/C region with the severity of liver disease [17]. A recent study from India has shown that chronic and fulminant hepatitis B is not associated with precore or core HBV mutants [24]. However, several studies have reported association between the severity of liver disease and the occurrence of A1896 mutations [36], [37], [38] and A1896 mutant has been detected frequently in HBeAg-negative asymptomatic carriers [39], [40]. In this study, there was no correlation between the presence of A1896 mutation and the presence of cirrhosis or elevated transaminase coinciding with previous reports of a lack of correlation between this mutation and liver disease [41], [42]. Thus, A1896 mutation alone appears to have no direct pathogenic role.

The prevalence of mutations at nt.1762 and 1764 in the core promoter and nt.1896 in the precore region increased proportionately with increased disease severity in patients with acute HBV infection. Thus, our results indicate that mutations in the core promoter and precore regions, together or independently, are associated with fulminant or severe acute hepatitis and that HBV strains with such mutations cannot direct the production of HBeAg. A low prevalence of HBeAg or anti-HBe in patients with fulminant and severe acute hepatitis B has been also noted. The precore mutant variants have also been reported in HBeAg-positive patients, ranging from 0%–80% [5], [43]. The BCP T1762/A1764 double mutations located at the HBV X gene diminishes HBeAg production, and is associated with more active liver disease [2], [44].

It is well known that the double mutation (T1762/A1764) in BCP is associated with an increased risk of liver disease. For instance, the frequency of double mutation (T1762/A1764) increased with advancing clinical status in Taiwanese patients (3%, 11%, 32% and 64% in ASC, LC, CH, and HCC groups, respectively) [45]. A recent report from China has also demonstrated that the incidence of double mutation increased along with the progression of liver disease; the percentage of the double mutation was 33%, 56% and 85% in CH, LC, and HCC groups, respectively [46]. In Indian patients, however, the T1762/A1764 double mutation was increased in CH from 20.7% to 38.5% in LC and 44.9% in HCC (Table 2). In the present study, detection of BCP double mutation T1762/A1764 was high in patients of FHF, LC and HCC, respectively; and had shown association with advanced form of liver diseases. Moreover, no significant difference (p = 0.866) was observed between the frequency of BCP double mutation in patients with HBeAg positive and HBeAg-negative phenotypes. Other studies have also shown a relationship between BCP double mutations and the clinical manifestations of HBV infection [5], [47]. In addition, analysis of the nucleotide at position 1753 showed that a T-to-V (A/G/C) mutation increased to 34.6% in LC from 18.9% in CH, but dramatically decreased in HCC (21.2%; Table 2), suggesting that this mutation is associated with liver cirrhosis rather than HCC. In contrast, analysis of sera or plasma from Japanese subjects with AC, CH, LC and HCC infected with HBV genotype C showed that the percentage of T1753V mutation increased with progression of liver disease [Takahashi et al., 1999]. It is also reported that T1753V mutation was higher in HCC (53.2%) compared with LC (18.8%) and CH (9.8%) [45]. These results were inconsistent with the present study, particularly in LC and HCC. These discrepancies might be due to the reason that most of the samples analyzed in the previous reports were HBV genotype C, whereas most of samples in the present study were HBV genotype D.

Our data also showed that viral mutations at nt. 1753 was more frequently observed in FH patients with fulminant hepatitis than in patients with acute hepatitis. T to C/A/G mutations at nt. 1753 was reported to be closely associated with progression of CH. These mutations were found in AT rich regions of the core promoter and can change the binding efficiency of transcription and translation factors.

The present study suggests that HBV genotype D and A were detected most frequently in HBV associated liver disease patients in India, and genotype D was predominant. There was an increased frequency of precore mutation and BCP double mutations amongst the patients studied. The study indicates that core mutations can be frequently detected in patients with chronic

HBV infection. It was observed that HBV genotype, as well as the serotype, may not be associated with an increased risk of HCC. The T1762/A1764 and T1753V mutations in BCP could be one of the indicators for progression of liver disease in India. Prospective studies on the sequence variations of the preC/C region of the HBV genome and the molecular mechanisms in relation to progression of liver disease would provide better understanding of the biological significance of HBV strains in India.

Author Contributions

Conceived and designed the experiments: PK SAH. Performed the experiments: AM DKS. Analyzed the data: AM. Contributed reagents/materials/analysis tools: PK SAH AA. Wrote the paper: AM.

References

1. Kao JH, Chen PJ, Lai MY, Chen DS (2002) Genotypes and clinical phenotypes of hepatitis B virus in patients with chronic hepatitis B virus infection. J Clin Microbiol 40: 1207–1209.
2. Hannoun C, Horal P, Lindh M (2000) Long-term mutation rates in the hepatitis B virus genome. J Gen Virol 81: 75–83.
3. Kidd-Ljunggren K, Miyakawa Y, Kidd AH (2002) Genetic variability in hepatitis B viruses. J Gen Virol 83: 1267–1280.
4. Kidd-Ljunggren K, Myhre E, Blackberg J (2004) Clinical and serological variation between patients infected with different Hepatitis B virus genotypes. J Clin Microbiol 42: 5837–5841.
5. Chen CH, Lee CM, Hung CH, Hu TH, Wang JH, et al. (2007) Clinical significance and evolution of core promoter and precore mutations in HBeAg-positive patients with HBV genotype B and C: a longitudinal study. Liver Int 27: 806–815.
6. Lin CL, Liu CH, Chen W, Huang WL, Chen PJ, et al. (2007) Association of pre-S deletion mutant of hepatitis B virus with risk of hepatocellular carcinoma. J Gastroenterol Hepatol 22: 1098–1103.
7. Seeger C, Mason WS (2000) Hepatitis B virus biology. Microbiol Mol Biol Rev 64(1): 51–68.
8. Tsai WL, Lo GH, Hsu PI, Lai KH, Lin CK, et al. (2008) Role of genotype and precore/basal core promoter mutations of hepatitis B virus in patients with chronic hepatitis B with acute exacerbation. Scand J Gastroenterol 43(2): 196–201.
9. Jammeh S, Tavner F, Watson R, Thomas HC, Karayiannis P (2008) Effect of basal core promoter and pre-core mutations on hepatitis B virus replication. J Gen Virol 89(Pt 4): 901–909.
10. Tong MJ, Blatt LM, Kao JH, Cheng JT, Corey WG (2007) Basal core promoter T1762/A1764 and precore A1896 gene mutations in hepatitis B surface antigen-positive hepatocellular carcinoma: a comparison with chronic carriers. Liver Int 27(10): 1356–1363.
11. Yuen MF, Tanaka Y, Shinkai N, Poon RT, But DY, et al (2008) Risk for hepatocellular carcinoma with respect to hepatitis B virus genotypes B/C, specific mutations of enhancer II/core promoter/precore regions and HBV DNA levels. Gut 57(1): 98–102.
12. Fang ZL, Sabin CA, Dong BQ, Ge LY, Wei SC, et al. (2008) HBV A1762T, G1764A mutations is a valuable biomarker for identifying a subset of male HBsAg carriers at extremely high risk of hepatocellular carcinoma: a prospective study. Am J Gastroenterol 103(9): 2254–2262.
13. Chen CH, Changchien CS, Lee CM, Hung CH, Hu TH, et al. (2008) Combined mutations in pre-s/surface and core promoter/precore regions of hepatitis B virus increase the risk of hepatocellular carcinoma: a case-control study. J Infect Dis 198(11): 1634–1642.
14. Tanaka Y, Mukaide M, Orito E, Yuen MF, Ito K, et al (2006) Specific mutations in enhancer II/core promoter of hepatitis B virus subgenotypes C1/C2 increase the risk of hepatocellular carcinoma. J Hepatol 45(5): 646–653.
15. Abbas Z, Muzaffar R, Siddiqui A, Naqvi SA, Rizvi SA (2006) Genetic variability in the precore and core promoter regions of hepatitis B virus strains in Karachi. BMC Gastroenterol: 6–20.
16. Rezende RE, Fonseca BA, Ramalho LN, Zucoloto S, Pinho JR, et al. (2005) The precore mutation is associated with severity of liver damage in Brazilian patients with chronic hepatitis. B J Clin Virol 32(1): 53–59.
17. Xu Y, Ren X, Liu Y, Li X, Bai S, et al. (2011) Association of hepatitis B virus mutations in basal core promoter and precore regions with severity of liver disease: an investigation of 793 Chinese patients with mild and severe chronic hepatitis B and acute-on-chronic liver failure. J Gastroenterol 46(3): 391–400.
18. Du H, Li T, Zhang HY, He ZP, Dong QM, et al. (2007) Correlation of hepatitis B virus (HBV) genotypes and mutations in basal core promoter/precore with clinical features of chronic HBV infection. Liver Int 27(2): 240–246.
19. Chen CH, Lee CM, Lu SN, Changchien CS, Wang JC, et al. (2006) Comparison of sequence changes of precore and core promoter regions in HBeAg-positive chronic hepatitis B patients with and without HBeAg clearance in lamivudine therapy. J Hepatol 44(1): 76–82.
20. Jain RC, Bhat SD, Sangle DS (1992) Prevalence of hepatitis surface antigen among rural population of Loni area in Ahmednagar district of Western Maharashtra. J Assoc Physicians India 40: 390–391.
21. Mital VN, Gupta OP, Nigam DK, Saxena PC, Kumar S (1980) Pattern of hepatitis B antigen-contact and carrier state in Northern India. J Indian Med Assoc 74: 105–107.
22. Thyagarajan SP, Jayaram S, Mohanavalli B (1996) Prevalence of HBV in general population of India. In S. K. Sarin and A. K. Singhal (eds). Hepatitis B in India: Problems and Prevention. CBS, New Delhi : 5–16.
23. Aggarwal R, Ghoshal UC, Naik SR (2003) Assessment of cost effectiveness of universal hepatitis B immunization in a low income country with intermediate endemicity using a Markov model. J Hepatol 38: 215–222.
24. Gandhe SS, Chadha MS, Walimbe AM, Arankalle VA (2003) Hepatitis B virus: Prevalence of precore/core promoter mutants in different clinical categories of Indian patients. J Viral Hepat 10: 367–382.
25. Ikeda KY, Arase SS, Kobayashi M, Someya T, Hosaka T, et al. (2006) Long-term outcome of HBV carriers with negative HBe antigen and normal aminotransferase. Am J Med 119: 977–985.
26. Irshad M, Sharma Y, I Dhar, J Singh, YK Joshi (2006) Transfusion-transmitted virus in association with hepatitis A-E viral infections in various forms of liver diseases in India. World J Gastroenterol 12(15): 2432–2436.
27. Trey C, Davidson CS (1970) The management of fulminant hepatic failure. In: Popper, H Scaffner, F, eds. Progress in liver failure. New york: Grune & Stratton. 282–98.
28. Xiao L, Zhou B, Gao H, Ma S, Yang G, et al. (2011) Hepatitis B virus genotype B with G1896A and A1762T/G1764A mutations is associated with hepatitis B related acute-on-chronic liver failure. J Med Virol. 83(9): 1544–1550.
29. Bruix J, Sherman M, Llovet JM, Beaugrand M, Lencioni R, et al. (2001) J. EASL Panel of Experts on HCC.
30. Tian Y, Xu Y, Zhang Z, Meng Z, Qin L, et al. (2007) The amino Acid residues at positions 120 to 123 are crucial for the antigenicity of hepatitis B surface antigen. J Clin Microbiol 45: 2971–2978.
31. Bartholomeusz A, Locarnini S (2006) Hepatitis B virus mutations associated with antiviral therapy. J Med Virol 78 (1): 52–55.
32. Angus P, Vaughan R, Xiong S, Yang H, Delaney W, et al. (2003) Resistance to adefovir dipivoxil therapy associated with the selection of a novel mutation in the HBV polymerase. Gastroenterology 125: 292–297.
33. Olinger CM, Weber B, Otegbayo JA, Ammerlaan W, Van der Taelem-Brule N, et al. (2007) Hepatitis B virus genotype E surface antigen detection with different immunoassays and diagnostic impact of mutations in the preS/S gene. Med Microbiol Immunol 196: 247–252.
34. Tatti KM, Korba BE, Stang HL, Peek S, Gerin JL, et al. (2002) Mutations in the conserved woodchuck hepatitis virus polymerase FLLA and YMDD regions conferring resistance to lamivudine. Antiviral Res 55: 141–150.
35. Frank T, Christina G, Tom L, Albert H, Michael P, et al. (2004) Basal Core Promoter and Precore Mutations in the Hepatitis B Virus Genome Enhance Replication Efficacy of Lamivudine-Resistant Mutants. J Virol 78(16): 8524–8535.
36. Liang TJ, Hasegawa K, Rimon N, Wands JR, Ben-Porath E (1991) A hepatitis B virus mutant associated with an epidemic of fulminant hepatitis. N Engl J Med 324: 1705–1709.
37. Akahane Y, Yamanaka T, Suzuki H, Sugai Y, Tsuda F, et al. (1990) Chronic active hepatitis with hepatitis B virus DNA and antibody against e antigen in the serum. Disturbed synthesis and secretion of e antigen from hepatocytes due to a point mutation in the precore region. Gastroenterology 99:1113–1119.
38. Okamoto H, Yotsumoto S, Akahane Y, Yamanaka T, Miyazaki Y, et al. (1990) Hepatitis B viruses with precore region defects prevail in persistently infected

hosts along with seroconversion to the antibody against e antigen. J Virol 64: 1298–1303.

39. Akarka US, Greene S, Lok ASF (1994) Detection of pre-core hepatitis B virus mutants in asymptomatic HBsAg-positive family members. Hepatology 19: 1366–1370.

40. Chan HLY, Hussain M, Lok ASF (1999) Different hepatitis B virus genotypes are associated with different mutations in the core promoter and precore regions during hepatitis B e antigen seroconversion. Hepatology 29: 976–984.

41. Chan HLY, Leung NWY, Hussain M, Wong ML, Lok ASF (2000) Hepatitis B e antigen-negative chronic hepatitis B in Hong Kong. Hepatology 31: 763–768.

42. Brunetto MR, Oliveri F, Coco B, Leandro G, Colombatto P, et al. (2002) Outcome of anti-HBe positive chronic hepatitis B in alpha-interferon treated and untreated patients: a long term cohort study. J Hepatol 36: 263–270.

43. Kao JH, Chen PJ, Lai MY, Chen DS (2003) Basal core promoter mutations of hepatitis B virus increase the risk of hepatocellular carcinoma in hepatitis B carriers. Gastroenterology 124: 327–334.

44. Kim BK, Revill PA, Ahn SH (2011) HBV genotypes: relevance to natural history, pathogenesis and treatment of chronic hepatitis B. Antivir Ther 16(8): 1169–1186.

45. Wang Z, Tanaka Y, Huang Y, Kurbanov F, Chen J, et al. (2007) Clinical and virological characteristics of hepatitis B virus subgenotypes Ba, C1, and C2 in China. J Clin Microbiol 45: 1491–1496.

46. Chen CH, Lee CM, Lu SN, Changchien CS, Eng HL, et al. (2005) Clinical significance of hepatitis B virus (HBV) genotypes and precore and core promoter mutations affecting HBV e antigen expression in Taiwan. J Clin Microbiol 43: 6000–6006.

47. Takahashi K, Ohta Y, Kanai K, Akahane Y, Iwasa Y, et al. (1999) Clinical implications of mutations C-to-T1653 and T-to-C/A/G1753 of hepatitis B virus genotype C genome in chronic liver disease. Arch Virol 144: 1299–1308.

5

A Genetic Validation Study Reveals a Role of Vitamin D Metabolism in the Response to Interferon-Alfa-Based Therapy of Chronic Hepatitis C

Christian M. Lange[1,2]*, Stephanie Bibert[3], Zoltan Kutalik[4], Philippe Burgisser[1], Andreas Cerny[5], Jean-Francois Dufour[6], Andreas Geier[7], Tilman J. Gerlach[8], Markus H. Heim[9], Raffaele Malinverni[10], Francesco Negro[11], Stephan Regenass[7], Klaus Badenhoop[2], Jörg Bojunga[2], Christoph Sarrazin[2], Stefan Zeuzem[2], Tobias Müller[12], Thomas Berg[13], Pierre-Yves Bochud[3], Darius Moradpour[1]*, the Swiss Hepatitis C Cohort Study Group[¶]

1 Division of Gastroenterology and Hepatology, Centre Hospitalier Universitaire Vaudois, University of Lausanne, Lausanne, Switzerland, 2 Medizinische Klinik 1, Klinikum der J. W. Goethe-Universität Frankfurt a.M., Frankfurt a.M., Germany, 3 Division of Infectious Diseases, Centre Hospitalier Universitaire Vaudois, University of Lausanne, Lausanne, Switzerland, 4 Division of Medical Genetics, Centre Hospitalier Universitaire Vaudois, University of Lausanne, Lausanne, Switzerland, 5 Liver Unit, Ospedale Moncucco, Lugano, Switzerland, 6 University Clinic of Visceral Surgery and Medicine, Inselspital, Bern, Switzerland, 7 Division of Gastroenterology and Hepatology, University Hospital Zürich, Zürich, Switzerland, 8 Division of Gastroenterology, Kantonsspital St. Gallen, St. Gallen, Switzerland, 9 Division of Gastroenterology and Hepatology, University Hospital Basel, Basel, Switzerland, 10 Hôpital Neuchâtelois, Neuchâtel, Switzerland, 11 Division of Gastroenterology and Hepatology, University Hospital Geneva, Geneva, Switzerland, 12 Medizinische Klinik mit Schwerpunkt Hepatologie und Gastroenterologie, Charité Campus Virchow Klinikum, Berlin, Germany, 13 Klinik für Gastroenterologie und Rheumatologie, Sektion Hepatologie, Universitätsklinikum Leipzig, Leipzig, Germany

Abstract

Background: To perform a comprehensive study on the relationship between vitamin D metabolism and the response to interferon-α-based therapy of chronic hepatitis C.

Methodology/Principal Findings: Associations between a functionally relevant polymorphism in the gene encoding the vitamin D 1α-hydroxylase (*CYP27B1-1260* rs10877012) and the response to treatment with pegylated interferon-α (PEG-IFN-α) and ribavirin were determined in 701 patients with chronic hepatitis C. In addition, associations between serum concentrations of 25-hydroxyvitamin D_3 (25[OH]D_3) and treatment outcome were analysed. *CYP27B1-1260* rs10877012 was found to be an independent predictor of sustained virologic response (SVR) in patients with poor-response *IL28B* genotypes (15% difference in SVR for rs10877012 genotype AA *vs.* CC, p = 0.02, OR = 1.52, 95% CI = 1.061–2.188), but not in patients with favourable *IL28B* genotype. Patients with chronic hepatitis C showed a high prevalence of vitamin D insufficiency (25[OH]D_3<20 ng/mL) during all seasons, but 25(OH)D_3 serum levels were not associated with treatment outcome.

Conclusions/Significance: Our study suggests a role of bioactive vitamin D (1,25[OH]$_2$$D_3$, calcitriol) in the response to treatment of chronic hepatitis C. However, serum concentration of the calcitriol precursor 25(OH)D_3 is not a suitable predictor of treatment outcome.

Editor: Stephen J. Polyak, University of Washington, United States of America

Funding: This work was supported by the Swiss National Science Foundation (3100A0-122447 to DM, 32003B-127613 to PYB as well as 3347C0-108782/1 and 33CSC0-108782/2 to SCCS), the Leenaards Foundation (to PYB), the European Community's FP7 (grant agreement 260844 to PYB; and grant agreement 241447 to KB), and the Santos-Suarez Foundation (to PYB). CML is the recipient of a Research Fellowship from the Deutsche Forschungsgemeinschaft (LA 2806/1-1). The funders had no role in study design, data collection and analysis, decision to publish, or preparation of the manuscript.

Competing Interests: The authors have declared that no competing interests exist.

* E-mail: Christian.Lange@chuv.ch (CL); Darius.Moradpour@chuv.ch (DM)

¶ Membership of the Swiss Hepatitis C Cohort Study Group is provided in the Acknowledgments.

Introduction

Chronic hepatitis C is one of the most serious infectious diseases worldwide [1]. Less than 50% of all patients infected with hepatitis C virus (HCV) genotype 1 and 4 as well as ~80% of those infected with genotype 2 and 3 can be cured with a combination therapy of pegylated interferon-α (PEG-IFN-α) and ribavirin [2]. The adjunction of directly acting antivirals (DAA), namely the NS3-4A protease inhibitors telaprevir and boceprevir, results in

substantially increased rates of sustained virologic response (SVR) in both treatment-naïve and treatment-experienced patients infected with HCV genotype 1 [3–7]. However, such triple therapy regimens are burdened with additional adverse events and their efficacy in prior null-responders (<2 log$_{10}$ reduction in HCV RNA after 12 weeks of PEG-IFN-α and ribavirin) remains limited [7,8]. Therefore, despite enormous progress, there is still a need to optimize IFN-α-based (or IFN-α-free) treatment regimens for chronic hepatitis C, and the establishment of algorithms (including, for example, on-treatment viral kinetics and *IL28B* genotype) to select appropriate treatment regimens for individual patients remains highly relevant [9–15]. The importance of host genetics in the prediction of treatment outcome has been impressively demonstrated by the discovery of the *IL28B* locus as determinant of spontaneous as well as of treatment-induced clearance from HCV infection [11,13]. The minor allele of *IL28B* (e. g. rs12979860 T allele) has a an adverse effect on both spontaneous and treatment-induced clearance, and it was shown that for example the adverse *IL28B* rs12979860 CT/TT genotype is one of the strongest baseline predictors of treatment failure [14].

Recently, vitamin D insufficiency (defined by a 25-hydroxyvitamin D [25(OH)D$_3$] serum concentration <20 ng/mL) has been proposed as a predictor of failure of treatment of chronic hepatitis C with PEG-IFN-α and ribavirin [16,17]. Moreover, severe vitamin D deficiency is a common feature of chronic hepatitis C, even in the absence of advanced liver fibrosis [18]. These findings may have important implications for the management of chronic hepatitis C, as vitamin D status is a potentially modifiable determinant of treatment outcome. However, it is currently unknown whether vitamin D itself affects response to IFN-α-based therapy or whether it is only a surrogate marker of treatment outcome.

A number of genetic polymorphisms in the vitamin D pathway have been shown to affect vitamin D signaling, and stratification according to such polymorphisms has already being implemented in randomized controlled clinical intervention studies [19–22]. Therefore, we believe that analyzing the impact of functionally relevant genetic polymorphisms in the vitamin D cascade on SVR may provide stronger evidence on an intrinsic role of vitamin D metabolism in the pathogenesis and treatment of chronic hepatitis C than analyzing exclusively vitamin D serum levels, which are affected by various parameters, including season, sunlight exposure, nutrition, and the metabolic syndrome [23,24]. Recently, some of us have observed an association of the 1α-hydroxylase promoter polymorphism *CYP27B1-1260* rs10877012 with SVR in a relatively small group of patients (n = 110) [18]. In the present study, we aimed to validate this association in 701 patients selected from a well-characterized patient cohort, the Swiss Hepatitis C Cohort Study (SCCS). In addition, we further characterized the relationship between 25(OH)D$_3$ serum levels and chronic hepatitis C as well as its treatment.

Methods

Objectives

The primary objective of the present study was to evaluate whether *CYP27B1 1260* rs10877012 genotype, a genetic marker of biologically active vitamin D, is associated with outcome of IFN-α based therapy of chronic hepatitis C. Secondary objectives were to characterize the frequency and determinants of vitamin D deficiency in patients with chronic hepatitis C, and whether serum levels of the calcitriol precursor 25(OH)D$_3$ are suitable for the prediction of treatment outcome as well.

Participants

Patients were followed within the framework of the SCCS, a multicenter study pursued at 8 major Swiss hospitals and their local affiliated centers, including a total of 3,648 patients with chronic or resolved HCV infection [25]. For the present retrospective analysis, two primary variables were analyzed: outcome of treatment with PEG-IFN-α and ribavirin (SVR *vs.* failure to achieve SVR) and 25(OH)D$_3$ serum concentration (as

continuous variable). Patients were included in the analysis of treatment response if they had treatment-naïve chronic hepatitis C, had provided written informed consent for genetic testing, had genomic DNA available for testing, were treated under clinical practice conditions with either PEG-IFN-α2a or PEG-IFN-α2b in combination with weight-based ribavirin, with standard treatment durations (48 weeks for HCV genotype 1 and 4, 24 weeks for HCV genotype 2 and 3), and if they had received ≥80% of the recommended dose of both agents during the first 12 weeks of therapy. Patients who received antiviral therapy not according to these pre-defined criteria were excluded from the analyses. Serum concentrations of 25(OH)D$_3$ were determined in all patients in whom a plasma sample at baseline of antiviral therapy was available. Moreover, 25(OH)D$_3$ serum levels were determined in additional patients from the SCCS in whom a plasma sample at the time of a liver biopsy was available.

Demographic and clinical characteristics including age, sex, HCV genotype, HCV viral load, histological grade and stage, alanine aminotransferase (ALT) serum levels, chronic hepatitis C treatment, alcohol consumption, body mass index (BMI), and presence or absence of diabetes were extracted from the SCCS database. SVR was defined as HCV RNA below the limit of detection in a sensitive assay ≥24 weeks after treatment completion, and all patients who failed to achieve SVR were classified as nonresponders. Data on rapid, early, and end-of-treatment virologic response were not available. High alcohol intake was defined as consumption >40 g per day over a period of ≥5 years. Liver biopsies were evaluated by experienced local pathologists. Liver fibrosis was classified according to the METAVIR score. Necroinflammatory activity was stratified into two groups, absent to mild activity *vs.* moderate to high activity. Steatosis was classified as absent or present.

Description of Investigations Undertaken

Serum levels of 25(OH)D$_3$ were measured as described previously [18]. Concentrations <20 ng/mL and <10 ng/mL were defined as vitamin D insufficiency and deficiency, respectively, whereas concentrations ≥20 ng/mL were considered as normal [24].

Genotyping for the *CYP27B1-1260* rs10877012 single nucleotide polymorphism (SNP) was performed using a TaqMan SNP Genotyping Assay (Applied Biosystems, Foster City, CA) and the ABI 7500 Fast Real-Time thermocycler, according to manufacturer's recommendations. TaqMan probes and primers were designed and synthesized by Applied Biosystems: rs10877012 forward 5′-AACAGAGAGAGGGCCTGTCT-3′, reverse 5′-GGGAGTAAGGAGCAGAGAGGTAAA-3′, Vic probe 5′-CTGTGGGAGATTCTTTTAT-3′, Fam probe 5′-TGTGGGA-GATTATTTTAT-3′. Automated allele calling was performed using SDS Software from Applied Biosystems. Positive and negative controls were used in each genotyping assay. *IL28B* rs12979860 genotyping was performed as described [26].

Ethics

The study was approved by local ethical committees of each hospital (Universitätsspital Basel, Basel; Inselspital, Bern; University Hospital Geneva, Geneva; CHUV, Lausanne; Ospedale Moncucco, Lugano; Hôpital Neuchâtelois, Neuchatel; Kantonsspital St. Gallen, St. Gallen; Universitätsspital Zürich, Zürich), and written informed consent was received from all participants.

Statistical Analyses

Testing for Hardy-Weinberg equilibrium was performed with the genhw package in Stata (version 9.1, StataCorp, College

Table 1. Baseline and demographic characteristics.

	Response to therapy		25(OH)D3 serum concentration (n = 496)
	SVR (n = 449)	Non-Response (n = 252)	
Sex			
Male, n (%)	276 (61)	170 (67)	314 (63)
Missing, n	0	0	0
Age, years			
Mean (range)	44 (23–78)	46 (21–70)	45 (21–76)
Missing, n	79	53	73
HCV genotype, n (%)			
1	140 (31)	170 (68)	203 (47)
2	70 (16)	11 (4)	44 (10)
3	206 (46)	43 (17)	148 (34)
4	32 (7)	26 (10)	41 (9)
Missing	1	2	60
Diabetes, n (%)			
Yes	26 (6)	26 (10)	32 (6)
Missing	0	0	0
HCV RNA, log_{10} IU/mL			
Mean (range)	5.77 (1–8)	5.00 (1–8)	5.66 (1–8)
Missing, n	0	0	3
Fibrosis stage, n (%)			
0	27 (9)	12 (7)	31 (10)
1	77 (26)	31 (18)	95 (31)
2	99 (33)	58 (34)	79 (26)
3	36 (12)	33 (19)	44 (15)
4	57 (19)	38 (22)	54 (18)
Missing	153	80	193
Steatosis, n (%)			
Yes	221 (72)	122 (76)	208 (73)
Missing, n	144	91	210
Activity, n (%)			
None-mild	227 (77)	137 (79)	237 (78)
Moderate-high	67 (23)	36 (21)	66 (22)
Missing, n	155	79	193
BMI, kg/m^2			
Mean (range)	24 (16–42)	25 (18–40)	24 (16–40)
Missing, n	106	70	171
ALT, U/L			
Mean (range)	94 (8–693)	107 (18–617)	121 (8–720)
Missing, n	106	70	171

Univariate P values for SVR *vs.* nonresponse are shown in Table 2. ALT, alanine aminotransferase; BMI, body mass index; HCV, hepatitis C virus; SVR, sustained virologic response. Of the 496 patients in whom 25(OH)D3 serum concentrations were measured, 269 were subsequently treated with pegylated interferon-α and ribavirin and assessed for treatment outcome.

Station, TX). Associations of *CYP27B1-1260* rs10877012 SNP with dichotomic variables (SVR *vs.* nonresponse) were assessed in logistic regression models. After univariate analyses, multivariate analyses were performed for significant associations. Multivariate models were obtained by backward selection, using a *P* value >0.15 for removal from the model. Sex, age, and *CYP27B1-1260* rs10877012 genotype were forced into the model. Only patients with complete data for the remaining covariates were included in multivariate analyses. SNPs were analyzed using an additive model (none, one or two copies of the minor allele were coded 0, 1 and 2, respectively, assuming greater effect with increased copy number of the minor allele), unless otherwise specified. Group differences (e.g. *CYP27B1-1260* rs10877012 AA *vs.* AC *vs.* CC)

Table 2. Genotype frequencies of the 1α-hydroxylase promoter polymorphism *CYP27B1-1260* rs10877012 in patients who received treatment with pegylated interferon-α and ribavirin.

	All, n (%)*	HCV gt 1/4, n (%)	HCV gt 2/3, n (%)
AA	63 (9)	34 (9)	29 (9)
CA	293 (42)	153 (42)	139 (42)
CC	345 (49)	181 (49)	162 (49)

The distribution of homozygous and heterozygous carriers corresponded to the expectations from the Hardy-Weinberg equilibrium (P = 0.35).
*This includes 3 patients with unknown HCV genotype. gt, genotype; HCV, hepatitis C virus.

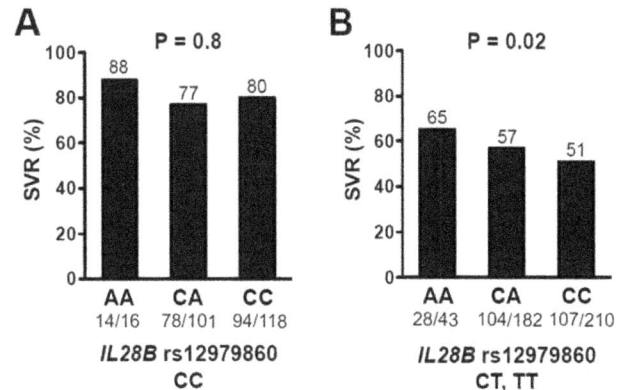

Figure 1. Treatment response according to *CYP27B1-1260* rs10877012 genotype. Overall sustained virologic response (SVR) rates across all HCV genotypes are shown for patients (**A**) with *IL28B* rs12979860 genotype CC and for (**B**) patients with *IL28B* rs12979860 genotype CT or TT. Numbers above bars indicate SVR rates in percent. Numbers below bars indicate absolute numbers of patients with SVR/all patients.

were assessed by means of χ^2 contingency tables or Wilcoxon-Mann-Whitney-U-tests, as appropriate.

Results

Patient Characteristics

Out of a total of 3,648 patients enrolled in the SCCS, 701 patients were included in the analysis of treatment response based on the selection criteria defined above. Of these, 269 patients had a plasma sample at baseline of antiviral therapy available for measurement of 25(OH)D$_3$ level. Moreover, 25(OH)D$_3$ serum concentrations were determined in an additional 227 patients from the SCCS in whom a plasma sample at the time of a liver biopsy was available. Thus, 25(OH)D$_3$ serum levels were determined in a total of 496 patients. Epidemiological and clinical characteristics of patients are summarized in Table 1.

CYP27B1-1260 rs10877012 and Response to Treatment of Chronic Hepatitis C

The *CYP27B1-1260* rs10877012 genotype was chosen as the primary variable to be assessed for associations with treatment outcome because this functional polymorphism in the promoter of the 1α-hydroxylase affects tissue concentrations of calcitriol (the C

allele results in reduced calcitriol synthesis), thereby being a well-characterized determinant of biologically active vitamin D [20,27]. rs10877012 genotype frequencies of the present cohort are shown in Table 2. They were largely comparable to those previously observed in the general population [18].

In a pooled analysis across all HCV genotypes, there was a progressive decrease in SVR rates according to *CYP27B1-1260* rs10877012 genotype (73% SVR for genotype AA, 65% for AC and 62% for CC), suggesting an additive effect of the SNP. However, the association was not significant (P = 0.11, OR = 1.22, 95% CI = 0.954–1.552). Significance level increased in a multivariate model, after adjustment for HCV genotype, age, sex, baseline viral load, BMI, ALT, diabetes, and *IL28B* rs12979860 genotype (P = 0.06, OR = 1.33, CI = 0.988–1.796, Table 3) or when comparing rs10877012 CC carriers to AA carriers (P = 0.04). When the association of *CYP27B1-1260* rs10877012 with SVR was examined in patients stratified according to *IL28B*

Table 3. Factors associated with sustained virologic response.

Variable	P value, univariate	P value, multivariate	Odds ratio (95% CI), multivariate
Age (years, continuous)	<0.001	<0.001	0.96 (0.94–0.98)
HCV RNA (log$_{10}$ IU/mL, continuous)	<0.001	<0.001	0.38 (0.29–0.50)
ALT (U/L, continuous)	0.05		
BMI (kg/m^2, continuous)	0.08		
Male sex	0.10	1.0	0.85 (0.57–1.28)
HCV genotype 2/3 *vs.* 1/4	<0.001	<0.001	8.99 (4.21–19.19)
Diabetes	0.03		
Fibrosis, F0–F1 *vs.* F2–F4	0.03		
Steatosis	0.47		
Necroinflammatory activity	0.71		
Alcohol (40 g/d ≥5 years)	0.28		
IL28B rs12979860	<0.001	<0.001	0.27 (0.17–0.43)
CYP27B1 rs10877012	0.11	0.06	1.33 (0.99–1.80)

ALT, alanine aminotransferase; BMI, body mass index; CI, confidence interval; HCV, hepatitis C virus.

Table 4. Factors associated with sustained virologic response in patients with unfavorable *IL28B* rs12979860 genotype CT or TT.

Variable	P value, univariate	P value, multivariate	Odds ratio (95% CI), multivariate
Age (years, continuous)	<0.001	0.001	0.96 (0.94–0.98)
HCV RNA (log$_{10}$ IU/mL, continuous)	<0.001	<0.001	0.35 (0.25–0.50)
ALT (U/L, continuous)	0.10		
BMI (kg/m^2, continuous)	0.16		
Male sex	0.11	0.11	0.97 (0.59–1.60)
HCV genotype 2/3 *vs*.1/4	<0.001	<0.001	12.4 (5.01–30.9)
Diabetes	0.05		
Fibrosis, F0–F1 *vs*. F2–F4	0.001		
Steatosis	0.82		
Necroinflammatory activity	0.86		
Alcohol (>40 g/d ≥5 years)	0.30		
CYP27B1 rs10877012	0.06	0.02	1.52 (1.06–2.19)

ALT, alanine aminotransferase; BMI, body mass index; CI, confidence interval; HCV, hepatitis C virus.

rs12979860 genotype CT and TT *vs*. CC, as shown in Figure 1, *CYP27B1-1260* rs10877012 was an independent predictor of SVR in patients with the poor-response genotype CT or TT (65% *vs*. 57% *vs*. 51% SVR in *CYP27B1-1260* rs10877012 AA *vs*. AC *vs*. CC, respectively; univariate P = 0.06; multivariate P = 0.02, OR = 1.52, 95% CI = 1.061–2.188, Table 4) but not in those with the good-response genotype CC (P = 0.8).

A similar impact of *CYP27B1-1260* rs10877012 on SVR was observed when patients infected with genotype 1 and 4 were analysed exclusively. Again, *CYP27B1-1260* rs10877012 genotype had no significant influence on SVR in patients with good-response *IL28B* rs12979860 genotype (SVR rates 88% *vs*. 65% *vs*. 73% for AA *vs*. CA *vs*. CC, respectively; P = 0.62). However, SVR rates in HCV genotype 1 and 4 patients with poor-response *IL28B* rs12979860 genotype were 42% *vs*. 39% *vs*. 30% in *CYP27B1-1260* rs10877012 AA *vs*. AC *vs*. CC, respectively (univariate P = 0.11; multivariate P = 0.09, OR = 1.46, 95% CI = 0.940–2.288), but the association formally lost statistical significance, most likely due to the low number (n = 24) of HCV genotype 1 and 4 patients with *CYP27B1-1260* rs10877012 AA and poor-response *IL28B* rs12979860 genotype. With respect to the low frequency of the beneficial minor A allele, *CYP27B1-1260* rs10877012 does not appear to be a suitable parameter for clinical decision making. Nevertheless, our genetic analyses point to a relevant role of

vitamin D metabolism in the response to treatment with PEG-IFN-α and ribavirin of chronic hepatitis C.

Serum Concentrations of 25-hydroxyvitamin D in Patients with Chronic Hepatitis C

Serum concentrations of 25(OH)D$_3$ were determined in 496 patients at baseline of treatment with PEG-IFN-α and ribavirin (n = 269) or at the time of liver biopsy in patients who were not treated (n = 227). Mean and median 25(OH)D$_3$ serum concentrations were 15.6 and 13.4 ng/mL (SD = 9.07; range 3.8–76.9 ng/mL), respectively, which are significantly lower than those determined in the general population (e. g. 22.2 and 20 ng/mL in Reusch et al., n>6.000) [24,28]. Among patients with chronic hepatitis C, 32%, 42%, and 26% had 25(OH)D$_3$ serum levels <10, ≥10 to <20, and ≥20 ng/mL, respectively. Because of the seasonal fluctuation of 25(OH)D$_3$ serum levels, we calculated median 25(OH)D$_3$ serum levels separately for each month. Although season had a substantial impact on median 25(OH)D$_3$ serum levels, at least 50% of HCV-infected individuals suffered from vitamin D insufficiency (<20 ng/mL) even during summer, while approximately 50% suffered from vitamin D deficiency (<10 ng/mL) between November and April (Figure 2).

In a univariate analysis, age, male sex, infection with HCV genotype 3, excessive alcohol consumption, presence of diabetes, advanced liver fibrosis, and season of blood sampling were significantly associated with low 25(OH)D$_3$ serum levels (< median; Table 5). In logistic regression analyses, age, advanced liver fibrosis, presence of diabetes, and season of blood sampling were independent and significant predictors of low 25(OH)D$_3$ serum levels (Table 5).

Serum Concentrations of 25-hydroxyvitamin D and Treatment Outcome

Since 25(OH)D$_3$ serum concentrations were only available in a subgroup of all treated patients included in this study (n = 269), we analyzed their relationship to treatment outcome separately from the above-described *CYP27B1* candidate gene study. In univariate analyses, no significant associations between SVR and 25(OH)D$_3$ serum levels either as continuous variable (p = 0.13, OR = 0.98, 95% CI = 0.95–1.01), or 25(OH)D$_3$ serum levels ≥10 ng/mL (p = 0.3, OR = 0.74, 95% CI = 0.43–1.30) and ≥20 ng/mL

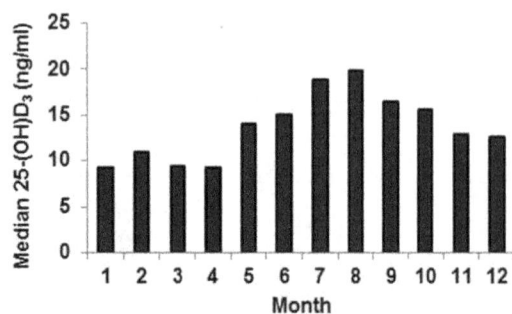

Figure 2. Seasonal variation of 25(OH)D$_3$ serum levels in patients with chronic hepatitis C. Median 25(OH)D$_3$ serum levels are shown for each month.

Table 5. Factors associated with 25-hydroxyvitamin D serum levels ($\geq$ median) in patients with chronic hepatitis C.

Variable	P value, univariate	P value, multivariate	Odds ratio (95% CI), multivariate
Age (years, continuous)	0.2	0.013	1.06 (1.01–1.12)
HCV RNA ($\log_{10}$ IU/mL, continuous)	0.3		
ALT (U/L, continuous)	0.6		
BMI (kg/m^2, continuous)	0.4		
IL28B rs12979860	0.3		
Male sex	0.003	0.5	0.77 (0.33–1.80)
HCV genotype 1,2,4 vs. 3[1]	0.034		
HIV coinfection	0.6		
Diabetes	0.049	0.01	0.17 (0.04–0.66)
Alcohol (>40 g/d $\geq$5 years)	0.010		
Fibrosis, F0–F1 vs. F2–F4	0.009	0.018	0.31 (0.12–0.82)
Necroinflammatory activity	0.9		
Steatosis	0.07		
Season of blood sampling	<0.0001	<0.0001	6.49 (2.71–15.6)

[1]Genotype 1, 2 and 4 were grouped vs. genotype 3 in this analysis, as the latter has been associated with metabolic disturbances (insulin resistance, steatosis) and more rapid fibrosis progression [37,38]. ALT, alanine aminotransferase; BMI, body mass index; CI, confidence interval; HCV, hepatitis C virus.

(p = 0.08, OR = 0.61, 95% CI = 0.36–1.10) were observed. Formally, these associations may be even interpreted as a statistical trend towards an inverse correlation between 25(OH)D$_3$ serum levels and SVR after treatment with PEG-IFN-α and ribavirin. However, in multivariate models adjusted for other predictors of treatment outcome (age, sex, IL28B rs12979860 genotype, HCV genotype, HCV RNA levels, presence of diabetes, BMI, and liver fibrosis), 25(OH)D$_3$ serum levels were clearly not associated with treatment outcome (p = 0.9 for 25[OH]D$_3$$\geq$20 ng/mL). These findings were similar when HCV genotype 1/4 or 2/3 patients were analyzed separately (data not shown).

Discussion

The results of the present genetic validation study suggest, in line with our previously published findings [18], an association between the CYP27B1-1260 promoter SNP rs10877012 and SVR to treatment of chronic hepatitis C with PEG-IFN-α and ribavirin. In the present study, this association was found only in patients with a poor-response IL28B genetic background, whereas CYP27B1-1260 rs10877012 was not significantly associated with SVR in patients with good-response IL28B genotype. CYP27B1-1260 rs10877012 is a functional polymorphism in the promoter of the 1α-hydroxylase, the enzyme required for the bioactivation of 25(OH)D$_3$ to 1,25(OH)$_2$D$_3$ (calcitriol) [20]. It has been shown that the CC genotype of CYP27B1-1260 rs10877012 impairs the expression of the 1α-hydroxylase, which results in reduced concentrations of bioactive vitamin D [18,27]. Consistently, the CC genotype of CYP27B1 is associated with poor response to interferon-α-based treatment of chronic hepatitis C in the present and in our previous study [18], as well as with the risk of bone disease or autoimmune disorders such as multiple sclerosis or type 1 diabetes [19,20,27,29]. Importantly, 1α-hydroxylase is expressed not only in the kidney but also in inflamed tissue and even in immune cells, were it serves as a local, inducible producer of calcitriol [30]. Bioactive vitamin D is an important immune modulator, as for example T cells and macrophages crucially depend on calcitriol in various conditions [31–33]. Thus, one may speculate that the "poor-response" CYP27B1-1260 rs10877012

genotype CC may result in lower local concentrations of calcitriol in the HCV-infected liver, resulting in reduced responsiveness to IFN-α or impaired adaptive immune responses. This may be especially relevant in patients with unfavourable IL28B genotype, who in general poorly respond to IFN-α.

The present study confirms that patients with chronic hepatitis C patients have a high prevalence of vitamin D insufficiency. However, in our study, 25(OH)D$_3$ serum levels were not associated with treatment outcome in a subgroup of 269 patients with available baseline serum samples before antiviral treatment. In fact, 25(OH)D$_3$ serum levels were even somewhat lower in patients who subsequently achieved SVR as compared to those who failed to respond to treatment. In two previous studies, including 167 and 211 patients treated with IFN-α-based therapy, a weak but significant correlation between 25(OH)D$_3$ serum levels and SVR was observed [16,34]. In our previous analysis we did not observe any significant association between 25(OH)D$_3$ serum levels and SVR to IFN-α-based therapy in a cohort of 317 HCV genotype 1-infected patients, but a significant association in a cohort of 156 patients infected with genotype 2 or 3 [18]. Two studies in HCV-HIV-coinfected patients found no correlation between 25(OH)D$_3$ serum levels and treatment outcome as well [35,36]. The reasons for these discrepancies remain unclear at the moment, but apparently 25(OH)D$_3$ serum levels cannot be considered as an established predictor of treatment outcome at the moment.

Importantly, it is well-known that 25(OH)D$_3$ serum levels correlate poorly with calcitriol serum concentrations, and 25(OH)D$_3$ serum levels are therefore not a suitable marker for bioactive vitamin D or vitamin D receptor signaling, especially not for local calcitriol levels during inflammatory conditions [24]. Thus, the lacking lack of an association between 25(OH)D$_3$ serum levels and SVR may simply reflect the limited biological relevance of 25(OH)D$_3$ serum levels. Unfortunately, there are no reliable methods to quantify serum levels of the bioactive vitamin D metabolite calcitriol, and the majority of clinical trials assessing the vitamin D status of patients focus on the calcitriol precursor 25(OH)D$_3$ [24]. Therefore, despite the lack of an association between 25(OH)D_3 serum levels and SVR, the replicated association between SVR and a functionally relevant genetic polymorphism in the vitamin D cascade, *CYP27B1-1260* rs10877012, suggests a role of vitamin D in the response to treatment of chronic hepatitis C. In line with this notion, we have recently identified an interaction between the vitamin D receptor and IFN-α-induced signaling through the Jak-STAT pathway, which results in a synergistic effect of calcitriol and INF-α on interferon-stimulated gene expression as well as on HCV replication *in vitro* (CML, MHH and DM, unpublished data). Therefore, the question as to whether optimization of the patients' vitamin D status may be beneficial before or during antiviral therapy remains open.

In conclusion, the present study suggests a role of vitamin D metabolism in the response to treatment of chronic hepatitis C, especially in patients with poor-response *IL28B* genotype, but importantly 25(OH)D_3 serum levels are not a reliable marker of treatment outcome.

Limitations

Several limitations of our study have to be acknowledged. First, the association between *CYP27B1-1260* rs10877012 and SVR is statistically relatively weak, as it might be expected from the moderate impact of this variation on calcitriol synthesis [20,27]. In line with this notion, we did not observe any significant association between *CYP27B1-1260* genotype and acute clearance from HCV infection in a cohort of 112 patients (data not shown). Therefore, *CYP27B1-1260* rs10877012 genotype does not appear to be a suitable marker for clinical decision making, and even larger sample sizes may be required to fully confirm the association between *CYP27B1* and SVR. Nevertheless, we believe that the

importance of this genetic validation study lies in the identification of vitamin D signaling as an intrinsic player in IFN-α-based therapy of chronic hepatitis C. Second, 25(OH)D_3 serum levels were available only for a subgroup of treated patients (n = 269), and significant associations might be identified in larger sample sizes. Furthermore, we cannot exclude a possible selection bias due the availability of serum in only a limited proportion of patients included in the primary analysis of *CYP27B1* genotype. Finally, incomplete datasets in some of our patients may be an additional source of bias, which represents a limitation inherent to cohort studies as compared to randomized controlled trials.

Acknowledgments

The members of the Swiss Hepatitis C Cohort Study Group are Francesco Negro (Chairman), Antoine Hadengue (Chairman of Scientific Committee), Laurent Kaiser, Laura Rubbia-Brandt (Geneva); Darius Moradpour, Cristina Cellerai (Lausanne); Martin Rickenbach (Lausanne Data Center); Andreas Cerny, Gladys Martinetti (Lugano); Jean-François Dufour, Meri Gorgievski, Virginie Masserey Spicher (Berne); Markus Heim, Hans Hirsch (Basel); Beat Müllhaupt, Beat Helbling, Stephan Regenass (Zurich); Raffaele Malinverni (Neuchatel); David Semela, Guenter Dollenmaier (St Gallen); Gieri Cathomas (Liestal).

Author Contributions

Conceived and designed the experiments: CML KB CS SZ PYB DM. Performed the experiments: CML SB ZK PYB. Analyzed the data: CML SB ZK PYB DM. Contributed reagents/materials/analysis tools: CML SB PB AC JFD AG TJG MHH RM FN SR JB TM TB PYB DM. Wrote the paper: CML SB ZK PB AC JFD AG TJG MHH RM FN SR KB JB CS SZ TM TB PYB DM SCCS.

References

1. Davis GL, Alter MJ, El-Serag H, Poynard T, Jennings LW (2010) Aging of hepatitis C virus (HCV)-infected persons in the United States: a multiple cohort model of HCV prevalence and disease progression. Gastroenterology 138: 513–521.

2. Zeuzem S, Berg T, Moeller B, Hinrichsen H, Mauss S, et al. (2009) Expert opinion on the treatment of patients with chronic hepatitis C. J Viral Hepat 16: 75–90.

3. Bacon BR, Gordon SC, Lawitz E, Marcellin P, Vierling JM, et al. (2011) Boceprevir for previously treated chronic HCV genotype 1 infection. N Engl J Med 364: 1207–1217.

4. Jacobson IM, McHutchison JG, Dusheiko G, Di Bisceglie AM, Reddy KR, et al. (2011) Telaprevir for previously untreated chronic HCV virus infection. N Engl J Med 364: 2405–2416.

5. Poordad F, McCone J, Bacon BR, Bruno S, Manns MP, et al. (2011) Boceprevir for untreated chronic HCV genotype 1 infection. N Engl J Med 364: 1195–1206.

6. Sherman KE, Flamm SL, Afdhal NH, Nelson DR, Sulkowski MS, et al. (2011) Response-guided telaprevir combination treatment for hepatitis C virus infection. N Engl J Med 365: 1014–1024.

7. Zeuzem S, Andreone P, Pol S, Lawitz E, Diago M, et al. (2011) Telaprevir for retreatment of HCV infection. N Engl J Med 364: 2417–2428.

8. Lange CM, Sarrazin C, Zeuzem S (2010) Review article: specifically targeted anti-viral therapy for hepatitis C - a new era in therapy. Aliment Pharmacol Ther 32: 14–28.

9. Berg T, Sarrazin C, Herrmann E, Hinrichsen H, Gerlach T, et al. (2003) Prediction of treatment outcome in patients with chronic hepatitis C: significance of baseline parameters and viral dynamics during therapy. Hepatology 37: 600–609.

10. Clark PJ, Thompson AJ, McHutchison JG (2010) IL28B genomic-based treatment paradigms for patients with chronic hepatitis C infection: the future of personalized HCV therapies. Am J Gastroenterol 106: 38–45.

11. Ge D, Fellay J, Thompson AJ, Simon JS, Shianna KV, et al. (2009) Genetic variation in IL28B predicts hepatitis C treatment-induced viral clearance. Nature 461: 399–401.

12. Lange CM, von Wagner M, Bojunga J, Berg T, Farnik H, et al. (2010) Serum lipids in European chronic HCV genotype 1 patients during and after treatment with pegylated interferon-alpha-2a and ribavirin. Eur J Gastroenterol Hepatol 22: 1303–1307.

13. Lange CM, Zeuzem S (2011) IL28B single nucleotide polymorphisms in the treatment of hepatitis C. J Hepatol 55: 962–701.

14. Thompson AJ, Muir AJ, Sulkowski MS, Ge D, Fellay J, et al. (2010) Interleukin-28B polymorphism improves viral kinetics and is the strongest pretreatment predictor of sustained virologic response in genotype 1 hepatitis C virus. Gastroenterology 139: 120–129 e118.

15. Lange CM, Kutalik Z, Morikawa K, Bibert S, Cerny A, et al. (2012) Serum ferritin levels are associated with a distinct phenotype of chronic hepatitis C poorly responding to pegylated interferon-alpha and ribavirin therapy. Hepatology 55: 1038–47.

16. Petta S, Camma C, Scazzone C, Tripodo C, Di Marco V, et al. (2010) Low vitamin D serum level is related to severe fibrosis and low responsiveness to interferon-based therapy in genotype 1 chronic hepatitis C. Hepatology 51: 1158–1167.

17. Abu Mouch S, Fireman Z, Jarchovsky J, Zeina AR, Assy N (2011) Vitamin D supplement improves sustained virologic response in chronic hepatitis C (genotype 1)-naive patients. World J Gastroenterol 17: 5184–5190.

18. Lange CM, Bojunga J, Ramos-Lopez E, von Wagner M, Hassler A, et al. (2011) Vitamin D deficiency and a CYP27B1–1260 promoter polymorphism are associated with chronic hepatitis C and poor response to interferon-alfa based therapy. J Hepatol 54: 887–893.

19. Bailey R, Cooper JD, Zeitels L, Smyth DJ, Yang JH, et al. (2007) Association of the vitamin D metabolism gene CYP27B1 with type 1 diabetes. Diabetes 56: 2616–2621.

20. Cooper JD, Smyth DJ, Walker NM, Stevens H, Burren OS, et al. (2011) Inherited variation in vitamin D genes is associated with predisposition to autoimmune disease type 1 diabetes. Diabetes 60: 1624–1631.

21. Dong LM, Ulrich CM, Hsu L, Duggan DJ, Benitez DS, et al. (2009) Vitamin D related genes, CYP24A1 and CYP27B1, and colon cancer risk. Cancer Epidemiol Biomarkers Prev 18: 2540–2548.

22. Martineau AR, Timms PM, Bothamley GH, Hanifa Y, Islam K, et al. (2011) High-dose vitamin D(3) during intensive-phase antimicrobial treatment of pulmonary tuberculosis: a double-blind randomised controlled trial. Lancet 377: 242–250.

23. Bouillon R, Auwerx J, Dekeyser L, Fevery J, Lissens W, et al. (1984) Serum vitamin D metabolites and their binding protein in patients with liver cirrhosis. J Clin Endocrinol Metab 59: 86–89.

24. Rosen CJ (2011) Clinical practice. Vitamin D insufficiency. N Engl J Med 364: 248–254.

25. Prasad L, Spicher VM, Zwahlen M, Rickenbach M, Helbling B, et al. (2007) Cohort Profile: the Swiss Hepatitis C Cohort Study (SCCS). Int J Epidemiol 36: 731–737.

26. Lange CM, Moradpour D, Doehring A, Lehr HA, Mullhaupt B, et al. (2011) Impact of donor and recipient IL28B rs12979860 genotypes on hepatitis C virus liver graft reinfection. J Hepatol 55: 322–327.

27. Clifton-Bligh RJ, Nguyen TV, Au A, Bullock M, Cameron I, et al. (2011) Contribution of a common variant in the promoter of the 1-alpha-hydroxylase gene (CYP27B1) to fracture risk in the elderly. Calcif Tissue Int 88: 109–116.

28. Reusch J, Ackermann H, Badenhoop K (2009) Cyclic changes of vitamin D and PTH are primarily regulated by solar radiation: 5-year analysis of a German (50 degrees N) population. Horm Metab Res 41: 402–407.

29. Sundqvist E, Baarnhielm M, Alfredsson L, Hillert J, Olsson T, et al. (2010) Confirmation of association between multiple sclerosis and CYP27B1. Eur J Hum Genet 18: 1349–1352.

30. Zehnder D, Bland R, Williams MC, McNinch RW, Howie AJ, et al. (2001) Extrarenal expression of 25-hdydroxyvitamin d(3)-1 alpha-hydroxylase. J Clin Endocrinol Metab 86: 888–894.

31. Liu PT, Stenger S, Li H, Wenzel L, Tan BH, et al. (2006) Toll-like receptor triggering of a vitamin D-mediated human antimicrobial response. Science 311: 1770–1773.

32. Ramagopalan SV, Heger A, Berlanga AJ, et al. (2010) A ChiP-seq defined genome-wide map of vitamin D receptor binding: Associations with disease and evolution. Genome Research 20: 1352–1360.

33. von Essen MR, Kongsbak M, Schjerling P, Olgaard K, Odum N, et al. (2010) Vitamin D controls T cell antigen receptor signaling and activation of human T cells. Nat Immunol 11: 344–349.

34. Bitetto D, Fattovich G, Fabris C, Ceriani E, Falleti E, et al. (2011) Complementary role of vitamin D deficiency and the IL-28B rs12979860 C/T polymorphism in predicting antiviral response in chronic hepatitis C. Hepatology.

35. Milazzo L, Mazzali C, Bestetti G, Longhi E, Foschi A, et al. (2011) Liver-related factors associated with low vitamin D levels in HIV and HIV/HCV coinfected patients and comparison to general population. Curr HIV Res 9: 186–193.

36. Terrier B, Carrat F, Geri G, Pol S, Piroth L, et al. (2011) Low 25-OH vitamin D serum levels correlate with severe fibrosis in HIV-HCV co-infected patients with chronic hepatitis. J Hepatol 55: 756–761.

37. Bochud PY, Cai T, Overbeck K, Bochud M, Dufour JF, et al. (2009) Genotype 3 is associated with accelerated fibrosis progression in chronic hepatitis C. J Hepatol 51: 655–666.

38. Hofer H, Bankl HC, Wrba F, Steindl-Munda P, Peck-Radosavljevic M, et al. (2002) Hepatocellular fat accumulation and low serum cholesterol in patients infected with HCV-3a. Am J Gastroenterol 97: 2880–2885.

Serum Vitamin D Levels Are Not Predictive of the Progression of Chronic Liver Disease in Hepatitis C Patients with Advanced Fibrosis

Kathleen E. Corey[1,4], Hui Zheng[2], Jorge Mendez-Navarro[1], Aymin Delgado-Borrego[3], Jules L. Dienstag[1,4], Raymond T. Chung[1,4]*, the HALT-C Trial Group

1 Gastrointestinal Unit, Massachusetts General Hospital, Boston, Massachusetts, United States of America, 2 Massachusetts General Hospital Biostatistics Center, Massachusetts General Hospital, Boston, Massachusetts, United States of America, 3 Division of Pediatric Gastroenterology, University of Miami, Miami, Florida, United States of America, 4 Department of Medicine, Harvard Medical School, Boston, Massachusetts, United States of America

Abstract

In animal models and human cross-sectional studies, vitamin D deficiency has been associated with liver disease progression. Vitamin D supplementation has been suggested as a treatment to prevent disease progression. We sought to evaluate the role of vitamin D levels in predicting chronic liver disease development. We conducted a nested case-control study of vitamin D levels in subjects with (cases) and without (controls) liver histologic progression or clinical decompensation over the course of the HALT-C Trial. Vitamin D levels were measured at 4 points over 45 months. 129 cases and 129 aged-matched controls were included. No difference in baseline vitamin D levels were found between cases and controls. (44.8 ng/mL vs. 44.0 ng/mL, P = 0.74). Vitamin D levels declined in cases and controls over time (P = 0.0005), however, there was no difference in the level of decline (P = 0.37). Among study subjects with diabetes mellitius, baseline vitamin D levels were higher in cases, 49.9 ng/mL, than controls, 36.3 ng/mL. (P = 0.03) In addition, baseline vitamin D levels were higher in black case subjects, 32.7 ng/mL, than in black control subjects, 25.2 ng/mL (P = 0.08) No difference in vitamin D levels was found between patients with and without progression of hepatitis C-associated liver disease over 4 years. Our data do not suggest any role for vitamin D supplementation in patients with advanced chronic hepatitis C and raise the possibility that higher vitamin D levels may be associated with disease progression.

Editor: Fu-Sheng Wang, Beijing Institute of Infectious Diseases, China

Funding: This work was principally supported by a grant from the American College of Gastroenterology. Additional support was provided by the National Institute of Diabetes & Digestive & Kidney Diseases, the National Institute of Allergy and Infectious Diseases, the National Cancer Institute, the National Center for Minority Health and Health Disparities and by General Clinical Research Center and Clinical and Translational Science Center grants from the National Center for Research Resources, National Institutes of Health. The content is solely the responsibility of the authors and does not necessarily represent the official views of the National Center for Research Resources or the National Institutes of Health. Additional funding to conduct this study was supplied by Hoffmann-La Roche, Inc., through a Cooperative Research and Development Agreement with the National Institutes of Health. Additional grants and contracts supporting the HALT-C Study are listed in the Acknowledgement section. The funders had no role in study design, data collection and analysis, decision to publish, or preparation of the manuscript.

Competing Interests: The authors have declared that no competing interests exist.

* E-mail: rtchung@partners.org

Introduction

Hepatic fibrosis results from wound healing following acute and chronic liver injury. In response to chronic hepatic inflammation, parenchymal cells release extracellular matrix proteins including type I collagen, resulting in the progressive deposition of, and accumulation of, fibrosis. Ultimately, fibrotic tissue can replace hepatocytes and disrupt lobular architecture, the hallmark of cirrhosis, which, in turn, results eventually in hepatic dysfunction. [1]

Emerging data suggest that vitamin D is an important modulator of both the inflammatory response and wound healing. [2,3] Vitamin D may modulate the inflammatory response and subsequent fibrosis via inhibition of TNF-α, a cytokine that plays a central role in the regulation of the immune response [4,5] and by inhibiting the development of fibrosis directly through suppression of TGF-β, a multifunctional cytokine that may influence fibrosis progression [6].[7].[8].

The importance of vitamin D in immune modulation and deposition of fibrosis may extend to the liver, which plays an important role in vitamin D homeostasis. The liver is the site of the conversion of vitamin D3 to 25-hydroxy-vitamin D (25-OH-vitamin D) and may be a site of vitamin D storage. [9] In addition, vitamin D receptors exist on hepatocytes and other hepatic parenchymal cells, including hepatic stellate cells. As in the kidney, vitamin D is postulated to play an antiinflammatory and antifibrotic role in the liver via binding to promoters of target genes, leading to down-regulation of TNF-α and TGF-β production.

Cross-sectional population data suggest that vitamin D deficiency is common in persons with advanced liver disease. [10,11] For example, Fisher et al. [12] evaluated vitamin D levels in 100 patients with liver disease, 51 with cirrhosis and 49 without cirrhosis, including 38 patients with chronic hepatitis C. The prevalence of vitamin D deficiency was significantly higher in cirrhotic than noncirrhotic subjects (86.3% versus 49.0%, p = 0.0001). Moreover, vitamin D levels decreased with advancing Child class; vitamin D levels were significantly lower in subjects with Child class C (22.7 nmol/L) than in those with Child class A (45.8 nmol/L, p<0.001). Such studies, however, are limited by their cross-sectional nature. Thus, while an association between vitamin D deficiency and advancing liver disease has been noted, the potential that vitamin D deficiency could be a predictor for progressive liver disease has not been explored.

Recently, vitamin D has been evaluated as a potential immunomodulator of hepatitis C virus (HCV), and preliminary data suggest that the addition of vitamin D to standard antiviral therapy may improve treatment response rates. [13] This observation lends further weight to the potential immunomodulatory role of vitamin D in liver disease.

The progression of hepatic fibrosis occurs over years, hampering the study of processes that affect fibrosis. On the other hand, the Hepatitis C Antiviral Long-term Treatment against Cirrhosis (HALT-C) Trial provided a unique opportunity to study fibrosis longitudinally over several years. [14] The HALT-C Trial was a 10-clinical center randomized, controlled trial to evaluate the benefit of long-term (3.5-years) peginterferon therapy in patients with histologically advanced (Ishak fibrosis stage ≥3) but clinically compensated chronic hepatitis C who had failed to respond previously to antiviral therapy. While the HALT-C Trial was a negative study, showing that such maintenance antiviral therapy was ineffective, the trial's study design, including sequential liver biopsies spanning 4 years rendered the trial population ideally suited for the study factors that might influence fibrosis progression. Therefore, we conducted a nested case-control study of vitamin D levels in subjects with and without liver histologic progression or clinical decompensation over the course of the HALT-C Trial.

Results

Baseline Characteristics of Cases and Controls

One hundred twenty-nine cases met the inclusion criteria and 129 aged matched controls were selected. (Table 1). Cases with progression were defined (as the primary outcomes in the HALT-C Trial) as subjects with Ishak fibrosis stage 3 or 4 who experienced (1) progression of fibrosis over the study period, defined by an increase in Ishak fibrosis score of ≥2 stages, (2) an increase in the Child-Turcotte-Pugh (CTP) score to ≥7 on two successive study visits (3 months apart), (3) hepatic decompensation, defined by the presence of ascites, hepatic encephalopathy, variceal hemorrhage, spontaneous bacterial peritonitis, or (4) death. Controls were subjects with stage 3 or 4 fibrosis who did not experience any of the primary study endpoints by the end of 4-years in the trial (a 24-week lead-in phase when all participants received full-dose peginterferon alfa-2a and weight-based ribavirin and a 3-½-year randomized phase of half-dose maintenance peginterferon therapy or observation).

The mean age was 49.5 years in the cases and 50.0 years in the controls, the mean BMI was 30.5 in the cases and 29.5 in the controls (P = 0.16), genotype 1 was predominant in both groups, and the mean viral load was 6.4 and 6.5 $\log_{10}$ IU/ml in cases and controls, respectively. Histologic Activity Index did not differ significantly between the two groups (P = 0.15). However, the cases had a significantly higher baseline ALT levels than controls (136.4 versus 103.8, P = 0.013). In addition, cases had more steatosis than controls (p = 0.002). 50.4% of control patients and 46.5% of case patients received pegylated interferon during the HALT-C trial (P = 0.53).

To further ensure that our cases and controls were appropriately selected we analyzed end of study levels of albumin, prothrombin time and platelets. Cases had significantly lower platelets than control patients (131.1 vs 180.7, p<0.0001) and significantly lower albumin level (3.77 vs 4.06, p<0.0001) and higher prothrombin times (1.09 vs 1.03, p<0.0001) suggesting that cases were correctly classified as having progressive disease.

When evaluated by HALT-C treatment status (pegylated interferon versus placebo) there was no difference in the distribution of gender, ethnicity, age, BMI, steatosis, HAI, glucose, HOMA-IR, ALT, genotype, average drinks per day, prevalence of diabetes, albumin, platelet count, total bilirubin. Subjects who received pegylated interferon had statistically lower baseline HCV RNA log (6.19 IU/mL vs 6.42 IU/mlL, p = 0.01).

Over the duration of the HALT-C Trial, 97.7% (n = 126) of cases had a ≥2-point increase in Ishak fibrosis score, and 17.1% (n = 22) had an increase in CTP score to ≥7. Encephalopathy developed in 6.2% (n = 8) of cases, ascites in 7.8% (n = 10), variceal hemorrhage in 2.3% (n = 3), and spontaneous bacterial peritonitis in 1.6% (n = 2) of patients. The death rate among cases was 5.4% (n = 7) and 3.1% among controls (n = 4), which was not statistically different (p − 0.51).

Factors Associated with Vitamin D Deficiency

Two vitamin D measurements were made in this study, vitamin D3 and vitamin D2 levels. Vitamin D3 levels reflect endogenous vitamin D while vitamin D2 levels reflect exogenous vitamin D (or vitamin from supplements). Total vitamin D is the sum of the vitamin D2 and Vitamin D3 levels.

Vitamin D levels have been shown to vary by latitude and season with higher vitamin D levels found in summer months and at latitudes closer to the equator. [15] Thus, we evaluated whether our cases and controls differed by latitude of HALT-C site and season during which blood was drawn.

We found no difference in the months of blood draws between cases and controls (P = 0.53) or in the season when evaluating winter (October to April) compared to summer (May to September) (P = 0.44). In addition, there was no difference in the location of clinical center between cases and controls. In the control group 27.8% of subjects and 27.1% of subjects in the case group came from latitudes of 35 degrees or less compared to 72.2% at latitudes greater than or equal to 35 degrees in the controls and 72.9% of cases. (P = 0.91)

In addition, we evaluated the difference in vitamin D levels based on HALT-C treatment status. No significant difference in vitamin D level was seen between subjects who received pegylated interferon and those who received placebo (34.7 mg/dL vs 35.7 mg/dl, p = 0.61). When further divided by cases and controls there was again no difference between subjects who received pegylated interferon and those who received placebo. Among cases who received pegylated interferon, mean vitamin D level was 34.7 mg/dL compared to 36.4 mg/dL in the placebo group (p = 0.52). Among controls who received pegylated interferon mean vitamin D level was 34.7 mg/dL compared to 35.0 mg/dL in the pacebo group p = 093).

A low vitamin D level was associated independently with black race (P<0.0001). (Table 2) Vitamin D levels were also significantly associated with the month of blood draw (P<0.0001). These remained significant when adjusted for the age, gender, BMI, HCV RNA level, diabetes, HAI, race, site of draw, month of draw and genotype. Clinical trial site was associated with vitamin D level with sites at latitudes of 35 degrees or below having significantly higher vitamin D levels than those above 35 degrees (40.1 mg/dL vs 46.0 mg/dL, P = 0.02) but was not significant

Table 1. Baseline characteristics of the cases and controls in the nested analysis.

	Case N (%)	Controls N (%)	P Value
N	129	129	
Male (%)	89 (69.0)	100 (77.5)	0.16
Female (%)	40 (31.0)	29 (22.5)	
Non-Hispanic White (%)	99 (76.7)	91 (70.5)	0.34
Black (%)	19 (14.7)	27 (20.9)	
Hispanic (%)	8 (6.2)	5 (3.9)	
Other (%)	3 (2.3)	6 (4.7)	
Mean Age (± SD)	49.5±6.5	50.0±7.3	0.54
Mean BMI (± SD)	30.5±5.4	29.5±5.0	0.16
BMI Profile (%)			0.19
- <18.5	0(0)	1(0.78%)	
- 18.5–24.9	14(10.85%)	20(15.50%)	
- 25–29.9	52(40.31%)	62(48.06%)	
- 30–34.9	48(37.21%)	31(24.03%)	
- 35–39.9	10(7.75%)	8(6.20%)	
- >40	5(3.88%)	7(5.43%)	
HCV Genotype 1	119(92.3)	124 (96.1)	0.28
HCV Genotype other	10 (7.8)	5 (3.9)	
HCV RNA Log_{10} IU/ml (± SD)	6.4±0.5	6.5±0.5	0.33
Mean Ishak Histologic Activity Index (± SD)	7.4±2.1	7.0±1.9	0.15
ALT (U/L)	136.4±125.7	103.8±77.6	0.013
Steatosis (%)			0.002
0	20(15.50%)	28(21.71%)	
1	38(29.46%)	62(48.06%)	
2	46(35.66%)	28(21.71%)	
3	21(16.28%)	10(7.75%)	
4	4(3.10%)	1(0.78%)	
Mean Glucose mg/dL (+/−SD)	113±46	105±35	0.12
Mean Insulin (+/−SD)	54.6±39.7	43.1±45.4	0.06
Mean HOMA-IR	16.8±16.6	12.6±17.7	0.09
Average Number of drinks per year (± SD)	683.7±1056.2	641.2±875.0	0.73
Average grams of ETOH per day (± SD)	22.5±34.7	21.1±28.7	0.73
Diabetes (%)	27 (20.9)	16 (12.4)	0.09
Pegylated Interferon Treatment	60 (46.5)	65 (50.4)	0.53
Blood drawn during winter months (out of 1023 draws)	284 (48.8)	298 (51.2)	0.44

when adjusted for the remaining variables. Vitamin D level was also found to be higher in patients with genotype 1 compared to non-genotype 1 patients (+10.75 mg/dL, p = 0.04) but is limited by only 15 patients being non-genotype 1. This association was not significant on multivariate analysis (p = 0.09) Vitamin D levels were not related to age, gender, BMI, HCV RNA level, presence of diabetes mellitus, Histologic Activity Index, or ALT when multivariate analysis was performed.

Are Vitamin D Levels Predictive of the Progression of Chronic Liver Disease?

Vitamin D levels were assessed at the time of HALT-C Trial screening, randomization to peginterferon or placebo (week 24), at month 27, and month 45 (Table 3). Baseline total vitamin D levels were 44.8 ng/mL in the cases and 44.0 ng/mL in the controls

(P = 0.74). Levels in both groups declined over the study period, falling to 44.4 ng/mL in cases and in 44.2 ng/mL controls at the time of randomization (P = 0.91), to 40.5 ng/mL in cases and 39.2 ng/mL in controls at month 27 (P = 0.59), and to 38.8 ng/mL in cases and 40.9 ng/mL in controls at month 45 (P = 0.32). While vitamin D levels declined significantly in both cases and controls over time (P = 0.0011), no difference emerged in the level of the decline between the case and control groups (−5.6 ng/mL versus −3.3 ng/mL respectively, P = 0.77). In addition, the levels of vitamin D2 (exogenous vitamin D derived from supplement use) and vitamin D3 (endogenous) did not differ between cases and controls at any time point during the study.

The prevalence of vitamin D deficiency, defined as is standard by a vitamin D level ≤30 ng/ml, was indistinguishable between cases, 24.6%, and controls, 23.8% (P = 0.88). Similarly, extreme

Table 2. Factors associated with vitamin D level (univariate).

Baseline Characteristics	P Value
HCV RNA level	0.45
BMI	0.73
Age	0.06
Gender	0.89
ALT U/L	0.61
Diabetes mellitus	0.81
Average alcoholic drinks per year	0.13
Race	0.0001
HCV Genotype	0.04
Diabetes or blood sugar >126 mg/dL	0.73
Month of blood draw	<0.0001
Site of blood draw	0.006

vitamin D deficiency, defined by a vitamin D level ≤20 ng/mL, was found in 7.1% of cases and 10.4% of controls (P = 0.38).

We suspected that while vitamin D levels may not be significantly different in our cohort as a whole, vitamin D deficiency may be higher in cases and controls in certain subgroups, diabetic subjects and black subjects, at higher risk for vitamin D deficiency. We found that in subjects with an established diagnoses of diabetes mellitius or an elevated fasting glucose >126, baseline vitamin D levels were higher in cases, 47.9 ng/mL, than controls, 36.3 ng/mL (P = 0.03) (Table 4 and 5). In addition, baseline vitamin D levels were higher in black subjects who had progressive liver disease, 32.7 ng/mL, than in black control subjects, 25.2 ng/mL (P = 0.08) (Table 6). These findings suggest, contrary to our belief, that increased serum vitamin D levels may be associated with a risk of liver-disease progression in specific groups with other risk factors.

Vitamin D Supplement Use

The self-reported use of vitamin D supplements was not available from the HALT-C study. However, vitamin D supplement use was directly measured by assaying for vitamin D2 levels. Over the course of the four year study 118 subjects did not have a detectable vitamin D2 level at any of the four time points indicating no supplement use with the remainder having a detectable vitamin D2 level at at least one time point. There was no significant difference in this distribution between cases and controls. (P = 0.14).

We analyzed the mean total vitamin D levels, vitamin D3 and vitamin D2 levels in those subjects with detectable vitamin D2

levels on all four occasions to determine if supplement use was greater in control patients and could account for a lack of progression of chronic liver disease (n = 28). We noted that at baseline cases had significantly higher vitamin D3 levels (46.3 mg/dL vs 32.4 mg/dL, P = 0.03) and total vitamin D levels (60.0 mg/dL vs 43.3 mg/dL, P = 0.02) when compared to control patients. (Table 7) Vitamin D2 levels, indicative of supplement use, had a trend toward higher levels in cases compared to controls (13.7 mg/dL vs 10.9 mg/dL, P = 0.28) although this did not reach statistical significance. We did not find, however, the supplement use or higher total vitamin D levels were associated with improved outcomes and our findings suggest that higher vitamin D levels may be associated with progression of liver disease.

Further, we analyzed the baseline vitamin D levels in patients who were taking vitamin D supplements at the time of enrollment (N = 77). We found that total vitamin D levels were significantly higher in the cases (53.6 mg/dL) when compared to controls (44.7 mg/dL, P = 0.04). Cases had a non-significant increase in both vitamin D2 (10.5 mg/dL vs. 8.1 mg/dL, P = 0.10) and vitamin D3 levels (42.5 mg/dL vs. 36.6 mg/dL, P = 0.16) when compared to controls.

Discussion

In this study, we had the opportunity to evaluate longitudinally the impact of vitamin D levels on the progression of chronic liver disease. Our nested case control study suggests that vitamin D levels do not influence the progression of chronic liver disease. We found no difference in mean vitamin D levels in patients with and without progressive chronic liver disease during any point over 45 months. Vitamin D levels declined over time in both groups consistent with the known effect of aging on vitamin D levels but persons with progression of liver disease did not experience a greater decline than persons without disease progression. [16] The existing literature contains conflicting evidence on the relationship between vitamin D and chronic liver disease. Our findings are supported by several studies in the literature evaluating vitamin D levels in chronic viral liver disease. Duarte et al evaluated 100 persons with chronic hepatitis C and found no difference in mean vitamin D levels in those with and without cirrhosis. Their levels of vitamin D, 46.6 ng/mL in non-cirrhotic persons and 45.6 ng/mL in cirrhotic patients (P = NS), were similar to the levels in our study. [17] Gallego-Rojo et al found similar levels with Child's Class A cirrhotic patients having a non-significant increase in vitamin D when compared to healthy controls (48.1 ng/mL vs. 45.5 ng/mL, respectively). [18] However, in several studies decreasing vitamin D levels have been associated with progression of chronic liver disease. [10,12,19,20]. However, these studies have several important limitations in their design that may explain the different findings. First, these studies are universally cross

Table 3. Mean vitamin D (ng/mL) levels in cases and controls.

	Cases (n = 129)			Control (n = 129)			P value		
	Total	D2	D3	Total	D2	D3	Total	D2	D3
Month 0 (Screening)	44.8±19.4	3.0±6.1	41.6±18.3	44.0±19.7	2.5±4.7	41.4±19.9	0.74	0.47	0.94
Week 24 (Randomization)	44.4±19.8	3.1±5.8	41.4±20.2	44.2±19.7	2.2±4.3	41.2±19.0	0.91	0.17	0.92
Month 27	40.5±17.3	3.2±5.9	37.6±17.4	39.2±20.7	2.3±4.3	35.6±17.6	0.59	0.15	0.38
Month 45	38.8±18.4	3.2±5.6	35.6±18.3	40.9±13.8	3.4±5.7	37.6±14.1	0.32	0.87	0.33

Table 4. Baseline characteristics of diabetic cases and controls in the nested analysis.

	Case N (%)	Controls N (%)	P Value
N	27	16	
Male (%)	20(74%)	15(94%)	0.11
Female (%)	7(26%)	1(6%)	
Non-Hispanic White (%)	20(74.07%)	6(37.50%)	0.04
Black (%)	5(18.52%)	8(50%)	
Hispanic (%)	1(3.70%)	2(12.50%)	
Other (%)	1(3.70%)	0(0%)	
Mean Age (± SD)	52±7.0	52±6.4	0.88
BMI Profile (%)			0.55
- <24.9	2(7.41%)	4(25%)	
- 25–29.9	11(40.74%)	7(43.75%)	
- 30–34.9	9(33.33%)	3(18.75%)	
- 35–39.9	2(7.41%)	1(6.25)	
- >40	3(11.11)	1(6.25)	
Mean Ishak Histologic Activity Index (± SD)	6.44±1.65	7.25±1.61	0.12
ALT (U/L)	103.7±67.9	84.1±51.7	0.33
Steatosis (%)			
0	6(22.22%)	6(37.50%)	0.34
1	9(33.33%)	8(50%)	
2	7(25.93%)	1(6.25%)	
3	4(14.81%)	1(6.25%)	
4	1(3.70%)	0(0%)	
Average Number of drinks per year (± SD)	653±758	652±823	0.99

sectional in nature, capturing the relationship between vitamin D and liver disease at only a single point in time and therefore are unable to assess changes in vitamin D temporally with the progression of liver disease. [10,12,19,20]. In addition, control subjects have in large part consisted of healthy controls introducing potentially confounders. Vitamin D levels have been found to be decreased in persons with a number of chronic diseases including hypertension, diabetes mellitus, nephritic syndrome and chronic kidney disease and further vitamin D level is considered an excellent marker of overall general health. [21,22] Thus, vitamin D deficiency may be the result of the chronic disease state rather than specifically the result of chronic liver disease which would not be highlighted by the use of healthy controls. Our study design, however, allows for controlling for the presence of chronic disease by choosing controls with chronic liver disease. By controlling for chronic disease we found that no difference was apparent in vitamin D levels.

Several advantages exist in the design of our study when compared to previously published works on vitamin D in chronic liver disease. First, our study was a nested case control rather than a traditional case control study. Nested case control studies have a distinct advantage from traditional case control studies because both cases and controls are chosen from the same, well-defined source population, in this study from the HALT-C study population where all patients had chronic hepatitis C infection with chronic liver disease. This is in contrast to other recently published works of cross-sectional case control studies where controls were uninfected healthy subjects. [20] Further, the traditional disadvantage of nested case control studies, which the cases and controls differ due to a higher death rate or loss to follow-up in the controls was not seen in HALT-C where no patients were lost to follow-up and only 21 deaths occurred.

In this study we also found that in specific subgroups, diabetic patients and black patients, cases had higher vitamin D levels than

Table 5. Mean baseline vitamin D (ng/mL) levels by in patients by diabetes status.

	Cases	Controls	P value
Diabetes	47.9±19.4	36.3±16.0	P=0.03
Non-DM	43.7±19.4	45.4±20.1	P=0.53

Table 6. Mean baseline vitamin D (ng/mL) levels by race.

	Cases	Controls	P Value
African Americans	32.7±15.8	25.2±12.4	0.08
White	47.2±19.7	49.7±18.5	0.36
Hispanic	48.8±13.6	53.8±15.2	0.54
Other	32.1±17.1	32.0±5.6	0.99

Table 7. Analysis of vitamin D levels in patients with detectable vitamin D2 at all time points.

	Cases (n = 16)			Control (n = 12)			P value		
	Total	D2	D3	Total	D2	D3	Total	D2	D3
Month 0 (Screening)	60.0±15.9	13.7±6.6	46.3±15.7	43.3±19.0	10.9±6.6	32.4±17.2	0.02	0.28	0.03
Week 24 (Randomization)	44.5±14.0	11.8±5.7	32.7±12.2	50.8±15.2	9.5±5.7	41.3±16.4	0.27	0.30	0.12
Month 27	41.6±12.9	12.3±5.3	30.7±10.7	39.0±7.9	9.4±3.7	29.6±8.5	0.54	0.12	0.77
Month 45	41.6±14.6	11.9±6.2	29.7±12.7	43.3±13.8	10.7±5.6	32.7±13.7	0.75	0.60	0.57

This is publication #59 of the HALT-C Trial.

controls suggesting that elevated levels of vitamin D may be harmful in these subgroups. Diabetic and black patients may be more susceptible to fibrosis progression, a progression that may be exacerbated by elevated levels of vitamin D. [20,23,24,25] While our study was not designed to evaluate the effect of vitamin D on fibrosis in these specific subgroups further study the suggestion of an association between elevated levels of vitamin D and accelerated disease progression in these groups warrants further evaluation.

Our study has several important limitations. First, in three quarters of our study subjects, the mean vitamin D levels were normal. This high proportion of normal vitamin D levels may be the result of the high supplement use among this group. Over the course of this study 140 subjects (54.7%) had detectable vitamin D2 levels, evidence of supplement use. In addition, subjects willing to participate in this rigorous long term trial may be highly motivated and have increased outdoor exercise and sun exposure leading to higher vitamin D levels. If the benefit of vitamin D were limited to vitamin D-deficient subjects, our study would have been underpowered to detect such an effect of vitamin D. On the other hand, in the two subgroups that did show a difference in vitamin D levels between cases and control, diabetics and black patients, vitamin D levels were higher in cases with histologic and/or clinical progression than in stable controls. Furthermore, in black subjects, mean vitamin D levels were in the deficiency range (mean 28.6 ng/mL); yet, vitamin D levels were higher in cases and then in controls.

In addition, our study is limited by its evaluation of only patients in the HALT-C study. The HALT-C study was limited to subjects who did not achieve sustained virologic response (SVR) to standard therapy. Low SVR rates have been associated with low vitamin D levels and suggest that at interaction between normal or high vitamin D levels may impact SVR. The patients in HALT-C, non-responders to therapy, may be a select group who do not benefit from normal or increased vitamin D levels and whose disease progression is not impacted by vitamin D.

In addition, in our study, we limited our evaluation to patients with Ishak fibrosis stage 3–4. Potentially, the benefits of vitamin D elevation (and supplementation) are negligible once this degree of fibrosis has occurred; our study group would not have revealed whether vitamin D may be beneficial in patients with no or early-stage fibrosis. On the contrary, by focusing on patients with stage 3–4 hepatic fibrosis, we were targeting patients with a high risk of disease progression, a group in which we would have expected to see the greatest potential benefit. In addition, we evaluated only patients with hepatitis C-induced liver disease and did not evaluate the role of vitamin D in other forms of chronic liver disease. Potentially, the impact of vitamin D levels in other types of chronic liver disease might be different.

Finally, while the HALT-C study had more than 4 years of follow-up this may still be insufficient follow-up time to adequately assess our desired outcomes. As was recently seen in an extended cohort of HALT-C, maintenance interferon therapy was associated with a reduced risk of HCC in cirrhotic patients. [26] Thus, vitamin D may be a predictor of longer term outcomes that cannot be assessed in the original HALT-C study.

In conclusion, we found no difference in vitamin D levels between patients with and without progression of hepatitis C-associated chronic liver disease over the course of nearly 4 years. Although we have not conducted a randomized trial of vitamin-D supplementation, our data do not suggest any role for vitamin D supplementation in patients with histologically advanced chronic hepatitis C and even raise the possibility that vitamin D supplementation may be harmful. Of course, vitamin D supplementation has been linked with a myriad of other health benefits, and our data are insufficient to support withholding vitamin D from these patients. On the side of caution, however, further study is needed in to evaluate the role of vitamin D supplementation in patients with chronic liver disease who are diabetic or black.

Methods

This ancillary study was approved by the Partners Human Research Committee. The HALT-C Trial was approved by institutional review boards at each of the participating sites, and all study subjects provided written informed consent. Participating sites included University of Massachusetts Medical School, Worcester, MA; University of Connecticut Health Center, Farmington, CT; Saint Louis University, Saint Louis, MO, Partners Healthcare, Boston, MA; University of Colorado Health Sciences, Aurora, CO; University of California, Irvine, Ivine, CA; Long Beach VAMC Research Health Care Group, Long Beach, California; University of Texas Southwestern Medical Center, Dallas, TX; University of Southern California Health Sciences Campus, Los Angeles, CA; University of Michigan Medical School, Ann Arbor, MI; Virginia Commonwealth University, Richmond, VA; National Institute of Diabetes and Digestive and Kidney Diseases National Institutes of Health, Bethesda, MD.

Study Design

This was a case-control study to evaluate the association of serum 25-OH-vitamin D levels with fibrosis progression. Cases with progression were defined (as the primary outcomes in the HALT-C Trial) as subjects with Ishak fibrosis stage 3 or 4 who experienced (1) progression of fibrosis over the study period, defined by an increase in Ishak fibrosis score of ≥2 stages, (2) an increase in the Child-Turcotte-Pugh (CTP) score to ≥7 on two successive study visits (3 months apart), (3) hepatic decompensation, defined by the presence of ascites, hepatic encephalopathy, variceal hemorrhage, spontaneous bacterial peritonitis, or (4) death. Controls were subjects with stage 3 or 4 fibrosis who did not experience any of the primary study endpoints by the end of 4-years in the trial (a 24-week lead-in phase when all participants received full-dose peginterferon alfa-2a and weight-based ribavirin and a 3-½-year randomized phase of half-dose maintenance peginterferon therapy or observation). We chose to expand our primary endpoint beyond fibrosis progression alone to limit the impact of the sampling variability of needle-liver biopsy as well as to include clinically significant outcomes. Controls and cases were matched for age (age less than 49 years of age or age equal to or greater than 49 years of age) Because hepatocellular carcinoma (HCC) may have independent effects on vitamin D homeostasis, we excluded patients in whom HCC developed. [27]

Inclusion Critieria

To be included as a case or a control in the nested case-control study, HALT-C Trial participants had to have (1) liver histopathology available at study entry and study cessation (baseline and 4 years [biopsies were done at baseline, year 2 and year 4]), (2) stored serum available for 25-OH-vitamin D assay, and (3) Ishak fibrosis stage 3 or 4 at study entry. Subjects with Ishak Fibrosis stage 5 or 6 at study entry, absence of serial liver biopsies, and those in whom HCC developed during the study period were excluded. Two hundred fifty-eight subjects from the HALT-C Trial met these inclusion criteria including 129 cases and 129 controls.

Endpoints

The primary endpoint was the mean vitamin D level at study entry; secondary endpoints were vitamin D levels at randomization (trial-week 24), month 27, and month 45. −Total 25-OH-Vitamin D was calculated from the sum of 25-OH vitamin D3 (endogenously produced vitamin D) and 25-OH-vitamin D2 (derived from supplements). Serum samples were aliquoted and frozen immediately at −70°C at each of the 10 clinical centers, then shipped on dry ice and stored at a central contract repository site. For the measurement of vitamin D levels deuterated stable isotope [d3-25-hydroxyvitamin D] was added to a 200 uL serum specimen as an internal standard. The specimen was then deproteinated by acetonitrile precipitation. 25-hydroxyvitamin D2, 25-hydroxyvitamin D3, and internal standard in the organic supernate were purified by a liquid chromatography system. Purified hydroxyvitamin D2, 25-hydroxyvitamin D3, and internal standard are ionized at atmospheric pressure and injected into a tandem mass spectrometer and quantified relative to calibrators prepared in charcoal-stripped human serum. The limit of quantitation for 25-hydroxyvitamin D2 is 2 ng/mL [CV = 15%] and for 25-hydroxyvitamin D3 is 3 ng/mL [CV = 25%]. The between-run CV for a quality control serum containing a total vitamin D concentration of 23 ng/mL is 7.5%. Storage time, up to 24 years, has shown to have no effect on vitamin D levels in stored serum. [28]

Statistical Analysis

We evaluated serum vitamin D levels in cases and controls as continuous variables. Baseline was defined as time of randomization. For those patients whose information was missing at randomization, information at screening was used as baseline. The cases and controls were weakly matched by age only. As a result, the correlation between case and control were very weak and the two groups can be considered independent. Student's t test

or Wilcoxon rank sum test was used as appropriate. Fisher's exact test or Chi-square test was used for bivariate analyses of categorical variables whenever appropriate. In addition, we evaluated serum 25-OH-vitamin D levels as categorical variables (binary: deficient and normal value as well as in quartiles) with the chi square test to create an odds ratio for the progression of fibrosis based on vitamin D levels. We performed multivariate modeling to evaluate the impact of vitamin D levels as well as other known variables that influence fibrosis (age, estimated duration of HCV infection, body mass index [BMI], diabetes mellitus, hypertension, alcohol use) on fibrosis progression. In addition, we performed a linear regression analysis to evaluate the impact of vitamin D levels on HCV RNA levels. With a sample size of 129 subjects per study arm, we had an 80% power to detect a mean difference of 0.3 times the standard deviation of the mean between groups at the 5% level of significance. Statistical analysis was performed with SAS software (SAS 9.1.3 Cary, NC).

Acknowledgments

In addition to the authors of this manuscript, the following individuals were instrumental in the planning, conduct and/or care of patients enrolled in this study at each of the participating institutions as follows:

University of Massachusetts Medical Center, Worcester, MA: (Contract N01-DK-9-2326) Gyongyi Szabo, MD, Barbara F. Banner, MD, Maureen Cormier, RN, Donna Giansiracusa, RN

University of Connecticut Health Center, Farmington, CT: (Grant M01RR-06192) Herbert L. Bonkovsky, MD, Gloria Borders, RN, Michelle Kelley, RN, ANP

Saint Louis University School of Medicine, St Louis, MO: (Contract N01-DK-9-2324) Adrian M. Di Bisceglie, MD, Bruce Bacon, MD, Brent Neuschwander-Tetri, MD, Elizabeth M. Brunt, MD, Debra King, RN

Massachusetts General Hospital, Boston, MA: (Contract N01-DK-9-2319, Grant M01RR-01066; Grant 1 UL1 RR025758-01, Harvard Clinical and Translational Science Center) Andrea E. Reid, MD, Atul K. Bhan, MD, Wallis A. Molchen, David P. Lundmark

University of Colorado Denver, School of Medicine, Aurora, CO: (Contract N01-DK-9-2327, Grant M01RR-00051, Grant 1 UL1 RR 025780-01), Gregory T. Everson, MD, Thomas Trouillot, MD, Marcelo Kugelmas, MD, S. Russell Nash, MD, Jennifer DeSanto, RN, Carol McKinley, RN

University of California - Irvine, Irvine, CA: (Contract N01-DK-9-2320, Grant M01RR-00827) Timothy R. Morgan, MD, John C. Hoefs, MD, John R. Craig, MD, M. Mazen Jamal, MD, MPH, Muhammad Sheikh, MD, Choon Park, RN

University of Texas Southwestern Medical Center, Dallas, TX: (Contract N01-DK-9-2321, Grant M01RR-00633, Grant 1 UL1 RR024982-01, North and Central Texas Clinical and Translational Science Initiative) William M. Lee, MD, Thomas E. Rogers, MD, Peter F. Malet, MD, Janel Shelton, Nicole Crowder, LVN, Rivka Elbein, RN, BSN, Nancy Liston, MPH

University of Southern California, Los Angeles, CA: (Contract N01-DK-9-2325, Grant M01RR-00043) Karen L. Lindsay, MD, MMM, Sugantha Govindarajan, MD, Carol B. Jones, RN, Susan L. Milstein, RN

University of Michigan Medical Center, Ann Arbor, MI: (Contract N01-DK-9-2323, Grant M01RR-00042, Grant 1 UL1 RR024986, Michigan Center for Clinical and Health Research) Anna S. Lok, MD, Robert J. Fontana, MD, Joel K. Greenson, MD, Pamela A. Richtmyer, LPN, CCRC, R. Tess Bonham, BS

Virginia Commonwealth University Health System, Richmond, VA: (Contract N01-DK-9-2322, Grant M01RR-00065) Mitchell L. Shiffman, MD, Richard K. Sterling, MD, MSc, Melissa J. Contos, MD, A. Scott Mills, MD, Charlotte Hofmann, RN, Paula Smith, RN

Liver Diseases Branch, National Institute of Diabetes and Digestive and Kidney Diseases, National Institutes of Health, Bethesda, MD: Marc G. Ghany, MD, T. Jake Liang, MD, David Kleiner, MD, PhD, Yoon Park, RN, Elenita Rivera, RN, Vanessa Haynes-Williams, RN

National Institute of Diabetes and Digestive and Kidney Diseases, Division of Digestive Diseases and Nutrition, Bethesda, MD: James E.

Everhart, MD, Leonard B. Seeff, MD, Patricia R. Robuck, PhD, Jay H. Hoofnagle, MD, Elizabeth C. Wright, PhD

University of Washington, Seattle, WA: (Contract N01-DK-9-2318) Chihiro Morishima, MD, David R. Gretch, MD, PhD, Minjun Chung Apodaca, BS, ASCP, Rohit Shankar, BC, ASCP, Natalia Antonov, M. Ed.

New England Research Institutes, Watertown, MA: (Contract N01-DK-9-2328) Kristin K. Snow, MSc, ScD, Anne M. Stoddard, ScD, May Yang, MPH

Armed Forces Institute of Pathology, Washington, DC: Zachary D. Goodman, MD, PhD

References

1. Friedman SL (2008) Mechanisms of hepatic fibrogenesis. Gastroenterology 134: 1655–1669.
2. Saggese G, Federico G, Balestri M, Toniolo A (1989) Calcitriol inhibits the PHA-induced production of IL-2 and IFN-gamma and the proliferation of human peripheral blood leukocytes while enhancing the surface expression of HLA class II molecules. J Endocrinol Invest 12: 329–335.
3. Peterlik M, Cross HS (2005) Vitamin D and calcium deficits predispose for multiple chronic diseases. Eur J Clin Invest 35: 290–304.
4. Shany S, Levy Y, Lahav-Cohen M (2001) The effects of 1alpha,24(S)-dihydroxyvitamin D(2) analog on cancer cell proliferation and cytokine expression. Steroids 66: 319–325.
5. Cohen ML, Douvdevani A, Chaimovitz C, Shany S (2001) Regulation of TNF-alpha by 1alpha,25-dihydroxyvitamin D3 in human macrophages from CAPD patients. Kidney Int 59: 69–75.
6. Czaja MJ, Weiner FR, Flanders KC, Giambrone MA, Wind R, et al. (1989) In vitro and in vivo association of transforming growth factor-beta 1 with hepatic fibrosis. J Cell Biol 108: 2477–2482.
7. Tan X, Li Y, Liu Y (2007) Therapeutic role and potential mechanisms of active Vitamin D in renal interstitial fibrosis. J Steroid Biochem Mol Biol 103: 491–496.
8. Zhang Z, Sun L, Wang Y, Ning G, Minto AW, et al. (2008) Renoprotective role of the vitamin D receptor in diabetic nephropathy. Kidney Int 73: 163–171.
9. Holick MF (2007) Vitamin D deficiency. N Engl J Med 357: 266–281.
10. Chen CC, Wang SS, Jeng FS, Lee SD (1996) Metabolic bone disease of liver cirrhosis: is it parallel to the clinical severity of cirrhosis? J Gastroenterol Hepatol 11: 417–421.
11. Bonkovsky HL, Hawkins M, Steinberg K, Hersh T, Galambos JT, et al. (1990) Prevalence and prediction of osteopenia in chronic liver disease. Hepatology 12: 273–280.
12. Fisher L, Fisher A (2007) Vitamin D and parathyroid hormone in outpatients with noncholestatic chronic liver disease. Clin Gastroenterol Hepatol 5: 513–520.
13. Abu-Mouch S, Fireman Z, Jarchovsky J (2009) The Beneficial Effect of Vitamin D with Combined Peg Interferon and Ribavirin for Chronic HCV Infection. AASLD Boston, MA 2009 Abstract LB20.
14. Di Bisceglie AM, Shiffman ML, Everson GT, Lindsay KL, Everhart JE, et al. (2008) Prolonged therapy of advanced chronic hepatitis C with low-dose peginterferon. N Engl J Med 359: 2429–2441.
15. Moosgaard B, Vestergaard P, Heickendorff L, Melsen F, Christiansen P, et al. (2005) Vitamin D status, seasonal variations, parathyroid adenoma weight and bone mineral density in primary hyperparathyroidism. Clin Endocrinol (Oxf) 63: 506–513.
16. Holick MF, Matsuoka LY, Wortsman J (1989) Age, vitamin D, and solar ultraviolet. Lancet 2: 1104–1105.
17. Duarte MP, Farias ML, Coelho HS, Mendonca LM, Stabnov LM, et al. (2001) Calcium-parathyroid hormone-vitamin D axis and metabolic bone disease in chronic viral liver disease. J Gastroenterol Hepatol 16: 1022–1027.
18. Gallego-Rojo FJ, Gonzalez-Calvin JL, Munoz-Torres M, Mundi JL, Fernandez-Perez R, et al. (1998) Bone mineral density, serum insulin-like growth factor I, and bone turnover markers in viral cirrhosis. Hepatology 28: 695–699.
19. Masuda S, Okano T, Osawa K, Shinjo M, Suematsu T, et al. (1989) Concentrations of vitamin D-binding protein and vitamin D metabolites in plasma of patients with liver cirrhosis. J Nutr Sci Vitaminol (Tokyo) 35: 225–234.
20. Petta S, Camma C, Di Marco V, Alessi N, Barbaria F, et al. (2008) Retinol-binding protein 4: a new marker of virus-induced steatosis in patients infected with hepatitis c virus genotype 1. Hepatology 48: 28–37.
21. Thomas MK, Lloyd-Jones DM, Thadhani RI, Shaw AC, Deraska DJ, et al. (1998) Hypovitaminosis D in medical inpatients. N Engl J Med 338: 777–783.
22. Pittas AG, Dawson-Hughes B (2010) Vitamin D and diabetes. J Steroid Biochem Mol Biol 121: 425–9.
23. Foxton MR, Quaglia A, Muiesan P, Heneghan MA, Portmann B, et al. (2006) The impact of diabetes mellitus on fibrosis progression in patients transplanted for hepatitis C. Am J Transplant 6: 1922–1929.
24. Muzzi A, Leandro G, Rubbia-Brandt L, James R, Keiser O, et al. (2005) Insulin resistance is associated with liver fibrosis in non-diabetic chronic hepatitis C patients. J Hepatol 42: 41–46.
25. Svegliati-Baroni G, Ridolfi F, Di Sario A, Casini A, Marucci L, et al. (1999) Insulin and insulin-like growth factor-1 stimulate proliferation and type I collagen accumulation by human hepatic stellate cells: differential effects on signal transduction pathways. Hepatology 29: 1743–1751.
26. Lok AS, Everhart JE, Wright EC, Di Bisceglie AM, Kim HY, et al. (2011) Maintenance peginterferon therapy and other factors associated with hepatocellular carcinoma in patients with advanced hepatitis C. Gastroenterology 140: 840–849. quiz e812.
27. Azam Z AZ, Saleem U, Jafri W (2008) Vitamin D Levels in Cirrhosis and Hepatocellular Carcinoma. Gastroenterology: A-824-A-825 AASLD Abstract T1931.
28. Agborsangaya C, Toriola AT, Grankvist K, Surcel HM, Holl K, et al. (2010) The effects of storage time and sampling season on the stability of serum 25-hydroxy vitamin D and androstenedione. Nutr Cancer 62: 51–57.

Data and Safety Monitoring Board Members: (Chair) Gary L. Davis, MD, Guadalupe Garcia-Tsao, MD, Michael Kutner, PhD, Stanley M. Lemon, MD, Robert P. Perrillo, MD

Author Contributions

Conceived and designed the experiments: KEC RTC JLD ADB HZ. Performed the experiments: KEC HZ. Analyzed the data: KEC RTC ADB JMN HZ JLD. Contributed reagents/materials/analysis tools: KEC RTC ADB JMN HZ JLD. Wrote the paper: KEC RTC JLD.

Reproductive Status Is Associated with the Severity of Fibrosis in Women with Hepatitis C

Erica Villa[1][¶]*, Ranka Vukotic[1][¶], Calogero Cammà[2], Salvatore Petta[2], Alfredo Di Leo[3], Stefano Gitto[1], Elena Turola[1][¶], Aimilia Karampatou[1][¶], Luisa Losi[4][¶], Veronica Bernabucci[1][¶], Annamaria Cenci[5], Simonetta Tagliavini[5], Enrica Baraldi[5], Nicola De Maria[1], Roberta Gelmini[6], Elena Bertolini[1][¶], Maria Rendina[3][¶], Antonio Francavilla[7]

1 Department of Gastroenterology, Azienda Ospedaliero-Universitaria & University of Modena and Reggio Emilia, Modena, Italy, 2 Sezione di Gastroenterologia, Di.Bi.M.I.S., University of Palermo, Palermo, Italy, 3 Department of Gastroenterology, University of Bari, Bari, Italy, 4 Department of Pathology, Azienda Ospedaliero-Universitaria, Modena, Italy, 5 Department of Clinical Pathology, NOCSAE, Modena, Italy, 6 Department of General Surgery, Azienda Ospedaliero-Universitaria, Modena, Italy, 7 Istituto di Ricovero e Cura "Saverio de Bellis", Castellana Grotte, Italy

Abstract

Introduction: Chronic hepatitis C is the main cause of death in patients with end-stage liver disease. Prognosis depends on the increase of fibrosis, whose progression is twice as rapid in men as in women. Aim of the study was to evaluate the effects of reproductive stage on fibrosis severity in women and to compare these findings with age-matched men.

Materials and Methods: A retrospective study of 710 consecutive patients with biopsy-proven chronic hepatitis C was conducted, using data from a clinical database of two tertiary Italian care centers. Four age-matched groups of men served as controls. Data about demographics, biochemistry, liver biopsy and ultrasonography were analyzed. Contributing factors were assessed by multivariate logistic regression analysis.

Results: Liver fibrosis was more advanced in the early menopausal than in the fully reproductive (P<0.0001) or premenopausal (P = 0.042) group. Late menopausal women had higher liver fibrosis compared with the other groups (fully reproductive, P<0.0001; premenopausal, P = <0.0001; early menopausal, P = 0.052). Multivariate analyses showed that male sex was independently associated with more severe fibrosis in the groups corresponding to premenopausal (P = 0.048) and early menopausal (P = 0.004) but not late menopausal pairs. In women, estradiol/testosterone ratio decreased markedly in early (vs. reproductive age: P = 0.002 and vs. premenopausal: P<0.0001) and late menopause (vs. reproductive age: P = 0.001; vs. premenopausal: P<0.0001). In men age-matched with menopausal women, estradiol/testosterone ratio instead increased (reproductive age group vs. early: P = 0.002 and vs. late M: P = 0.001).

Conclusions: The severity of fibrosis in women worsens in parallel with increasing estrogen deprivation and estradiol/testosterone ratio decrease. Our data provide evidence why fibrosis progression is discontinuous in women and more linear and severe in men, in whom aging-associated estradiol/testosterone ratio increase occurs too late to noticeably influence the inflammatory process leading to fibrosis.

Editor: Naglaa H. Shoukry, University of Montreal, Canada

Funding: The study was supported by an unrestricted grant by Merck & Co (Whitehouse Station, NJ, USA). The funding source had no role in the design of the study; collection, analysis, and interpretation of the data; drafting of the manuscript or decision to submit the manuscript for publication.

Competing Interests: The study was supported by an unrestricted grant by Merck & Co (Whitehouse Station, NJ, USA). The funding source had no role in the design of the study; collection, analysis, and interpretation of the data; drafting of the manuscript or decision to submit the manuscript for publication.

* E-mail: erica.villa@unimore.it

¶ On behalf of the Research Network "Women_in_Hepatology"

Introduction

Chronic hepatitis C (CHC) is the primary cause of death in patients with end-stage liver disease [1]. Its prognosis depends on the accumulation of fibrosis over time due to various mechanisms of tissue damage caused by viral infection, ultimately leading to the development of cirrhosis and related complications. The development of hepatic fibrosis is most directly correlated with necro-inflammation, and several other host and viral factors have been associated with the rate of fibrosis progression [2], including older age, alcohol consumption, duration of infection, viral co-infections, steatosis, insulin resistance, and vitamin D deficiency [3].

Studies of large cohorts of patients with CHC have also found that high levels of estrogens (as observed during pregnancy) [4] are associated with decreased inflammatory activity in HCV women and that the progression of fibrosis in CHC is twice as rapid in men as in women [5,6]. This difference has been attributed to the protective role of estrogens and has been supported by experimental and clinical data. Experimentally, estrogens were shown to have a relevant fibrosuppressive role in a rat model of dimethylnitrosamine- or pig-serum-induced liver fibrosis [7,8]. Clinically, Di Martino et al. [9] and Codes et al. [10] showed that the progression of fibrosis increased significantly in women after menopause, whereas prolonged periods of hormone replacement therapy (HRT) were able to maintain this progression at a level similar to that in premenopausal women. In women, menarche initiates a long period of estrogen exposure that begins to decline in the premenopausal period, often leading to undetectable estrogen levels in early and late menopause. In women with CHC, this reduction in estrogen levels is accompanied by consensual fluctuation in the levels of pro-inflammatory [11,12] and anti-inflammatory [12] cytokines that could interfere with the course of necro-inflammation and the progression of fibrosis. Much less is known about this process in men: pro-inflammatory cytokines do not fluctuate in age subgroups corresponding to female reproductive stages [11], but it remains unknown whether a relationship exists with changes in sex hormone balance in men.

Thus, the aim of our study was to evaluate the effects of differential hormonal exposure on the severity of fibrosis in men and women: we therefore compared women with CHC in different reproductive phases (reproductive age, premenopause, early menopause, late menopause) with four age-matched groups of men and investigated the correlations between fibrosis and the respective Estradiol and Testosterone levels.

Materials and Methods

Between January 2002 and December 2008, 1000 consecutive patients with CHC were recruited to receive standard antiviral treatment at the Gastrointestinal and Liver Units of the University Hospitals of Modena and Bari, Italy. Eligible patients were ≥18 years of age, had compensated liver disease due to chronic hepatitis C virus (HCV) infection (any fibrosis stage, including compensated cirrhosis), detectable plasma HCV RNA levels, and had received no previous treatment for hepatitis C. Patients were excluded if they were co-infected with human immunodeficiency virus or hepatitis B virus or had any other cause of liver disease, severe depression or psychiatric disorder, or active substance or alcohol consumption >20 g/day in the last five years, as evaluated by a questionnaire. Women who had been using hormone replacement therapy were not included in the analysis. The detailed demographic characteristics of this cohort of patients have been reported previously [11].

Within this cohort, four groups of women were selected according to reproductive stage:

Group 1: full reproductive age (i.e., regular menses); Group 2: premenopausal; women included in this group entered menopause (defined as no menstrual period for 12 consecutive months) within 5 years from enrollment in the study; Group 3: early menopausal (menopause was present at the time of enrollment for less than 5 years); Group 4: late menopausal (menopause was present at the time of enrollment for at least 10 years).

Four groups of men contained patients that were pair-matched by age (1:1) with the female cohort.

This study was approved by the institutional review boards of the two hospitals and was conducted in accordance with the provisions of the Declaration of Helsinki and Good Clinical Practice guidelines (ClinicalTrials.gov identifier: NCT01402583).

Clinical and Laboratory Assessment

All patients had undergone liver biopsy within 1 year before enrollment. Portal vein diameter (mm) was determined by color Doppler ultrasonography before liver biopsy. The following data were collected at the time of liver biopsy: age, sex, weight, height, and body mass index (BMI); serum levels of alanine aminotransferase (ALT), γ-glutamyl transpeptidase (GGT), glucose insulin; and platelet count. Insulin resistance was determined using the homeostasis model assessment (HOMA). HCV RNA was quantified by Abbott RealTime HCV assay (Abbott Molecular Inc., Des Plaines, IL, USA) and genotyped by INNO-LiPA assay (Innogenetics, Gent, Belgium). All biopsy specimens were reviewed and scored according to Ishak et al. [13] by a single pathologist (LL) who was blinded to the patients' identities and histories. The percentage of hepatocytes containing macrovesicular fat was determined for each 10× field, and steatosis was classified as absent, mild (<5%), moderate (5–20%), or severe (≥20%).

Hormone Assays

Estradiol and testosterone. Blood samples were obtained from all patients by venipuncture and processed within 2 h after withdrawal. Serum was stored at $-20°C$ and assayed to determine estradiol and testosterone levels. Serum samples were subjected to chemiluminescent microparticle immunoassays (CMIA) to determine 17β-estradiol and testosterone levels using commercially available kits and a c4000 Architect system (Abbott Diagnostic Division, Abbott Laboratories, Abbott Park, IL, USA). Estradiol was additionally quantitated using the Abbott Architect Estradiol Assay 200 (rev. 2004) one-step CMIA. Assay sensitivity was <10 pg/mL for estradiol and 50 pg/mL for testosterone. The intra- and inter-assay coefficients of variation were 5.6% and 4.9% for estradiol, and 4% and 4.6% for testosterone.

Anti-Müllerian hormone. Serum anti-Müllerian hormone (AMH) levels were assessed in female patients by enzyme-linked immunosorbent assay (AMH Gen II ELISA; Beckman Coulter, Inc., Brea, CA, US). The sensitivity of the assay was 0.08 ng/mL. Intra- and interassay coefficients of variation were <5% and <7%, respectively.

Statistical Analysis

Continuous variables are summarized as mean (SD) and categorical variables as frequency (%). Continuous variables within each group were compared by the nonparametric Mann–Whitney U-test. Categorical data were compared by the chi-square test. Multiple logistic regression models were used to assess the relationship between severe fibrosis (Ishak staging ≥3) and the demographic, metabolic, and histological characteristics of patients in the individual groups and in each male–female pair group. In the statistical models, dependent variables were coded as 1 (present) or 0 (absent).

Regression analyses were performed using PROC LOGISTIC, PROC REG, and subroutines in SAS (SAS Institute, Inc., Cary, NC) [14].

Results

The detailed epidemiological, virological, laboratorial, histological, and ultrasonographic results of each male–female pair group are presented in Tables S1 and S2. Women in each group were selected according to reproductive status (full reproductive age, premenopausal, early menopausal, late menopausal), and data from the female groups were compared with those from age-matched male groups (intragroup analysis, Mann-Whitney U test).

Characteristics of Reproductive Status–Stratified Female Groups

We identified 123 women of full reproductive age [mean (SD), 36.7 (6.9) years; range, 18–45 years], 38 premenopausal women [mean (SD), 47.6 (1.8) years; range, 46–50 years], 50 women in the early menopausal stage [mean (SD), 53.8 (3.6) years; range, 47–60 years], and 144 women of late menopausal stage [mean (SD), 62.3 (3.2) years; range, 55–73 years].

The detailed comparison between the various groups is reported in Tables S3 and S4. Women in the first two cohorts (full reproductive age, premenopausal) showed similar moderately severe disease states, as indicated by liver necro-inflammatory activity (P = 0.42; Table S3) and staging (P = 0.062; Table S3, Figure 1). No significant difference in mean BMI was observed between these two groups (P = 0.118). Severe steatosis was more prevalent in premenopausal women (3/38, 8.0%) than in women of full reproductive age (4/123, 3.2%) although the difference did not reach significance (Table S4). The presence of cirrhosis in both groups at the time of enrollment was negligible.

The comparison of reproductive-aged women (full reproductive age, premenopausal) with those in early menopause revealed significant differences in several variables. The estimated duration of HCV infection was significantly longer in early menopausal women than in fully reproductive (P<0.0001) or premenopausal (P = 0.017) women. All indicators of disease severity were significantly worse in early menopausal women in comparison with the two reproductive-aged groups (early menopause vs. full reproductive age: grading, P = 0.020; staging, P<0.0001; early menopause vs. premenopause: grading, P = 0.014; staging, P = 0.042; Figure 1, Table S3). BMI did differ significantly among women in early menopause vs. full reproductive age (P = 0.039) but not between early menopause vs. premenopausal women (P = 0.90). A significantly higher percentage of early menopausal women had cirrhosis compared with reproductive-aged women (P = 0.039, Table S3).

In the late menopausal group, grading did not differ significantly in comparison with the reproductive-aged and premeno-

pausal groups, but was significantly lower than that in the early menopausal group (P = 0.004). Staging at the time of liver biopsy was significantly higher in late menopausal women than in full reproductive age and premenopausal groups (P<0.0001 for both) while it was of borderline significance vs. early menopause (P = 0.052) (Table S3, Figure 1). Accordingly, cirrhosis was more prevalent in late menopausal women than in fully reproductive (P = 0.004) or premenopausal (P = 0.026) women; however, prevalence was not significantly different between late and early menopausal women (P = 0.25; Table S3). BMI, insulin resistance, and presence of steatosis did not differ significantly between any pair of female groups.

Multivariate analysis showed that necro-inflammation (OR: 1.506; 95% confidence interval (CI), 1.181–1.922, P = 0.001), steatosis (0 vs. >20%) (OR: 3.029; CI 1.154–7.951, P = 0.024), circulating estradiol levels (OR: 0.973, CI 0.947–0.999), P = 0.041), ALT (OR: 1.011, CI 0.003–1.019, P = 0.009) and portal vein diameter (OR: 2.644, CI 1.657–4.220, P<0.0001) were independently associated with the severity of fibrosis (Table 1). Neither age nor estimated length of HCV infection or estimated age of acquisition of infection was significantly related with severity of fibrosis.

Comparison of Reproductive Status–Stratified Female and Male Groups

The results of the comparison of each male–female group pair are reported in Table S1. The estimated duration of HCV infection did not differ significantly between each male–female group pair. Men in groups paired with the first three female groups (reproductive age, premenopause, early menopause) showed remarkably more severe liver disease, as indicated by mean stage of fibrosis (P<0.0001 for all 3 groups; Table S1 and Figure 1), but no significant difference in fibrosis was found between women in the late menopausal group and age-matched men. Similarly, no significant difference in the presence of cirrhosis was observed between male–female pairs correlating with full reproductive age and late menopause, whereas the

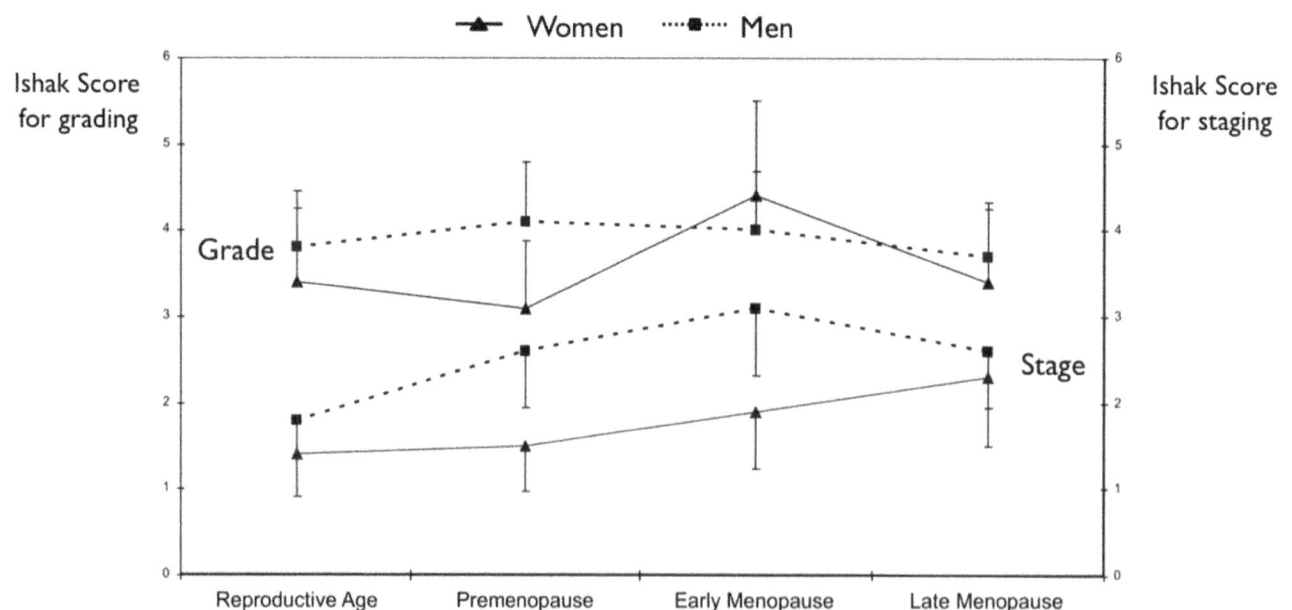

Figure 1. Mean necro-inflammation and fibrosis scores in the four subgroups of female and age-matched male patients with chronic hepatitis (Women: triangles; Men: squares). Levels of significance of the intra- and inter-group comparison are reported in the text.

Table 1. Univariate and multivariate analysis for fibrosis in the women with chronic hepatitis C.

	Univariate		Multivariate	
	OR (95% CI)	P	OR (95% CI)	P
Age (years)	1.089 (1.040–1.140)	0.000	1.028 (0.939–1.126)	0.553
Duration of HCV infection (years)	1.118 (1.037–1.205)	0.004	1.015 (0.884–1.166)	0.833
HCV infection's Acquisition Age	1.036 (1.015–1.057)	0.001	1.000 (0.879–1.139)	0.996
Necro-inflammation	1.458 (1.277–1.665)	0.000	1.506 (1.181–1.1.922)	0.001
Steatosis (0 vs. >20%)	1.775 (1.018–3.095)	0.043	3.029 (1.154–7.951)	0.024
Circulating Estradiol (pgml)	0.977 (0.963–0.991)	0.001	0.973 (0.947–0.999)	0.041
Baseline HCV RNA (IU/mL)	1.000 (1.000–1.000)	0.024	1.000 (1.000–1.000)	0.578
ALT (IU/L)	1.009 (1.004–1.013)	0.000	1.011 (0.003–1.019)	0.009
GGT (IU/L)	1.028 (1.016–1039)	0.000	1.008 (0.992–1.025)	0.327
Platelet count (×10³/mm³)	0.970 (0.969–0.981)	0.000	0.988 (0.974–1.002)	0.099
Portal vein diameter (mm)	2.392 (1.804–3.171)	0.000	2.644 (1.657–4.220)	0.0001

Only factors found to be significant by univariate analysis are reported.

incidence of cirrhosis was significantly lower in the two intermediate groups of women than in age-matched groups of men (P = 0.003 for both; Table S1). In contrast, no difference in grading or steatosis was observed between male–female group pairs.

GGT levels were significantly lower in women than in men in all group pairs (full reproductive age, P<0.0001; premenopause, P = 0.001; early menopause, P = 0.007; late menopause, P = 0.017; Table S1). BMI differed significantly between men and women in all group pairs except the early menopause pair (full reproductive age, P<0.0001; premenopause, P = 0.045; late menopause, P = 0.0012; Table S1).

No difference in the severity of liver necro-inflammation was observed between men and women in each group pair (Table S1).

Multivariate analysis in the whole male and female cohort, reported in Table 2, showed that sex (OR: 0.460, CI 0.236–0.896, P = 0.023), necro-inflammation (OR: 1.401, CI 1.239–1.584,

P<0001), circulating estradiol levels (OR: 0.980, CI 0.962–0.999, P = 0.040), platelets count (OR: 0.974, 0.967–0.981, P<0.0001) and portal vein diameter (OR: 1.903, CI 0.539–2.354, P<0.0001) were independently related with severe fibrosis.

Results of multivariate analysis in the whole cohort, stratified in the four reproductive subgroups, are reported in Table 3. Male sex was independently associated with the severity of fibrosis in the premenopausal [male as reference: odds ratio (OR), 0.074; 95% confidence interval (CI), 0.007–0.834; P = 0.048] and early menopausal (OR, 0.037; 95% CI, 0.004–0.344; P = 0.004) group pairs, but not in the reproductive-aged or late menopausal group pairs (Table 3).

Hormone Assays

Serum concentrations of AMH in the four female groups are shown in Figure 2. Mean values were 2.4 (1.8) ng/mL in reproductive-aged women and 0.5 (0.3) ng/mL in premenopausal

Table 2. Univariate and multivariate analysis for fibrosis in the whole cohort of patients with chronic hepatitis C.

	Univariate		Multivariate	
	OR (95% CI)	P	OR (95% CI)	P
Sex*	0.406 (0.254–0.649)	0.000	0.460 (0.236–0.896)	0.023
Age (years)	1.049 (1.027–1.072)	0.000	1.031 (1.000–1.062)	0.050
Duration of HCV infection (years)	1.064 (1.023–1.107)	0.002	0.989 (0.941–1.039)	0.654
Necro-inflammation	1.427 (1.312–1.553)	0.000	1.401 (1.239–1.584)	0.0001
Steatosis (0 vs. >20%)	1.469 (1.062–2.032)	0.020	1.301 (0.840–2.016)	0.239
Circulating Estradiol (pg/ml)	0.982 (0.972–0.991)	0.000	0.980 (0.962–0.999)	0.040
Blood Iron (ng/mL)	1.010 (1.003–1.017)	0.006	1.018 (0.993–1.043)	0.170
Ferritin (ng/mL)	1.002 (1.000–1.003)	0.031	1.001 (0.995–1.006)	0.784
ALT (IU/L)	1.008 (1.005.011)	0.000	1.002 (0.998–1.006)	0.279
GGT (IU/L)	1.016 (1.010–1021)	0.000	1.003 (0.996–1.010)	0.387
Platelet count (x10³/mm³)	0.973 (0.967–0.979)	0.000	0.974 (0.967–0.981)	0.0001
Portal vein diameter (mm)	2.233 (1.901–2.622)	0.000	1.903 (0.539–2.354)	0.000

Only factors found to be significant by univariate analysis are reported.
*Male as reference. HCV, hepatitis C virus; BMI, body mass index; ALT, alanine aminotransferase; GGT, γ-glutamyl transpeptidase; OR, odds ratio; CI, confidence interval.

Table 3. Comparison of the baseline independent predictive factors for fibrosis in the four cohorts of patients with chronic hepatitis C.

	Reproductive-aged women/age-matched men (n=123)				Premenopausal women/age-matched men (n=38)				Early menopausal women/age-matched men (n=50)				Late menopausal women/age-matched men (n=144)			
	Univariate		Multivariate		Univariate		Multivariate		Univariate		Multivariate		Univariate		Multivariate	
	OR (95% CI)	P	OR (95% CI)	P	OR (95% CI)	P	OR (95% CI)	P	OR (95% CI)	P	OR (95% CI)	P	OR (95% CI)	P	OR (95% CI)	P
Sex*	0.231 (0.075–0.706)	0.010	0.869 (0.161–4.667)	0.870	0.071 (0.009–0.594)	0.015	0.074 (0.007–0.834)	**0.048**	0.112 (0.030–0.419)	0.001	0.037 (0.004–0.344)	**0.004**	0.794 (0.425–1.485)	0.471	§
Age (years)	1.061 (0.998–1.127)	0.058	1.113 (0.931–1.332)	0.240	1.027 (0.676–1.560)	0.902	§		0.966 (0.857–1.089)	0.572	§		1.077 (0.983–1.181)	0.110	§
Estimated duration of HCV infection (years)	0.930 (0.809–1.069)	0.305	§		1.062 (0.913v1.236)	0.434	§		1.046 (0.959–1.40)	0.309	§		1.048 (0.992–1.106)	0.094	§
Mean BMI (kg/m²)	0.954 (0.814–1.111)	0.544	§		1.032 (0.874–1.217)	0.711	§		1.119 (0.982–1.274)	0.090	0.997 (0.789–1.260)	0.981	0.974 (0.900–1.054)	0.512	§
Necro-inflammation	1.370 (1.155–1.625)	0.000	1.448 (1.092–1.922)	**0.010**	1.433 (1.083–1.896)	0.012	1.501 (1.003–2.248)	**0.048**	1.556 (1.254–1.930)	0.000	1.727 (1.238–2.410)	**0.001**	1.407 (1.254–1.579)	0.000	1.566 (1.295–1.894)	**0.0001**
Steatosis (0 vs. >20%)	2.782 (0.854–9.055)	0.089	1.874 (0.402–8.729)	0.424	2.038 (1.216–3.415)	0.007	5.242 (0.402–68.421)	0.206	1.455 (0.517–4.391)	0.478	§		1.177 (0.711–1.947)	0.527	§
Blood Iron (ng/mL)	1.012 (1.001–1.024)	0.038	1.018 (0.993–1.043)	0.170	1.013 (0.987–1.038)	0.333	§		1.011 (0.998–1.025)	0.089	§		1.002 (0.987–1.017)	0.796	§
Ferritin (ng/mL)	1.002 (1.000–1.005)	0.047	1.001 (0.995–1.006)	0.784	1.044 (0.995–1.013)	0.422	§		1.004 (1.000–1.009)	0.046	0.993 (0.978–1.008)	0.376	1.000 (0.997–1.002)	0.805	§
ALT (IU/L)	1.007 (1.003–1.010)	0.001	1.002 (0.995–1.010)	0.549	1.010 (0.995–1.025)	0.178	§		1.008 (1.002–1.014)	0.006	0.999 (0.989–1.010)	0.880	1.010 (1.005–1.014)	0.000	1.006 (0.999–1.001)	0.102
GGT (IU/L)	1.021 (1.011–1031)	0.000	1.013 (1.000–1.026)	**0.045**	1.013 (0.998–1.028)	0.092	0.997 (0.979–1.015)	0.713	1.028 (1.010–1.046)	0.002	0.997 (0.982–1.012)	0.653	1.011 (1.004–1.018)	0.001	1.001 (0.993–1.009)	0.800
Platelet count (×10³/mm³)	0.976 (0.967–0.986)	0.000	0.982 (0.969–0.997)	**0.015**	0.972 (0.956–0.988)	0.001	0.973 (0.954–0.992)	**0.005**	0.971 (0.956–0.985)	0.000	0.975 (0.955–0.996)	**0.022**	0.972 (0.962–0.981)	0.000	0.967 (0.954–0.981)	**0.002**
Portal vein diameter (mm)	1.888 (1.416–2.516)	0.000	1.394 (0.5919–2.114)	0.118	3.822 (1.874–7.794)	0.000	4.611 (0.891–11.245)	**0.001**	2.111 (1.455–3.061)	0.000	2.316 (1.204–4.455)	**0.012**	5.960 (2.665–3.326)	0.000	4.729 (1.524–14.679)	**0.007**

Only factors found by univariate analysis to be significant in at least one of the four groups are reported.
*Male as reference; § Not included in multivariate model because not significant in univariate analysis.
HCV, hepatitis C virus; BMI, body mass index; ALT, alanine aminotransferase; GGT, γ-glutamyl transpeptidase; OR, odds ratio; CI, confidence interval.

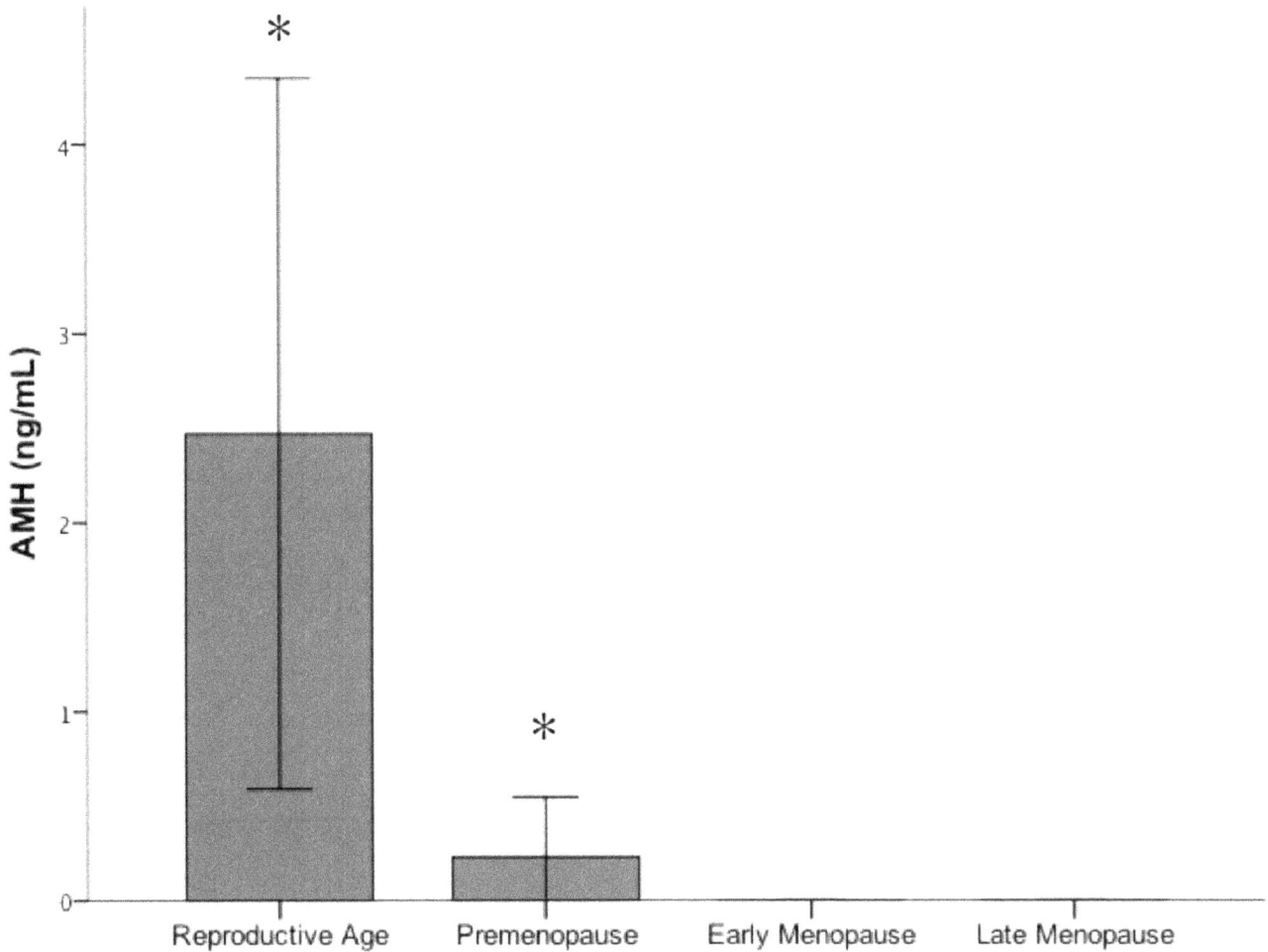

Figure 2. Mean serum levels of anti-müllerian hormone (AMH) in women divided according to reproductive phases. AMH levels were significantly lower in premenopausal women in comparison with women in full reproductive age (p<0.0001) and became undetectable in menopausal women (both early and late).

women (Mann–Whitney U-test, P<0.0001). AMH levels were undetectable in early and late menopausal women.

Serum concentrations of estradiol and testosterone in the four group pairs are shown in Figures 3A and 3B, respectively, and the estradiol/testosterone ratio [E2/T; estradiol (pg/mL)/testosterone (ng/mL)] is reported in Figure 3C. Estradiol concentrations changed significantly in both men and women with age, with a marked difference observed in both sexes at the age corresponding to female menopausal onset. In particular, estradiol levels were significantly higher in reproductive-aged and premenopausal women than in early (reproductive age: P<0.0001; premenopausal: P<0.0001) and late menopausal women (reproductive age: P<0.0001; premenopausal: P<0.0001), whereas males exhibited a significant change in the opposite direction at corresponding ages (reproductive vs. early menopause: P = 0.003, vs. late menopause: P = 0.05; premenopausal groups vs. early: P = 0.001, vs. late P = 0.005). Testosterone levels changed significantly only in women, who showed significantly higher levels in the full reproductive age group than in the other groups (reproductive vs. premenopausal P = 0.44; vs. early menopausal P = 0.006; vs. late menopausal P = 0.013). Although a decline in testosterone levels was observed in the two older groups of men, this difference was not significant. The E2/T ratio changed significantly with age in both men and women. In women, the E2/T ratio decreased

markedly in early (vs. reproductive age: P = 0.002 and vs. premenopausal: P<0.0001) and late menopause (vs. reproductive age: P = 0.001 and vs. premenopausal: P<0.0001). The opposite change occurred in men (reproductive age group vs. early menopause group: P = 0.002 and vs. late: P = 0.001) (Figure 3C).

Discussion

In this cross-sectional study comparing a large cohort of women with CHC who were grouped, according to reproductive status, with age-matched men with CHC, we found that hormonal phases were differently associated with the histological severity of liver disease.

A few clinical studies [8,9] have found that estrogens exert a beneficial effect on liver disease by slowing the progression of fibrosis; however, this effect has previously been evaluated in terms of lifetime exposure, rather than according to different reproductive stages. To overcome this limitation, we divided a cohort of 355 women with CHC into four groups according to reproductive status. The allocation of patients to these groups was substantiated using AMH levels, because this glycoprotein is a more accurate indicator of ovarian reserve than is age or other conventional serum marker (follicle stimulating hormone, estradiol, inhibin B) [14–16]. The AMH levels obtained in our study were in

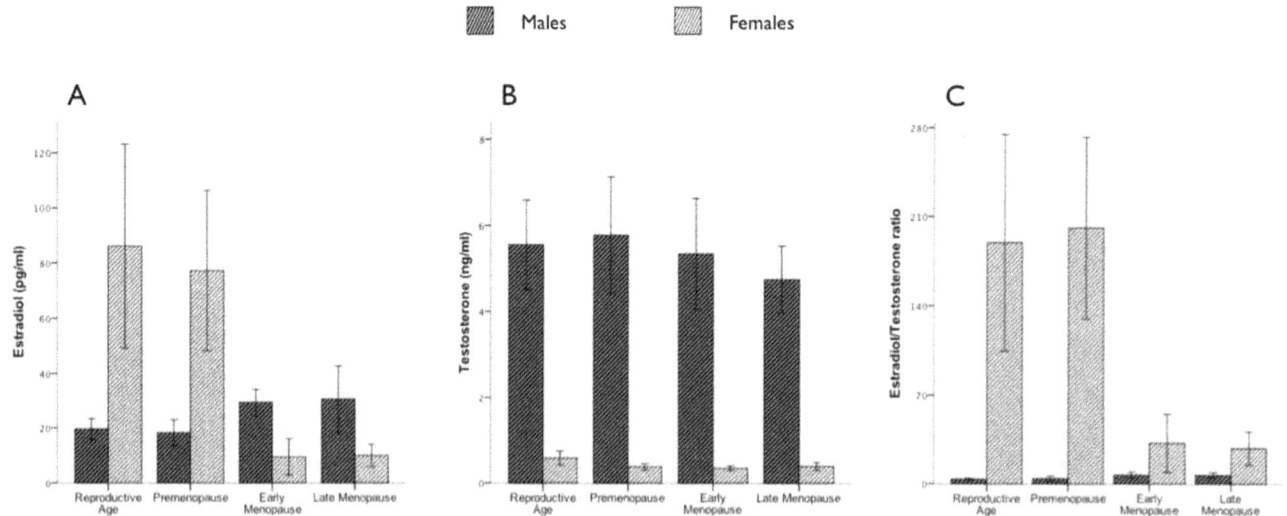

Figure 3. Estradiol and Testosterone serum levels and E2/T ratio in men and women divided according to women's reproductive phases as described in Methods. Values (reported as mean±SD) were compared by Mann-Whitney test. The levels of significance are reported in the text.

agreement with those reported for reproductive age, premenopause, and established menopause [17,18], and thus validated the composition of the four groups.

The results of our study support the concept that the progression of fibrosis in women is a discontinuous process: very slow during reproductive age and accelerating rapidly after menopause. We found that disease severity at the time of liver biopsy, as measured by the severity of liver necro-inflammation and fibrosis, was very low in women of reproductive age and in premenopausal ones while it became higher among early menopausal women; the severity of fibrosis was found to be even higher among late menopausal women. Further support for the protective role of estrogens toward development of fibrosis comes from the multivariate analysis of risk factors for severe fibrosis: neither estimated duration of HCV infection nor the age of acquisition of HCV infection was independently associated with fibrosis while levels of circulating estradiol was.

The impact of hormonal exposure on fibrosis became even more complex when the female groups were compared with their age-matched male counterparts. Although the estimated duration of HCV infection was similar in all group pairs and age was equivalent by definition, women had less severe fibrosis than men in all but the late menopausal group pair. Female sex appeared to be independently associated with a lower prevalence of severe fibrosis in the premenopausal and early menopausal group pairs [19].

These findings may be explained by the observed changes in hormone levels according to reproductive status. The high estradiol levels observed in the reproductive-aged groups (full reproductive, premenopause) likely provided protection against the development of severe liver injury. However, an independent correlation between fibrosis and sex was found only in the premenopausal and early menopausal group pairs, and not in the fully reproductive group pair. This finding may be due to the short duration of infection and to the very mild stage of disease present in both sexes in the reproductive-aged group pair.

In contrast, menopausal women exhibited greater disease severity than those in the reproductive-aged and premenopausal group pairs, probably due to the decline in estradiol levels that occurs rapidly with menopause development. We have already

shown that a marked up-regulation of inflammatory cytokines, especially interleukin-6 (IL-6), occurs in close temporal relationship with the onset of menopause [11,12], when for the first time in a woman's life E2/T ratio dramatically decreases: this is associated with a sharp increase in necro-inflammatory activity and is eventually followed (as the change in fibrosis score between early and menopausal women shows) by a significant increase in fibrosis in late menopausal women. As the late menopausal male-female group comparison indicates, at this stage women lose the advantage that they had in earlier reproductive stages: fibrosis and percentage of cirrhosis are no longer significantly different from males and only subtle indicators of disease progression (like portal vein diameter and platelets count) are still better in females. A further element that may play a relevant role in reducing differences in disease severity between genders in the late groups is the significant increase of estradiol levels and E2/T ratio that was observed in males of the early and late menopausal groups. This increase did not result in a change in necro-inflammation, but was associated with a significant reduction in fibrosis severity in men in group 4 (group 4 vs. group 3, P = 0.010). This is in agreement with the recently reported positive correlation between testosterone levels and increased risk of both advanced hepatic fibrosis and advanced hepatic inflammatory activity in HCV-infected men [20]: although this study evaluated only absolute Testosterone levels and not Estradiol or the E2/T ratio, it is relevant that higher unopposed levels of Testosterone related with higher severity of disease. In our cohort, the late inversion of the E2/T ratio in males coincided with the first and only improvement in fibrosis score in males.

These findings not only reinforce the view that the lengthy period of exposure to estrogens in women plays a favorable role in the progression of chronic liver disease in comparison with men, but also suggest that this protective effect is reversible and strictly dependent on estrogen levels. When the process of hormonal aging leads to an inversion in the E2/T balance characteristic of full reproductive age, women lose the favorable estrogen effect and show patterns similar to those of men. Accordingly, male sex is constantly and independently associated with a higher degree of fibrosis in cohorts whose mean age coincides with the full reproductive stage (i.e., <50 years of age) [5,6]. In contrast, cohorts with higher mean ages (>50 years; a surrogate indicator of menopause in women) show similar patterns of fibrosis progression in men and women, and male sex is no longer a predictor of severe fibrosis progression [6,21,22].

Although our study was not designed to clarify the pathogenesis of the association between reproductive phase and the severity of fibrosis in women, previous studies have provided several hypotheses. Many experimental data have shown that estradiol inhibits transforming growth factor (TGF)-β1 expression and hepatic stellate cell (HSC) activation, thereby suppressing the induction of hepatic fibrosis [8,23,24]. Estradiol is also known to induce the down-regulation of tumor necrosis factor (TNF) alpha, IL-6, and IL-1β [25–27], mediators contributing to hepatic necro-inflammation and the activation of HSCs. The favorable role of estrogens in men has also been suggested by two case reports, in which different pathological conditions required prolonged estrogen treatment in two young men, one with hepatitis C [28] and the other with nonalcoholic steatohepatitis (NASH) [29]. In the first case, the addition of estradiol reduced disease activity and maintained viral loads at lower levels than observed before treatment [28]. In the second case, it reversed hepatic steatosis and insulin resistance [28].

In this study of a cohort of women with CHC classified by reproductive phase and compared with age-matched men with CHC, we found that the severity of fibrosis in women is strictly related with Estradiol levels and E2/T ratio. Progression of fibrosis follows the sharp rise of necro-inflammatory activity occurring in coincidence with estrogen deprivation in early menopause [11]. This finding explains the discontinuous rate of fibrosis progression in women and the more linear rate observed in men, in whom the modification of sex hormone balance determined by aging-associated Estradiol increase occurs very late in life and thus may have only a limited beneficial effect on hepatic condition.

References

1. Yen T, Keeffe EB, Ahmed A (2003) The epidemiology of hepatitis C virus infection. J Clin Gastroenterol 36: 47–53.
2. George SL, Bacon BR, Brunt EM, Mihindukulasuriya KL, Hoffmann J, et al. (2009) Clinical, virologic, histologic, and biochemical outcomes after successful HCV therapy: a 5-year follow-up of 150 patients. Hepatology 49: 729–738.
3. Petta S, Amato M, Cabibi D, Cammà C, Di Marco V, et al. (2010) Visceral Adiposity Index is Associated with Histological Findings and with High Viral Load in Patients with Chronic Hepatitis C Due to Genotype 1. Hepatology 52: 1543–1552.
4. Conte D, Fraquelli M, Prati D, Colucci A, Minola E. (2000) Prevalence and Clinical Course of Chronic Hepatitis C Virus (HCV) Infection and Rate of HCV Vertical Transmission in a Cohort of 15,250 Pregnant Women. Hepatology; 31: 751–5.
5. Poynard T, Bedossa P, Opolon P (1997) Natural history of liver fibrosis progression in chronic hepatitis C. Lancet 349: 825–832.
6. Deuffic-Burban S, Poynard T, Valleron AJ (2002) Quantification of fibrosis progression in patients with chronic hepatitis C using a Markov model. J Viral Hepat 9: 114–122.
7. Yasuda M, Shimizu I, Shiba M, Ito S (1999) Suppressive effects of estradiol on dimethylnitrosamine-induced fibrosis of the liver in rats. Hepatology 29: 719–727.
8. Shimizu I, Mizobuchi Y, Yasuda M, Shiba M, Ma YR, et al. (1999) Inhibitory effect of estradiol on activation of rat hepatic stellate cells in vivo and in vitro. Gut 44: 127–136.
9. Di Martino V, Lebray P, Myers RP, Pannier E, Paradis V, et al. (2004) Progression of liver fibrosis in women infected with hepatitis C: long-term benefit of estrogen exposure. Hepatology 40: 1426–1433.
10. Codes L, Asselah T, Cazals-Hatem D, Tubach F, Vidaud D, et al. (2007) Liver fibrosis in women with chronic hepatitis C: evidence for the negative role of the menopause and steatosis and the potential benefit of hormone replacement therapy. Gut 56: 390–395.
11. Villa E, Karampatou A, Cammà C, Di Leo A, Luongo M, et al. (2011) Early menopause is associated with lack of response to antiviral therapy in women with chronic hepatitis C. Gastroenterology 140: 818–829.
12. Pfeilschifter J, Köditz R, Pfohl M, Schatz H. Changes in proinflammatory cytokine activity after menopause 2002 Endocr Rev 23: 90–119.
13. Ishak K, Baptista A, Bianchi L, Callea F, De Groote J, et al. (1995) Histological grading and staging of chronic hepatitis. J Hepatol 22: 696–699.
14. SAS Technical Report, SAS/STAS software (1992): changes & enhance- ment, release 6. 07. Vol. 7. Cary, NC: SAS Institute Inc.
15. Van Disseldorp J, Faddy MJ, Themmen AP, De Jong FH, Peeters PH, et al. (2008) Relationship of serum antimullerian hormone concentration to age at menopause. J Clin Endocrinol Metab 93: 2129–2134.
16. Riggs RM, Duran EH, Baker MW, Kimble TD, Hobeika E, et al. (2008) Assessment of ovarian reserve with anti-Mullerian hormone: a comparison of the predictive value of anti-Mullerian hormone, follicle-stimulating hormone, inhibin B, and age. Am J Obstet Gynecol 199: 202. e1–8.
17. La Marca A, Broekmans FJ, Volpe A, Fauser BC, Macklon NS, et al. (2009) Anti-Mullerian hormone (AMH): what do we still need to know? Hum Reprod 24: 2264–2275.
18. Seifer DB, Baker VL, Leader B (2011) Age-specific serum anti-Mullerian hormone values for 17,120 women presenting to fertility centers within the United States. Fertil Steril 95: 747–750.
19. Sweeting MJ, De Angelis D, Neal KR, Ramsay ME, Irving WL, et al. (2006) Estimated progression rates in three United Kingdom hepatitis C cohorts differed according to method of recruitment. J Clin Epidemiol 59: 144–152.
20. White DL, Tavakoli-Tabasi S, Kuzniarek J, Pascua R, Ramsey DJ, et al. (2012) Higher serum testosterone is associated with increased risk of advanced hepatitis C-related liver disease in males. Hepatology 55: 759–768.
21. Miyaaki H, Ichikawa T, Taura N, Miuma S, Shibata H, et al. (2011) Predictive value of the fibrosis scores in patients with chronic hepatitis C associated with liver fibrosis and metabolic syndrome. Intern Med 50: 1137–1141.
22. Hoefs JC, Shiffman ML, Goodman ZD, Kleiner DE, Dienstag JL, et al. (2011) Rate of progression of hepatic fibrosis in patients with chronic hepatitis c: results from the HALT-C trial. Gastroenterology 141: 900–908.
23. Xu JW, Gong J, Chang XM, Luo JY, Dong L, et al. (2002) Estrogen reduces CCl4-induced liver fibrosis in rats. World J Gastroenterol 8: 883–887.
24. Itagaki T, Shimizu I, Cheng X, Yuan Y, Oshio A, et al. (2005) Opposing effects of oestradiol and progesterone on intracellular pathways and activation processes in the oxidative stress-induced activation of cultured rat hepatic stellate cells. Gut 54: 1782–1789.
25. Friedman SL (2008) Hepatic stellate cells: protean, multifunctional, and enigmatic cells of the liver. Physiol Rev 88: 125–172.

Limitations

The main limitation of this study lies in its cross-sectional design, which prevented the evaluation of fibrosis progression in individual patients according to baseline reproductive status and reproductive transitions. A further methodological question is the potentially limited external validity of the results for different populations and settings, because our study included a cohort of Italian subjects enrolled at a tertiary care center.

Supporting Information

Table S1 Comparison between female and age-matched male patients with chronic hepatitis.

Table S2 Comparison between female and age-matched male patients with chronic hepatitis.

Table S3 Comparison between the four groups of female patients with chronic hepatitis C.

Table S4 Comparison between the four groups of female patients with chronic hepatitis C.

Author Contributions

Conceived and designed the experiments: EV RV CC SP. Performed the experiments: RG LS AC ST EB. Analyzed the data: EV CC ADL NDM AF. Contributed reagents/materials/analysis tools: ADL SG AK ET LL VB AC ST EB MR. Wrote the paper: EV RV CC AF.

26. Kireev RA, Tresguerres AC, Garcia C, Borras C, Ariznavarreta C, et al. (2010) Hormonal regulation of pro-inflammatory and lipid peroxidation processes in liver of old ovariectomized female rats. Biogerontology 11: 229–243.
27. Rogers A, Eastell R (2001) The effect of 17 β-estradiol on production of cytokines in cultures of peripheral blood. Bone 29: 30–34.
28. Shimizu I, Omoya T, Kondo Y, Kusaka Y, Tsutsui A, et al. (2001) Estrogen therapy in a male patient with chronic hepatitis C and irradiation-induced testicular dysfunction. Intern Med 40: 100–104.
29. Maffei L, Murata Y, Rochira V, Tubert G, Aranda C, et al. (2004) Dysmetabolic syndrome in a man with a novel mutation of the aromatase gene: effects of testosterone, alendronate, and estradiol treatment. J Clin Endocrinol Metab 89: 61–70.

Cancer-Associated Carbohydrate Antigens as Potential Biomarkers for Hepatocellular Carcinoma

Chen-Shiou Wu[1,5◑], Chia-Jui Yen[3,4◑], Ruey-Hwang Chou[2,6], Shiou-Ting Li[5], Wei-Chien Huang[1,2], Chien-Tai Ren[5], Chung-Yi Wu[1,5]*, Yung-Luen Yu[1,2,6]*

1 The Ph.D. Program for Cancer Biology and Drug Discovery, China Medical University, Taichung, Taiwan, 2 Graduate Institute of Cancer Biology and Center for Molecular Medicine, China Medical University, Taichung, Taiwan, 3 Graduate Institute of Clinical Medicine, National Cheng Kung University, Tainan, Taiwan, 4 Division of Hematology/Oncology, Department of Internal Medicine, National Cheng Kung University Hospital, Tainan, Taiwan, 5 Genomics Research Center, Academia Sinica, Taipei, Taiwan, 6 Department of Biotechnology, Asia University, Taichung, Taiwan

Abstract

Hepatocellular carcinoma (HCC) is one of the most common human malignancies. Therefore, developing the early, high-sensitivity diagnostic biomarkers to prevent HCC is urgently needed. Serum a-fetoprotein (AFP), the clinical biomarker in current use, is elevated in only ~60% of patients with HCC; therefore, identification of additional biomarkers is expected to have a significant impact on public health. In this study, we used glycan microarray analysis to explore the potential diagnostic value of several cancer associated carbohydrate antigens (CACAs) as biomarkers for HCC. We used glycan microarray analysis with 58 different glycan analogs for quantitative comparison of 593 human serum samples (293 HCC samples; 133 chronic hepatitis B virus (HBV) infection samples, 134 chronic hepatitis C virus (HCV) infection samples, and 33 healthy donor samples) to explore the diagnostic possibility of serum antibody changes as biomarkers for HCC. Serum concentrations of anti-disialosyl galactosyl globoside (DSGG), anti-fucosyl GM1 and anti-Gb2 were significantly higher in patients with HCC than in chronic HBV infection individuals not in chronic HCV infection patients. Overall, in our study population, the biomarker candidates DSGG, fucosyl GM1 and Gb2 of CACAs achieved better predictive sensitivity than AFP. We identified potential biomarkers suitable for early detection of HCC. Glycan microarray analysis provides a powerful tool for high-sensitivity and high-throughput detection of serum antibodies against CACAs, which may be valuable serum biomarkers for the early detection of persons at high risk for HCC.

Editor: Erica Villa, University of Modena & Reggio Emilia, Italy

Funding: This work was supported by National Science Council of Taiwan grants NSC99-2320-B-039-030-MY3, NSC99-2632-B-039-001-MY3, NSC100-2321-B-039-004, and The University of Texas MD Anderson-China Medical University and Hospital Sister Institution Fund DMR-101-115. The funders had no role in study design, data collection and analysis, decision to publish, or preparation of the manuscript.

Competing Interests: The authors have declared that no competing interests exist.

* E-mail: cyiwu@gate.sinica.edu.tw (CYW); ylyu@mail.cmu.edu.tw (YLY)

◑ These authors contributed equally to this work.

Introduction

Hepatocellular carcinoma (HCC) is the fifth most common cancer worldwide, with China and North America showing a continuous increase in the incidence and mortality rate [1]. HCC nearly always develops in the setting of chronic hepatitis virus infection or liver cirrhosis [2–4]. The prognosis for patients with HCC remains poor, and the 5-year survival rate after diagnosis OR for most patients is less than 5%, mainly because the disease is often diagnosed in an advanced stage [5]. For patients with a diagnosis of HCC at an early stage, the survival rate can be improved significantly by surgical resection, liver transplantation, and other curative therapies such as ablative treatments [6,7]. Moreover, surveillance of at-risk patients improves detection and potentially the curative effect of treatments for small tumors. Therefore, early prognostic markers are crucial for effective treatment and prevention of HCC.

The most common HCC biomarker used to screen patients with liver cirrhosis is serum a-fetoprotein (AFP), which is measured at 6-month intervals [8]. Nevertheless, AFP levels are often elevated in some patients with chronic liver disease who do not have cancer, and AFP levels are not elevated in 30–40% of patients with liver cancer [9]. The serum AFP test has low sensitivity, and about one-third of patients with early-stage HCC and small tumors (<3 cm) have the same level of AFP as that in normal individuals, which makes the AFP test insufficient for the early detection of HCC in at-risk populations [10]. In addition, the AFP test has a high false-positive rate of ~20% among patients with chronic hepatitis and 20–50% among those with liver cirrhosis [5,11]. In this regard, there is an urgent need to identify more sensitive and reliable serum biomarkers for the detection of HCC [12,13].

Oncogenesis is often associated with changes in the expression of cell surface carbohydrates. In some instances, the carbohydrate pattern may be specific to the disease type [14]. In other instances, levels of anti-carbohydrate antibodies may be markedly enhanced with the onset of disease [15]. Previous studies have shown that cellular glycosylation profiles change significantly during carcinogenesis [14]. Carbohydrates play crucial roles in various biological events such as cell recognition [16], inter- and intracellular signaling, embryonic development, cell adhesion [17], and cell-cell interactions [18]. Currently, glycan marker discovery with glycan microarray analysis presents great potential for identifying biomarkers relevant for the diagnosis of breast cancer [19].

Glycan microarrays allow direct characterization of carbohydrate-protein interactions [20]. Microarray techniques are effective and sensitive methods for the rapid analysis of the specificity of protein-carbohydrate interactions and the characterization of differentiation processes pertaining to the onset of cancer at the molecular level [21]. In addition, the attachment of sugars to surfaces can effectively mimic the presentation of these compounds on the membrane of cells and thus can be used to bind antibodies [20]. In this report, we focused on glycans that are known to be cancer-associated carbohydrate antigens (CACAs) in many cancers but that have not been studied in HCC. We used glycan microarray analysis to explore the diagnostic possibility of serum antibody changes as biomarkers for HCC. In addition, we compared the accuracy of the biomarkers we identified with the conventional AFP biomarker for HCC.

Results

Patient Characteristics

A total of 593 participants including 293 HCC patients, 133 chronic hepatitis B virus (HBV) infection patients, 134 chronic hepatitis C virus (HCV) infection patients, and 33 normal subjects were recruited into this study (**Table 1**). There were no significant differences of age and sex between cases and controls. In addition, the HCC group and the healthy controls group had statistically different laboratory results for albumin, aspartate aminotransferase (AST), alanine aminotransferase (ALT) and total bilirubin (BIL-T) (p<0.05). The pathological staging (AJCC) of HCC was grade I in 96 cases (41.3%), grade II in 80 cases (34.5%), grade III in 48 cases (20.7%), and grade IV in 8 cases (3.4%).

Detection of Serum Antibodies Against Carbohydrate Antigens with Glycan Microarray Analysis

We tested serum from patients with HCC for antibodies that bind to glycan fragments. Glass slides printed in microarray format with glycan compounds 1–58 (**Figure S1**) were incubated with serum samples, and bound antibodies were detected using Cy3-labeled goat anti–human IgG secondary antibody (**Figure 1**). The

fluorescent scans were processed to quantify the intensity of each spot. The resulting data were represented as the mean relative fluorescence intensity from replicates of each sample. We noted that the background intensity of carbohydrate antigen binding from healthy individuals could be the result of non-specific binding; therefore, mean fluorescence intensities of <35,000 were removed from the analysis. This approach provided a rationale for the development of a glycan microarray to detect the presence of 47 different glycan antibodies in the serum of patients (after removal of sample numbers 2, 3, 5, 7, 16, 20, 23, 24, 30, 31, and 47).

We examined serum samples from 155 patients with HCC and 33 healthy individuals for antibodies that bound to carbohydrate antigens on the glycan microarray. The fluorescence data reflecting antibody reactivity to each glycan were normalized to Gb5 for each sample, and the relative fluorescence intensities for IgG antibodies from patients with HCC and healthy individuals are presented as mean glycan:Gb5 IgG ratios (**Figure 2**). Antibodies that bound to Gb5 were detected in patients with HCC and healthy donors. We observed that the levels of IgG against glycan numbers 4 (SLacNAc $6SO_3$), 15 (disialosyl galactosyl-globoside; DSGG), 18 (fucosyl GM1), 35 (Gb3), 36 (Gb2), 42 (B19), and 56 (Man7) were significantly higher in patients with HCC than in healthy individuals.

Comparison of the Levels of Seven Anti-glycan Antibodies Among Female and Male Patients with HCC and Healthy Individuals

In a previous study [22], men had a higher incidence of HCC than women. In our current study, we increased the HCC samples numbers up to 293 patients and stratified our results by gender to determine whether anti-glycan antibody levels varied by gender. Among females, levels of IgG against glycan numbers 15, 18, and 35 were significantly higher in patients with HCC than in healthy individuals (P<0.01) (**Figure 3A**). Among males, levels of IgG against glycan numbers 15, 18, 35, 36, and 42 were significantly higher in patients with HCC than in healthy individuals (P<0.05) (**Figure 3B**). Interestingly, we observed similar results for glycan numbers 15, 18 and 35 between two groups.

Comparison of the Level of Select Anti-glycan Antibodies from HCC and Chronic Liver Disease (CLD) by Gender

Worldwide, more than 52% of HCC cases are associated with chronic HBV infection, and 25% of HCC cases are associated with HCV infection [23]. Known HBV or HCV infection may increase the risk of developing HCC [7]. To examine differences in HCC patients with HBV or HCV infection, we divided patients into the HBV-positive HCC (HBV-HCC; n = 132) or HCV-positive HCC (HCV-HCC; n = 65) to compare chronic liver disease (HBV-CLD; n = 133 and HCV-CLD; n = 134). For both genders, levels of IgG against glycans 15, 18, and 36 for females and males were higher in HBV patients with HCC from those patients without HCC (P<0.05) (**Figure 4A and B**). There were no significant differences in anti-glycan levels between patients with HCV-HCC and chronic HCV patients (**Figure 5A and B**).

We next compared detection of glycan analogs and AFP for their diagnostic sensitivity for HCC from CLD and Healthy. For a patient with a history of liver disease, consensus for the diagnosis of HCC can be achieved with an elevated AFP level (≥200 ng/dL), along with a dynamic imaging study showing a hepatic tumor. In Taiwan, the cutoff value of serum AFP level for HCC diagnosis is set at 200 ng/ml, and according to the guidelines of clinical diagnosis and staging criteria for HCC. Therefore, we change cutoff value of AFP. When AFP_{200} (AFP at a cutoff value of

Table 1. Summary of clinical details of subjects used for glycan microarray analysis.

	Healthy (n = 33)	CLD (HBV) (n = 133)	CLD (HCV) (n = 134)	HCC (N–293)
Men, n (%)	22 (66.7)	89 (66.9)	73 (54.5)	223 (76.1)
Laboratory values mean(SD)				
ALBUMIN(g/dL)	4.3 (0.2)	3.9 (0.6)	3.9 (0.5)	4.1 (0.6)
AST(U/L)	27.6 (10.3)	106.1 (144.8)	162.2 (514.6)	136.3 (241.3)
ALT(U/L)	29.3 (19.6)	152.2 (223.6)	185.2 (391.9)	119.4 (232.6)
BIL-T(mg/dL)	0.5 (0.1)	1.2 (1.7)	1.4(3.1)	0.7 (0.6)
Pathological staging(AJCC) (n = 232), n (%)				
I				96 (41.3)
II				80 (34.5)
III				48 (20.7)
IV				8 (3.4)

(CLD: chronic liver disease).

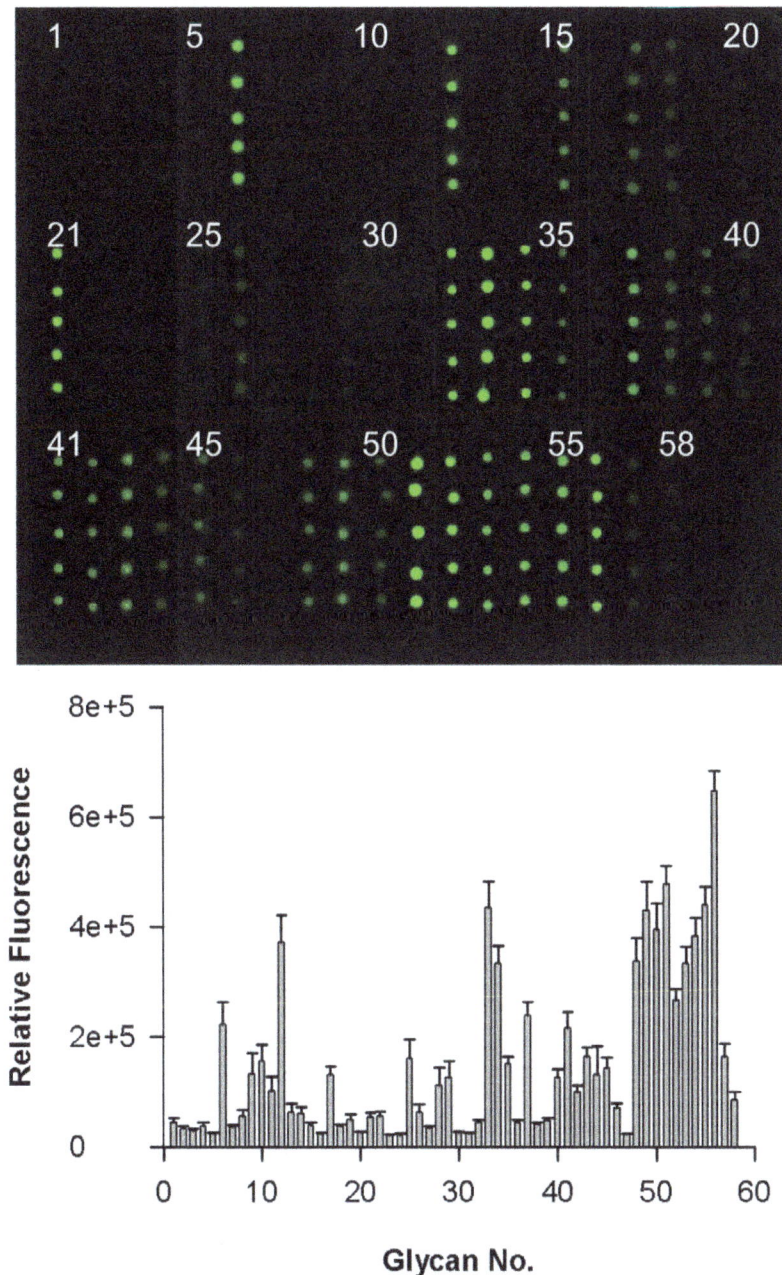

Figure 1. Detection of antibodies to 58 carbohydrate antigens in serum from patients with HCC. (A) A representative slide image obtained from a fluorescence scan after detection of IgG in serum samples. Each grid was printed with glycan numbers 1–20 in the top row, 21–40 in the middle row, and 41–58 in the bottom row. (B) Mean ± standard deviation binding specificity of antibodies to glycan numbers 1–58 in serum samples from patients with HCC. Relative fluorescence intensities were calculated for each spot (containing 100 µM glycan) in the glycan microarray.

>200 ng/ml) was used to predict the HCC stage, a sensitivity of 33.33% (10 of 30) was obtained for females, and 24.51% (25 of 102) was obtained for males (**Table 2**). We observed that the sensitivity of 3 anti-glycan numbers (15, 18, and 36) were better than that of AFP to 63.33% (19 of 30)/42.16% (43 of 102), 56.67% (17 of 30)/35.29% (36 of 102), and 43.33% (13 of 30)/45.1% (46 of 102), respectively, in female/male. (**Table 2**). To test whether the sensitivity of classification could be increased by including clinical data, AFP values were included in the analysis. As seen in Table 2, inclusion of AFP values and 3 anti-glycan markers increased sensitivity of the correct classification of HCC

states to 80% (24 of 30) and 74.5% (76 of 102), respectively, in female and male.

The Diagnostic Value of Three Anti-glycan Antibodies for HCC

To evaluate whether serum anti-glycan levels can be used as a potential diagnostic marker for HCC, Receiver operating characteristics (ROC) curve analyses were performed. It was revealed that serum 3 anti-glycan markers plus AFP levels was a potential marker for discriminating HBV-positive HCC patients from healthy controls with an AUC (the areas under the ROC curve)

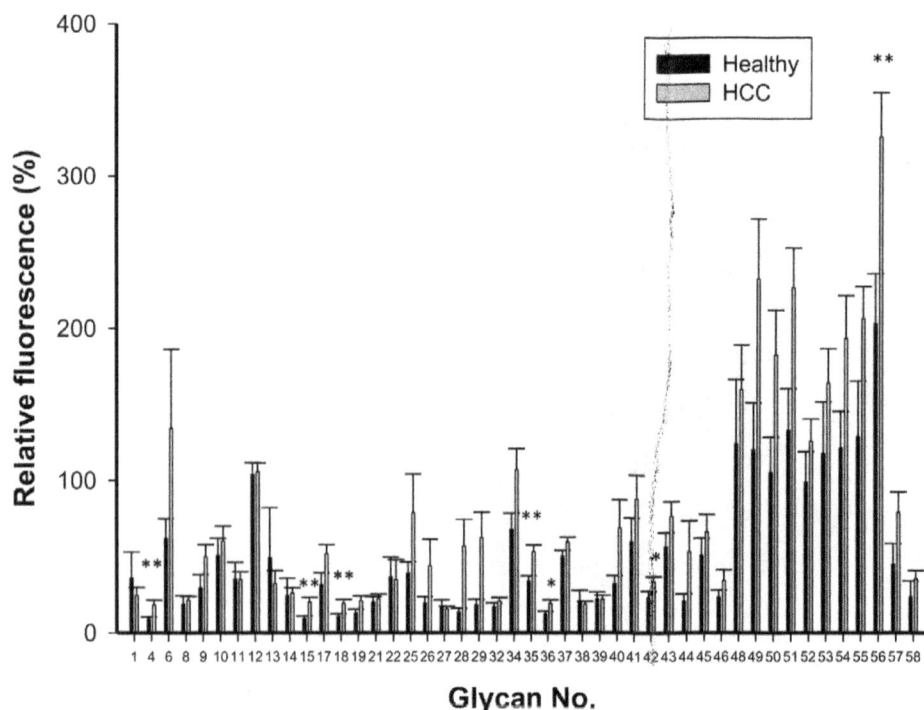

Figure 2. Ratio of anti-glycan IgG levels to anti-Gb5 levels in serum from healthy individuals and patients with HCC. Relative fluorescence ratios were calculated as the relative fluorescence intensity of each glycan analog divided by the relative fluorescence intensity of Gb5, and they are expressed as percentages in the figure. The figure shows the mean ratio ± standard deviation for each glycan. Asterisks indicate glycans in which the mean glycan:Gb5 IgG ratio was significantly higher in serum from patients with HCC (n = 155) than in serum from healthy individuals (n = 33). The p values were calculated with a Student's t-test (*$p<0.05$; **$p<0.01$).

of 0.6843 (95% CI: 0.5882–0.7805) (**Figure 6A**). At the cut-off value of 0.4974, the sensitivity and specificity for this marker was 46.21% and 84.85%. The AUC of serum 3 anti-glycan markers plus AFP levels for discriminating HBV-positive HCC from chronic HBV was 0.6923 (95% CI: 0.6215–0.7631) (**Figure 6B**). At the cut-off value of 0.5268, the sensitivity and specificity for this marker was 57.58% and 82.43%. This result suggests that these 3 anti-glycan markers plus AFP may be applicable to the diagnosis of HBV-related HCC.

Discussion

Tumor markers in the serum of patients with HCC can be used as diagnostic tools, prognostic factors, and treatment parameters [24]. Using our glycan microarray, we examined serum to search for antibodies that could distinguish between patients with HCC and healthy individuals. This study has demonstrated the potential of a glycan microarray for identifying CACAs biomarker candidates in serum from patients with HCC. In our current study, the differences in serum antibody levels between patients with HCC and healthy individuals were substantial, with antibody levels for 7 of 58 glycans differentially abundant (p<0.01). These glycans were SLacNAc 6SO$_3$, DSGG, fucosyl GM1, Gb3, Gb2, B19, and Man7. Alterations in glycosylation in cancer, as well as other diseases, have attracted much interest and have shown potential both as a source of disease markers and as targets for immunotherapy of tumors [15]. Changes in glycosyltransferase expression levels commonly lead to an increase in the size and branching of N-linked glycans, which creates additional sites for terminal sialic acid residues [25]. A corresponding increase in sialyltransferase expression ultimately leads to an overall increase in sialylation [26]. Overexpression of

the glycosyltransferases that are involved in linking terminal residues to glycans leads to overexpression of certain terminal glycan epitopes such as SLacNAc 6SO$_3$, DSGG, and fucosyl GM1 on tumors [27–29].

We found that anti-DSGG levels distinguished between patients with HCC and CLD. DSGG is a disialyl glycosphingolipid with a globo-series core structure [27]. In a previous study, DSGG was identified as an adhesion molecule expressed on renal cell carcinoma, and its relationship to metastatic cancer was demonstrated [27]. Our data are the first to suggest that DSGG is highly expressed in HCC.

Interestingly, a gender difference has been described for HCC in almost all study populations, with a male:female ratio for the incidence of HCC averaging between 2:1 and 4:1 [30]. One mechanism that may explain the gender disparity observed in the incidence of HCC is the increased activity of estrogens in female patients, which may offer protection from hepatocarcinogenesis [22]. In addition, there are probably other cellular regulatory molecules involved in the gender disparity in the incidence of HCC. In our current study, we observed a gender disparity in levels of slightly different anti-carbohydrate antibodies. Levels of anti-fucosyl GM1 differed in patients with HCC and chronic HBV or healthy individuals. Fucosyl GM1 belongs to one kind of gangliosides [28]. In a previous study, fucosyl GM1 was strongly associated with small-cell cancer of the lung, and this tumor-associated antigen was detected with high sensitivity and specificity using an immunofluorescence method [28]. The role of this glycan in cancer is unclear. The glycosylation of hormone receptors has been suggested as an explanation for gender disparities in coronary heart disease and prostate cancer [31,32]. Although how general these observations are to populations with a more

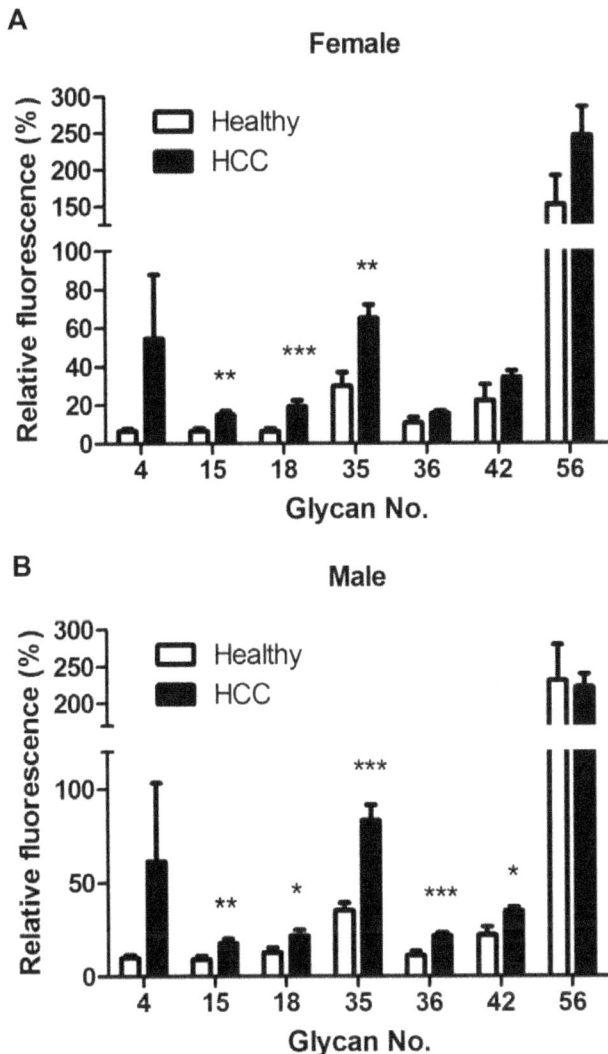

Figure 3. Comparison of the level of seven anti-glycan antibodies in serum from healthy individuals and patients with HCC for females and males. Relative fluorescence ratios were calculated as the fluorescence intensity for each glycan analog divided by the fluorescence intensity for Gb5, and they are expressed as percentages in the figures. The figure shows the mean ratio ± standard deviation for each glycan. (A) The glycan:Gb5 IgG ratios for glycan numbers 15, 18, and 35 were significantly higher in serum from female patients with HCC (n = 70) than in serum from healthy females (n = 11). (B) The glycan:Gb5 IgG ratios for glycan numbers 15, 18, 35, 36 and 42 were significantly higher in serum from male patients with HCC (n = 223) than in serum from healthy males (n = 22). Asterisks indicate glycans in which the mean glycan:Gb5 IgG ratio was significantly higher in serum from patients with HCC than in serum from healthy individuals. The p values were calculated with a Student's t-test (*P<0.01).

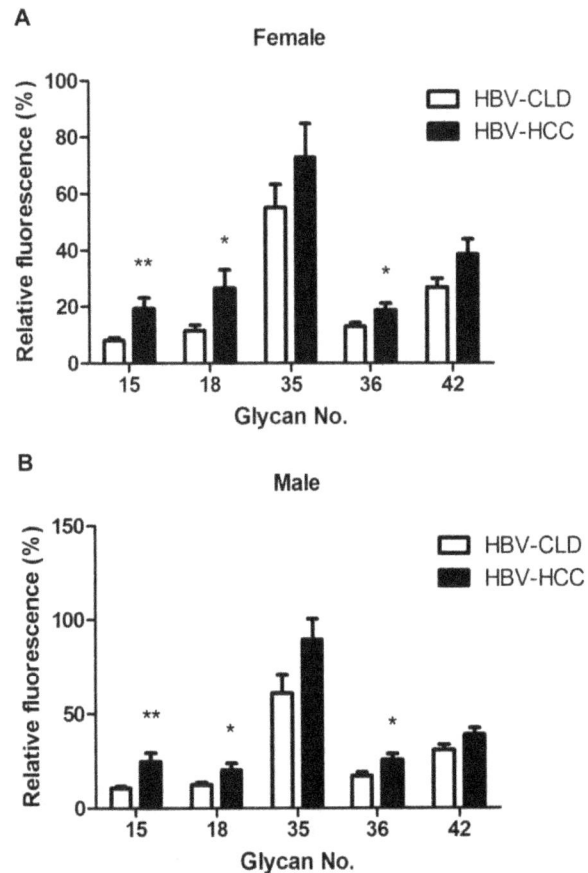

Figure 4. Comparison of the level of select anti-glycan antibodies from HBV-related HCC and CLD by gender. Relative fluorescence ratios were calculated as the fluorescence intensity for each glycan analog divided by the fluorescence intensity for Gb5, and they are expressed as percentages in the figures. The figure shows the mean ratio ± standard deviation for each glycan. The ratios for glycan numbers 15, 18, and 36 were significantly higher from HBV-related HCC than CLD (HBV) in females (n = 30 and 44, separately) (A) and males (n = 102 and 89, separately) (B). The p values were calculated with a Student's t-test (*P<0.05, **P<0.01, ***P<0.001).

heterogeneous disease etiology remains to be examined, the results presented here on potential glycan biomarkers seem quite encouraging. Recently, large-scale analytical methods have been developed for the human serum glycoproteome, which is also a powerful tool for the discovery of diagnostic and therapeutic targets. Using lectin-based glycoproteomic analysis, glycoprotein (GP) 73 was found to be a novel tumor marker for HCC [33]. Serum GP73 levels were significantly increased in patients with HCC, even in HCC patients with serum AFP levels less than 20 ng/ml [24]. Fucosylation of GP73 is reported to be increased in patients with HCC [33]. A previous study suggested that fucosylation plays an important role in the interaction between interleukin-8 and its receptor, thereby inducing the migration of cancer cells in HCC [34]. Our current results suggest that fucosyl GM1 is a candidate hepatic CACAs biomarkers.

HCC is associated with HBV infection in approximately 50% of cases [35]. In this study, we observed that five types of anti-glycan antibodies were increased in patients with HCC and HBV infection. Therefore, we extrapolate that the increase in antibodies and HBV infection are related. Woodchucks are used as a preferred animal model of chronic HBV infection [36]. This model recapitulates the disease progression of HBV infection to HCC and has documented similarities in protein glycosylation with human HCC [36]. As HCC usually takes years to develop as a result of chronic HBV infection, investigation of early events in the woodchuck model of HBV infection may provide helpful information about potential biomarkers for the prognosis of HCC. The biological influences driving these changes require further examination.

A

Female

B

Male

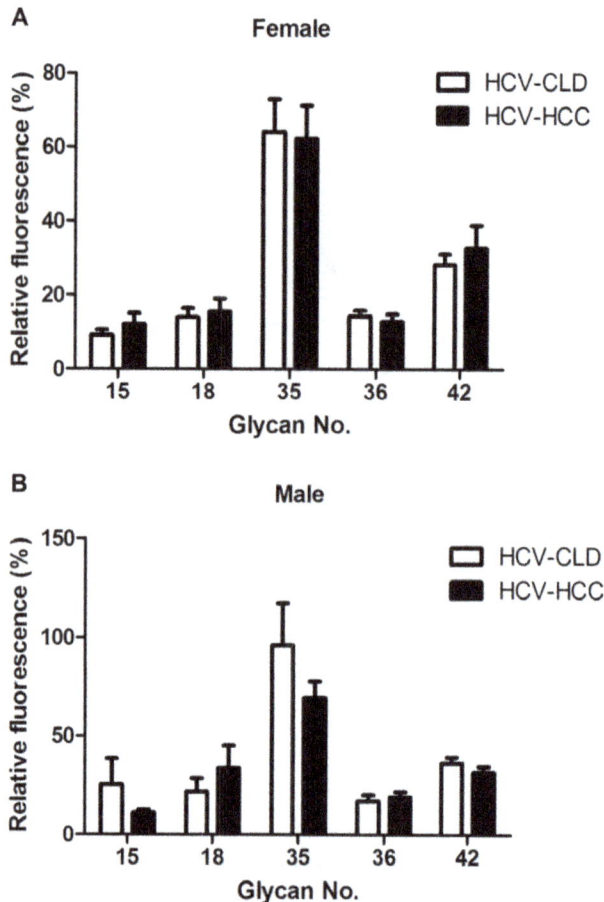

Figure 5. Comparison of the level of select anti-glycan antibodies from HCV-related HCC and CLD by gender. Relative fluorescence ratios were calculated as the fluorescence intensity for each glycan analog divided by the fluorescence intensity for Gb5, and they are expressed as percentages in the figures. The figure shows the mean ratio ± standard deviation for each glycan. The ratios for glycan numbers 15, 18, 35, 36 and 42 were no significant difference between HCV-related HCC and CLD (HCV) in females (n = 18 and 61, separately) (A) and males (n = 47 and 73, separately) (B). ($P > 0.05$).

Table 2. Comparison of the sensitivity of select anti-glycan antibodies and AFP for the diagnosis of HBV-positive HCC in females and males.

Glycan female	Sensitivity (%)	Glycan male	Sensitivity (%)
15(DSGG)	63.33%	15(DSGG)	42.16%
18(Fucosyl GM1)	56.67%	18(Fucosyl GM1)	35.29%
36(Gb2)	43.33%	36(Gb2)	45.10%
AFP_{200}	33.33%	AFP_{200}	24.51%
(15)+(18)+(36)+AFP_{200}	80%	(15)+(18)+(36)+AFP_{200}	74.51%

NOTE: AFP_{200}, AFP at a cutoff value >200 ng/ml.

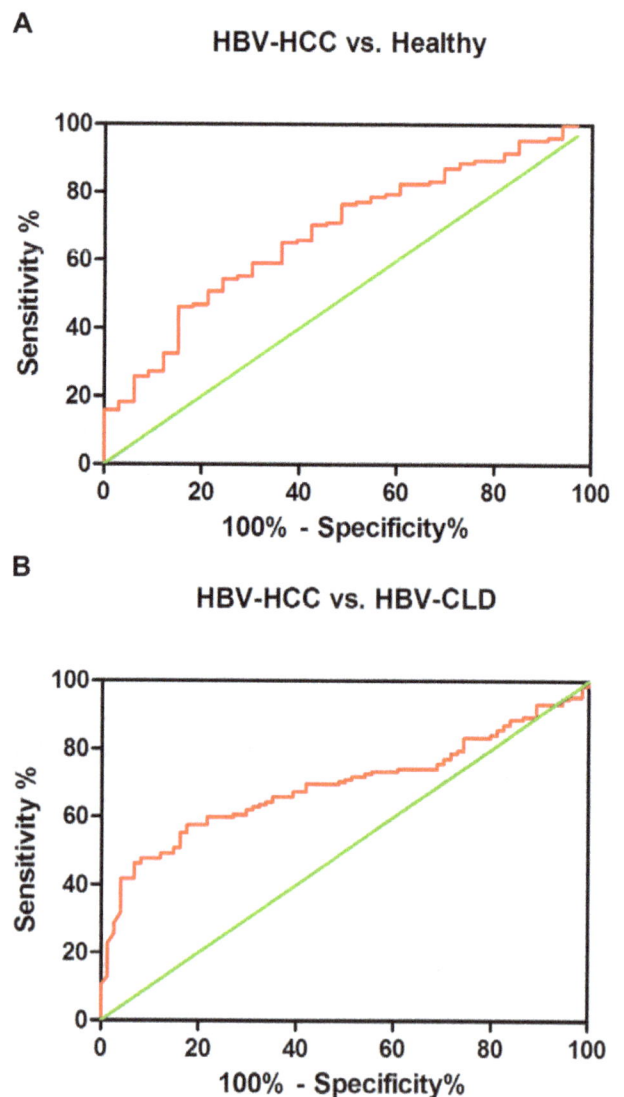

A

HBV-HCC vs. Healthy

B

HBV-HCC vs. HBV-CLD

Figure 6. ROC curve analysis using serum anti-glycan antibodies for discriminating HCC patients from HBV-CLD patients and healthy controls. These 3 anti-glycan antibodies yielded an AUC (the areas under the ROC curve) of 0.6843 (95% CI: 0.5882–0.7805) with 46.21% sensitivity and 84.85% specificity for discriminating HCC patients from healthy controls (A), and an AUC of 0.6923 (95% CI: 0.6215–0.7631) with 57.58% sensitivity and 82.43% specificity for discriminating HCC from HBV-CLD patients (B).

AFP is the only serological marker currently used for clinical detection of HCC. Although AFP improves the detection of HCC, a significant number of patients with HCC do not have elevated AFP levels, and thus, additional biomarkers are needed to increase the sensitivity of HCC detection [37,38]. In past research, AFP has shown limited sensitivity (41–65%) in the diagnosis of HCC [39]. Therefore, there is an urgent need to discover additional biomarkers for the screening and diagnosis of HCC. Our study compared patients with HCC and CLD plus healthy, and these 3 glycan provided better sensitivity than AFP. Moreover, the sensitivity of 3 anti-carbohydrate antibodies plus AFP provided better diagnosis sensitivity.

In addition, there was no correlation between levels of these 3 anti-glycan antibodies and the tumor stage (data not shown). Therefore, we suggest that the 3 anti-carbohydrate antibodies may be as biomarkers for the initiation of tumor formation, but not tumor progression. Further examination using a larger patient group and a validation process that includes prospectively collected patient samples are needed to verify our observations. These new CACAs biomarkers, in combination with other existing serologic biomarkers, can be valuable in the diagnosis of HCC.

Based on our results, we suggest that combining glycan microarray analysis with AFP measurements will provide a much better tool for HCC diagnosis than the use of AFP alone.

Biomarkers have long been sought for their diagnostic, prognostic, and therapeutic uses. However, there are no reliable biomarkers for most solid tumors, including HCC. The methods described in our current study are useful for identifying possible biomarkers of disease. The development of a glycan microarray has enabled high-sensitivity and high-throughput analysis of carbohydrate-protein interactions and has contributed to significant advances in glycomics. This approach provides both a powerful tool for basic research and a promising technique for medical diagnosis and the detection of pathogens and cancers [20]. This method requires very small amounts of material and is more effective and sensitive than the traditional ELISA method; thus, it provides another platform to monitor the immune response to carbohydrate epitopes at different stages during differentiation, metastasis, and treatment [21]. Our current research identified five CACAs biomarkers for HCC diagnosis that need to be evaluated further in future work. Identification of CACAs will be useful in the development of new cancer therapies such as generation of vaccines or antibodies targeting CACAs [14,19,40–42]. We believe that the glycan microarray is a viable method for clinical diagnosis of HCC. This method should improve prognosis and may offer insights into the development of novel therapeutic approaches for other cancers. New glycan antigens may prove to be useful targets of existing carbohydrate vaccines and those in development.

In conclusion, we have shown that glycan microarray analysis used to identify new candidate glycan biomarkers for HCC may be useful in the screening of serum biomarkers for HCC. The biomarker candidates we identified using glycan microarray analysis showed good predictive sensitivity in the study population, and in general, they were superior to AFP. Addition of the above results to the conventional liver function tests may indeed enhance the diagnostic accuracy of liver diseases. Glycan microarray analysis provides a powerful tool for high-sensitivity and high-throughput detection of serum antibodies against CACAs, and the identified serum biomarkers may be useful for early detection of HCC in high-risk populations.

Materials and Methods

Ethics Statement

The study protocol was approved by the Institutional Review Board of Human Subjects Research Ethics Committee of Cheng Kung University Hospital in Taiwan (No. ER-99-176). Additionally, written informed consent was obtained from participants for the use of their blood in this study.

Serum Samples

Serum samples from healthy individuals (n = 33), chronic HBV (n = 133), chronic HCV (n = 134) and patients with HCC (n = 293) were collected at the National Cheng Kung University Hospital in Tainan, Taiwan. Samples were encrypted to protect patient confidentiality and were used under a protocol approved by the Institutional Review Board of Human Subjects Research Ethics Committee of Cheng Kung University Hospital in Tainan, Taiwan. The patients were diagnosed using a combination of data (clinical, laboratory, and imaging findings and/or biopsy). All samples were stored at −20°C until use.

General Methods

NEXTERION slide H were purchased from SCHOTT North America. The coating on the SCHOTT NEXTERION Slide H consists of a cross-linked, multi-component polymer layer activated with N-hydroxysuccinimide (NHS) esters to provide covalent immobilization of amine groups. The general procedure for the synthesis of glycans was conducted as reported [20,21,43].

Glycan Microarray Fabrication

Microarrays were printed (BioDot; Cartesian Technologies) with a robotic pin (SMP3; TeleChem International) with a deposition of ≈ 0.7 nL of various concentrations of amine-containing glycans in printing buffer (300 mM phosphate buffer [pH 8.5] containing 0.005% Tween-20) from a 96-well microtiter plate onto NHS-coated glass slides. The slides were spotted with 50 uM solutions of each glycan, with two rows from bottom to top and five vertical replicates in each subarray. Each slide was designed for 14 grids. Printed slides were allowed to react in an atmosphere of 80% humidity for 1 h followed by desiccation overnight. The slides were stored at room temperature in a desiccator until use. Before the binding assay, the slides were blocked with ethanolamine (50 mM ethanolamine in 50 mM borate buffer [pH 9.2]) and then washed twice with water and phosphate buffer saline (PBS) (pH 7.4).

Microarray Analysis of Serum Samples

Serum samples from patients with HCC and healthy individuals were diluted 1:20 with a buffer consisting of 0.05% Tween 20 and 3% BSA in PBS (pH 7.4), applied to the grids of the glycan microarrays, and then incubated in a humidified chamber with shaking for 1 h. The slides then were washed three times each with 0.05% Tween 20 in PBS (pH 7.4), PBS (pH 7.4), and H_2O. Next, Cy3-conjugated goat anti–human IgG antibody (Jackson ImmunoResearch) was added to the slides, as described above, and the slides were incubated under a coverlid in a humidified chamber with shaking for 1 h. The slides were washed three times each with 0.05% Tween 20 in PBS (pH 7.4), PBS (pH 7.4), and H_2O, and then dried. The slides were scanned at 532 nm (for Cy3-conjugated secondary antibody) with a microarray fluorescence chip reader (arrayWoRx microarray reader).

Data Analysis

The software GenePix Pro (Axon Instruments) was used for the fluorescence analysis of the extracted data. The local background was subtracted from the signal at each antibody spot. The "medians of ratios" from replicate spots were averaged within the same array. To obtain the relative binding intensities of glycans in human sera, we set the binding intensity for Gb5 to 100% and normalized the relative binding intensities of each glycan analog for each serum sample. The ratio of anti-glycan: anti-Gb5 in sera was calculated by dividing the mean relative binding intensity for glycan replicates by the mean relative binding intensity for Gb5 replicates, and the results were expressed as percentages. Sensitivity was calculated as the ratio of the number of HCC samples that were classified correctly as HCC (true positives) to the total number of HCC samples. Finally, statistical analysis of IgG levels in patients with HCC and healthy individuals was performed using an unpaired Student's t-test. Receiver operating characteristic (ROC) curves were constructed and the area under the curve (AUC) was calculated to evaluate the specificity and sensitivity of predicting cases and controls. Data analysis was done using Prism 5 (GraphPad Software, Inc.) and SigmaPlot 9.0 software (SigmaPlot).

Author Contributions

Conceived and designed the experiments: YLY CYW. Performed the experiments: CSW CJY. Analyzed the data: YLY CYW CSW. Contributed reagents/materials/analysis tools: RHC STL WCH CTR. Wrote the manuscript: YLY.

References

1. Parkin DM, Bray F, Ferlay J, Pisani P (2005) Global cancer statistics, 2002. CA Cancer J Clin 55: 74–108.
2. Beasley RP (1988) Hepatitis B virus. The major etiology of hepatocellular carcinoma. Cancer 61: 1942–1956.
3. Caporaso N, Romano M, Marmo R, de Sio I, Morisco F, et al. (1991) Hepatitis C virus infection is an additive risk factor for development of hepatocellular carcinoma in patients with cirrhosis. J Hepatol 12: 367–371.
4. el-Refaie A, Savage K, Bhattacharya S, Khakoo S, Harrison TJ, et al. (1996) HCV-associated hepatocellular carcinoma without cirrhosis. J Hepatol 24: 277–285.
5. Hao K, Luk JM, Lee NP, Mao M, Zhang C, et al. (2009) Predicting prognosis in hepatocellular carcinoma after curative surgery with common clinicopathologic parameters. BMC Cancer 9; 389.
6. El-Serag HB, Marrero JA, Rudolph L, Reddy KR (2008) Diagnosis and treatment of hepatocellular carcinoma. Gastroenterology 134: 1752–1763.
7. Pang RW, Joh JW, Johnson PJ, Monden M, Pawlik TM, et al. (2008) Biology of hepatocellular carcinoma. Ann Surg Oncol 15: 962–971.
8. Bruix J, Sherman M, Llovet JM, Beaugrand M, Lencioni R, et al. (2001) Clinical management of hepatocellular carcinoma. Conclusions of the Barcelona-2000 EASL conference. European Association for the Study of the Liver. J Hepatol 35: 421–430.
9. Chen DS, Sung JL, Sheu JC, Lai MY, How SW, et al. (1984) Serum alpha-fetoprotein in the early stage of human hepatocellular carcinoma. Gastroenterology 86: 1404–1409.
10. Chen L, Ho DW, Lee NP, Sun S, Lam B, et al. (2010) Enhanced detection of early hepatocellular carcinoma by serum SELDI-TOF proteomic signature combined with alpha-fetoprotein marker. Ann Surg Oncol 17: 2518–2525.
11. Bruix J, Sherman M (2005) Management of hepatocellular carcinoma. Hepatology 42: 1208–1236.
12. Luk JM, Lam CT, Siu AF, Lam BY, Ng IO, et al. (2006) Proteomic profiling of hepatocellular carcinoma in Chinese cohort reveals heat-shock proteins (Hsp27, Hsp70, GRP78) up-regulation and their associated prognostic values. Proteomics 6: 1049–1057.
13. Yi X, Luk JM, Lee NP, Peng J, Leng X, et al. (2008) Association of mortalin (HSPA9) with liver cancer metastasis and prediction for early tumor recurrence. Mol Cell Proteomics 7: 315–325.
14. Shriver Z, Raguram S, Sasisekharan R (2004) Glycomics: a pathway to a class of new and improved therapeutics. Nat Rev Drug Discov 3: 863–873.
15. Kobata A, Amano J (2005) Altered glycosylation of proteins produced by malignant cells, and application for the diagnosis and immunotherapy of tumours. Immunol Cell Biol 83: 429–439.
16. Varki A (1993) Biological roles of oligosaccharides: all of the theories are correct. Glycobiology 3: 97–130.
17. Isaji T, Gu J, Nishiuchi R, Zhao Y, Takahashi M, et al. (2004) Introduction of bisecting GlcNAc into integrin alpha5beta1 reduces ligand binding and down-regulates cell adhesion and cell migration. J Biol Chem 279: 19747–19754.
18. Stanley P (2002) Biological consequences of overexpressing or eliminating N-acetylglucosaminyltransferase-TIII in the mouse. Biochim Biophys Acta 1573: 363–368.
19. Wang CC, Huang YL, Ren CT, Lin CW, Hung JT, et al. (2008) Glycan microarray of Globo H and related structures for quantitative analysis of breast cancer. Proc Natl Acad Sci U S A 105: 11661–11666.
20. Wu CY, Liang PH, Wong CH (2009) New development of glycan arrays. Org Biomol Chem 7: 2247–2254.
21. Huang CY, Thayer DA, Chang AY, Best MD, Hoffmann J, et al. (2006) Carbohydrate microarray for profiling the antibodies interacting with Globo H tumor antigen. Proc Natl Acad Sci U S A 103: 15–20.
22. Wands J (2007) Hepatocellular carcinoma and sex. N Engl J Med 357: 1974–1976.
23. Liaw YF (2005) Prevention and surveillance of hepatitis B virus-related hepatocellular carcinoma. Semin Liver Dis 25 Suppl 1: 40–47.
24. Marrero JA, Romano PR, Nikolaeva O, Steel L, Mehta A, et al. (2005) GP73, a resident Golgi glycoprotein, is a novel serum marker for hepatocellular carcinoma. J Hepatol 43: 1007–1012.
25. Dennis JW, Laferte S, Waghorne C, Breitman ML, Kerbel RS (1987) Beta 1–6 branching of Asn-linked oligosaccharides is directly associated with metastasis. Science 236: 582–585.
26. Kim YJ, Varki A (1997) Perspectives on the significance of altered glycosylation of glycoproteins in cancer. Glycoconj J 14: 569–576.
27. Satoh M, Handa K, Saito S, Tokuyama S, Ito A, et al. (1996) Disialosyl galactosylgloboside as an adhesion molecule expressed on renal cell carcinoma and its relationship to metastatic potential. Cancer Res 56: 1932–1938.
28. Brezicka FT, Olling S, Nilsson O, Bergh J, Holmgren J, et al. (1989) Immunohistological detection of fucosyl-GM1 ganglioside in human lung cancer and normal tissues with monoclonal antibodies. Cancer Res 49: 1300–1305.
29. Chandrasekaran EV, Chawda R, Rhodes JM, Xia J, Piskorz C, et al. (2001) Human lung adenocarcinoma alpha1,3/4-L-fucosyltransferase displays two molecular forms, high substrate affinity for clustered sialyl LacNAc type 1 units as well as mucin core 2 sialyl LacNAc type 2 unit and novel alpha1,2-L-fucosylating activity. Glycobiology 11: 353–363.
30. Montalto G, Cervello M, Giannitrapani L, Dantona F, Terranova A, et al. (2002) Epidemiology, risk factors, and natural history of hepatocellular carcinoma. Ann N Y Acad Sci 963: 13–20.
31. Nealen ML, Vijayan KV, Bolton E, Bray PF (2001) Human platelets contain a glycosylated estrogen receptor beta. Circ Res 88: 438–442.
32. de Leoz ML, An HJ, Kronewitter S, Kim J, Beecroft S, et al. (2008) Glycomic approach for potential biomarkers on prostate cancer: profiling of N-linked glycans in human sera and pRNS cell lines. Dis Markers 25: 243–258.
33. Block TM, Comunale MA, Lowman M, Steel LF, Romano PR, et al. (2005) Use of targeted glycoproteomics to identify serum glycoproteins that correlate with liver cancer in woodchucks and humans. Proc Natl Acad Sci U S A 102: 779–784.
34. Wu LH, Shi BZ, Zhao QL, Wu XZ (2010) Fucosylated glycan inhibition of human hepatocellular carcinoma cell migration through binding to chemokine receptors. Glycobiology 20: 215–223.
35. Liaw YF (2005) The current management of HBV drug resistance. J Clin Virol 34 Suppl 1: S143–146.
36. Lattova E, McKenzie EJ, Gruwel ML, Spicer V, Goldman R, et al. (2009) Mass spectrometric study of N-glycans from serum of woodchucks with liver cancer. Rapid Commun Mass Spectrom 23: 2983–2995.
37. Marrero JA (2005) Screening tests for hepatocellular carcinoma. Clin Liver Dis 9: 235–251, vi.
38. Zhang BH, Yang BH, Tang ZY (2004) Randomized controlled trial of screening for hepatocellular carcinoma. J Cancer Res Clin Oncol 130: 417–422.
39. Filmus J, Capurro M (2004) Glypican-3 and alphafetoprotein as diagnostic tests for hepatocellular carcinoma. Mol Diagn 8: 207–212.
40. Henry CJ, Buss MS, Hellstrom I, Hellstrom KE, Brewer WG, et al. (2005) Clinical evaluation of BR96 sFv-PE40 immunotoxin therapy in canine models of spontaneously occurring invasive carcinoma. Clin Cancer Res 11: 751–755.
41. Brandlein S, Pohle T, Ruoff N, Wozniak E, Muller-Hermelink HK, et al. (2003) Natural IgM antibodies and immunosurveillance mechanisms against epithelial cancer cells in humans. Cancer Res 63: 7995–8005.
42. Ouerfelli O, Warren JD, Wilson RM, Danishefsky SJ (2005) Synthetic carbohydrate-based antitumor vaccines: challenges and opportunities. Expert Rev Vaccines 4: 677–685.
43. Tseng SY, Wang CC, Lin CW, Chen CL, Yu WY, et al. (2008) Glycan arrays on aluminum-coated glass slides. Chem Asian J 3: 1395–1405.

9

Natural Killer Cells Are Characterized by the Concomitantly Increased Interferon-γ and Cytotoxicity in Acute Resolved Hepatitis B Patients

Juanjuan Zhao[1]9, Yonggang Li[2]9, Lei Jin[3], Shuye Zhang[3], Rong Fan[3], Yanling Sun[3], Chunbao Zhou[3], Qinghua Shang[4], Wengang Li[3], Zheng Zhang[3]*, Fu-Sheng Wang[1,3]*

1 Center for Infection and Immunity, Institute of Biophysics, Chinese Academy of Science, Beijing, China, 2 Integrative Medicine Center, Beijing 302 Hospital, Beijing, China, 3 Research Center for Biological Therapy, Institute of Translational Hepatology, Beijing 302 Hospital, Beijing, China, 4 Department of Liver Disease, Tai-An 88 Hospital, Tai-An, Shan Dong Province, China

Abstract

Natural killer (NK) cells are abundant in the liver and have been implicated in inducing hepatocellular damage in patients with chronic hepatitis B virus (HBV) infection. However, the role of NK cells in acute HBV infection remains to be elucidated. We comprehensively characterized NK cells and investigated their roles in HBV clearance and liver pathology in 19 chronic hepatitis B (CHB) patients and 21 acute hepatitis B (AHB) patients as well as 16 healthy subjects. It was found that NKp46$^+$ NK cells were enriched in the livers of AHB and CHB patients. We further found that peripheral NK cells from AHB patients expressed higher levels of activation receptors and lower levels of inhibitory receptors than those from CHB patients and HC subjects, thus displaying the increased cytolytic activity and interferon-γ production. NK cell activation levels were also correlated positively with serum alanine aminotransferase levels and negatively with plasma HBV DNA levels in AHB patients, which is further confirmed by the longitudinal follow-up of AHB patients. Serum pro-inflammatory cytokine and chemokine levels were also increased in AHB patients as compared with CHB and HC subjects. Thus, the concomitantly increased interferon-γ and cytotoxicity of NK cells were associated with liver injury and viral clearance in AHB patients.

Editor: Johan K. Sandberg, Karolinska Institutet, Sweden

Funding: This study was funded in full by the National Natural Science Foundation of China (30972752, 81172779), in part by the National Key Basic Research Program of China (No. 2012CB519005) and the National Grand Program on Key Infectious Disease (No. 2012ZX10002007-002). The funders had no role in study design, data collection and analysis, decision to publish, or preparation of the manuscript.

Competing Interests: The authors have declared that no competing interests exist.

* E-mail: fswang302@163.com (F-SW); zhangzheng1975@yahoo.com.cn (ZZ)

9 These authors contributed equally to this work.

Introduction

Hepatitis B virus (HBV) infection is a major human threat that affects approximately 400 million people worldwide. While HBV infection in utero or early in life results in chronic infection, adults infected with this virus usually develop an acute self-limited infection [1]. Particularly, acute hepatitis B (AHB) is difficult to diagnose in the clinic because 90% of adult patients enter the convalescence period without obvious clinical manifestations by the time the patient first presents to the physician. Therefore, little is known about the early events in acute HBV infection.

The host immune response is generally considered to drive disease progression of HBV infection [1]; however, the relevant immunological factors that determine different outcomes of HBV infection are unknown [2,3]. Generally, HBV-specific T cell responses are thought to be of considerable importance in viral control and immune-mediated liver damage [4]. During acute HBV infection, virus-specific T cell responses are often readily detectable and multi-specific [5–7]; while in chronic HBV infections, virus-specific T cell responses are generally weak and display functional exhaustion as a result of the upregulation of programmed death-1 [8,9], T cell attrition through Bcl2 signaling

[10] and impaired T cell receptor signaling through the ζ-chain [11]. Despite the associations between the adaptive T cell responses, viral clearance and liver damage during acute and chronic HBV infection, the innate immune effector mechanisms that are responsible for viral clearance and liver pathogenesis remained obscure [12].

Innate immune cells, for example natural killer (NK) cells, are predominantly enriched into the human liver [13,14]. NK cell activation is generally regulated by a set of activation and inhibitory receptors that are expressed on the cell surface [15]. The intensity and quality of NK cell responses also depend on the cytokine microenvironment. Type I interferon (IFN), interleukin (IL)-12, IL-15 and IL-18 are potent activators of NK cell function [16]. Several recent studies have reported the role of NK cells in liver injury in chronic Hepatitis C virus (HCV) [17,18] and HBV infections [18–21], in which NK cells are biased towards cytolytic activity but without a concomitant increase in IFN-γ production. In contrast, in acute HBV infection, early NK cell responses are likely to contribute to the initial control of infection and to allow timely development of an efficient adaptive immune response [7,22]. However, this early activation and IFN-γ production by NK cells can be transiently inhibited by a surge of IL-10 during peak viremia [23]. Although NK cells are known to be functionally involved in liver pathogenesis in chronic HBV-infected patients [18–21], limited data are available regarding the immune status and clinical significance of these cells in acute HBV infected patients with longitudinal follow-up.

This study comprehensively characterized NK cells in a cohort of acute HBV-infected patients with longitudinal follow-up, and found that increased IFN-γ production by NK cells may play a role in HBV control, and the increased cytolytic capacity of these cells may promote liver injury. Our findings may facilitate the rational development of immunotherapeutic strategies to enhance viral control while limiting or abolishing liver injury in HBV infection.

Results

Increased CD56^{bright} NK subsets, but reduced CD56^{dim} NK subsets in patients with acute and chronic HBV infection

Analysis of the frequencies of circulating total NK cells (CD3$^-$CD56$^+$) and NK subsets (CD3$^-$CD56^{bright} and CD3$^-$CD56^{dim}) in all enrolled subjects (Figure 1A) revealed that the total NK cell frequencies were significantly decreased in both CHB and AHB patients compared with those in HC subjects (both $P<0.05$; Figure 1B). The contribution of the two NK subsets to the total NK cell frequency was investigated in these individuals. It was observed that CD3$^-$CD56^{bright} NK cells were significantly expanded in both CHB and AHB patients compared to the HC group. In contrast, CD3$^-$CD56^{dim} NK cells were greatly reduced in CHB and AHB patients compared with the HC group (Figure 1B). We further analyzed the correlation between the frequencies of total NK cells and NK cell subsets and clinical parameters such as viral load and ALT levels in AHB patients. There were no significant associations between the frequencies of NK cell subsets with HBV load or serum ALT levels (data not shown). These data indicate a re-distribution in peripheral NK cell compartments in patients with acute and chronic HBV infections.

NK cells were enriched in patients with acute and chronic HBV infections

The distribution of hepatic CD3$^+$, CD56$^+$ and NKp46$^+$ (a unique NK marker) cells were investigated by immunohistochemical staining (Figure 1C). Few CD3$^+$, CD56$^+$ and NKp46$^+$ cells were present in the livers of healthy donors. In contrast, numerous CD3$^+$, CD56$^+$ and NKp46$^+$ cells were frequently seen in the livers of CHB and AHB patients. Quantitative analysis of hepatic CD3$^+$, CD56$^+$ and NKp46$^+$ cell counts in both portal and lobular areas further confirmed this observation (Figure 1D). Notably, more CD56$^+$ and NKp46$^+$ cells were found to be accumulated in the moderately and severely inflamed lobular areas of liver in AHB patients, where hepatocyte necrosis is usually observed. These data indicate that NK cells were also enriched in the livers of AHB and CHB patients.

AHB patients were characterized by the increased activation of both NK and T cells in peripheral blood

Expression of CD69, CD38 and HLA-DR was analyzed to assess the activation state of NK cells and conventional T cells in CHB and AHB patients (Figure 2A). It was observed that the frequencies of activation markers, CD38 and HLA-DR but not CD69 were significantly increased on NK cells in both AHB and CHB patients compared with HC subjects (Figure 2B). A similar pattern was observed for the MFI of CD38, CD69 and HLA-DR expression on total NK cells (Figure 2C). Interestingly, the expression levels of these activation markers on total T cells were also significantly increased in AHB patients but not in CHB patients as compared with that in HC subjects (data not shown). The further investigation demonstrate a clear discrimination between these three groups of subjects on the basis of HLA-DR MFI levels: HC, NK^{low} T^{low}; CHB: NK^{high} T^{low} and AHB: NK^{high} T^{high} (Figure 2D). Correlation analysis further confirmed that the percentage HLA-DR expression on total NK cells correlated positively with serum ALT levels and negatively with HBV DNA levels (both $P<0.05$; Figure 2E). These data suggest that the presence of activated NK cells is closely associated with liver necroinflammation and HBV clearance in AHB patients.

NK cells displayed abnormal NK receptor expression in AHB patients

We further analyzed NK cell receptor expression including activation receptors NKp30, NKp44 and NKp46, NKG2D and NKG2C and inhibitory receptors NKG2A, CD158a and CD158b, as well as TRAIL expression which has been demonstrated previously to be up-regulated on NK cells in CHB patients [20,21] in the three groups (Figure 3A). A significant upregulation of activation receptors NKp30, NKp44, NKp46, NKG2C but not NKG2D was observed on total NK cells (Figure 3B) as well as CD56^{bright} (Figure 3C) and CD56^{dim} (Figure 3D) subsets in AHB and CHB patients as compared with HC subjects. A similar increase of TRAIL on NK subsets was also observed in AHB and CHB patinets as compared with HC subjects (Figure 3B–3D). However, the inhibitory receptors CD158a and CD158b as well as NKG2A on total and NK subsets were significantly downregulated in HBV infected individuals compared with HC subjects. Interestingly, it was observed that NKp46 and NKG2C expression levels were further upregulated by peripheral NK subsets in AHB patients compared with CHB subjects, and inhibitory receptors CD158a, CD158b and NKG2A were further downregulated on NK subsets in AHB patients compared with CHB patients (Figure 3B–3D). Thus, activation receptor-expressing NK cells were preferentially enriched in AHB patients, while the inhibitory receptor-expressing NK cells were further reduced in AHB patients compared with CHB patients.

NK cells from AHB patients displayed the increased cytolytic activity and IFN-γ responses

The functional properties of NK cell subsets were investigated by monitoring intracellular IFN-γ production and CD107a expression in response to major histocompatibility complex (MHC)-devoid target cells (K562 cells), cytokine IL-12 and IL-18 and mitogenic PMA/ionomycin stimulation (Figure 4A). It was observed that both CD56^{bright} and CD56^{dim} NK cells responded to stimulation with PMA/ionomycin, IL-12/IL18 and MHC-devoid K562 cells. Differently, PMA/ionomycin induced high levels of IFN-γ and CD107a in both CD56^{bright} and CD56^{dim} NK cell subsets. IL-12/IL-18 induced high and median levels of IFN-γ production by CD56^{bright} and CD56^{dim} NK cell subsets respectively, but induced low levels of CD107a in both subsets. However, following stimulation by MHC-devoid K562 cells, CD107a expression was upregulated in the CD56^{dim} NK cell subset but not in the CD56^{bright} NK cell subset. IFN-γ was produced by both CD56^{bright} and CD56^{dim} NK cell subsets at low levels (Figure 4A).

IFN-γ and CD107a production was then compared in total NK cells, CD56^{bright} and CD56^{dim} NK cell subsets among the three groups. The ability of total NK cells and CD56^{dim} NK cells to produce both IFN-γ and CD107a expression in response to PMA/

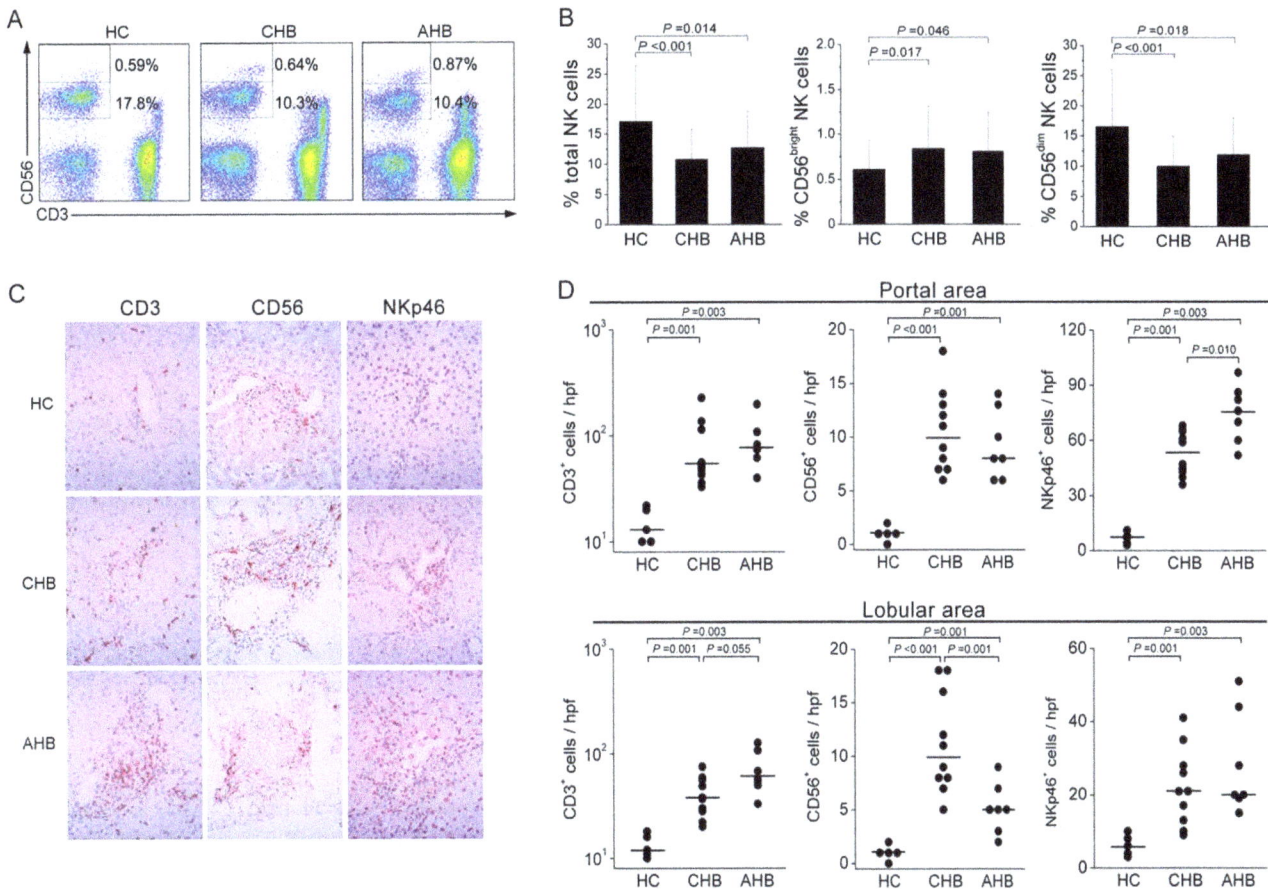

Figure 1. Increased CD56^bright NK subsets in patients with acute and chronic HBV infection. (A) Flow cytometric analysis of CD3 and CD56 expression by peripheral blood mononuclear cells (PBMCs) after application of a lymphocyte gate. Values indicate the percentages of CD3⁻CD56^bright and CD3⁻CD56^dim NK cell subset among lymphocytes. (B) Pooled data showing the frequencies of total NK, CD56^bright and CD56^dim NK cells in HC subjects (n = 16) and CHB (n = 19) and AHB patients (n = 21). The data represent the mean ± SD. P-values are shown. (C) Immunohistochemical detection of CD3⁺, CD56⁺ and NKp46⁺ cells in the liver tissues of CHB (n = 10) and AHB patients (n = 7) and HC donors (n = 5) (magnification, ×400). Positively stained cells appear red and were present in both portal and lobular areas in the livers. (D) Pooled data showing CD3⁺, CD56⁺ and NKp46⁺ cell counts in both portal and lobular areas in CHB (n = 10) and AHB patients (n = 7) and HC donors (n = 5). Each dot represents one subject. Horizontal lines illustrate the median percentiles. P-values are shown. HC, healthy controls; CHB, chronic hepatitis B; AHB, acute hepatitis B. (B and D), Multiple comparisons were first made among the three groups using the Kruskal-Wallis *H* non-parametric test. Then the comparisons between two groups were performed using the Mann-Whitney *U* test.

ionomycin was similar in the three groups of subjects. In contrast, CD56^bright NK cells have more potential to produce IFN-γ and CD107a in AHB and CHB patients in response to PMA/ionomycin stimulation, as compared with those from HC subjects (Figure 4B).

Notably, the expression of IFN-γ and CD107a by total NK was significantly elevated in AHB patients as compared with CHB patients and HC subjects following the stimulation with IL-12/IL-18 and K562 cells respectively (Figure 4B). Furthermore, CD107a expression by the CD56^bright subset and both IFN-γ and CD107a expression by the CD56^dim NK cell subset were also significantly increased in response to IL-12/IL-18 in AHB patients. IFN-γ production by the CD56^dim NK cell subset was also significantly increased in response to K562 cells in AHB patients. No significant differences in IFN-γ and CD107a expression by NK subsets were detected between CHB patients and HC subjects with the exception of CD107a expression by total NK cells and the CD56^bright subset, which was higher in CHB patients compared with HC subjects. These data suggest that the increased NK cell

activity indicated by IFN-γ and CD107a upregulation in AHB patients compared with CHB patients and HC subjects.

Increased levels of plasma pro-inflammatory cytokines and chemokines in AHB patients

Plasma levels of the pro-inflammatory cytokines (IL-1Ra, IL-12p70 and IFN-γ), chemokines (IL-8, RANTES, IP-10, MIP-1β and eotaxin) and growth factors (VEGF, GM-CSF and PDGF-BB) were significantly increased in AHB patients compared with those of CHB patients and HC subjects (Figure 5). No significant changes of these markers were observed between CHB patients and HC subjects, with the exception of IFN-γ, IL-1ra, IP-10 and PDGF-bb, which were also increased in CHB patients compared with HC subjects (Figure 5). Other cytokine levels in plasma including IL-1β, IL-2, IL-4, IL-5, IL-6, IL-7, IL-8, IL-9, IL-10, IL-13, IL-15, IL-17, basic FGF, G-CSF, MIP-1α, and TNF-α were not compared among these three groups due to undetectable levels. These data indicate higher levels of systemic inflammation in AHB patients compared with CHB patients.

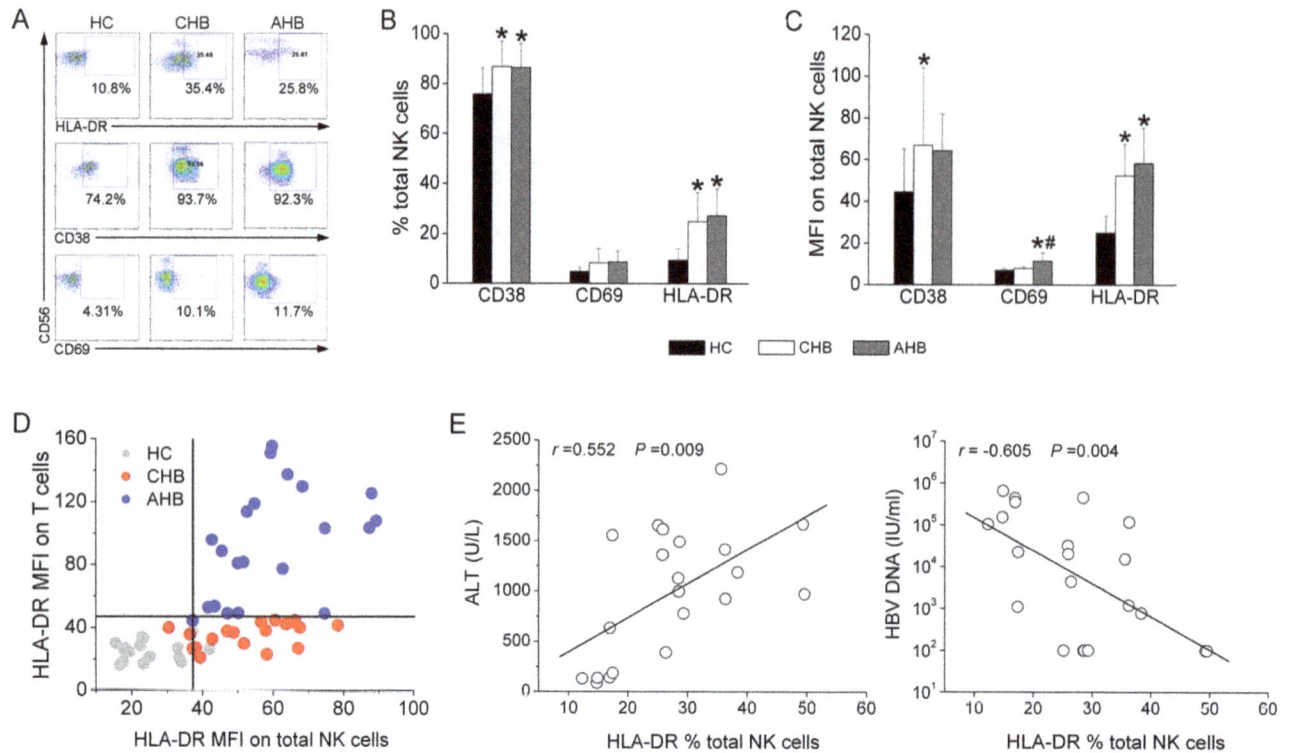

Figure 2. NK cells displayed an increased activation status in AHB patients in vivo. (A) Representative dot plots depict the expression of activation markers CD69, CD38 and HLA-DR on total NK cells among HC subjects and CHB and AHB patients. CD3⁻CD56⁺ NK cells were gated. Values in quadrants represent the percentages of CD3⁻CD56⁺ NK cells that express activation markers. (B and C) Pooled data showed the percentages and MFI of CD69, CD38 and HLA-DR expression by total NK cells from the HC (n = 16), CHB (n = 19) and AHB (n = 21) groups. Multiple comparisons were first made among the three groups using the Kruskal-Wallis H non-parametric test. Then the comparisons between two groups were performed using the Mann-Whitney U test. *$P<0.05$ compared with HC subjects; #$P<0.05$ compared with CHB patients. (D) Scatter plots show the HLA-DR MFI on NK cells and T cells simultaneously in HC (n = 16), CHB (n = 19) and AHB (n = 21) subject groups. (E) Correlation analysis between HLA-DR percentages on total NK cells and plasma ALT and HBV DNA levels in AHB patients (n = 21). Correlations between the two variables were evaluated using the Spearman rank correlation test. r, correlation coefficient; P-values are shown.

Longitudinal detection of NK cell activation in AHB patients

The plasma ALT and HBV load and NK cell frequency, activation markers HLA-DR and CD38 and TRAIL expression were longitudinally detected at acute (median 2 weeks since the clinical onset, range [1 week–3 weeks]) and convalescence phases (median 15 weeks since the clinical onset, range [5 weeks–27 weeks]) in 10 of AHB patients (Figure 6A). It was found that the serum HBV loads and ALT levels were both reduced to undetectable levels or normal levels (<40 U/L) from the acute phase to convalescence phase in these AHB patients (Figure 6B). Interestingly, the percentages of total NK cells and CD3⁻CD56^dim NK cells were slightly increased at convalescence phase as compared with acute phase in these AHB patients; in contrast, the CD3⁻CD56^bright frequency remained stable during the process (Figure 6C). More important, we observed that NK cell activation indicated by HLA-DR and CD38 expression as well as TRAIL expression were all significantly reduced at convalescence phase as compared with acute phase in these AHB patients (Figure 6D). These data indicated that NK cell activation was decreased with the disease recovery in AHB patients.

Discussion

The current study characterized NK cell subsets during the early and convalescence phase of in a cohort of AHB patients and demonstrated that NK cells are preferentially activated at the acute phase but decreased at the convalescence phase, thus associating with both liver injury and simultaneous viral clearance. These findings clearly demonstrated the immune status of NK cells in vivo and defined the double-edged roles of NK cells in viral clearance and liver injury in patients with acute HBV infection.

Similar to NK cells from immune activation (IA) patients with chronic HBV infection [20], AHB patients exhibited decreased total NK frequencies and increased NK activation status. Interestingly, NK cells from AHB patients displayed several unique properties that differed from those of CHB patients. NK cells in AHB patients displayed a greater potential to produce IFN-γ and CD107a compared with that in CHB patients. The increased IFN-γ may associate with HBV clearance via a non-cytolytic mechanism [24,25]; while the increased CD107a expression by NK cells may be associated with hepatocyte injury in AHB patients. In contrast, as described in our previous report [20], NK cells exhibited an enhanced cytolytic activity without concomitant IFN-γ production, which may result in liver damage but favor viral persistence in CHB patients. TRAIL up-regulation may further aggravate the liver injury as like in CHB patients [21]. The role of NK cells in viral clearance in acute HBV infection was also supported by several previous reports in which early large quantities of IFN-γ production by NK cells may contribute to the initial control of infection and allow timely development of an adaptive immune response [7,22]. These findings, in combination

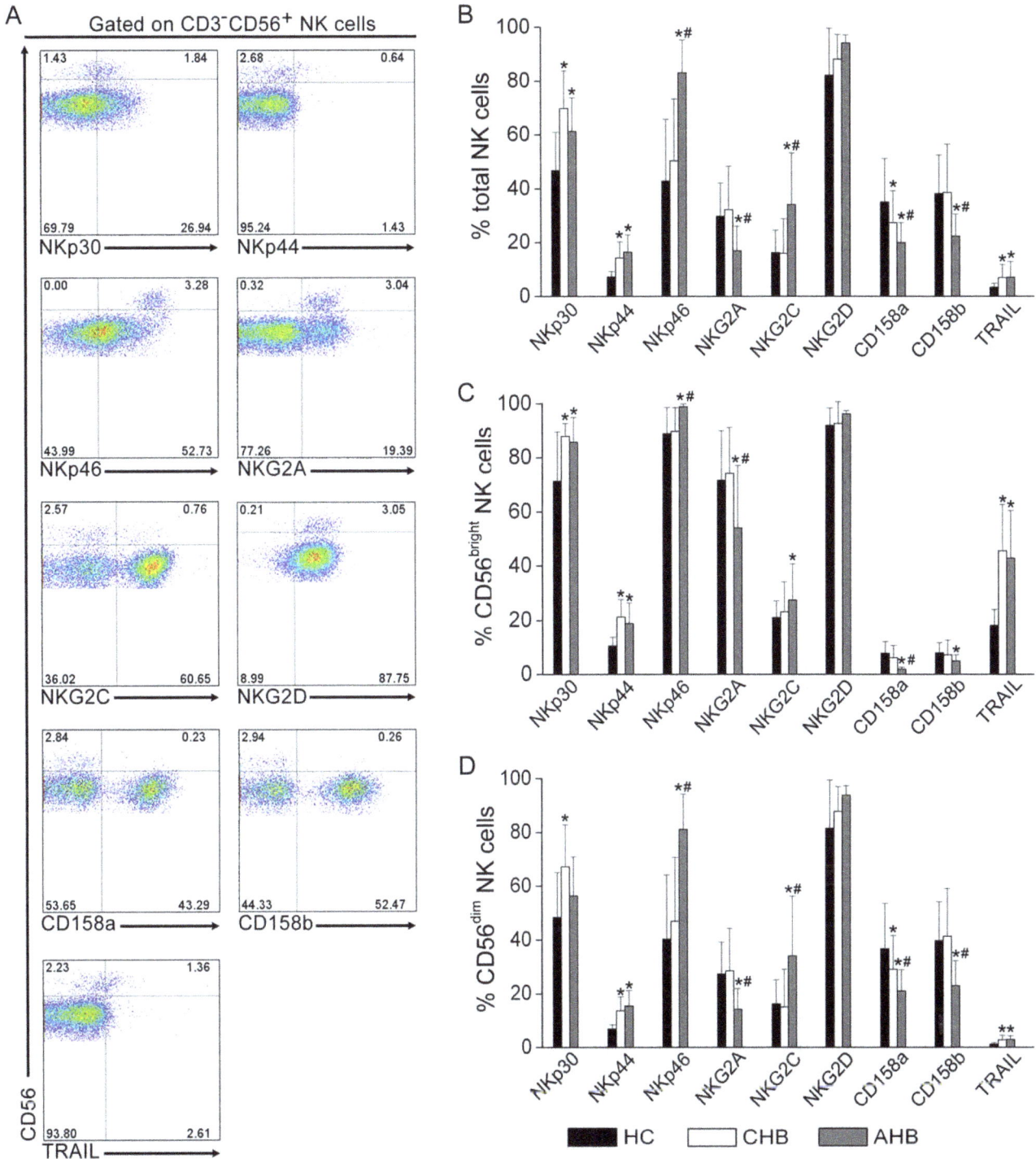

Figure 3. NK cells displayed abnormal NK receptor expression in AHB patients. (A) Representative dot plots depict the expression of NK activation receptors (NKp30, NKp44, NKp46, NKG2D and NKG2C) and inhibitory receptors (CD158a, CD158b and NKG2A) and TRAIL in an AHB patient. CD3⁻CD56⁺ NK cells were gated. Values in quadrants represent the percentages of CD3⁻CD56⁺ NK cells that express NK receptors. (B–D) Pooled data show the frequencies of total (B), CD56^{bright} (C) and CD56^{dim} (D) NK cell subsets expressing NK activation receptors (NKp30, NKp44, NKp46, NKG2D and NKG2C) and inhibitory receptors (CD158a, CD158b and NKG2A) and TRAIL in HC (n = 16), CHB (n = 19) and AHB (n = 21) groups. Multiple comparisons were first made among the three groups using the Kruskal-Wallis H non-parametric test. Then the comparisons between two groups were performed using the Mann-Whitney U test. The data represent the mean ± SD. * $P<0.05$ compared with HC subjects; # $P<0.05$ compared with CHB patients.

with recent studies of CHB patients [18] and chronic HCV infection [17], support the concept that the enhanced NK cytolytic activity may mediate liver injury in acute and chronic hepatitis virus infection, whereas sufficient IFN-γ production by NK cells may also be sufficient to achieve viral clearance in acute viral infection. In particular, NKp46⁺ NK cells were enriched in the

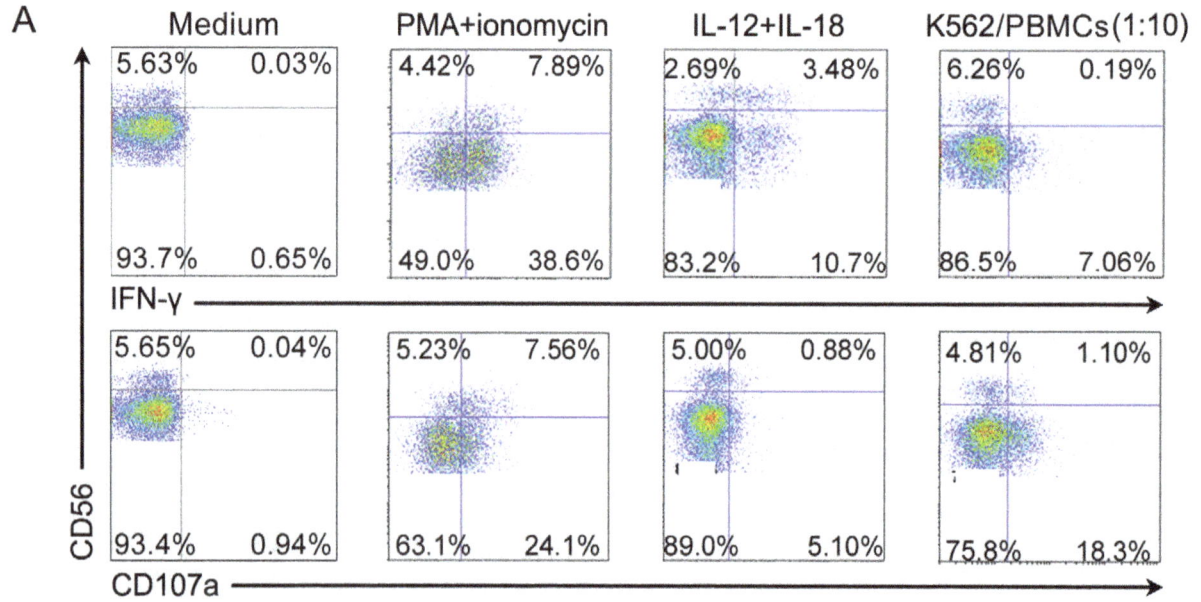

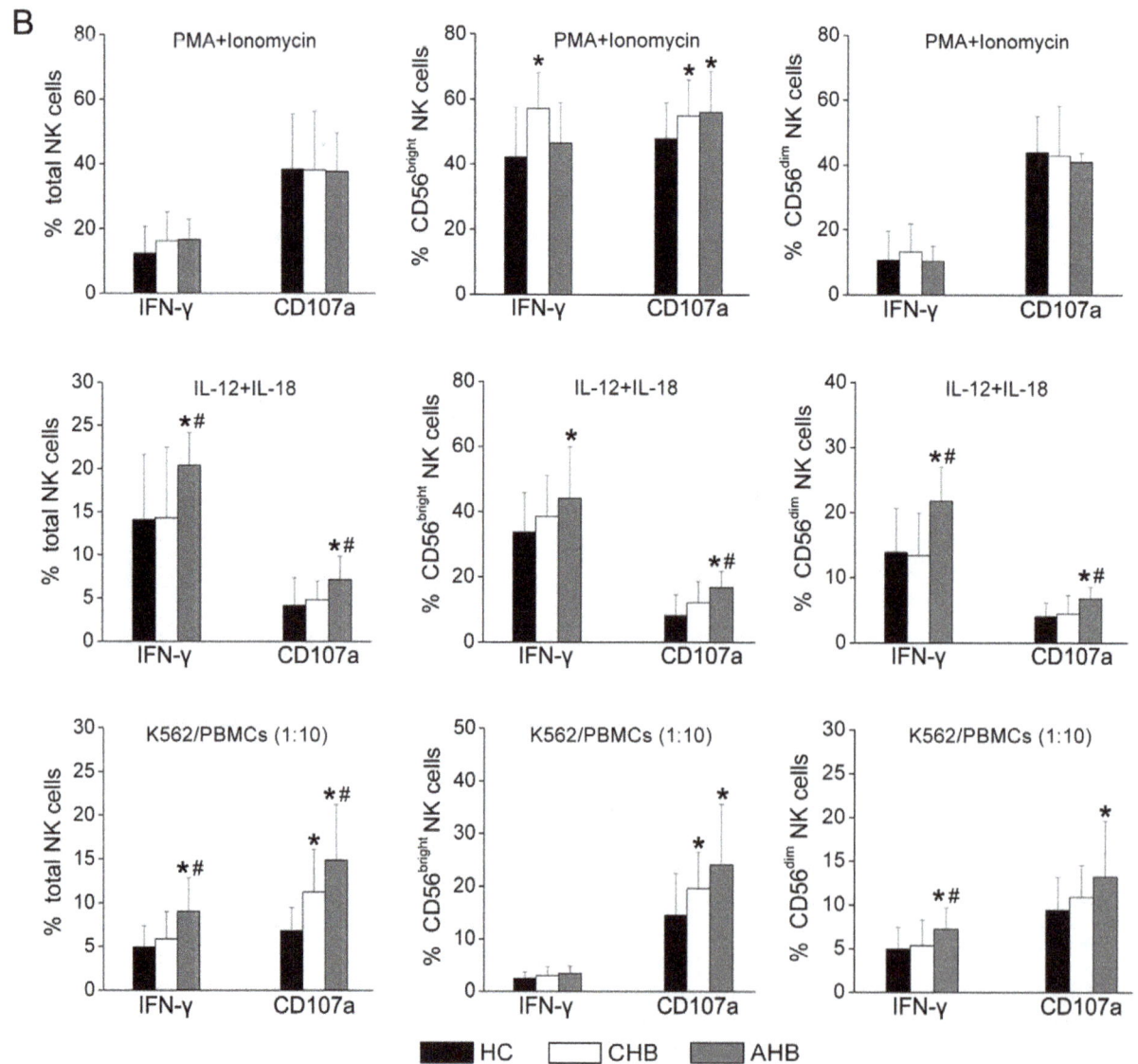

Figure 4. IFN-γ production and CD107a expression by NK cells were concurrently increased in AHB patients. (A) Representative dot plots depict IFN-γ and CD107a expression by NK subsets from an HC subject following PMA/ionomycin, IL-12/IL-18 and K562 stimulation. CD3⁻CD56⁺ cells were gated. Values in the quadrants represent the percentages of CD3⁻CD56⁺ NK cells that express IFN-γ or CD107a. (B) Pooled data show the proportion of IFN-γ⁺ and CD107a⁺ NK cell subsets in response to three stimulation conditions in HC (n = 16), CHB (n = 19) and AHB (n = 16) groups. Multiple comparisons were first made among the three groups using the Kruskal-Wallis *H* non-parametric test. Then the comparisons between two groups were performed using the Mann-Whitney *U* test. The data represent the mean ± SD. *$P<0.05$ compared with HC subjects; # $P<0.05$ compared with CHB patients.

livers of AHB and CHB patients may further strengthen their antiviral and hepatocytic effects because several recent studies have identified that NKp46⁺ NK cells were characterized by both IFN-γ production and high cytolytic activity and have the potential to control HCV replication and to kill hepatic stellate cells [26–28]. Their impact on the liver disease progression in HBV infection will be of interest.

The mechanisms underlying the differential regulation of NK activity in AHB and CHB patients remain to be elucidated but may include variation in expression profiles of NK receptor/ligands and cytokines [29]. In this regard, the present study showed that there are more types of activation receptors were upregulated (such as NKp46, NKG2C) and more types of inhibitory receptors (CD158a, CD158b and NKG2A) were

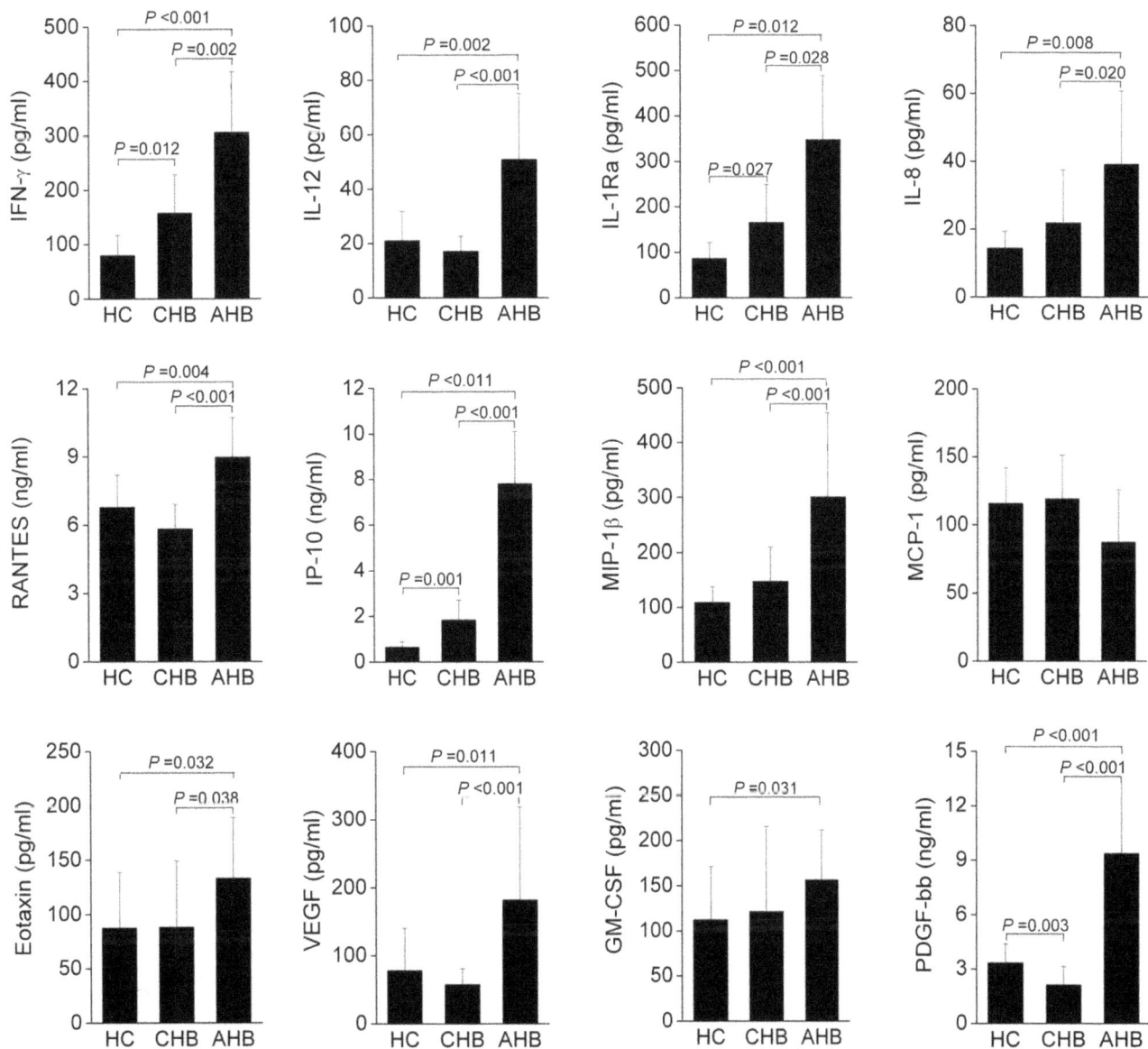

Figure 5. Plasma cytokine levels were significantly increased in AHB patients. Plasma cytokine levels including inflammatory cytokines IL-12p70, IL-1Ra and IFN-γ, chemokines including RANTES, IP-10, MIP-1β, MCP-1, IL-8 and eotaxin, and growth factors including GM-CSF, VEGF and PDGF-bb in HC (n = 10), CHB (n = 10) and AHB (n = 10) groups are shown. Multiple comparisons were first made among the three groups using the Kruskal-Wallis *H* non-parametric test. Then the comparisons between two groups were performed using the Mann-Whitney *U* test. The data represent the mean ± SD. *P*-values are shown.

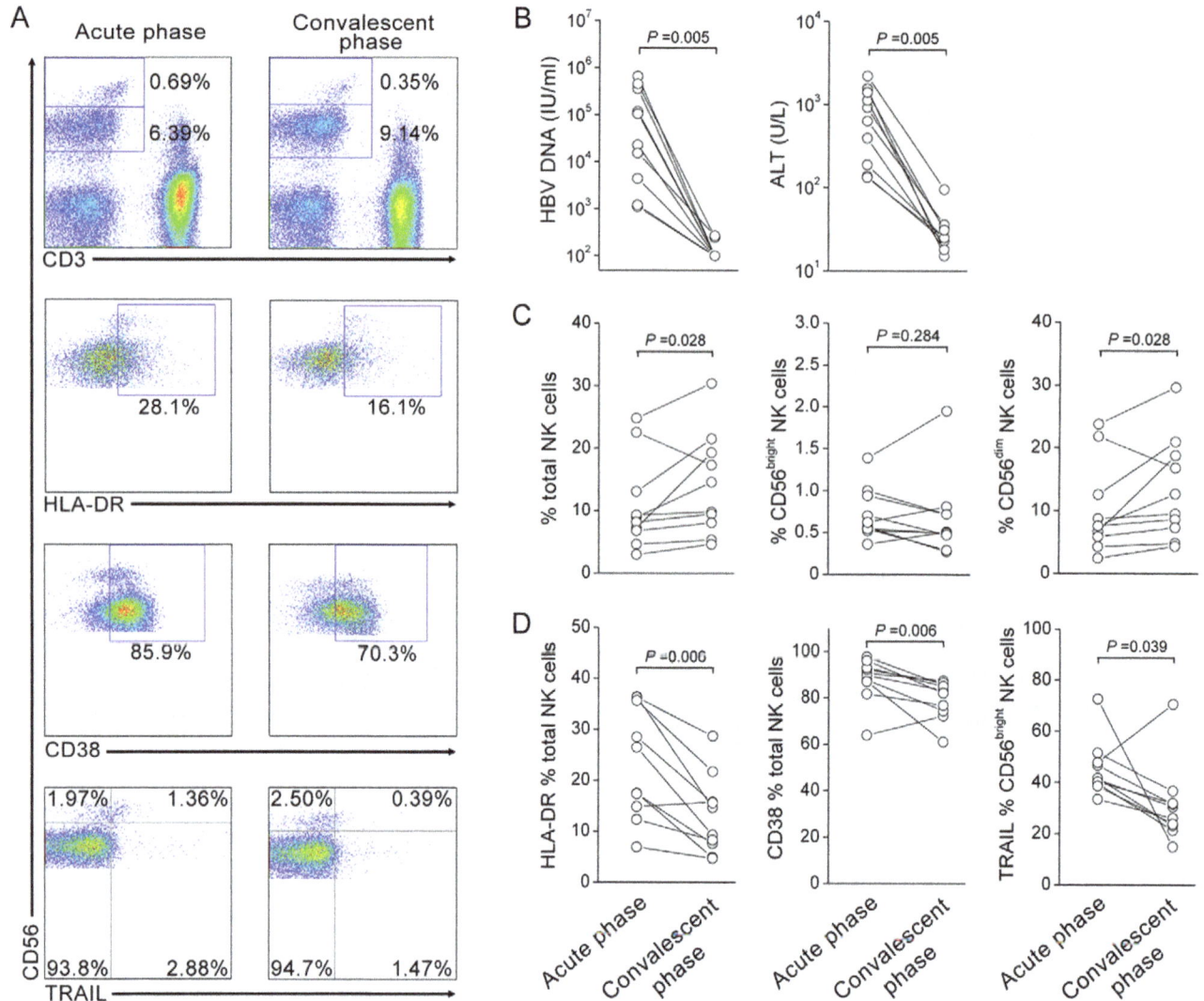

Figure 6. Dynamic expression of clinical and immunological parameters in AHB patients (n = 10). (A) The representative dot plots indicate the NK subsets frequencies and activation markers HLA-DR and CD38 as well as TRAIL expression on NK cells in AHB patients at acute and convalescent phases of illness. Values indicate the percentages of HLA-DR, CD38 and TRAIL among CD3$^-$CD56$^+$ NK cells. (B–D) The dynamic change of HBV DNA and serum ALT levels (B), the percentages of total, CD56^{bright} and CD56^{dim} NK cells (C) and HLA-DR, CD38 and TRAIL expression on NK cell subsets (D) were analyzed in AHB patients at the acute and convalescent phases of illness, respectively. P values are shown. The comparisons were performed using the Wilcoxon matched pairs T test.

downregulated by NK cells from AHB patients compared with those from CHB patients. Furthermore, the expression levels of the activation receptors NKp46 and NKG2C were significantly higher and those of inhibitory receptors CD158a, CD158b and NKG2A were significantly lower in NK cell subsets from AHB patients compared with those from CHB patients. This significant bias in activation and inhibitory receptor expression may partially explain the increased activity of NK cells in AHB patients compared with CHB patients. Furthermore, expression profiles of cytokines such as IFN-α and IL-12/IL-15/IL-18 may also be involved in the regulation of NK cell activity in chronic HCV and HBV infection [20,30]. In this study, significantly increased plasma levels of multiple cytokines, including IL-12 and chemokines, including MIP-1β, IP-10, IL-8, RANTES and eotaxin as well as the growth factors GM-CSF, PDGF-BB and VEGF in AHB patients suggested an increased systematic inflammation in AHB patients. Further studies are required to

elucidate the regulatory roles of these altered cytokine and chemokine profiles on NK cell activity in AHB patients.

Another important finding of this study was the activation of both NK cells and T cells in AHB patients, while in contrast only NK cells were activated and T cells deactivated in CHB patients. Previous studies have shown that T cells are often readily activated and multi-clonal in acute HBV infection [5–7,31]. However, in chronic HBV infection, virus-specific T cell responses are generally weak and exhibit functional exhaustion, also indicated by deactivation of T cells. Thus, the activation of both innate immunity and adaptive immunity may favor viral clearance [32]. However, activation of innate immunity such as NK cell activation mediates relatively poor viral clearance, but has the potential to mediate liver injury. This notion was further confirmed in longitudinal detection of NK cells in AHB patients who displayed a decrease in NK cell activation and an increase in NK cell percentages at the convalescence phase as compared with that at acute phase; this process was accompanied by HBV clearance and the recovery of liver injury in these patinets. This finding also suggested that NK activation combined with T cell activation serves as a marker to distinguish acute hepatitis and the acute exacerbation of chronic hepatitis, although this requires confirmation in further prospective studies.

This study was limited by the lack of access to samples from the incubation phase of acute HBV infection. During this initial phase after viral entry, there appears to be a temporary block to HBV replication and spread [33]. It can be speculated that this is partially mediated by innate immune mechanisms, as suggested by elevated IL-15 and NK activation/function just before the expansion phase in some patients [23]. Another study also showed activation of NK and NKT cells within 72 hours of experimental infection with woodchuck hepadnavirus, resulting in transient suppression of viral replication [34]. Another limitation in our study was the absence of the detection of NK cell function in the intrahepatic compartment, which is the site of viral replication, although NK cell distribution was just detectable in liver biopsies through IHC staining using our previously stored samples [35]. However, changes in the circulation have been found to closely mirror those in the liver in acute HBV infection in chimpanzees [36]. In accordance with this, we have previously demonstrated NK activation in the liver of patients with chronic HBV infection [20].

In conclusion, this study indicates that NK cells are activated and exhibit concomitantly increased cytolytic activity and IFN-γ production in the acute phase, which was subsequently decreased at the the convalescence phase as companied by the HBV clearance and the recovery of liver injury in these AHB patinets. This study, therefore, highlights the roles of NK cells in liver immunopathogenesis in acute HBV infection and will facilitate the rational development of immunotherapeutic strategies that decrease NK cytolytic capacity while enhancing IFN-γ production in chronic HBV infection.

Materials and Methods

Ethics Statement

The study protocol was approved by the Ethics Committee of Beijing 302 Hospital. The individual in this manuscript has given written informed consent (as outlined in the PLoS consent form) to publish these case details.

Study subjects

Twenty-one AHB and 19 CHB patients were recruited into this study. All patients were diagnosed according to previously described criteria [20,35] and had not received antiviral therapy or immunosuppressive drugs within 6 months of the start of sampling. Sixteen age- and sex-matched healthy individuals were enrolled as controls (HC). Individuals with concurrent HCV, human immunodeficiency virus infections, autoimmune liver diseases or alcoholic liver disease were excluded. All of these subjects enrolled in the study are hepatitis D virus negative except one CHB patient who displayed HDV-specific IgG and antigen positive. The basic characteristics of these enrolled subjects are listed in Table 1.

For AHB patients, alanine aminotransferase (ALT) levels at clinical onset were at least 10-fold greater than the upper limit of the normal level and first detection of serum hepatitis B surface antigen (HBsAg) and immunoglobulin (Ig) M anti-hepatitis B core antigen (HBcAg) [5,6,35]. The detailed clinical descriptions of acute phase at the onset of sampling were shown in the Table 2.

Table 1. Characteristics of subjects at the sampling time in the study.

	HC	CHB	AHB
Case	16	19	21
Age	30 (25–45)	38 (22–65)	37 (17–56)
Gender (M/F)	12/4	15/4	15/6
ALT (U/L)	NA	242 (42–1298)	974 (88–2216)*
HBV DNA (IU/ml)	NA	1.5×10^7 (4.94×10^2–4.17×10^8)	2.01×10^4 (<100–6.51×10^5)*

Data are shown as median and range. * $P<0.05$ versus CHB patients; HC: healthy controls; CHB, chronic hepatitis B; AHB, acute hepatitis B. NA: not applicable.

Among these 21 AHB patients, 10 of patients were also followed-up for immunological detection at the convalescent phases.

Peripheral blood mononuclear cells (PBMCs) were isolated from all enrolled subjects. Liver biopsies were collected from AHB patients (n = 7), CHB patients (n = 10) and healthy donors (n = 5), which have been used in our previous studies [20,35]. These healthy liver tissue samples, were obtained from the healthy donors whose livers were used for transplantation after receiving the informed consent from each donor. For pathological evaluation, liver biopsy specimens were embedded in Tissue Tek for in situ immunohistochemical staining.

FACS analysis

All antibodies were purchased from BD Biosciences (San Jose, CA, USA) with the exception of phycoerythrin (PE)-conjugated anti-NKG2A, anti-NKG2C, anti-NKG2D, anti-NKp30 and anti-NKp46 antibodies, which were purchased from R&D Systems (Minneapolis, MN). Peripheral NK subset frequencies and NK receptor expression were analyzed according to previously described protocols [20,37]. For detection of NK cell activation, PBMCs were incubated with PE-conjugated anti-CD3, APC-conjugated anti-CD56 and PerCP-conjugated anti-HLA-DR, or FITC-conjugated anti-CD69 or FITC-conjugated anti-CD38. For intracellular IFN-γ and CD107a staining, cells were permeabilized and stained with the corresponding intracellular antibodies. Cells were then analyzed using FACSCalibur and Flowjo software (TreeStar, Ashand, OR, USA). At least 200,000 events were acquired per run.

Degranulation of NK cells and IFN-γ detection

CD107a degranulation is now widely used to assess NK cell cytotoxic potential [35] Briefly, freshly isolated PBMCs (5×10^5) were directly stimulated with PMA (100 ng mL-1) and ionomycin (1 μg mL-1), IL-12 (10 ng mL-1) in combination with IL-18 (10 ng mL-1; Biovision, PA, CA) or K562 cells at an effector to target ratio (E:T) of 10:1. Unstimulated PBMCs served as negative controls. Anti-CD107a and GolgiStop were added directly into the medium and incubated for 5 h. Cells were then collected and stained with surface antibodies and stained intracellularly with anti-IFN-γ.

Immunohistochemical staining

Paraform-fixed liver biopsy sections (5 μm) were incubated with anti-CD3 (clone F7.2.38, Dako Company, Denmark), anti-CD56 (clone 123C3, Dako Company) antibodies and anti-NKp46 (clone

Table 2. The baseline clinical data of the enrolled AHB patients.

Pt No	Sampling weeks since clinical onset	Age (years)	Gender	sAg/sAb/eAg/eAb/cAb	ALT (U/L)	HBV DNA (IU/ml)
1	1w	19	male	+/−/+/+/+	1415	1200
2	3w	51	female	+/−/−/+/+	1188	779
3	1w	35	male	+/+/−/+/+	974	100
4	1w	34	male	−/+/−/+/+	132	104000
5	2w	17	female	+/−/+/+/+	1617	20100
6	2w	19	male	+/−/+/−/+	2216	15100
7	1w	36	male	+/−/+/−/+	1491	100
8	1w	26	female	+/−/+/+/+	1656	100
9	2w	43	male	+/−/+/−/+	1669	100
10	3w	37	male	+/−/−/+/+	141	436000
11	3w	37	male	−/+/−/+/+	88	153000
12	2w	30	male	+/−/+/+/+	1360	31800
13	3w	46	male	+/−/+/+/+	779	100
14	3w	38	male	+/+/−/+/+	635	353000
15	1w	56	female	−/−/−/+/+	997	100
16	1w	38	male	+/+/−/+/+	1557	1100
17	1w	26	female	+/−/+/−/+	1128	449000
18	3w	39	male	−/−/−/−/+	188	22400
19	3w	39	male	−/−/−/+/+	137	651000
20	2w	43	female	+/−/−/+/+	392	4380
21	2w	49	male	+/−/−/−/+	925	117000

195314, R&D Systems) overnight at 4°C, respectively, after blocking endogenous peroxidase activity with 0.3% H_2O_2. 3-Amino-9-ethyl-carbazole (red color) was used for single staining. High powered fields (hpf, ×400) were used for counting positive cells according to previously described protocols [20,35]. Positive cells were counted in three different fields by two independent observers. Results are expressed as the median and range of all tested patients in each group.

Luminex

Plasma cytokines were detected using a Luminex Bio-Plex ProTm Human Cytokine Standard Group I 27-Plex kit (Cat No: 5021099, including IL-1β, IL-1ra, IL-2, IL-4, IL-5, IL-6, IL-7, IL-8, IL-9, IL-10, IL-12p70, IL-13, IL-15, IL-17, Eotaxin, basic FGF, G-CSF, GM-CSF, IFN-γ, IP-10, MCP-1, MIP-1α, MIP-1β, PDGF-BB, RANTES, TNF-α and VEGF) on a Luminex 100 System (BioRad, Hercules, CA, USA) according to the protocol provided by the manufacturer.

Virological assessment

The virological assay protocol was performed as previously described [20,35] with a cut-off value of 100 IU ml-1.

Statistical analysis

All data were analyzed using SPSS 13.0 for Windows software (SPSS Inc., Chicago, IL, USA). Multiple comparisons were made among the different groups using the Kruskal-Wallis H non-parametric test. Comparisons between various individuals were performed using the Mann-Whitney U test; while comparisons between the same individual were performed using the Wilcoxon matched pairs T test. Correlations between variables were evaluated using the Spearman rank correlation test. For all tests, two-sided $P < 0.05$ was considered to be significant.

Acknowledgments

We thank Songshan Wang for his excellent technical support and all patients, study-site staff, and all participating consultants for their contributions, which made this study possible.

Author Contributions

Conceived and designed the experiments: JJZ ZZ YGL F-SW. Performed the experiments: JJZ YGL LJ SYZ RF YLS CBZ. Analyzed the data: JJZ ZZ CBZ SYZ. Contributed reagents/materials/analysis tools: JJZ CBZ QHS. Wrote the paper: JJZ ZZ F-SW. Enrolled patients: YGL JL RF YLS QHS WGL. Sampled: YGL JL RF YLS QHS.

References

1. Rehermann B, Nascimbeni M (2005) Immunology of hepatitis B virus and hepatitis C virus infection. Nat Rev Immunol 5: 215–229.
2. Zhang Z, Zhang JY, Wang LF, Wang FS (2012) Immunopathogenesis and prognostic immune markers of chronic hepatitis B virus infection. J Gastroenterol Hepatol 27: 223–230.
3. Wang FS, Zhang Z (2009) Host immunity influences disease progression and antiviral efficacy in humans infected with hepatitis B virus. Expert Rev Gastroenterol Hepatol 3: 499–512.
4. Thimme R, Wieland S, Steiger C, Ghrayeb J, Reimann KA, et al. (2003) CD8(+) T cells mediate viral clearance and disease pathogenesis during acute hepatitis B virus infection. J Virol 77: 68–76.
5. Boettler T, Panther E, Bengsch B, Nazarova N, Spangenberg HC, et al. (2006) Expression of the interleukin-7 receptor alpha chain (CD127) on virus-specific CD8+ T cells identifies functionally and phenotypically defined memory T cells during acute resolving hepatitis B virus infection. J Virol 80: 3532–3540.

6. Urbani S, Boni C, Missale G, Elia G, Cavallo C, et al. (2002) Virus-specific CD8+ lymphocytes share the same effector-memory phenotype but exhibit functional differences in acute hepatitis B and C. J Virol 76: 12423–12434.

7. Webster GJ, Reignat S, Maini MK, Whalley SA, Ogg GS, et al. (2000) Incubation phase of acute hepatitis B in man: dynamic of cellular immune mechanisms. Hepatology 32: 1117–1124.

8. Chang JJ, Thompson AJ, Visvanathan K, Kent SJ, Cameron PU, et al. (2007) The phenotype of hepatitis B virus-specific T cells differ in the liver and blood in chronic hepatitis B virus infection. Hepatology 46: 1332–1340.

9. Boni C, Fisicaro P, Valdatta C, Amadei B, Di Vincenzo P, et al. (2007) Characterization of hepatitis B virus (HBV)-specific T-cell dysfunction in chronic HBV infection. J Virol 81: 4215–4225.

10. Lopes AR, Kellam P, Das A, Dunn C, Kwan A, et al. (2008) Bim-mediated deletion of antigen-specific CD8 T cells in patients unable to control HBV infection. J Clin Invest 118: 1835–1845.

11. Das A, Hoare M, Davies N, Lopes AR, Dunn C, et al. (2008) Functional skewing of the global CD8 T cell population in chronic hepatitis B virus infection. J Exp Med 205: 2111–2124.

12. Das A, Maini MK (2010) Innate and adaptive immune responses in hepatitis B virus infection. Dig Dis 28: 126–132.

13. Racanelli V, Rehermann B (2006) The liver as an immunological organ. Hepatology 43: S54–62.

14. Gao B, Jeong WI, Tian Z (2008) Liver: An organ with predominant innate immunity. Hepatology 47: 729–736.

15. Lanier LL (2005) NK cell recognition. Annu Rev Immunol 23: 225–274.

16. Vivier E, Tomasello E, Baratin M, Walzer T, Ugolini S (2008) Functions of natural killer cells. Nat Immunol 9: 503–510.

17. Ahlenstiel G, Titerence RH, Koh C, Edlich B, Feld JJ, et al (2010) Natural killer cells are polarized toward cytotoxicity in chronic hepatitis C in an interferon-alfa-dependent manner. Gastroenterology 138: 325–335 e321–322.

18. Oliviero B, Varchetta S, Paudice E, Michelone G, Zaramella M, et al. (2009) Natural killer cell functional dichotomy in chronic hepatitis B and chronic hepatitis C virus infections. Gastroenterology 137: 1151-1160, 1160 e1151–1157.

19. Bonorino P, Ramzan M, Camous X, Dufeu-Duchesne T, Thelu MA, et al. (2009) Fine characterization of intrahepatic NK cells expressing natural killer receptors in chronic hepatitis B and C. J Hepatol 51: 458–467.

20. Zhang Z, Zhang S, Zou Z, Shi J, Zhao J, et al. (2011) Hypercytolytic activity of hepatic natural killer cells correlates with liver injury in chronic hepatitis B patients. Hepatology 53: 73–85.

21. Dunn C, Brunetto M, Reynolds G, Christophides T, Kennedy PT, et al. (2007) Cytokines induced during chronic hepatitis B virus infection promote a pathway for NK cell-mediated liver damage. J Exp Med 204: 667–680.

22. Fisicaro P, Valdatta C, Boni C, Massari M, Mori C, et al. (2009) Early kinetics of innate and adaptive immune responses during hepatitis B virus infection. Gut 58: 974–982.

23. Dunn C, Peppa D, Khanna P, Nebbia G, Jones M, et al. (2009) Temporal analysis of early immune responses in patients with acute hepatitis B virus infection. Gastroenterology 137: 1289–1300.

24. Yang PL, Althage A, Chung J, Maier H, Wieland S, et al. (2010) Immune effectors required for hepatitis B virus clearance. Proc Natl Acad Sci U S A 107: 798–802.

25. Stacey AR, Norris PJ, Qin L, Haygreen EA, Taylor E, et al. (2009) Induction of a striking systemic cytokine cascade prior to peak viremia in acute human immunodeficiency virus type 1 infection, in contrast to more modest and delayed responses in acute hepatitis B and C virus infections. J Virol 83: 3719–3733.

26. Golden-Mason L, Stone AE, Bambha KM, Cheng L, Rosen HR (2012) Race- and genderrelated variation in NKp46 expression associated with differential anti-HCV immunity. Hepatology doi: 10.1002/hep.25771.

27. Kramer B, Korner C, Kebschull M, Glassner A, Eisenhardt M, et al. (2012) NKp46(High) expression defines a NK cell subset that is potentially involved in control of HCV replication and modulation of liver fibrosis. Hepatology doi: 10.1002/hep.25804.

28. Heeg M, Thimme R (2012) NK cells and hepatitis C; NKp46 expression linked to antiviral and antifibrotic activity. Hepatology.

29. Mondelli MU, Varchetta S, Oliviero B (2010) Natural killer cells in viral hepatitis: facts and controversies. Eur J Clin Invest 40: 851–863.

30. Edlich B, Ahlenstiel G, Azpiroz AZ, Stoltzfus J, Noureddin M, et al. (2012) Early changes in interferon signaling define natural killer cell response and refractoriness to interferon-based therapy of hepatitis C patients. Hepatology 55: 39–48.

31. Sprengers D, van der Molen RG, Kusters JG, De Man RA, Niesters HG, et al. (2006) Analysis of intrahepatic HBV-specific cytotoxic T-cells during and after acute HBV infection in humans. J Hepatol 45: 182–189.

32. Gujar SA, Jenkins AK, Guy CS, Wang J, Michalak TI (2008) Aberrant lymphocyte activation precedes delayed virus-specific T-cell response after both primary infection and secondary exposure to hepadnavirus in the woodchuck model of hepatitis B virus infection. J Virol 82: 6992–7008.

33. Bertoletti A, Ferrari C (2003) Kinetics of the immune response during HBV and HCV infection. Hepatology 38: 4–13.

34. Guy CS, Mulrooney-Cousins PM, Churchill ND, Michalak TI (2008) Intrahepatic expression of genes affiliated with innate and adaptive immune responses immediately after invasion and during acute infection with woodchuck hepadnavirus. J Virol 82: 8579–8591.

35. Zhang Z, Zhang JY, Wherry EJ, Jin B, Xu B, et al. (2008) Dynamic programmed death 1 expression by virus-specific CD8 T cells correlates with the outcome of acute hepatitis B. Gastroenterology 134: 1938–1949, 1949 e1931–1933.

36. Guidotti LG, Rochford R, Chung J, Shapiro M, Purcell R, et al. (1999) Viral clearance without destruction of infected cells during acute HBV infection. Science 284: 825–829.

37. Cai L, Zhang Z, Zhou L, Wang H, Fu J, et al. (2008) Functional impairment in circulating and intrahepatic NK cells and relative mechanism in hepatocellular carcinoma patients. Clin Immunol 129: 428–437.

10

Clinical Usefulness of Measuring Red Blood Cell Distribution Width in Patients with Hepatitis B

YuFeng Lou, ManYi Wang, WeiLin Mao*

Department of Clinical Laboratory, First Affiliated Hospital, Zhejiang University School of Medicine, Hangzhou, Zhejiang Province, People's Republic of China

Abstract

Background: Red blood cell distribution width (RDW), an automated measure of red blood cell size heterogeneity (*e.g.*, anisocytosis) that is largely overlooked, is a newly recognized risk marker in patients with cardiovascular diseases, but its role in persistent viral infection has not been well-defined. The present study was designed to investigate the association between RDW values and different disease states in hepatitis B virus (HBV)-infected patients. In addition, we analyzed whether RDW is associated with mortality in the HBV-infected patients.

Methodology/Principal Findings: One hundred and twenty-three patients, including 16 with acute hepatitis B (AHB), 61 with chronic hepatitis B (CHB), and 46 with chronic severe hepatitis B (CSHB), and 48 healthy controls were enrolled. In all subjects, a blood sample was collected at admission to examine liver function, renal function, international normalized ratio and routine hematological testing. All patients were followed up for at least 4 months. A total of 10 clinical chemistry, hematology, and biochemical variables were analyzed for possible association with outcomes by using Cox proportional hazards and multiple regression models. RDW values at admission in patients with CSHB (18.30±3.11%, $P<0.001$), CHB (16.37±2.43%, $P<0.001$) and AHB (14.38±1.72%, $P<0.05$) were significantly higher than those in healthy controls (13.03±1.33%). Increased RDW values were clinically associated with severe liver disease and increased 3-month mortality rate. Multivariate analysis demonstrated that RDW values and the model for end-stage liver disease score were independent predictors for mortality (both $P<0.001$).

Conclusion: RDW values are significantly increased in patients with hepatitis B and associated with its severity. Moreover, RDW values are an independent predicting factor for the 3-month mortality rate in patients with hepatitis B.

Editor: Anand S. Mehta, Drexel University College of Medicine, United States of America

Funding: The work was supported by grants from Health Department of Zhejiang Province (2011KYA058). URL http://www.zjwst.gov.cn/The funders had no role in study design, data collection and analysis, decision to publish, or preparation of the manuscript.

Competing Interests: The authors have declared that no competing interests exist.

* E-mail: mao_wei_lin@163.com

Introduction

Red cell distribution width (RDW) is an automated measure of the heterogeneity of red blood cell (RBC) sizes (*e.g.* anisocytosis) and routinely performed as part of a complete blood cell counts [1–3]. RDW is used in the differential diagnosis of anemia [4]. Recently, a series of studies have demonstrated that RDW can serve as a novel, independent predictor of prognosis in patients with cardiovascular diseases (*e.g.* heart failure [5–7], stable coronary diseases [8], acute myocardial infarction [9], strokes [10], and pulmonary hypertension [11]). Elevated RDW values were also shown to be associated with increased risk of mortality in the general population [12–14]. However, to our knowledge, the role of RDW values in persistent viral infection has not been well-defined. More importantly, whether RDW values are associated with different disease states of hepatitis B virus (HBV) infection such as acute hepatitis B (AHB), chronic hepatitis B (CHB) and chronic severe hepatitis B (CSHB) remains unknown. The present study was designed to investigate the association between RDW values and different disease states in HBV-infected patients. In addition, we analyzed whether RDW is associated with mortality in the HBV-infected patients.

Materials and Methods

Subjects

Adult HBV-infected patients admitted to the First Affiliated Hospital of Zhejiang University School of Medicine and diagnosed with AHB, CHB or CSHB were consecutively recruited between August 1, 2010 and August 1, 2011. In the present study, whereas there were no exclusions for age/sex, patients who received any anti-HBV agents or steroids 6 months before admission were excluded. Patients with a concurrent infection of HCV, hepatitis D virus, hepatitis G virus, and/or human immunodeficiency virus and any autoimmune liver disease were also excluded. During the same time period, age- and sex-matched healthy individuals were recruited as controls at a patient/control ratio of 3:1.

Blood samples were collected from all HBV-infected patients within 24 hours after admission, and blood samples were taken from 48 healthy individuals at the time of recruitment. After discharge, all patients were followed up monthly by phone conversation, and every three months by patient's visit to the hospital. Blood samples were collected at each visit for laboratory tests including the detection of HBsAg. Neither the technician who performed the laboratory tests nor the investigator who followed up the patients knew the diagnosis of the patients.

The study was approved by the Ethics Committee of the First Affiliated Hospital of Zhejiang University School of Medicine, and written informed consent for participation was obtained from each study participant.

Clinical Diagnosis

The diagnostic criteria for AHB, CHB and CSHB were in accordance with the 2000 Xi'an Viral Hepatitis Management Guidelines recommended by the Chinese Society of Infectious Diseases and Parasitology, and the Chinese Society of Hepatology, of the Chinese Medical Association [15]. Briefly, viral hepatitis B is classified into three major clinical types, namely AHB, CHB and CSHB. AHB is defined as when hepatitis B surface Ag (HBsAg)-negative conversion occurs within 6 months after the initial onset of symptoms due to HBV infection. CHB is defined as when a HBV carrier requires a clinical course of hepatitis B infection for more than 6 months and may have exhibited symptoms or signs of hepatitis and abnormal hepatic function, or with histological changes. CSHB is defined as when there is a history of CHB or liver cirrhosis with serum HBsAg positivity of more than 6 months and a serum total bilirubin level of more than 10 times the normal level (i.e. 171 μmol/L), with at least one of the following five liver failure indexes: prothrombin activity of less than 40%, hepatic encephalopathy, ascites, progressive reduction in liver size, and hepatorenal syndrome. In addition, the diagnosis of liver cirrhosis was made on the basis of clinical (e.g. physical stigmata of cirrhosis), biochemical (e.g. decreased serum albumin and increased serum globulin levels), and ultrasonographic or computed tomography (e.g. nodular liver surface, coarsened echogenicity of liver parenchyma, enlarged spleen, and/or ascites) findings [16,17].

Laboratory Methods

RDW, hemoglobin level, and mean corpuscular volume (MCV) were determined using the XE-2100 automated hematology analyzer (Sysmex Corp, Kobe, Japan), as one part of a complete blood cell count. The normal reference range for RDW in the laboratory of our hospital is 11.6% −15.0%. Serum creatinine, serum albumin, total protein, total bilirubin and alanine transaminase levels were measured using the Hitachi 704 Analyzer (Boehringer Mannheim Diagnostics), and the international normalized ratio (INR) was generated by the Sysmex CA1500 full-automatic analyzer (Sysmex Corp, Hyogo, Japan). At baseline, demographic and clinical characteristics, including the model for end-stage liver disease (MELD) score (with higher scores indicating more severe illness), were collected.

MELD Score

Liver disease severity at admission was evaluated via the MELD score, which uses the patient's serum bilirubin and creatinine levels and the INR for prothrombin time to predict survival. The MELD score was calculated using the web site calculator (http://www.mayoclinic.org/gi-rst/mayomodel7.html).

Statistical Analysis

All continuous variables were expressed as mean value ± standard deviation (SD), and categorical data as percentages. We used SPSS version 15.0 (SPSS, Inc., Chicago, IL) to perform statistical procedures. The Kruskal-Wallis H test and Mann-Whitney nonparametric U test were used for comparison between groups. Categorical data were evaluated by the χ^2-test or Fisher's exact test, as appropriate. A multivariable stepwise logistic regression test was used to evaluate independent clinical parameters predicting mortality. The receiver operating characteristic (ROC) curve was obtained and area under the curve (AUC) was calculated to identify the best RDW to predict mortality in patients with HBV infection. A value of $P<0.05$ was considered statistically significant.

Results

Increased RDW Values in HBV-infected Patients

A total of 123 HBV-infected patients, 16 with AHB, 61 with CHB, and 46 with CSHB, as well as 48 healthy individuals, were recruited during the study period (Table 1).

The RDW values of HBV-infected patients at admission ranged from 12.0% to 27.3%. The values in patients with CSHB patients (18.30±3.11%, $P<0.001$), CHB patients (16.37±2.43%, $P<0.001$) and AHB patients (14.38±1.72%, $P<0.05$) were significantly higher than those in healthy controls (13.03±1.33%). Moreover, CSHB patients had higher RDW values than CHB and AHB patients (both $P<0.001$), and CHB patients had higher RDW values than AHB patients ($P<0.05$) (Figure 1).

Baseline Characteristics and Baseline Factors Related with RDW

Patients were divided into three groups based on their RDW values: group A (RDW ≤15.0%), group B (>15.0%, but <20.0%) and group C (≥20.0%). Differences in clinical and laboratory characteristics among the three groups of RDW are listed in Table 2. Patients with higher values of RDW tended to be older, were more likely to have severe liver disease, had lower levels of hemoglobin, total protein, and serum albumin, and had higher INR and total bilirubin. The serum creatinine, gender and MCV were not significantly different among the three groups.

The MELD score in groups A, B, and C were 10.7±4.2, 15.1±4.7 and 19.8±4.4, respectively. There was a stepwise increase in MELD scores with increasing values of RDW ($P<0.001$ between groups A and B, and between groups B and C) (Figure 2, left).

Association of RDW with 3-month Mortality in HBV-infected Patients

The median follow-up period was 72 days (range, 21–128 days). During the follow-up, 41 patients died, none of whom were patients with AHB, six were with CHB and 35 were with CSHB.

There was a significantly increase in the 3-month mortality rate following increasing RDW values, with 12.7% in group A, 35.8% in group B and 69.6% in group C ($P<0.01$ between groups A and B, and between groups B and C) (Figure 2, right).

To evaluate the values for RDW and MELD score to predict mortality, ROC curves were drawn (Figure 3). The AUCs were calculated as 0.847±0.034 for the MELD score and 0.664±0.049 for RDW (both $P<0.001$). When RDW and MELD were combined, the AUC was 0.905±0.019 ($P<0.001$). The multivariate logistic regression analysis showed that only the RDW values and MELD score were independent factors predicting mortality rate (Table 3).

Discussion

RDW reflects the variability in circulating RBC size. It is based on the width of the RBC volume distribution curve, with larger values indicating greater variability [18]. RDW is elevated when there is increased red cell destruction, or, more commonly,

Table 1. Clinical characteristics of studied subjects.

	AHB (n = 16)	CHB (n = 61)	CSHB (n = 46)	Healthy controls (n = 48)
Age (year) *	39.8±13.0	44.5±12.1	49.9±13.5	43.3±10.9
Gender (male/female)	11/5	46/15	36/10	36/12
Total bilirubin (μmol/L) *	107±54	65±13	304±150	12±5
Alanine aminotransferase (U/L) *	1027±818	111±146	123±118	24±11
International normalized ratio*	1.39±0.44	1.13±0.23	2.23±1.18	0.91±0.21
HBsAg positive	16	61	46	0
HBeAg positive	7	61	20	0
HBcAb IgM positive	16	0	0	0
HBV DNA positive	10	61	22	0
Mortality	0	6	35	0

*Data are expressed as mean ± standard deviation.
AHB, Acute hepatitis B; CHB, Chronic hepatitis B; CSHB, Chronic severe hepatitis B; HBsAg, Hepatitis B surface Antigen; HBeAg, Hepatitis B e Antigen; HBcAb, Hepatitis B core Antibody; HBV, Hepatitis B virus.

ineffective red cell production. RDW may represent a nutritional deficiency (*e.g.* iron, vitamin B12, or folic acid), bone marrow depression, or chronic inflammation [19–21]. These conditions are often present in patients with liver disease, correlate with the severity of the disease, and are associated with a worse prognosis [22]. In our study, patients with hepatitis B had significantly higher RDW values compared with healthy subjects and CSHB patients had the highest RDW values among the patients. Thus, we speculate that this difference is an important factor that influences the disease progression, and may present an important marker for patients with HBV infection.

The most significant finding from our study is that increasing RDW values can serve as an independent predictor of mortality in HBV-infected patients. Over the past decade, the MELD score has emerged as the most widely used model for organ allocation in liver transplantation. This model, which includes variables related to both liver and renal function, was implemented in the USA in 2002 and is currently being used in many countries to classify patients with cirrhosis awaiting transplantation according to the severity of their liver disease [23]. Our previous study reported that the MELD score was related to the prognosis of the patients with HBV-related acute-on-chronic liver failure [24]. In the

present study, we reported that RDW can be used for predicting HBV-infected patients mortality, although the prediction power of RDW was relatively lower (AUC = 0.664±0.049 $P<0.001$) than that of MELD score (AUC = 0.847±0.034, $P<0.001$). Moreover, combining RDW with the MELD score further added to prediction power of predicting mortality (AUC = 0.905±0.019, $P<0.001$). This is more relevant to patients with CSHB. The present study included 16 patients with AHB, 61 with CHB and 46 with CSHB. It is well-known that AHB patients are relatively less commonly observed in the clinical setting because 90–95% of adult patients generally have a spontaneously self-limited acute hepatitis without obvious manifestation and often develop the convalescence period through a short-term acute phase before they see doctors. Thus, a 3-month mortality rate is relatively low in patients with AHB. Indeed, in the present study, we found that none of patients with AHB died, whereas six patients with CHB and 35 patients with CSHB died before the 3-month follow-up period.

The mechanisms underlying the association between RDW and severity of hepatitis and its role in predicting mortality in HBV-infected patients are unclear. Recently, in a large unselected cohort of patients, RDW showed a strong and graded association

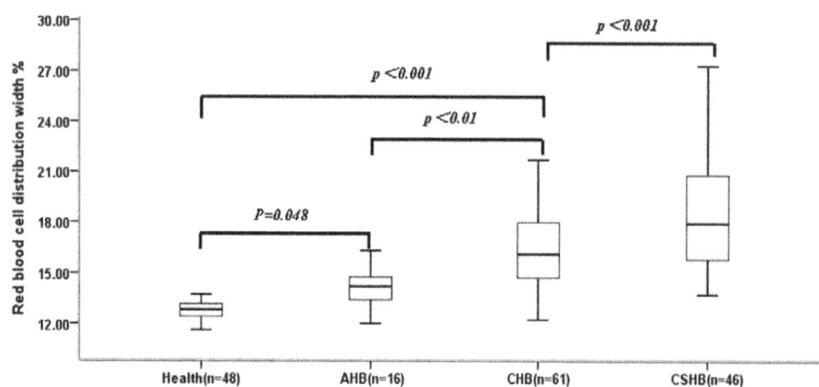

Figure 1. The association between red cell distribution width (RDW) values and different disease states in HBV-infected patients. Data are expressed as box plots, in which the horizontal lines illustrate the 25th, 50th, and 75th percentiles of the values of RDW. The vertical lines represent the 5th and 95th percentiles. AHB, Acute hepatitis B; CHB, Chronic hepatitis B; CSHB, Chronic severe hepatitis B.

Table 2. Clinical and laboratory characteristics among patients with different red blood cell distribution width (RDW) values at admission.

	Group A (RDW≤15.0%, n = 47)	Group B (15.0<RDW<20.0%, n = 53)	Group C (RDW≥20.0%, n = 23)	P
RDW (%)*	13.95±0.94	17.05±1.41	21.70±1.59	<0.001
Age (year) *	41.8±13.2	48.7±12.1	54.7±11.5	0.003
Gender (male/female)	39/8	44/9	16/7	0.077
MCV (fL) *	92.8±5.2	92.5±8.2	89.8±13.2	0.087
Hemoglobin (g/dL) *	133.8±16.3	115.6±18.6	94.4±21.8	<0.001
Total Protein (g/L) *	65.7±6.2	61.2±6.1	59.0±5.9	<0.001
Albumin (g/L) *	38.8±6.2	33.7±5.0	32.9±2.9	<0.001
Alanine aminotransferase (U/L) *	433.1±658.1	128.9±143.1	66.8±31.5	0.003
International normalized ratio *	1.33±0.41	1.53±0.47	1.99±0.63	<0.001
Creatinine(mmol/L) *	63.4±14.9	65.7±17.8	68.9±33.5	0.544
Total bilirubin (μmol/L) *	105.7±115.3	164.7±140.5	250.1±198.7	0.001
MELD score *	10.7±4.2	15.1±4.7	19.8±4.4	<0.001
Hepatic cirrhosis (yes/no)	5/42	20/33	19/4	<0.001
Ascites (yes/no)	2/45	12/41	18/5	<0.001
mortality (yes/no)	6/41	19/34	16/7	<0.01

*Data are expressed as mean±standard deviation.
MCV, mean corpuscular volume; MELD score, model for end-stage liver disease score; RDW, red cell distribution width.

with inflammatory markers, which was independent of ferritin, age, sex, and other haematological variables [25]. Inflammation might contribute to increased RDW values not only by impairing iron metabolism but also by inhibiting the production of or response to erythropoietin or by shortening RBC survival [26,27]. Indeed, a number of studies have shown that proinflammatory cytokines suppress erythropoietin gene expression, inhibit proliferation of erythroid progenitor cells, down-regulate erythropoietin receptor expression, and reduce erythrocyte life-span [27]. Inflammation in a HBV-infected liver is proven to be mediated by cytokines that play a pivotal role in the pathogenesis of chronic HBV infection [28,29]. A number of cytokines are released from macrophages or monocytes in response to stimulation by endotoxins, and these cytokines affect disease status [30]. We hypothesize that the association of RDW with an increased mortality risk may, in part, be due to an effect of inflammation on

anisocytosis and risk. Moreover, as shown in the present study, we also found an association between RDW and the severity of the liver disease, and patients with higher values of RDW tended to be older, had lower levels of hemoglobin, total protein, and serum albumin, and had higher INR and total bilirubin. Meanwhile, a typical anemia with a high RDW was found in liver cirrhosis principally in relation to the disease severity [31]. Several studies of the RBC mass and plasma volume in cirrhosis have shown that there is an expanded plasma volume in the presence of portal hypertension, leading to low hematcrit [32], and that RBC survival is also reduced in cirrhotic patients, especially those with anemia, although blood loss may partly contribute to the reduced RBC survival [33]. Hemolysis appears to be the major cause of anemia in advanced cirrhosis, in which an enlarged spleen sequesters and destroys blood cells efficiently, leading to macro-normoblastic bone marrow [34].

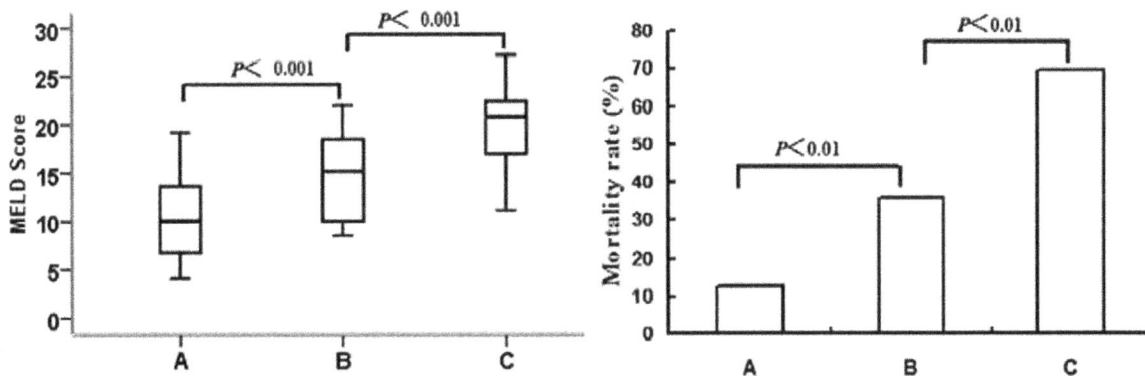

Figure 2. Comparisons of the Model for End-stage liver disease (MELD) score (left) and mortality rate (right) among patients with different red cell distribution width (RDW) values. Patients were divided into three groups based on serum RDW values: group A (≤15.0%), B (>15.0%, but <20.0%) and C (≥20.0%).

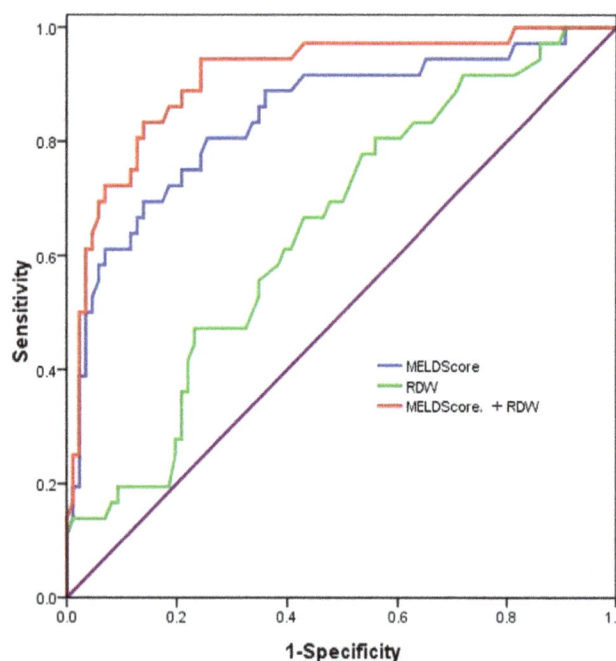

Figure 3. Receiver operating characteristic (ROC) curve analysis for prediction of mortality by red cell distribution width (RDW) values (green line), Model for End-stage Liver Disease (MELD) scores (blue line) and their combination (red line) at admission.

Table 3. Independent predictors of mortality by multivariate logistic regression analysis.

Predictor	Odds ratio	95% CI	P
RDW (%)	1.973	1.290–2.173	0.027
MELD Score	2.474	1.980–3.047	0.005

Variables included in the analysis were sex, age, hemoglobin, RDW, mean corpuscular volume, MELD score, serum albumin, total protein, international normalized ratio, and total bilirubin.
MELD, model for end-stage liver disease; RDW, red cell distribution width.

support system is effective in some cases, the mortality rate of CSHB may still reach 80%–100% in patients with stage III–IV hepatic encephalopathy [46]. For these patients, orthotopic liver transplantation [47] might be the last option. Therefore, identification of novel predicting biomarkers is critical in therapeutical management for CSHB.

A few limitations warrant consideration. First, we did not investigate the causes of elevated RDW values, such as iron or vitamin B12 deficiency, which could confound the association between RDW values and adverse outcome. Second, this was a single-center study and thus our relatively small sample size may have posed a limitation to this study. Therefore, our findings need to be confirmed in multi-center and prospectively designed studies. Finally, RDW values were not dynamically observed, and thus, whether RDW values are stepwise elevated when patient's condition is progressively deteriorated remains unclear.

In conclusion, RDW values are significantly increased in patients with hepatitis B and associated with the severity. Moreover, RDW values are an independent predicting factor for the 3-month mortality rate in patients with hepatitis B. Because RDW values are easily attainable at no additional cost to the routine complete blood cell counts and is highly reproducible, it may serve as an important biomarker. The strength of RDW's association with mortality risk that we and others have observed compares favorably with established risk factors. It is unknown, however, whether the risk associated with RDW is modifiable or if RDW itself is modified by current therapies that alter prognosis.

Author Contributions

Conceived and designed the experiments: WM. Performed the experiments: YL. Analyzed the data: MW. Contributed reagents/materials/analysis tools: WM. Wrote the paper: WM.

It should be mentioned that, in the present study, AHB, CHB and CSHB were diagnosed in accordance with the 2000 Xi'an Viral Hepatitis Management Guidelines recommended by the Chinese Society of Infectious Diseases and Parasitology, and the Chinese Society of Hepatology of the Chinese Medical Association [15]. In China, the term 'CSHB' is usually used for the fatal form of chronic hepatitis, which resembles the term 'liver failure caused by chronic hepatitis B'' in Western countries. Although the term is not uniformly used globally, this chronic liver condition often demonstrates serious clinical courses with fatal consequences. Acute attacks may occur in some patients with CHB. Moreover, the disease may develop into liver failure (*i.e.* CSHB) due to various factors, such as HBV mutations [35,36], coinfection with other hepatotropic viruses [37–42], over-work, alcohol overdose [43], long-term corticosteroid treatment [44], and bacterial infections [45], during the long course of the disease. Although the application of newly developed drugs with an artificial liver

References

1. Perkins SL (2003) Examination of blood and bone marrow. In: Greer JP, Foerster J, Lukens JN, Paraksevas F, Glader BE, eds. Wintrobe's Clinical Hematology. UT: Lippincott Wilkins & Williams. pp 5–25.
2. Bessman JD, Hurley EL, Groves MR (1983) Nondiscrete heterogeneity of human erythrocytes: comparison of Coulter-principle flow cytometry and Soret-hemoglo-binometry image analysis. Cytometry 3: 292–295.
3. England JM, Down MC (1974) Red-cell-volume distribution curves and the measurement of anisocytosis. Lancet 1: 701–703.
4. Demir A, Yarali N, Fisgin T, Duru F, Kara A (2002) Most reliable indices in differentiation between thalassemia trait and iron deficiency anemia. Pediatr Int 44: 612–616.
5. Felker GM, Allen LA, Pocock SJ, Shaw LK, McMurray JJ, et al. (2007) CHARM Investigators. Red cell distribution width as a novel prognostic marker in heart failure: data from the CHARM Program and the Duke Databank. J Am Coll Cardiol 50: 40–47.
6. Förhécz Z, Gombos T, Borgulya G, Pozsonyi Z, Prohászka Z, et al. (2009) Red cell distribution width in heart failure: prediction of clinical events and relationship with markers of ineffective erythropoiesis, inflammation, renal function, and nutritional state. Am Heart J 158: 659–666.

7. Pascual-Figal DA, Bonaque JC, Redondo B, Caro C, Manzano-Fernandez S, et al (2009) Red blood cell distribution width predicts long-term outcome regardless of anaemia status in acute heart failure patients. Eur J Heart Fail 11: 840–846.
8. Tonelli M, Sacks F, Arnold M, Moye L, Davis B, et al. (2008) for the Cholesterol and Recurrent Events (CARE) Trial Investigators. Relation between red blood cell distribution width and cardiovascular event rate in people with coronary disease. Circulation 117: 163–168.
9. Dabbah S, Hammerman H, Markiewicz W, Aronson D (2010) Relation between red cell distribution width and clinical outcomes after acute myocardial infarction. Am J Cardiol 105: 312–317.
10. Ani C, Ovbiagele B (2009) Elevated red blood cell distribution width predicts mortality in persons with known stroke. J Neurol Sci 277: 103–108.
11. Hampole CV, Mehrotra AK, Thenappan T, Gomberg, Maitland M, et al. (2009) Usefulness of red cell distribution width as a prognostic marker in pulmonary hypertension. Am J Cardiol. 104: 868–872.
12. Perlstein TS, Weuve J, Pfeffer MA, Beckman JA (2009) Red blood cell distribution width and mortality risk in a community based prospective cohort. Arch Intern Med 169: 588–594.

13. Patel KV, Ferrucci L, Ershler WB, Longo DL, Guralnik JM (2009) Red blood cell distribution width and the risk of death in middle-aged and older adults. Arch Intern Med169: 515–523.
14. Chen PC, Sung FC, Chien KL, Hsu HC, Su TC, et al. (2010) Red blood cell distribution width and risk of cardiovascular events and mortality in a community cohort in Taiwan. Am J Epidemiol 171: 214–220.
15. Anonymous (2000) Management scheme of diagnostic and therapy criteria of viral hepatitis. Zhonghua Gan Zang Bing Za Zhi (Chinese J. Hepatol.) 6: 324–329.
16. Shakil AO, Kramer D, Mazariegos GV, Fung JJ, Rakela J (2000) Acute liver failure: clinical features, outcome analysis, and applicability of prognostic criteria. Liver Transpl 2000; 6: 163–169.
17. Jalan R, Williams R (2002) Acute-on-chronic liver failure: pathophysiological basis of therapeutic options. Blood Purif 2002; 20: 252–226.
18. Huo TI, Wu JC, Lin HC, Lee FY, Hou MC, et al. (2005) Evaluation of the increase in model for end-stage liver disease (DMELD) score over time as a prognostic predictor in patients with advanced cirrhosis: risk factor analysis and comparison with initial MELD and Child–Turcotte–Pugh score. J. Hepatol 42: 826–832.
19. Huo TI, Lin HC, Wu JC, Lee FY, Hou MC, et al. (2006) Proposal of a modified Child–Turcotte–Pugh scoring system and comparison with the model for end-stage liver disease for outcome prediction in patients with cirrhosis. Liver Transpl. 12: 65–71.
20. Karnad A, Poskitt TR (1985) The automated complete blood cell count. Use of the red blood cell volume distribution width and mean platelet volume in evaluating anemia and thrombocytopenia. Arch Intern Med 145: 1270–1272.
21. Thompson WG, Meola T, Lipkin M Jr., Freedman ML (1988) Red cell distribution width, mean corpuscular volume, and transferrin saturation in the diagnosis of iron deficiency. Arch Intern Med 148: 2128–2130.
22. Evans TC, Jehle D (1991) The red blood cell distribution width. J EmergMed 9(suppl 1): 71–74.
23. Aslan D, Gumruk F, Gurgey A, Altay C (2002) Importance of RDW value in differential diagnosis of hypochrome anemias. Am J Hematol 69: 31–33.
24. Bingham J (1960) The macrocytosis of hepatic disease. Thin macrocytosis. Blood 15: 244–254.
25. Freeman RB Jr., Wiesner RH, Harper A, McDiarmid SV, Lake J, et al. (2002) The new liver allocation system: Moving toward evidence-based transplantation policy. Liver Transpl 8: 851–858.
26. Mao W, Ye B, Lin S, Fu Y, Chen Y, et al. (2010) The Prediction Value of MELD scoring System on Prognosis in the Acute on Chronic Liver Failure Patients With Artificial Liver Support System. ASAIO 56: 475–478.
27. Lippi G, Targher G, Montagnana M, Salvagno GL, Zoppini G, et al. (2009) Relation between red blood cell distribution width and inflammatory biomarkers in a large cohort of unselected outpatients. Arch Pathol Lab Med 133: 628–632.
28. Douglas SW, Adamson JW (1975) The anemia of chronic disorders: studies of marrow regulation and iron metabolism. Blood 45: 55–65.
29. Weiss G, Goodnough LT (2005) Anemia of chronic disease. N Engl J Med 352: 1011–1023.
30. Chisari FV, Ferrari C (1995) Hepatitis B virus immunopathogesis. Ann Rev Immunol 13: 29–60.
31. Bertoletti A, D'Elios MM, Boni C, De Carli M, Zignego AL, et al. (1997) Different cytokine profiles of intrahepatic T cells in chronic hepatitis B and hepatitis C virus infections. Gastroenterology. 112: 193–199.
32. Mao WL, Chen Y, Chen YM, Li LJ (2011) Changes of Serum Cytokine Levels in Patients with Acute on Chronic Liver Failure Treated by Artificial Liver Support System. J Clin Gastroenterol 45: 551–555.
33. Lieberman FL, Reynolds TB (1967) Plasma volume in cirrhosis of the liver: its relation to portal hypertension, ascites, and renal failure. J Clin Invest 46: 1297–1308.
34. Maruyama S, Hirayama C, Yamamoto S, Koda M, Udagawa A, et al. (2001) Red blood cell status in alcoholic and non-alcoholic liver disease. J Lab Clin Med. 138: 332–337.
35. Katz R, Velasco M, Guzman C, Alessandri H (1964) Red cell survival estimated by radioactive chromium in hepatobiliary disease. Gastroenterology 46: 399–404.
36. Nunnally RM, Levine I (1961) Macronormoblastic hyperplasia of the bone marrow in cirrhosis. Am J Med 30: 972–975.
37. Okumura A, Ishikawa T, Yoshioka K, Yuasa R, Fukuzawa Y, Kakumu S (2001) Mutation at codon 130 in hepatitis B virus (HBV) core region increases markedly during acute exacerbation of hepatitis in chronic HBV carriers. J Gastroenterol 2001; 36: 103–110.
38. Asahina Y, Enomoto N, Ogura Y, Kurosaki M, Sakuma I, Izumi N, et al. (1996) Sequential changes in full-length genomes of hepatitis B virus accompanying acute exacerbation of chronic hepatitis B. J Hepatol 1996; 25: 787–794.
39. Lai YC, Hu RT, Yang SS, Wu CH (2002) Coinfection of TT virus and response to interferon therapy in patients with chronic hepatitis B or C. World J Gastroenterol 2002; 8: 567–570.
40. Chu CM, Lin SM, Hsieh SY, Yeh CT, Lin DY, Sheen IS, et al. (1999) Etiology of sporadic acute viral hepatitis in Taiwan: the role of hepatitis C virus, hepatitis E virus and GB virus-C/hepatitis G virus in an endemic area of hepatitis A and B. J Med Virol 1999; 50. 154–159.
41. Coursaget P, Buisson Y, N'Gawara MN, Van Cuyck-Gandre H, Roue R (1998) Role of hepatitis E virus in sporadic cases of acute and fulminant hepatitis in an endemic area (Chad). Am J Trop MedHyg 1998; 58: 330–334.
42. Xess A, Kumar M, Minz S, Sharma HP, Shahi SK (2001) Prevalence of hepatitis B and hepatitis C virus coinfection in chronic liver disease. Indian J Pathol Microbiol 2001; 44: 253–255.
43. Summerfield JA (2000) Virus hepatitis update. J R Coll Physicians Lond 2000; 34: 381–385.
44. Imperial JC (1999) Natural history of chronic hepatitis B and C. J Gastroenterol Hepatol 1999; 14(Suppl): S1–5.
45. Shiota G, Harada K, Oyama K, Udagawa A, Nomi T, Tanaka K, et al. (2000) Severe exacerbation of hepatitis after short-term corticosteroid therapy in a patients with "latent" chronic hepatitis B. Liver 2000; 20: 415–420.
46. Horney JT, Galambos JT (1977) The liver during and after fulminant hepatitis. Gastroenterology 1997; 73: 639–645.
47. Xue YL, Zhao SF, Luo Y, Li XJ, Duan ZP, Chen XP, et al. (2001) TECA hybrid artificial liver support system in treatment of acute liver failure. World J Gastroenterol 2001; 7: 826–829.
48. Tang ZY (2001) Hepatocellular carcinoma-cause, treatment and metastasis. World J Gastroenterol 2001; 7: 445–454.
49. Bramhall SR, Minford E, Gunson B, Buckels JA (2001) Liver transplantation in the UK. World J Gastroenterol 2001; 7: 602–611.

11

The Treatment Cascade for Chronic Hepatitis C Virus Infection in the United States: A Systematic Review and Meta-Analysis

Baligh R. Yehia[1,2,3]*, **Asher J. Schranz**[4], **Craig A. Umscheid**[1,2,3,5], **Vincent Lo Re III**[1,3]

1 Department of Medicine, University of Pennsylvania Perelman School of Medicine, Philadelphia, Pennsylvania, United States of America, 2 Leonard Davis Institute of Health Economics, University of Pennsylvania, Philadelphia, Pennsylvania, United States of America, 3 Center for Clinical Epidemiology and Biostatistics, Department of Biostatistics and Epidemiology, University of Pennsylvania Perelman School of Medicine, Philadelphia, Pennsylvania, United States of America, 4 Department of Medicine, New York University School of Medicine, New York, New York, United States of America, 5 Center for Evidenced-Based Practice, University of Pennsylvania Health System, Philadelphia, Pennsylvania, United States of America

Abstract

Background: Identifying gaps in care for people with chronic hepatitis C virus (HCV) infection is important to clinicians, public health officials, and federal agencies. The objective of this study was to systematically review the literature to provide estimates of the proportion of chronic HCV-infected persons in the United States (U.S.) completing each step along a proposed HCV treatment cascade: (1) infected with chronic HCV; (2) diagnosed and aware of their infection; (3) with access to outpatient care; (4) HCV RNA confirmed; (5) liver fibrosis staged by biopsy; (6) prescribed HCV treatment; and (7) achieved sustained virologic response (SVR).

Methods: We searched MEDLINE, EMBASE, and the Cochrane Database of Systematic Reviews for articles published between January 2003 and July 2013. Two reviewers independently identified articles addressing each step in the cascade. Studies were excluded if they focused on specific populations, did not present original data, involved only a single site, were conducted outside of the U.S., or only included data collected prior to 2000.

Results: 9,581 articles were identified, 117 were retrieved for full text review, and 10 were included. Overall, 3.5 million people were estimated to have chronic HCV in the U.S. Fifty percent (95% CI 43–57%) were diagnosed and aware of their infection, 43% (CI 40–47%) had access to outpatient care, 27% (CI 27–28%) had HCV RNA confirmed, 17% (CI 16–17%) underwent liver fibrosis staging, 16% (CI 15–16%) were prescribed treatment, and 9% (CI 9–10%) achieved SVR.

Conclusions: Continued efforts are needed to improve HCV care in the U.S. The proposed HCV treatment cascade provides a framework for evaluating the delivery of HCV care over time and within subgroups, and will be useful in monitoring the impact of new screening efforts and advances in antiviral therapy.

Editor: Stacey A. Rizza, Mayo Clinic, United States of America

Funding: This work was supported by the National Institutes of Health [K23 MH097647 to BRY and K01 AI070001 to VLR]. The funders had no role in study design, data collection and analysis, decision to publish, or preparation of the manuscript.

Competing Interests: BRY receives investigator-initiated research support (to the University of Pennsylvania) from Gilead Sciences; AJS has no such interests; CAU has no such interests; VLR receives investigator-initiated research support (to the University of Pennsylvania) from AstraZeneca, Bristol Myers-Squibb, Merck, and Gilead Sciences.

* Email: byehia@upenn.edu

Introduction

The HIV treatment cascade (diagnosis, linkage to care, retention in care, prescription of antiretroviral therapy, and viral suppression) is an effective tool for improving the health of people living with HIV (PLWH) and for achieving the public health benefits of antiretroviral therapy [1,2]. It has been used by federal, state, and local agencies to identify gaps in the delivery of care, prioritize and target resources, and monitor the United States (U.S.) *National HIV/AIDS Strategy* [2–6]. As different patient behaviors and health system mechanisms are required to successfully complete each step of the cascade, it also demonstrates the need for coordinated action to meet treatment goals [7].

Similar to PLWH, people with chronic hepatitis C virus (HCV) infection need to fulfill several steps along a care continuum to achieve optimal health outcomes [8,9]. First, individuals must be diagnosed and aware of their HCV infection and seek care [10]. Once in care, patients should have HCV RNA confirmation testing and undergo liver fibrosis staging to help inform prognosis and make decisions regarding HCV therapy [11]. Lastly, individuals must receive and adhere to HCV treatment to achieve a sustained virologic response (SVR) [12]. Throughout this continuum, patients should receive recommended screenings, vaccinations, and care as outlined by national guidelines [11,13].

This HCV treatment cascade aligns with the goals of the U.S. *Action Plan for the Prevention, Care, and Treatment of Viral Hepatitis,* which established early identification, linkage to care and treatment, and improved quality of care as top priorities for combating the silent epidemic of chronic HCV infection [14]. As antiviral therapy for chronic HCV advances to become more convenient, effective, and better-tolerated, monitoring the HCV treatment cascade will become increasingly important to clinicians, public health officials, and federal agencies [15]. This systematic review and meta-analysis builds on prior studies evaluating rates of HCV detection, referral to care, and treatment [16,17], and integrates published data to provide estimates of the number of chronic HCV-infected persons living in the U.S. completing each step along the HCV treatment cascade. These data will help identify key deficits in chronic HCV care that will be important for the development of programs to improve diagnosis, linkage to care, and management of this disease.

Methods

Data Sources and Searches

We examined data addressing 7 key steps along the HCV treatment cascade to identify the number of people with: (1) chronic HCV infection; and the proportion of chronic HCV-infected individuals: (2) diagnosed and aware of their infection; (3) with access to outpatient care; (4) HCV RNA confirmed; (5) disease staged by liver biopsy; (6) prescribed HCV treatment; and (7) achieving SVR [16,17]. We searched MEDLINE, EMBASE, and the Cochrane Database of Systematic Reviews for English language articles published between January 2003 and July 2013 using keywords and structured language representing each step along the HCV treatment cascade [18]. Details appear in **Table S1**.

Study Selection

Titles and abstracts were screened by a single reviewer (BRY or AS). Articles were selected for full-text review if they were relevant to HCV treatment cascade steps. Two independent reviewers (BRY and VLR) evaluated articles selected for full-text review using a standardized form. Disagreements were resolved by consensus.

Studies were included if they addressed one or more steps along the HCV treatment cascade, were conducted inside the U.S., presented original data, and used data collected after January 1, 2000. We intentionally focus on studies conducted inside the U.S., and not in other developed counties, as multiple steps in the treatment cascade are directly influenced by the healthcare delivery system and these systems vary widely across countries [19]. The use of data collected after January 1, 2000 corresponds with the introduction of dual therapy with a pegylated interferon and ribavirin for the treatment of chronic HCV infection that occurred in the early 2000 s, and was also selected to ensure the use of the most current data available. To improve generalizability, single site studies and those exclusively focusing on specific populations (e.g., only immigrants, injection drug users, those with HIV/HCV co-infection) were excluded. If multiple publications resulted from the same patient sample or longitudinal cohort, we selected the most inclusive and current study. Bibliographies of included studies were reviewed for additional studies, and three experts in chronic HCV infection were contacted to ensure no relevant studies were missed.

Data Extraction

Data from each included study were extracted by one author (BRY) into tables stratified by HCV treatment cascade step and verified by another author (VLR) for accuracy. Discrepancies were resolved through consensus. We extracted information on study design, period, population, sample size, definition of outcome measure(s), and raw data to permit calculation of estimates of chronic HCV-infected persons completing each cascade step.

Data Synthesis and Analysis

The number of chronic HCV-infected persons completing each step along the HCV treatment cascade was determined. After ascertaining the initial estimate of chronic HCV-infected persons in the U.S. (cascade step 1), we estimated the number of chronic HCV-infected persons diagnosed and aware of their infection (cascade step 2). Among those diagnosed and aware of their chronic HCV infection, we estimated the number with access to outpatient care (cascade step 3). Next, among chronic HCV-infected persons diagnosed and aware of their infection and with access to outpatient care, we estimated the number who had: HCV RNA confirmed (cascade step 4), underwent a liver biopsy (cascade step 5), and antiviral therapy prescribed (cascade step 6). Since cascade steps 4–6 had the same denominator, the proportion of persons prescribed HCV treatment was not conditioned on the number with HCV RNA confirmation and liver biopsy. Finally, among persons prescribed HCV treatment, we estimated the number that achieved a sustained virologic response (cascade step 7). Using the above estimates, we calculated the proportion of chronic HCV-infected persons completing each step along the HCV treatment cascade by dividing the number of people who completed each step (numerator) by the number of chronic HCV-infected persons in the U.S. (denominator, obtained from cascade step 1).

Since multiple studies were identified for HCV treatment cascade steps 5–7, we performed random-effects meta-analyses for these steps to determine pooled prevalence estimates with 95% confidence intervals (CIs). We assessed the heterogeneity between study results using the I^2 statistic. Significant heterogeneity was defined as an I^2 statistic $\geq 50\%$ [20]. Analyses were performed in OpenMeta[Analyst] [21].

The U.S. Veterans Health Administration (VA) is the largest single provider of HCV care in the U.S., currently caring for approximately 165,000 veterans with chronic HCV infection [13]. Because of differences in the prevalence of comorbid diseases, as well as the management and treatment of chronic HCV infection between U.S. Veterans and non-Veterans [13], we distinguished VA and non-VA studies. The primary analysis focused on non-VA studies. In a secondary analysis, we preferentially selected VA studies when available.

Results

Our literature search yielded 9,581 citations (excluding duplicates), of which 117 met eligibility for full text review (**Figure 1**). Of those, 107 were excluded because they did not address any of the study questions, were conducted outside of the U.S., did not present original data, only analyzed data collected prior to 2000, involved a single site, focused on special populations, or examined study subjects used in a more recent study. Among the remaining 10 articles [22–31], three focused exclusively on U.S. Veterans. Details on the study populations, periods, and sample sizes of included studies by cascade step are shown in **Table 1**.

Based on National Health and Nutrition Examination Survey (NHANES) data from 1999 through 2002, approximately 3.2 million people in the U.S. have chronic HCV infection [22]. Since NHANES did not sample high-risk groups, particularly incarcerated, homeless, or institutionalized individuals, the actual preva-

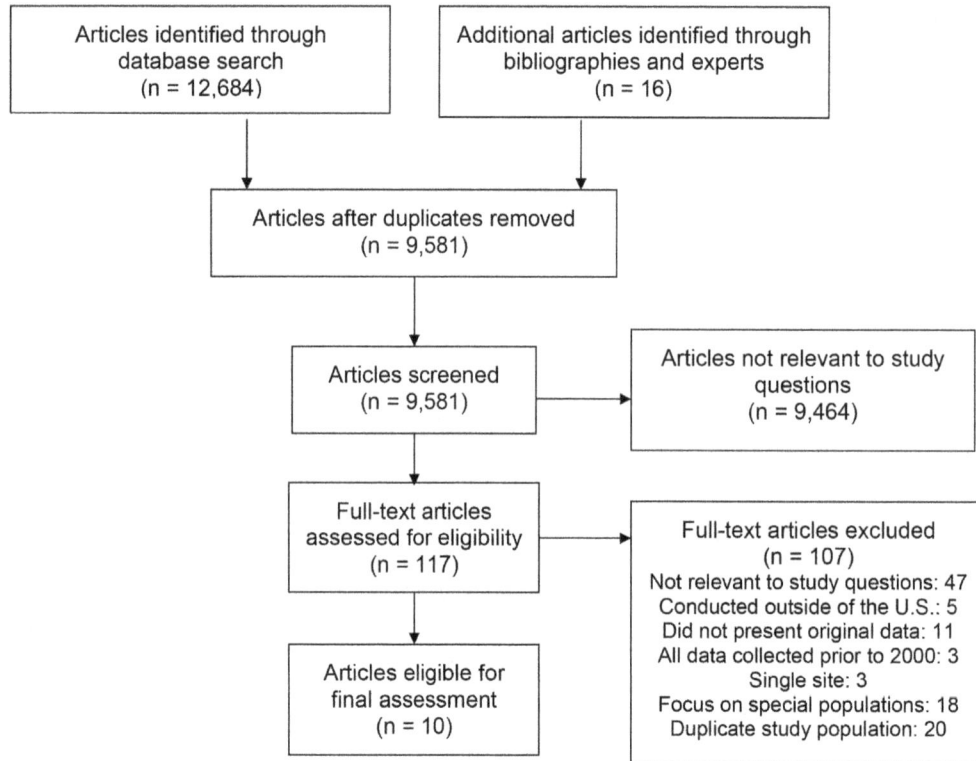

Figure 1. Summary of Article Search, Screening, and Selection Process.

Table 1. Evaluation of chronic hepatitis C virus treatment cascade studies eligible for final assessment.

Author, Year	Data Source	Time Period	Sample Size	Estimate (95% CI)	Pooled Prevalence Estimate (95% CI)*
Study Question 1: Number of people with chronic HCV infection					
Armstrong et al, 2006	NHAS	1999–2002	15,079	3,500,000 people	–
Study Question 2: Proportion aware of their infection					
Younossi et al, 2013	NHAS	2001–2010	203	49.8% (42.9–56.7)	–
Study Question 3: Proportion with access to healthcare, among those aware of their infection					
Younossi et al, 2013	NHAS	2001–2010	101	86.9% (80.3–93.5)	–
Study Question 4: Proportion HCV RNA confirmed, among those in care					
Moorman et al, 2013	4 HCOs	2001–2010	8,810	62.9% (61.9–63.9)	–
Study Question 5: Proportion disease staged by liver biopsy, among those in care					
Moorman et al, 2013	4 HCOs	2001–2010	8,810	38.4% (37.4–39.4)	–
Groessl et a, 2012	*VA*	*1996–2006*	*171,893*	*16.7% (16.5–16.9)*	
Study Question 6: Proportion prescribed HCV treatment, among those in care					
Moorman et al, 2013	4 HCOs	2001–2010	8,810	36.4% (35.4–37.4)	36.7% (35.8–37.6)
Kanwal et al, 2010	Insurance claims	2003–2006	2,893	37.5% (35.7–39.3)	
Kanwal et al, 2012	*VA*	*2003–2006*	*34,749*	*17.9% (17.5–18.3)*	–
Study Question 7: Proportion achieving SVR, among those in care and prescribed HCV treatment					
Mitra et al, 2010	Insurance claims	2002–2006	575	58.4% (54.4–62.4)	58.8% (56.1–61.5)
Arora et al, 2011	22 clinics	2004–2009	407	58.0% (53.2–62.8)	
Russell et al, 2012	Health system	2002–2008	259	60.1% (54.1–66.1)	
Backus et al, 2011	*VA*	*2001–2009*	*16,864*	*44.1% (43.4–44.9)*	–

Abbreviations: HCOs = healthcare organization; NHANES = National Health and Nutrition Examination Survey; VA = Veterans Administration.
*Obtained from meta-analyses. These estimates do not include Veterans Administration-based studies (*in italics*).

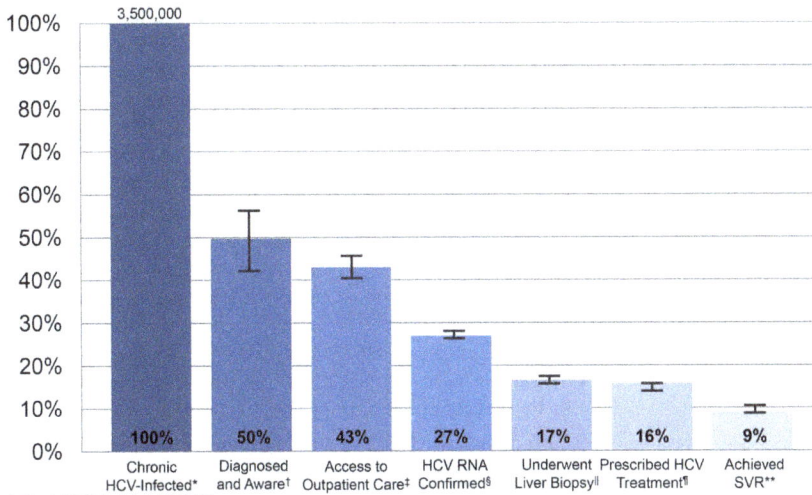

* Chronic HCV-Infected; N=3,500,000.
† Calculated as estimated number chronic HCV-infected (3,500,000) x estimated percentage diagnosed and aware of their infection (49.8%); n=1,743,000.
‡ Calculated as estimated number diagnosed and aware (1,743,000) x estimated percentage with access to outpatient care (86.9%); n=1,514,667.
§ Calculated as estimated number with access to outpatient care (1,514,667) x estimated percentage HCV RNA confirmed (62.9%); n=952,726.
‖ Calculated as estimated number with access to outpatient care (1,514,667) x estimated percentage who underwent liver biopsy (38.4%); n=581,632.
¶ Calculated as estimated number with access to outpatient care (1,514,667) x estimated percentage prescribed HCV treatment (36.7%); n=555,883.
** Calculated as estimated number prescribed HCV treatment (555,883) x estimated percentage who achieved SVR (58.8%); n=326,859.
Note: Only non-VA studies are included in the above HCV treatment cascade.

Figure 2. Treatment Cascade for People with Chronic Hepatitis C Virus (HCV) Infection, Prevalence Estimates with 95% Confidence Intervals. * Chronic HCV-Infected; N = 3,500,000. † Calculated as estimated number chronic HCV-infected (3,500,000) x estimated percentage diagnosed and aware of their infection (49.8%); n = 1,743,000. ‡ Calculated as estimated number diagnosed and aware (1,743,000) x estimated percentage with access to outpatient care (86.9%); n = 1,514,667. § Calculated as estimated number with access to outpatient care (1,514,667) x estimated percentage HCV RNA confirmed (62.9%); n = 952,726. ‖ Calculated as estimated number with access to outpatient care (1,514,667) x estimated percentage who underwent liver biopsy (38.4%); n = 581,632. ¶ Calculated as estimated number with access to outpatient care (1,514,667) x estimated percentage prescribed HCV treatment (36.7%); n = 555,883. ** Calculated as estimated number prescribed HCV treatment (555,883) x estimated percentage who achieved SVR (58.8%); n = 326,859. Note: Only non-VA studies are included in the above HCV treatment cascade.

lence of chronic HCV infection was estimated to be 3.5 million [22]. This estimate was used for cascade step 1 (**Figure 2**).

Among those living with chronic HCV, approximately 50% are unaware of their diagnosis based on data from the NHANES Hepatitis C Follow-Up Survey [31,32]. A total of 500 participants who tested positive for HCV RNA between 2001 and 2010 were asked if they were aware of their HCV status before being notified by NHANES. Half of the 203 respondents were unaware of their HCV status [31,32]. Thus, 1,743,000 chronic HCV-infected persons (49.8% [95% CI, 42.9–56.7%] of 3.5 million) are estimated to be diagnosed and aware of their infection (cascade step 2).

In this same study, participants who were aware of their chronic HCV status were also asked about their health insurance status [31,32]. Among those aware of their chronic HCV infection, 86.9% had health insurance compared to 60.4% of those unaware of their HCV infection. Thus, 1,514,667 persons (43.3% [95% CI, 39.9–46.6%] of 3.5 million) are estimated to be aware of their chronic HCV diagnosis and have access to outpatient healthcare (cascade step 3).

Once in care, measurement of HCV RNA is needed to confirm diagnosis of chronic HCV infection, and staging of liver disease is important for guiding HCV treatment decisions. Data from the Chronic Hepatitis B and C Cohort Study, which included 8,810 patients with chronic HCV receiving care at four health systems in the U.S. (Detroit, Michigan; Danville, Pennsylvania; Honolulu, Hawaii; and Portland, Oregon), reported that 5,540 (62.9%) of these patients had confirmatory HCV RNA testing, and 3,380 (38.4%) had hepatic fibrosis staging with a liver biopsy during 2001–2010 [29]. Based on these data, 952,726 persons (27.2% [95% CI, 26.8–27.7%] of 3.5 million) are estimated to be aware of their chronic HCV diagnosis, have access to healthcare, and

received confirmatory HCV RNA testing (cascade step 4) and 581,632 (16.6% [95% CI, 16.2–17.1%] of 3.5 million) are estimated to be aware of their chronic HCV diagnosis, have access to healthcare, and have underwent a liver biopsy for hepatic fibrosis staging (cascade step 5). In contrast, an evaluation of the national VA Hepatitis C Clinical Case Registry from 1997 to 2006 indicated that only 16.7% (28,677 of 171,893) of VA patients with chronic HCV received a liver biopsy [25]. Using these VA-based data, 252,949 persons (7.2% [95% CI, 7.1–7.3%] of 3.5 million) are estimated to be aware of their chronic HCV diagnosis, have access to healthcare, and received a liver biopsy (cascade step 5).

Two non-VA studies evaluated prescription of pegylated interferon plus ribavirin treatment among patients with chronic HCV infection [27,29]. Given the recent introduction of direct-acting antiviral agents, we did not identify any population-based studies evaluating these agents that met our selection criteria. Kanwal and colleagues examined prescription rates among 2,893 patients enrolled in one of the largest commercial health insurance carriers in the U.S. [27], while Moorman et al. focused on 8,810 patients receiving care within four U.S. health systems [29]. The proportion of chronic HCV-infected patients prescribed pegylated interferon plus ribavirin ranged from 36–38%, with a pooled proportion of 36.7% (95% CI, 35.8–37.6%; $I^2 = 4$%). Thus, 555,883 persons (15.9% [95% CI, 15.5–16.3%] of 3.5 million) are estimated to be aware of their chronic HCV diagnosis, have access to healthcare, and have received HCV therapy (cascade step 6). This estimate differed from data reported by the VA system, where 17.9% (6,224 of 34,749) of chronic HCV-infected patients have been prescribed pegylated interferon plus ribavirin treatment [26]. Using these VA-based data, 271,125 people (7.7% [95% CI, 7.6–7.9%] of 3.5 million) are estimated to be aware of their chronic

HCV diagnosis, have access to healthcare, and received HCV treatment (cascade step 6).

Three non-VA studies examined SVR rates among chronic HCV-infected patients who received antiviral therapy [23,28,30]. These included an analysis of 575 patients (71% HCV genotype 1, 29% HCV genotype 2/3) within 40 managed care plans [28]; a study of 407 patients (57% HCV genotype 1, 42% HCV genotype 2/3) in care within a network composed of 21 community clinics and one academic health center [23]; and an evaluation of 258 patients in an integrated health care system (55% HCV genotype 1/4/6, 45% HCV genotype 2/3) [30]. The proportion of treated chronic HCV-infected patients who achieved SVR varied by genotype, with a pooled proportion of 47.0% (95% CI, 42.0–52.1%; $I^2 = 0$%) for genotype 1, 75.1% (95% CI, 65.3–84.9%; $I^2 = 74$%) for genotype 2/3, and 58.8% (95% CI, 56.1–61.5%; $I^2 = 0$%) for all genotypes. Using the overall pooled proportion, 326,859 people (9.3% [95% CI, 8.9–9.8%] of 3.5 million) are estimated to be aware of their chronic HCV diagnosis, have access to healthcare, have been prescribed antiviral therapy, and achieved SVR (cascade step 7). In comparison, a national study of 16,864 chronic HCV-infected Veterans who received antiviral therapy (72% HCV genotype 1, 28% HCV genotype 2/3) reports an overall SVR rate of 44.1% [24]. Using these VA-based data, 245,144 people (7.0% [95% CI, 6.9–7.1%] of 3.5 million) are estimated to be aware of their chronic HCV diagnosis, have access to healthcare, received HCV treatment (based on the VA estimate reported above), and achieved SVR (cascade step 7).

Discussion

This review identifies large gaps between current practice and treatment goals for people with chronic HCV infection. It also highlights multiple opportunities for improving engagement along the HCV treatment cascade, particularly in the diagnosis and awareness of infection, prescription of antiviral therapy, and achievement of SVR. Our study confirms findings reported in a commentary by Holmberg *et al.* that only 5–6% of all people with chronic HCV infection in the U.S. successfully progressed from detection of HCV infection to achievement of SVR [16] and extends this work by rigorously reviewing and meta-analyzing the literature, highlighting differences between U.S. Veteran and non-Veteran populations. In addition, the proposed HCV treatment cascade provides a framework for evaluating the delivery of HCV care over time and within subgroups, which will be necessary to monitor the impact of new screening efforts [33,34] and advances in antiviral therapy [34,35] which will likely increase the number of people completing each step along the cascade.

In 2012, the Centers for Disease Control and Prevention recommended one-time HCV testing without prior ascertainment of risk for persons born between 1945 and 1965 - a group estimated to account for three-fourths of all HCV infections in the U.S. [34]. Implementation of this recommendation, which also calls for referral of newly identified HCV-infected persons for management, may improve the proportion of individuals diagnosed and aware of their infection and referred to care.

Hepatic fibrosis assessment via liver biopsy is not required for HCV therapy, as per current professional guidelines [11]. However, staging of liver fibrosis remains important for determining the urgency and timing of HCV therapy and for identification of cirrhosis, which should prompt screening for hepatocellular carcinoma and monitoring for the development of hepatic decompensation [36,37]. We therefore included hepatic fibrosis assessment as a step in the HCV treatment cascade. While liver biopsy has traditionally been the "gold standard" for assessing liver disease, noninvasive tests, including serum biochemical markers (e.g., aspartate aminotransferase-to-platelet ratio index, FIB-4, HCV FibroSure [LabCorp, Burlington, NC], Hepascore [San Juan Capistrano, CA], Fibrotest [Biopredictive, Paris, France]) and imaging modalities (e.g., transient elastometry [FibroScan, Echosens, Paris, France]), are increasingly playing a role in staging liver fibrosis screening [11,33,38]. As these noninvasive and more convenient tests evolve, it is likely that the number of patients undergoing hepatic fibrosis staging will increase.

The advent of new direct-acting antiviral agents will shorten treatment duration, likely increase the number of people offered treatment, and improve HCV cure rates (final two steps of the HCV treatment cascade) [15,35]. However, educating providers and the general public about HCV prevention, care, and treatment; ensuring access to providers skilled in the treatment of HCV infection; and addressing the high cost of these agents will be critical to maximizing the benefits of these new therapies [14,39]. In a recent cost-effectiveness simulation evaluating birth-cohort HCV screening and subsequent treatment of HCV-infected adults, Rein and colleagues note that birth-cohort screening followed by HCV treatment including direct-acting antiviral agents will increase quality-adjusted life-years (QALYs) by $532,200 and medical costs by $19.0 billion, for an incremental cost-effectiveness ratio of $35,700 per QALY saved (95% credible interval, $28,200 to $47,200) [40]. While these simulations accounted for common HCV-associated complications, funders, public health administrators, and providers should be aware of the financial burden of untreated HCV infection. Using data from the 2010 U.S. National Health and Wellness Survey, El Khoury et al. note that persons with untreated HCV infection had significantly ($p < 0.001$) higher annual productivity losses ($10,316 vs. $5,459 per employed person) and annual all-cause healthcare costs ($22,818 vs. $15,362 per person) compared to HCV-uninfected individuals. [41] Evaluating the trade-off between the benefits and costs of these new agents will be critical to scaling up HCV treatment [35].

Individuals' progression along the HCV treatment cascade varied widely, with large drop-offs occurring at diagnosis and awareness of infection, prescription of antiviral therapy, and achievement of SVR. Studies are needed to evaluate and compare the population-level benefits and costs of interventions, such as screening and treatment efforts, at each step. These data can further assist public health officials in allocating resources to increase the proportion of chronic HCV-infected patients completing the cascade steps. In addition, monitoring the HCV treatment cascade over time will be critically important to defining overall progress and identifying persistent barriers at individual steps.

Since the VA system is the largest single provider of HCV care in the U.S. and because of potential differences in the management of chronic HCV infection among U.S. Veterans [42], we conducted a separate analysis to estimate the numbers of chronic HCV-infected people completing steps 5–7 in the HCV treatment cascade using VA-specific data. Among chronic HCV-infected Veterans in care, the proportion of those who received hepatic fibrosis staging by liver biopsy and who were prescribed HCV treatment was 22% and 19% lower, respectively, compared to the general population. Similarly, among Veterans with chronic HCV infection who were prescribed pegylated interferon plus ribavirin, a smaller proportion achieved SVR compared to the general population (44% vs. 58%). These variations may be due to differences in patient populations or in VA provider practices. Prior studies indicate that Veterans with chronic HCV have higher rates of absolute and relative contraindications to HCV treatment than persons seen at non-VA clinics [43–45]. In addition, differences in medication adherence [12], provider management, and health system factors may contribute to the lower proportion of Veterans completing the final steps of the HCV treatment cascade. Future studies should evaluate how the HCV treatment cascade changes for Veterans and non-Veterans with the advancement of new direct-acting antiviral therapies.

This study has several potential limitations. First, our treatment cascade included seven steps, as identified by prior research [8,9], evaluated at one time point. Future studies should explore the addition (e.g. linkage to and retention in HCV care) and deletion (e.g., liver biopsy) of cascade steps to best assist public health officials in monitoring HCV care in the U.S. Further, since patients receive care over time, the studies included in this analysis may not have allowed sufficient time for certain steps in the HCV treatment cascade to take place. Monitoring the steps of the cascade over time may help to define overall progress toward population-based goals and barriers at individual steps. Second, our systematic review was limited by the relatively small number of studies identified, particularly for cascade steps 1–3. Many studies excluded prisoners and homeless individuals, populations heavily affect by chronic HCV infection. These exclusions may underestimate cascade steps, particularly access to outpatient care. Third, we broadly focused on estimating the number of chronic HCV-infected people in the general population. Estimates for each step in the HCV treatment cascade could not be determined by sex, race/ethnicity, socioeconomic status, injection drug use, and HIV status because these data were not available in the included studies. Future studies should determine the cascade within these subgroups. Fourth, HCV RNA confirmation in evaluated studies was restricted to patients' healthcare network. This may underestimate HCV RNA testing, particularly for patients who transfer care between providers. Similarly, liver biopsy was used as the marker for HCV disease staging; however, this may underestimate the number of people who were staged through the use of noninvasive tests. Fifth, not all patients immediately require or are eligible to receive antiviral therapy for chronic HCV, which may underestimate the proportion of patients treated. Further, failure to achieve SVR may be a consequence of biological factors, including HCV genotype, treatment efficacy and tolerability, or

adherence to therapy. Differentiating between these causes may be important because each requires a different intervention strategy. In addition, data on prescription and SVR rates of newer direct-acting anti-HCV medications were not available. Monitoring how these steps change as providers increasingly use these new therapies will be critical. Lastly, we present the treatment cascade for people with chronic HCV infection living in the U.S., but evaluating the treatment cascade in other countries will be important and may help identify models for improving HCV monitoring and public health in those areas.

In summary, our results suggest that continued efforts are needed to improve HCV care in the U.S. In a field that is changing rapidly, with increased attention on HCV screening and approval of new, effective direct-acting antiviral agents, this proposed HCV treatment cascade provides a framework for identifying gaps in care. This framework will be useful in monitoring the impact of new public health initiatives, care models, and treatments. Only by increasing the number of persons completing each step in the cascade can the goals of the U.S. *Action Plan for the Prevention, Care, and Treatment of Viral Hepatitis* be achieved.

Acknowledgments

We are grateful to Drs. K. Rajender Reddy, Jay R. Kostman, and Stacey Trooskin for their advice and support, and to Dr. Matthew D. Mitchell for his assistance with data analysis.

Author Contributions

Conceived and designed the experiments: BRY AJS CAU VLR. Performed the experiments: BRY AJS CAU VLR. Analyzed the data: BRY AJS CAU VLR. Wrote the paper: BRY AJS CAU VLR.

References

1. Gardner EM, McLees MP, Steiner JF, Del Rio C, Burman WJ (2011) The spectrum of engagement in HIV care and its relevance to test-and-treat strategies for prevention of HIV infection. Clin Infect Dis 52: 793–800.
2. Vital Signs (2011) HIV prevention through care and treatment–United States. MMWR Morb Mortal Wkly Rep 60: 1618–1623.
3. Hull MW, Wu Z, Montaner JS (2012) Optimizing the engagement of care cascade: a critical step to maximize the impact of HIV treatment as prevention. Curr Opin HIV AIDS 7: 579–586.
4. Mahle Gray K, Tang T, Shouse L, Li J, Mermin J, et al. (2013) Using the HIV surveillance system to monitor the National HIV/AIDS Strategy. Am J Public Health 103: 141–147.
5. Yehia B, Frank I (2011) Battling AIDS in America: an evaluation of the National HIV/AIDS Strategy. Am J Public Health 101: e4–8.
6. Fleishman JA, Yehia BR, Moore RD, Korthuis PT, Gebo KA, et al. (2012) Establishment, retention, and loss to follow-up in outpatient HIV care. J Acquir Immune Defic Syndr 60: 249–259.
7. Mugavero MJ, Amico KR, Horn T, Thompson MA (2013) The State of Engagement in HIV Care in the United States: From Cascade to Continuum to Control. Clin Infect Dis 57(8):1164–71.
8. Insitute of Medicine (2010) Hepatitis and Liver Cancer: A National Strategy for Prevention and Control of Hepatitis B and C. Washington, DC.
9. Edlin BR (2011) Perspective: test and treat this silent killer. Nature 474: S18–19.
10. Brau N (2013) Evaluation of the hepatitis C virus-infected patient: the initial encounter. Clin Infect Dis 56: 853–860.
11. Ghany MG, Strader DB, Thomas DL, Seeff LB, American Association for the Study of Liver Disease (2009) Diagnosis, management, and treatment of hepatitis C: an update. Hepatology 49: 1335–1374.

12. Lo Re V III, Teal V, Localio AR, Amorosa VK, Kaplan DE, et al. (2011) Relationship between adherence to hepatitis C virus therapy and virologic outcomes: a cohort study. Ann Intern Med 155: 353–360.
13. Yee HS, Chang MF, Pocha C, Lim J, Ross D, et al. (2012) Update on the management and treatment of hepatitis C virus infection: recommendations from the Department of Veterans Affairs Hepatitis C Resource Center Program and the National Hepatitis C Program Office. Am J Gastroenterol 107: 669–689; quiz 690.
14. US Department of Health and Human Services (2011) Combating the Silent Epidemic of Viral Hepatitis: Action Plan for the Prevention, Care & Treatment of Viral Hepatitis. Washington, DC. pp. 1–76.
15. Aghemo A, De Francesco R (2013) New horizons in Hepatitis C antiviral therapy with direct-acting antivirals. Hepatology 58(1):428–38.
16. Holmberg SD, Spradling PR, Moorman AC, Denniston MM (2013) Hepatitis C in the United States. N Engl J Med 368(20):1859–1861.
17. Kramer JR, Kanwal F, Richardson P, Mei M, El-Serag HB (2012) Gaps in the achievement of effectiveness of HCV treatment in national VA practice. J Hepatol 56: 320–325.
18. Umscheid CA (2013) A Primer on Performing Systematic Reviews and Meta-analyses. Clin Infect Dis 57: 725–734.
19. Cornberg M, Razavi HA, Alberti A, Bernasconi E, Buti M, et al. (2011) A systematic review of hepatitis C virus epidemiology in Europe, Canada and Israel. Liver Int 31 Suppl 2: 30–60.
20. Higgins JP, Thompson SG (2002) Quantifying heterogeneity in a meta-analysis. Stat Med 21: 1539–1558.
21. OpenMeta[Analyst] (2012). Accessed at http://www.cebm.brown.edu/open_meta. on Dec 15, 2013.

22. Armstrong GL, Wasley A, Simard EP, McQuillan GM, Kuhnert WL, et al. (2006) The prevalence of hepatitis C virus infection in the United States, 1999 through 2002. Ann Intern Med 144: 705–714.

23. Arora S, Thornton K, Murata G, Deming P, Kalishman S, et al. (2011) Outcomes of treatment for hepatitis C virus infection by primary care providers. N Engl J Med 364: 2199–2207.

24. Backus LI, Boothroyd DB, Phillips BR, Belperio P, Halloran J, et al. (2011) A Sustained Virologic Response Reduces Risk of All-Cause Mortality in Patients With Hepatitis C. Clin Gastroenterol Hepatol 9: 509–516.e501.

25. Groessl EJ, Liu L, Ho SB, Kanwal F, Gifford AL, et al. (2012) National patterns and predictors of liver biopsy use for management of hepatitis C. J Hepatol 57: 252–259.

26. Kanwal F, Hoang T, Chrusciel T, Kramer JR, El-Serag HB, et al. (2012) Process of care for hepatitis C infection is linked to treatment outcome and virologic response. Clin Gastroenterol Hepatol 10: 1270–1277.

27. Kanwal F, Schnitzler MS, Bacon BR, Hoang T, Buchanan PM, et al. (2010) Quality of care in patients with chronic hepatitis C virus infection: a cohort study. Ann Intern Med 153: 231–239.

28. Mitra D, Davis KL, Beam C, Medjedovic J, Rustgi V (2010) Treatment patterns and adherence among patients with chronic hepatitis C virus in a US managed care population. Value Health 13: 479–486.

29. Moorman AC, Gordon SC, Rupp LB, Spradling PR, Teshale EH, et al. (2013) Baseline characteristics and mortality among people in care for chronic viral hepatitis: the chronic hepatitis cohort study. Clin Infect Dis 56: 40–50.

30. Russell M, Pauly MP, Moore CD, Chia C, Dorrell J, et al. (2012) The impact of lifetime alcohol use on hepatitis C treatment outcomes in privately insured members of an integrated health care plan. Hepatology 56: 1223–1230.

31. Younossi ZM, Stepanova M, Afendy M, Lam BP, Mishra A (2013) Knowledge about infection is the only predictor of treatment in patients with chronic hepatitis C. J Viral Hepat 20: 550–555.

32. Denniston MM, Klevens RM, McQuillan GM, Jiles RB (2012) Awareness of infection, knowledge of hepatitis C, and medical follow-up among individuals testing positive for hepatitis C. National Health and Nutrition Examination Survey 2001–2008. Hepatology 55: 1652–1661.

33. Moyer VA, on behalf of the USPSTF (2013) Screening for Hepatitis C Virus Infection in Adults: U.S. Preventive Services Task Force Recommendation Statement. Ann Intern Med 159(5): 349–57.

34. Smith BD, Morgan RL, Beckett GA, Falck-Ytter Y, Holtzman D, et al. (2012) Recommendations for the identification of chronic hepatitis C virus infection among persons born during 1945–1965. MMWR Recomm Rep 61: 1–32.

35. Thomas DL (2012) Advances in the treatment of hepatitis C virus infection. Top Antivir Med 20: 5–10.

36. Garcia-Tsao G (2001) Current management of the complications of cirrhosis and portal hypertension: variceal hemorrhage, ascites, and spontaneous bacterial peritonitis. Gastroenterology 120: 726–748.

37. Bruix J, Sherman M, American Association for the Study of Liver D (2011) Management of hepatocellular carcinoma: an update. Hepatology 53: 1020–1022.

38. Chou R, Wasson N (2013) Blood tests to diagnose fibrosis or cirrhosis in patients with chronic hepatitis C virus infection: a systematic review. Ann Intern Med 158: 807–820.

39. Chan K, Lai MN, Groessl EJ, Hanchate AD, Wong JB, et al. (2013) Cost effectiveness of direct-acting antiviral therapy for treatment-naive patients with chronic HCV genotype 1 infection in the veterans health administration. Clin Gastroenterol Hepatol 11: 1503–1510.

40. Rein DB, Smith BD, Wittenborn JS, Lesesne SB, Wagner LD, et al. (2012) The cost-effectiveness of birth-cohort screening for hepatitis C antibody in U.S. primary care settings. Ann Intern Med 156: 263–270.

41. El Khoury AC, Vietri J, Prajapati G (2012) The burden of untreated hepatitis C virus infection: a US patients' perspective. Dig Dis Sci 57: 2995–3003.

42. Veterans Health Administration. (2009) The State of Care for Veterans with HIV/AIDS. Available: http://www.hiv.va.gov/provider/policy/state-of-care/. Accessed 2013 Dec 15.

43. Butt AA, Khan UA, Shaikh OS, McMahon D, Dorey-Stein Z, et al. (2009) Rates of HCV treatment eligibility among HCV-monoinfected and HCV/HIV-coinfected patients in tertiary care referral centers. HIV Clin Trials 10: 25–32.

44. Butt AA, Justice AC, Skanderson M, Good C, Kwoh CK (2006) Rates and predictors of hepatitis C virus treatment in HCV-HIV-coinfected subjects. Aliment Pharmacol Ther 24: 585–591.

45. Kanwal F, Hoang T, Spiegel BM, Eisen S, Dominitz JA, et al. (2007) Predictors of treatment in patients with chronic hepatitis C infection - role of patient versus nonpatient factors. Hepatology 46: 1741–1749.

12

Dynamic Changes of Lipopolysaccharide Levels in Different Phases of Acute on Chronic Hepatitis B Liver Failure

Calvin Pan[1,◊], Yurong Gu[2,◊], Wei Zhang[3], Yubao Zheng[2], Liang Peng[2], Hong Deng[2], Youming Chen[2], Lubiao Chen[2], Sui Chen[2], Min Zhang[2], Zhiliang Gao[2]*

1 Division of Liver Diseases, Department of Medicine, The Mount Sinai Medical Center, Mount Sinai School of Medicine, New York, New York, United States of America, 2 Department of Infectious Disease, The Third Affiliated, Hospital of Sun-Yet-Sen University, Guangzhou, China, 3 Department of Infectious Disease, Beijing Youan Hospital, Capital Medical University, Beijing, China

Abstract

Background: High serum levels of lipopolysaccharide (LPS) with LPS-MD-2/TLR4 complex activated NF-kb and cytokine cause hepatic necrosis in animal models. We investigated the dynamic changes of LPS levels in patients with acute on chronic hepatitis B liver failure (ACHBLF).

Methods: We enrolled ACHBLF patients for a 12-week study. Patients' LPS levels were measured along with 10 healthy controls. Patients on supportive care and recovered without intervention(s) were analyzed. Patients' LPS levels during the disease progression phase, peak phase, and remission phase were compared with healthy controls.

Results: Among 30 patients enrolled, 25 who received interventions or expired during the study period were excluded from the analysis, five patients on supportive care who completed the study were analyzed. Significant abnormal distributions of LPS levels were observed in patients in different phases (0.0168 ± 0.0101 in progression phase; 0.0960 ± 0.0680 in peak phase; 0.0249 ± 0.0365 in remission phase; and 0.0201 ± 0.0146 in controls; respectively, $p<0.05$). The highest level of LPS was in the peak phase and significantly elevated when compared to controls (0.0201 ± 0.0146 vs. 0.0960 ± 0.0680, $p=0.007$). There were no statistically significant differences in LPS levels between healthy controls and subjects in the progression phase or remission phase. Dynamic changes of LPS were correlated with MELD-Na in the progression phase ($p=0.01$, $R=0.876$) and in the peak phase ($p=0.000$, $R=-1.00$).

Conclusions: Significant abnormal distributions of LPS levels were observed in ACHBLF with the highest level in the peak phase. The dynamic changes of LPS were correlated with disease severity and suggested LPS causing secondary hepatic injury.

Editor: Sang-Hoon Ahn, Yonsei University College of Medicine, The Republic of Korea

Funding: This study was funded by the Natural Science Fund of Guangdong Province (No.10451008901004818), the National Natural Science Foundation of China (No.30971356), and the National Grant Program on Key Infectious Disease in the Treatment and Prevention of Infectious Diseases of AIDS and Viral Hepatitis (No. 2012ZX10002007). The funders had no role in study design, data collection and analysis, decision to publish, or preparation of the manuscript.

Competing Interests: The authors have declared that no competing interests exist.

* E-mail: zlgao99@hotmail.com

◊ These authors contributed equally to this work.

Introduction

Hepatitis B virus (HBV) infection is the most common cause of liver disease worldwide [1]. Approximately 400 million people are suffering from chronic hepatitis B (CHB) infection and may develop complications like cirrhosis, and hepatocellular carcinoma (HCC) [2]. Acute on chronic liver failure (ACLF) is an acute hepatic insult in patients who have chronic liver disease, manifesting as jaundice (serum bilirubin>5 mg/dl or 85 mol/L) and coagulopathy (INR>1.5 or prothrombin activity<40%), often complicated by ascites and/or encephalopathy within 4 weeks of the acute presentation [3]. The underlying chronic liver diseases in ACLF vary depending on the geographic region. Alcoholic hepatitis is common in western countries, whereas chronic hepatitis B or C infections are often seen in Asian countries. The common participating factors include viral hepatitis reactivation, alcohol, hepatotoxic drugs/herbs. In acute on chronic hepatitis B liver failure (ACHBLF), HBV reactivation is the major acute insults and precipitation liver failure [3]. It may occur after withdrawal of HBV antiviral treatment but more often, due to non- HBV treatment related events, which include disease reactivation either spontaneous or secondary to intensive chemotherapy/immunosuppressive therapy. Liver transplantation is the only curative therapeutic option for ACHBLF with a 5-year survival rate of 85% [4,5]. However, infectious complications often preclude transplant in patients with ACHBLF and many die on the waiting list due to the shortage of organs [6]. In 2008, the local standard of care for ACHBLF other than transplantation for ACHBLF was supportive care. Prior to the time we concluded this study, there was no prospective randomized control trial to support the effectiveness and safety use of antiviral therapy in patients with ACHBLF [7]. In addition, Lange et al reported that a significant portion of patients with high MELD scores and treated with entecavir developed lactic acidosis resulting in high mortality [8]. Thus, the local standard of care at that time required a detailed discussion with patients and obtaining the consent prior to the antiviral use in patients with ACHBLF. Due to the lacking of evidence on the use of antiviral for ACHBLF during our study period, two patterns of clinical practice were observed in our center: patients who believed the potential benefit of antiviral treatment were treated with nucleoside (tenofovir was not available in China), whereas, patients who believed that the antiviral had no role on hepatic regeneration during acute setting or unwilling to take the risk of lactic acidosis could defer the antiviral treatment until they recovered from the acute event, and then received antiviral treatment for CHB when their disease severity was improved (low MELD scores had less frequency of lactic acidosis). Our study was designed to capture those patients who deferred antiviral treatment but were able to recover spontaneously from ACHBLF without intervention.

The mechanism of ACHBLF remains unclear. It was speculated that pro-inflammatory cytokines mediated hepatic inflammation along with oxidative stress and the production of nitric oxide initiated the acute hepatic injury, followed by neutrophil dysfunction from circulating endotoxins (the cause of secondary liver damage), resulting in sepsis, multi-organ failure and impairment of liver regeneration [9,10,11,12,13]. LPS is an endotoxin derived from Gram-negative bacteria in the intestinal micro-flora. Evidently, trace amounts of LPS were measurable in serum samples from portal vein in normal healthy subjects since LPS may penetrate the intestinal mucosa. However, the majority of LPSs were cleared by liver filtration [10,14]. West et al demonstrated that about 40%–50% of an intravenous dose of LPS was cleared up by the liver filtration in animal models [13]. In addition to the filtration, hepatic and Kupffer cell (KC) uptake in the liver with detoxification played a key role in preventing high circulating levels of LPS [9]. In CHB patients, Sozinov et al observed that high incidence of Gram-negative bacteria overgrowth leads to the over production of LPS and results in higher serum levels of LPS [14]. On the other hand, several studies in animal models suggested that delayed clearance of LPS from the circulation occurred in chronic liver diseases because of the impaired phagocytosis of KC [15,16,17]. The persistence of endotoxinemia not only activated the liver immune cells with participating inflammatory process but also caused dysfunction of liver parenchymal cells and apoptosis [18]. Another theory on hepatic injury implied that LPS in the circulation interacted with toll like receptor 4 (TLR4) and mediated a signal transduction pathway, which included the formation of LPS-LBP-CD14-secreted protein MD-2-TLR4 receptor complex [19,20,21]. The complex combined with myeloid differentiation factor 88, then phosphorylated and activated a series of cell kinases [21]. The activated kinases collectively further activated the transcription factor, mainly nuclear factor κB (NF-κB) [19,22], which resulted in increased production of pro-inflammatory cytokines, and led to hepatic necrosis [19,20,21,22,23]. Lastly, LPS may also activate hepatic stellate cells (HSCs) to up-regulate gene expression of chemokines and adhesion molecules to induce liver injury [24,25,26].

Although the above theories on liver injury from LPS have been supported by animal models or a few in vivo studies, the

relationship between the circulating LPS levels and liver disease activity or severity has not been fully explored in patients with ACHBLF. Previous published studies have focused on compensated liver disease or acute liver failure, which showed a significant correlation between elevated serum levels of LPS and liver disease severity [11,14,27]. In animal models for ACLF, Han et al suggested that LPS circulating in the blood may reach a certain level and then triggered the secondary liver injury on top of primary chronic liver disease. However, this theory has not been fully explored in patients with ACHBLF [10]. We sought to investigate LPS levels in different disease stages of ACHBLF and the dynamic changes of LPS levels associated with the disease severity measured by clinical parameters in ACHBLF patients.

Study Design and Methods

This was a 12 week prospective, observational study with healthy controls that enrolled ACHBLF patients and healthy volunteers from a single tertiary care center, the Third Affiliated Hospital of Sun Yet-Sen University in China from October 2008 through April 2010. The study protocol and the inform consent form were both approved (IRB approval N0:2008-321) by the Ethical Committee Board of Sun Yet-Sen University. All subjects were (or their designated health care proxy holders) consented prior to the screening.

Study Population and Data Collection

Adult patients with ACHBLF who were willing to participate and consented to the study were screened for the following eligibility criteria: (1) age of 18–50 years; (2) meeting the diagnostic criteria of ACHBLF which included jaundice (serum bilirubin $\geqq 5$ mg/dl [85 umol/l]) and coagulopathy (INR $\geqq 1.5$ or prothrombin activity<40%), ascites and/or encephalopathy as determined by physical examination within 4 weeks of the disease onset, and previously diagnosed chronic hepatitis B. (3) exacerbation of CHB for the first time. Key exclusion criteria were the followings: the time point of acute onset of ACHBLF was more than 14 days prior to the enrollment date; clinical evidence of cirrhosis or documented stage IV fibrosis on liver biopsy (if available); co-infection with hepatitis A, C, D, E or HIV virus; pregnant woman; diagnosis of other liver diseases including autoimmune hepatitis and Wilson disease, or evidence of hepatic tumor; history of renal, cardiovascular, pulmonary, endocrine or neurological diseases; history of antiviral therapy prior to the onset of ACHBLF, history of drug abuse including alcohol abuse; treatment with immune modulator, antibiotic treatment, or Chinese herbal medicine within six months prior to the screening.

Patients enrolled were followed every week by research team until week 12. As per good clinical practice standard, further interventions for ACHBLF in addition to supportive care were allowed and decided by clinical team members who were blind to the protocol, which included referral for liver transplant, providing antiviral treatment or using antibiotic when sepsis developed. However, only patients who were on supportive care without interventions during the study period were analyzed to delineate the relationship between LPS levels and disease severity in ACHBLF. Total bilirubin (TBil) levels were used as the marker for disease phases in ACHBLF. According to the dynamic change of TBil, the phases of ACHBLF in this study were defined as the following: 1) progression phase, which was from the onset of ACHBLF (at the time of diagnosis of ACHBLF) to the point of peak level of TBil; 2) peak phase, which was the period when TBil level plateaued after reaching the peak; and 3) remission phase, which was from the point of decrease in TBil after plateauing to the return of TBil level to the baseline. Although clinical parameters were measured and LPS samples were obtained weekly, only 1–2 samples collected during each phase of ACHBLF (selected at the mid time point of the phase) were used to determine the LPS level in the individual phase.

Available serum and plasma samples were measured in our research laboratory. Patients' HBV DNA levels, HBeAg and HBsAg status, ALT, albumin, creatinine, prothrombin time, model for end stage liver disease scores with sodium (MELD-Na) were recorded in all subjects at one week interval. Data for healthy volunteers were also prospectively collected and their blood samples were measured for LPS levels and TBil level in the same laboratory. The standard of supportive care for ACHBLF at the study center was the following: patients routinely received high calorie diet (35–40 Cal/kg/day) with reduced glutathione. Patients also received proton pump inhibitors, enteral/parenteral nutrition, and albumin transfusion if needed.

Measurement of LPS and Parameters for Disease Severity

The primary measurement of this study was the followings: 1) measured serum LPS levels in three disease phases of ACHBLF and compared to those in the control group; 2) evaluated dynamic changes in LPS levels in ACHBLF by comparing the distribution pattern of LPS levels throughout all phases of ACHBLF. The secondary measurement was to assess the association between LPS levels and the disease severity indicated by MELD-Na scores. In addition to MELD-Na scores, serum total bilirubin levels were also selected as the main markers for the disease severity in this study. Other clinical parameters were also assessed, which included aspartate aminotransferase (AST), and alanine aminotransferase (ALT) albumin, creatinine (automatic biochemical analyzer, Olympus, Japan), prothrombin time (automatic hemostasis/thrombosis analyzer, STA compact).

All laboratory tests for patients in our center were performed in the hospital central laboratory. HBV serologies were tested by either CMIA (Abbott I 2000, USA) or ECL kits (Roche Laboratories, Germany). All serum samples for HBV DNA were tested by real-time quantitative PCR (Shanghai Kehua Bioengineering Co., Ltd., China) with the detection range of 500 copies –8 log10 copies/mL. Total bilirubin (TBIL), ALT (ULN = 40 U/L) and other biochemistry markers were tested by a Hitachi 7600 fully-automatic biochemical (Hitachi Co. Ltd., Tokyo, Japan). LPS concentrations in plasma were measured with the Limulus Amebocyte Lysate (LAL) test (Xiamen Houshiji, Ltd., Xiamen, China) according to the manufacturer's instructions. All the materials used were pyrogen free and LPS in the test samples was calculated by comparison to a standard curve. All samples were tested in duplicate and read at 450 nm for LPS in a Thermomax microplate reader (Molecular Devices, Sunnyvale, CA).

Statistics

Baseline characteristics and laboratory results were summarized for two groups by means of descriptive statistics. SPSS 15.0 software (SPSS, Inc., Chicago, IL) was used to analyze changes within groups during the study period. Statistical significance between two groups was calculated using a one-way Anova test or nonparametric Mann-Whitney test. Correlation used the Pearson correlation test. The evaluation on the normality and pattern of LPS level distribution among three disease phases of ACHBLF were performed with Kolmogorov-Smirnov test and compared to LPS levels in the healthy controls. For all analyses, a p-value equal to or less than 0.05 was considered significant.

Results

1. Clinical Characteristics and Baseline of Subjects

Among 58 consecutive ACHBLF patients who consented and were screened with the above criteria, 30 patients enrolled. 25 patients were excluded from final analysis for the following reasons: 11 patients with rapid disease progression and died in the first 4 weeks (mostly from sepsis) despite interventions; 10 patients were excluded because of using antibiotics for infection or receiving antiviral therapy. 1 patient with CHB and history of Grave's disease (history obtained after the enrollment) was suspected to have a flare of autoimmune hepatitis and received additional intervention; and 3 patients took herbs medication during the study period. A total of 5 patients who deferred antiviral treatment were included for the analysis and assigned to the ACHBLF group. These 5 patients had totally recovered from ACHBLF and were discharged after 12 to 16 weeks of hospitalization. A summary of patients' deposition is shown in Figure 1. Ten healthy volunteers between the ages of 18 and 50 were enrolled and assigned to the control group. The baseline assessments of study subjects from these two groups are shown in Table 1. All five patients with ACHBLF were male and 80% were HBeAg positive. Their mean HBV DNA levels were 6.27±2.24 log10 IU/mL and mean MELD-Na scores were 19.22±3.8 at the baseline. All were admitted and observed with supportive care in the hospital and achieved remission without further intervention within 12 weeks. In addition, two female and eight male healthy volunteers were prospectively enrolled as controls. The mean ages of subjects in the two study groups were well matched without statistical significance.

2. LPS Levels in Different Phases of ACHLF

In the ACHBLF group, the mean duration of disease progression from the onset of the disease to the peak phase was 31.24±2.77 days. The mean duration of the peak phase was 6.00±1.00 days. The mean duration of remission phase was 31.60±15.24 days. Significantly higher levels of LPS were observed in the peak phase compared to those in progression phase (0.0960±0.0680 vs. 0.0168±0.0101, p = 0.008) or those in remission phase (0.0960±0.0680 vs. 0.0249±0.0365, p = 0.021). When compared to the control group, LPS levels during the peak phase in ACHBLF were also significantly higher (0.0201±0.0146 vs. 0.0960±0.0680, P = 0.007). However, there were no statistically significant differences in LPS levels between controls and ACHBLF patients in progression phase (0.0168±0.0101 vs. 0.0201±0.0146, p = 0.618) or in remission phase (0.0249±0.0365 vs. 0.0201±0.0146, p = 0.706). The changes of LPS levels in different phases when compared to controls are shown in Figure 2.

3. The Dynamic Changes of LPS Levels and Disease Severity

The dynamic changes in mean levels of plasma LPS through the three phases of ACHBLF appeared to be a bell shape with a significant increase from the progressive phase to the peak phase, followed by a decrease or return to the baseline in the remission phase. Significantly abnormal distributions of LPS levels were observed during the phases of ACHBLF (Kolmogorov-Smirnov Test, P<0.05) when compared to healthy controls.

The highest MELD-Na mean scores in the ACHBLF group were observed in the peak phase and in parallel with the peak level of LPS. MELD-Na scores were correlated with LPS on progression phase (p = 0.01, R = 0.876) and peak phase (p = 0.000, R = −1.00). Although higher levels of TBil in patients

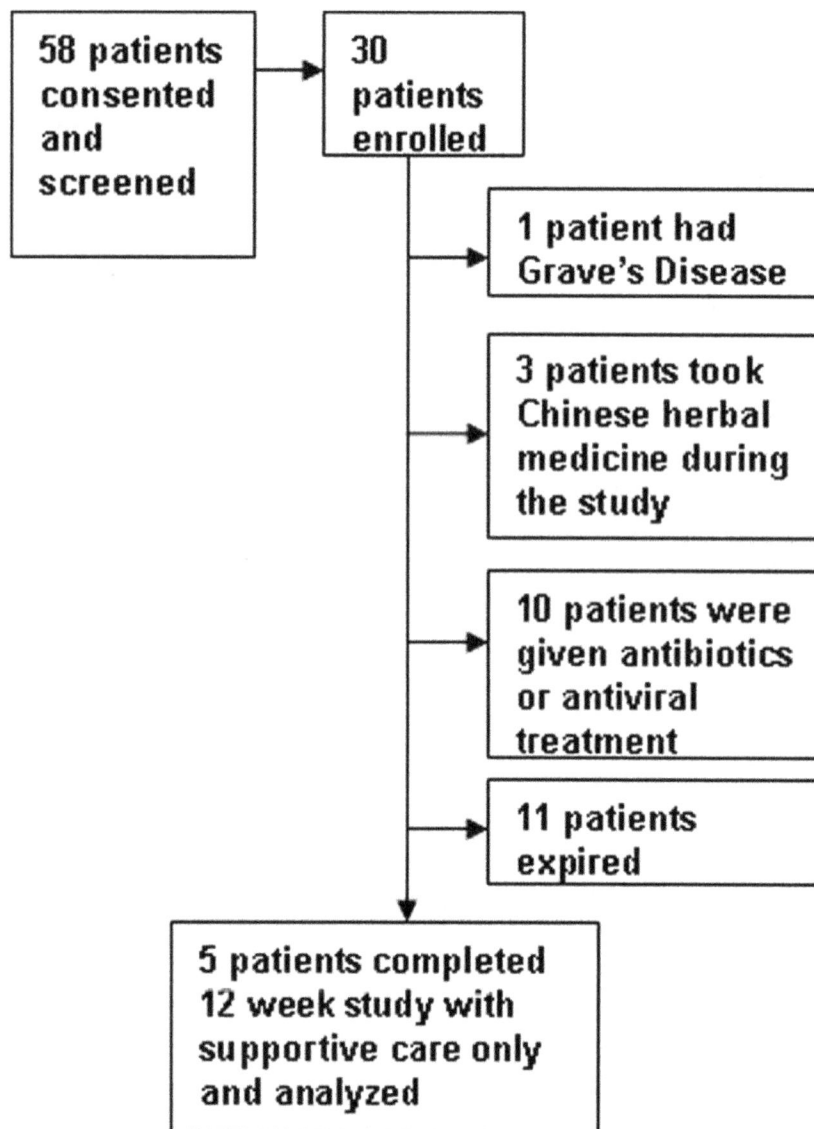

Figure 1. Patient selection and deposition.

with ACHBLF were observed in the peak phase and in parallel with the peak levels of LPS, the change of TBil were not statistically correlated with plasma LPS levels (p>0.05). The changes of LPS levels, Tbil and MELD-Na scores in the different phases of ACHBLF and their correlations are shown in Table 2.

Discussion

ACHBLF has significant morbidity and mortality with limited intervention unless liver transplant is offered [3,5,28]. However, even in the transplant center, majority of patients with ACHBLF die on the waiting list due to the shortage of organs or developed sepsis [3,6]. The first prospective randomized control trial for antiviral use in ACHBLF patients was published by Grag et al in 2011, which demonstrated that tenofovir could safely reduce short term mortality in these patients. Our study was concluded prior to the first aforementioned randomized control trial. Although antiviral treatment may provide some short term survival benefits, many patients died despite the significant reduction of HBV DNA [29]. Thus, our data remained relevant for the understanding of

disease mechanism and the future development of novel intervention. Previous studies have demonstrated that endotoxinemia and delayed clearance of LPS in the circulation resulted in the development of ACLF in alcoholic liver disease [18,30,31,32,33,34]. Although Han et al proposed that LPS played an important role in ACHBLF as a secondary liver injury on top of the CHB infection in animal models [10]. The changes of LPS levels and their roles on disease severity in patients with ACHBLF were not fully explored.

Our study showed that baseline LPS levels in ACHBLF patients did not differ from those in the healthy controls. However, significant elevation in LPS levels was observed in the peak phase of ACHBLF when compared to those in the progression or remission phase.

The abnormal distributions of LPS levels among different phases were statistically significant in ACHBLF. In addition, the changes in LPS levels were correlated with MELD-Na scores in the progression and the peak phase. To our knowledge, this is by far the first study in which detailed the dynamic changes of LPS

Table 1. Baseline assessments of ACHBLF patients and healthy subjects.

Mean ± SD	Control group(n = 10)	ACHBLF group(n = 5)	case 1	case 2	case 3	case 4	case 5
Male (M)	8	5	M	M	M	M	M
Age (year)*	32.30±4.30	34.2±8.23	28	37	25	35	46
HBeAg (%)		(80%)	+	+	+	-	+
HBV-DNA (log10 IU/mL)*		6.27±2.24	3.44	6.22	8.39	4.71	8.56
Serum bilirubin (umol/l)*	12.33±2.06	307.54±78.53	237.1	321.7	215.8	389.8	373.3
ALT (IU/l)*	20.70±5.33	867±1004.88	423	921	2579	337	75
AST (IU/l)*	19.40±3.37	829.4±885.32	293	1466	2071	144	173
Creatinine(mmol/l)*	47.69±3.63	76.44±18.46	57.8	76.0	70.1	71.1	107.2
Prothrobin time (Sec.)*	12.54±0.51	26.4±4.11	23.3	33.2	23.7	24.5	27.3
MELD-Na score		19.22±3.8	15.13	25.00	17.67	20.14	17.55
Serum LPS (EU/mL)	0.0201±0.0146	0.0183±0.012	0.0086	0.0350	0.0095	0.0271	0.0113

Test of normality is done by Kolmogorov-Smirnov Test.
*P>0.05.

levels in different phases of ACHBLF, and provided the evidence of acute liver injury in ACHBLF associated with increased LPS levels. Since MELD-Na scores were correlated with LPS levels in the progression and the peak phase, our data pointed to the direction of the secondary injury from LPS in chronic liver disease leading to liver failure, which was proposed by Han et al. in the study from animal model. Further studies with histology correlation to LPS are needed to confirm if the severity of liver injury actually is directly correlated with LPS levels in ACHBLF patients.

The findings in this study also implied a possible therapeutic intervention for ACHBLF by removing LPS from the serum.

Several studies done by Adachi et al observed that there was a positive correlation between the occurrence of bacterial translocation from the gut to portal system and liver dysfunction in alcoholic hepatitis [34,35]. Li et al demonstrated that elevation of endotoxin levels in the circulation from translocation of gut flora occurred during acute flares in patients with chronic hepatitis [27]. It is possible that the elevation of LPS level in CHB patients was due to bacterial translocations from the gut to portal circulation resulting in endotoxemia in the early phase (or progressive phase) of ACHBLF. On the other hand, the liver dysfunction in the early stage of ACHBLF probably further induced bacterial translocation from the gut leading to higher level of endotoxemia. In addition, in patients with liver dysfunction, the uptake of endotoxin by hepatic and Kupffer cells were compromised as compared to normal physical conditions, resulting in higher circulating levels of LPS [9,13,36]. High levels of LPS then induced the aggravations of liver injury through the LPS-MD-2/TLR4/NF-kb signal pathway and further negatively impacted on KC and hepatic clearance of endotoxin [33]. Thus, it is expected that the peak level of LPS was observed during the peak phase of ACHBLF. In our study, the dynamic changes of LPS were paralleled with the changes of TBil and MELD-Na in different phases of ACHBLF. The changes in LPS levels were correlated with MELD-Na scores in the progression and the peak phase, further indicated that the worsen disease severity was the result of LPS induced liver injury. The

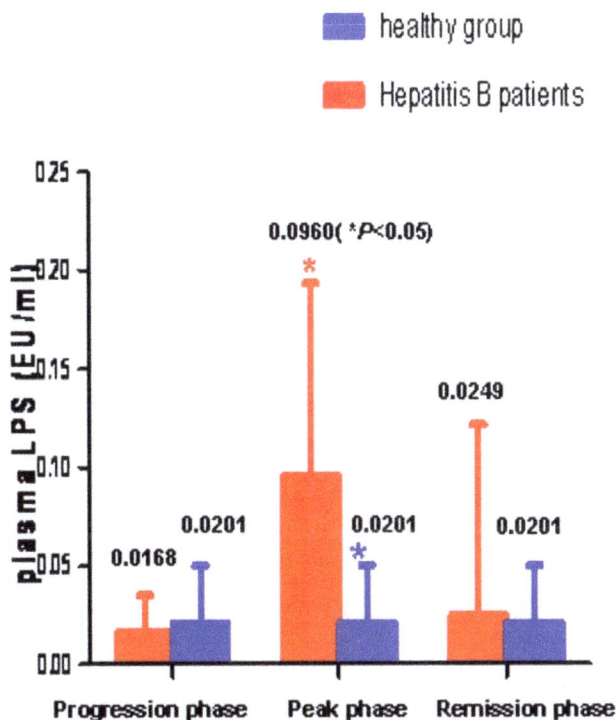

Figure 2. LPS levels in different disease phases compared to those in the healthy group.

Table 2. Total bilirubin, MELD-Na scores, and LPS levels in different phases of ACHBLF.

Mean ± SD	Progression phase	Peak phase	Remission phase
Serum TBIL(umol/l)	362.63±114.16	632.73±141.38	398.04±105.67
MELD-Na score	18.14±3.94*	26.35±18.23**	17.96±5.62
Plasma LPS(EU/ml)	0.0168±0.0101	0.096±0.068	0.0249±0.0365

MELD-Na score correlated with LPS in the progression phase (*p = 0.01, R = 0.876) and in the peak phase, (**p = 0.000, R = −1.00), respectively.

MELD-Na scores were not correlated with LPS levels in the remission phase. It is possible that the sample size of this study was too small to reflect such a correlation. Another possibility was that a delay on the improvement of MELD-Na scores occurred after the LPS level decreased by the buffering of LPS-binding substance produced in the remission phase. As suggested by previous studies, we presume that higher LPS levels were due to the production of LPS surpassed the phagocytic ability of kupffer cells rather than the decrease binding capacity of LPS-binding substances in acute phase [13,36]. As disease progressed, the buffering system of LPS-binding substances was activated and reached the peak level in remission phase. Thus, it is possible that the liver injury induced by LPS was establish in the progression and peak phase with fluctuating lower levels of LPS-binding substances [12,37]. Although our data was generated prospectively with control subjects, several limitations in this study are worth noting: 1) Patients included in the analysis were those who achieved spontaneous remission within 12 weeks on supportive care. The study result may not be applied to patients with prolonged peak phases and worsening disease activity or received additional intervention on top of supportive care; 2) Data analysis excluded patients expired during the study. Thus, the scale or levels of LPS in patients with severe liver necrosis remains uncertain. 3) For the feasibility of the study, we use healthy individuals as controls, which were less desirable than using CHB patients without ACHBLF. 4) A number of patients were not analyzed due to the intervention during the study period as required by the standard of care, such as antibiotic treatments for sepsis and antiviral use if patient consented to it. These patients were excluded because antibiotic may affect the gut flora and antiviral may influence the

LPS level, which was reported by Koh et al in patients with CHB or hepatitis C during antiviral treatment [38]. Due to the limited numbers of patients that were analyzed in this study, a future trial with the larger sample size is warranted to confirm our findings.

In conclusion, the peak levels of LPS occurred during the severe necrosis phase (peak phase) in ACHBLF patients. The abnormal distributions of LPS levels among different phases were statistically significant in ACHBLF when compared to the controls. The highest MELD-Na mean scores in the ACHBLF group were observed in the peak phase and in parallel with the peak level of LPS. MELD-Na scores were correlated with LPS on progression phase and peak phase. Our data demonstrated the dynamic changes of LPS in ACHBLF as well as the relationship between LPS levels and the disease severity indicated by MELD-Na scores. These findings are important and may serve as the concept for the future development of therapeutic agents with the capacity to reduce LPS production or improve LPS clearance, which may have a significant impact on the clinical outcome of patients with ACHBLF.

Acknowledgments

We'd like to thank Tom and Kristin Muneyyirci for proof-reading of the manuscript.

Author Contributions

Conceived and designed the experiments: CQP YG ZG DC LC HD YC. Performed the experiments: YG WZ LP YZ SC MZ. Analyzed the data: CQP YG ZG DC LC. Contributed reagents/materials/analysis tools: GQP YG ZG. Wrote the paper: CQP YG ZG.

References

1. Shepard CW, Simard EP, Finelli L, Fiore AE, Bell BP (2006) Hepatitis B virus infection: epidemiology and vaccination. Epidemiologic reviews 28: 112–125.
2. Liaw YF (2009) Natural history of chronic hepatitis B virus infection and long-term outcome under treatment. Liver Int 29 Suppl 1: 100–107.
3. Sarin SK, Kumar A, Almeida JA, Chawla YK, Fan ST, et al. (2009) Acute-on-chronic liver failure: consensus recommendations of the Asian Pacific Association for the study of the liver (APASL). Hepatol Int 3: 269–282.
4. Hessel FP, Bramlage P, Wasem J, Mitzner SR (2010) Cost-effectiveness of the artificial liver support system MARS in patients with acute-on-chronic liver failure. European journal of gastroenterology & hepatology 22: 213–220.
5. Zheng MH, Shi KQ, Fan YC, Li H, Ye C, et al. (2011) A model to determine 3-month mortality risk in patients with acute-on-chronic hepatitis B liver failure. Clinical gastroenterology and hepatology : the official clinical practice journal of the American Gastroenterological Association 9: 351–356 e353.
6. Merion RM, Sharma P, Mathur AK, Schaubel DE (2011) Evidence-based development of liver allocation: a review. Transpl Int 24: 965–972.
7. Garg H, Sarin SK, Kumar M, Garg V, Sharma BC, et al. (2011) Tenofovir improves the outcome in patients with spontaneous reactivation of hepatitis B presenting as acute-on-chronic liver failure. Hepatology 53: 774–780.
8. Lange CM, Bojunga J, Hofmann WP, Wunder K, Mihm U, et al. (2009) Severe lactic acidosis during treatment of chronic hepatitis B with entecavir in patients with impaired liver function. Hepatology research : the official journal of the Japan Society of Hepatology 05: 2001–2006.
9. Roth J, McClellan JL, Kluger MJ, Zeisberger E (1994) Attenuation of fever and release of cytokines after repeated injections of lipopolysaccharide in guinea-pigs. J Physiol 477 (Pt 1): 177–185.
10. Han DW (2002) Intestinal endotoxemia as a pathogenetic mechanism in liver failure. World J Gastroenterol 8: 961–965.
11. Li LJ, Wu ZW, Xiao DS, Sheng JF (2004) Changes of gut flora and endotoxin in rats with D-galactosamine-induced acute liver failure. World J Gastroenterol 10: 2087–2090.
12. Barclay GR (1995) Endogenous endotoxin-core antibody (EndoCAb) as a marker of endotoxin exposure and a prognostic indicator: a review. Prog Clin Biol Res 392: 263–272.
13. West MA, Heagy W (2002) Endotoxin tolerance: a review. Crit Care Med 30: S64–73.
14. Sozinov AS (2002) Systemic endotoxemia during chronic viral hepatitis. Bull Exp Biol Med 133: 153–155.
15. Nakao A, Taki S, Yasui M, Kimura Y, Nonami T, et al. (1994) The fate of intravenously injected endotoxin in normal rats and in rats with liver failure. Hepatology 19: 1251–1256.
16. Dambach DM, Watson LM, Gray KR, Durham SK, Laskin DL (2002) Role of CCR2 in macrophage migration into the liver during acetaminophen-induced hepatotoxicity in the mouse. Hepatology 35: 1093–1103.
17. Schafer SL, Lin R, Moore PA, Hiscott J, Pitha PM (1998) Regulation of type I interferon gene expression by interferon regulatory factor-3. J Biol Chem 273: 2714–2720.
18. Szabo G, Bala S (2010) Alcoholic liver disease and the gut-liver axis. World J Gastroenterol 16: 1321–1329.
19. Zhang G, Ghosh S (2000) Molecular mechanisms of NF-kappaB activation induced by bacterial lipopolysaccharide through Toll-like receptors. J Endotoxin Res 6: 453–457.
20. Backhed F, Hornef M (2003) Toll-like receptor 4-mediated signaling by epithelial surfaces: necessity or threat? Microbes Infect 5: 951–959.
21. Takeda K, Akira S (2004) TLR signaling pathways. Semin Immunol 16: 3–9.
22. Yu H, Wu SD (2008) Activation of TLR-4 and liver injury via NF-kappa B in rat with acute cholangitis. Hepatobiliary Pancreat Dis Int 7: 185–191.
23. Tsung A, McCoy SL, Klune JR, Geller DA, Billiar TR, et al. (2007) A novel inhibitory peptide of Toll-like receptor signaling limits lipopolysaccharide-induced production of inflammatory mediators and enhances survival in mice. Shock 27: 364–369.
24. Karaa A, Thompson KJ, McKillop IH, Clemens MG, Schrum LW (2008) S-adenosyl-L-methionine attenuates oxidative stress and hepatic stellate cell activation in an ethanol-LPS-induced fibrotic rat model. Shock 30: 197–205.
25. Paik YH, Schwabe RF, Bataller R, Russo MP, Jobin C, et al. (2003) Toll-like receptor 4 mediates inflammatory signaling by bacterial lipopolysaccharide in human hepatic stellate cells. Hepatology 37: 1043–1055.
26. Quiroz SC, Bucio L, Souza V, Hernandez E, Gonzalez E, et al. (2001) Effect of endotoxin pretreatment on hepatic stellate cell response to ethanol and acetaldehyde. J Gastroenterol Hepatol 16: 1267–1273.
27. Li L, Wu Z, Ma W, Yu Y, Chen Y (2001) Changes in intestinal microflora in patients with chronic severe hepatitis. Chin Med J (Engl) 114: 869–872.
28. Katoonizadeh A, Laleman W, Verslype C, Wilmer A, Maleux G, et al. (2010) Early features of acute-on-chronic alcoholic liver failure: a prospective cohort study. Gut 59: 1561–1569.
29. Garg H, Sarin SK, Kumar M, Garg V, Sharma BC, et al. (2011) Tenofovir improves the outcome in patients with spontaneous reactivation of hepatitis B presenting as acute-on-chronic liver failure. Hepatology 53: 774–780.
30. Wu D, Cederbaum AI (2009) Oxidative stress and alcoholic liver disease. Semin Liver Dis 29: 141–154.

31. Sen S, Davies NA, Mookerjee RP, Cheshire LM, Hodges SJ, et al. (2004) Pathophysiological effects of albumin dialysis in acute-on-chronic liver failure: a randomized controlled study. Liver Transpl 10: 1109–1119.
32. Mandrekar P, Szabo G (2009) Signalling pathways in alcohol-induced liver inflammation. J Hepatol 50: 1258–1266.
33. Bhonchal S, Nain CK, Taneja N, Sharma M, Sharma AK, et al. (2007) Modification of small bowel microflora in chronic alcoholics with alcoholic liver disease. Trop Gastroenterol 28: 64–66.
34. Adachi Y, Bradford BU, Gao W, Bojes HK, Thurman RG (1994) Inactivation of Kupffer cells prevents early alcohol-induced liver injury. Hepatology 20: 453–460.
35. Adachi Y, Moore LE, Bradford BU, Gao W, Thurman RG (1995) Antibiotics prevent liver injury in rats following long-term exposure to ethanol. Gastroenterology 108: 218–224.
36. Hoek JB (1999) Endotoxin and alcoholic liver disease: tolerance and susceptibility. Hepatology 29: 1602–1604.
37. Brenchley JM, Price DA, Schacker TW, Asher TE, Silvestri G, et al. (2006) Microbial translocation is a cause of systemic immune activation in chronic HIV infection. Nat Med 12: 1365–1371.
38. Koh C, Sandler NG, Roque A, Eccleston J, Kleiner DE, et al. (2011) Markers of Microbial Translocation Are Elevated in Hepatitis B (HBV) and Hepatitis C (HCV) Infection; A Window Into Biology and Surrogate Markers for Detecting Disease Progression. Gastroenterology 140: S-897.

The CXCR3(+)CD56Bright Phenotype Characterizes a Distinct NK Cell Subset with Anti-Fibrotic Potential That Shows Dys-Regulated Activity in Hepatitis C

Marianne Eisenhardt, Andreas Glässner, Benjamin Krämer, Christian Körner, Bernhard Sibbing, Pavlos Kokordelis, Hans Dieter Nischalke, Tilman Sauerbruch, Ulrich Spengler, Jacob Nattermann*

Department of Internal Medicine I, University of Bonn, Bonn, Germany

Abstract

Background: In mouse models, natural killer (NK) cells have been shown to exert anti-fibrotic activity via killing of activated hepatic stellate cells (HSC). Chemokines and chemokine receptors critically modulate hepatic recruitment of NK cells. In hepatitis C, the chemokine receptor CXCR3 and its ligands have been shown to be associated with stage of fibrosis suggesting a role of these chemokines in HCV associated liver damage by yet incompletely understood mechanisms. Here, we analyzed phenotype and function of CXCR3 expressing NK cells in chronic hepatitis C.

Methods: Circulating NK cells from HCV-infected patients (n = 57) and healthy controls (n = 27) were analyzed with respect to CXCR3 and co-expression of different maturation markers. Degranulation and interferon-γ secretion of CXCR3(+) and CXCR3($-$) NK cell subsets were studied after co-incubation with primary human hepatic stellate cells (HSC). In addition, intra-hepatic frequency of CXCR3(+) NK cells was correlated with stage of liver fibrosis (n = 15).

Results: We show that distinct NK cell subsets can be distinguished based on CXCR3 surface expression. In healthy controls CXCR3(+)CD56Bright NK cells displayed strongest activity against HSC. Chronic hepatitis C was associated with a significantly increased frequency of CXCR3(+)CD56Bright NK cells which showed impaired degranulation and impaired IFN-γ secretion in response to HSC. Of note, we observed intra-hepatic accumulation of this NK cell subset in advanced stages of liver fibrosis.

Conclusion: We show that distinct NK cell subsets can be distinguished based on CXCR3 surface expression. Intra-hepatic accumulation of the functionally impaired CXCR3(+)CD56Bright NK cell subset might be involved in HCV-induced liver fibrosis.

Editor: Johan K. Sandberg, Karolinska Institutet, Sweden

Funding: This work was supported by the German Research Foundation (DFG SFB/TRR 57), the H. W. and J. Hector Foundation [grant number M42], and by a grant from the BMBF (German Ministry for Science and Education) [01KI0791]. The funders had no role in study design, data collection and analysis, decision to publish, or preparation of the manuscript.

Competing Interests: The authors have declared that no competing interests exist.

* E-mail: jacob.nattermann@ukb.uni-bonn.de

Introduction

Hepatitis C Virus (HCV) is a major cause for chronic inflammatory liver disease with variable progression towards liver fibrosis/cirrhosis. Hepatic infiltration of immunocompetent cells, including lymphocytes, is a hallmark of HCV infection, and there is accumulating evidence that this inflammatory infiltrate pivotally modulates immunopathogenesis of hepatitis C.

Recruitment of lymphocytes to the liver is importantly regulated via chemokines and chemokine receptors. Chemokines are small molecules involved in the regulation of chemotaxis and tissue extravasation of lymphocytes as well as in modulation of leukocyte function. Leukocytes sense chemokine concentration gradients via their respective chemokine receptors and move towards increasing concentration gradients.

In hepatitis C the CXC-chemokine receptor CXCR3 and its ligands (CXCL9, CXCL10, CXCL11) have gained specific attention because various studies demonstrated elevated levels of CXCR3 ligand CXCL10 to be predictive of the failure to response to HCV therapy [1–4] and to be associated with stage of fibrosis [4–10].

For years it was an unsolved paradox of why a pro-inflammatory chemokine, responsible for the hepatic recruitment of activated lymphocytes, is a marker for treatment failure and advanced liver fibrosis. However, recently Casrouge and co-workers provided an interesting explanation of this phenomenon by showing that CXCL10 in the plasma of patients with chronic hepatitis C mainly exists in a truncated antagonist form [11]. This CXCL10 variant can bind to CXCR3 without signaling and competitively inhibit binding of the agonist form of CXCL10, thereby interfering with proper recruitment of CXCR3-expressing lymphocytes.

However, analyzing fibrotic livers from HCV-infected patients Zeremski et al. nicely showed that most intra-hepatic lymphocytes express CXCR3 [8]. Therefore, we speculated that the mechanism(s) how CXCR3/CXCR3 ligands modulate hepatic fibrogenesis may imply biological functions beyond immune cell recruitment. Regarding hepatic trafficking of leukocytes most studies focused on the potential role of CXCR3-expressing T lymphocytes [12,13]. However, CXCR3 is expressed on various immunocompetent cells including natural killer (NK) cells, which represent an important component of the intra-hepatic lymphocyte pool. In contrast to the peripheral blood which contains about 5–10% NK cells, intra-hepatic lymphocytes comprise about 30% NK cells, and the percentage of intra-hepatic NK cells may even increase in inflammatory liver diseases [11].

In mouse models NK cells have been shown to exert anti-fibrotic capacity [14,15] and dys-function of NK cells was associated with a more rapid progression of liver fibrosis [16]. Accordingly, in vitro activity of NK cells has been demonstrated to correlate with the degree of HCV-associated liver fibrosis [17,18].

However, it remained unclear whether distinct NK cell subsets differ regarding their anti-fibrotic activity.

Here, we compared phenotype and functional activity against primary human hepatic stellate cells of CXCR3(+) NK cell subsets in healthy individuals and chronic hepatitis C.

Results

CXCR3 Expression Dissects CD56Dim and CD56Bright NK Cells in Specific Subsets

First, we studied expression of CXCR3 on circulating NK cells obtained from healthy donors. Flowcytometric analysis revealed that CD56Dim and CD56Bright NK cells can clearly be separated into CXCR3(+) and CXCR3(−) NK cell subsets (Figure 1A) with frequency of CXCR3(+) NK cells being higher in the CD56Bright sub-population.

To further characterize CXCR3(+) and CXCR3(−) NK cell sub-populations we next studied the co-expression of known NK cell maturation/differentiation markers in peripheral NK cells obtained from HCV-negative individuals. As is shown in figure 1B we found CD27, CD62L, CD127, and CD94 to be highly expressed in circulating CXCR3(+)CD56Bright NK cells, indicating an immature phenotype of this NK cell subset. Interestingly, expression of these markers progressively decreased in CXCR3(−)CD56Bright, CXCR3(+)CD56Dim, and CXCR3(−)CD56Dim NK cells, with CXCR3(−)CD56Dim NK cells displaying lowest surface expression. These findings were confirmed when NK cells from HCV infected patients were analyzed (data not shown). Taken together, these data indicate that CXCR3 expression dissects both CD56Dim and CD56Bright NK cells in phenotypically different subsets.

CXCR3 Expression Correlates with NK Cell Activity Against Human Hepatic Stellate Cells

CXCR3/CXCR3 ligands have been suggested to play a role in HCV-associated hepatic fibrogenesis. Therefore, we next analyzed the functional activity of circulating CXCR3(+) and CXCR3(−) NK cells using primary human hepatic stellate cells (HSC) as targets. We found that peripheral CXCR3-positive NK cells from healthy individuals displayed significantly higher degranulation as compared to their CXCR3-negative counterparts following co-incubation with HSC (Figure 2A). To verify that this differential functional activity was correlated with CXCR3 expression we then studied CD56BrightCXCR3(+), CD56BrightCXCR3(−), CD56DimCXCR3(+), and CD56DimCXCR3(−) NK cells separately (Figure 2C). Of note, we observed a sequential decrease in degranulation in these four subsets with highest activity in CD56BrightCXCR3(+) NK cells (CD56BrightCXCR3(+) >

CD56BrightCXCR3(−) > CD56DimCXCR3(+) > CD56DimCXCR3(−).

Beyond direct killing of HSC NK cells have been suggested to mediate anti-fibrotic effects via release of IFN-γ, thereby inducing HSC cell cycle arrest and apoptosis [19]. Therefore, we next studied production of IFN-γ following co-incubation with activated NK cells. As is shown in figure 2D we found CXCR3-expressing NK cells to produce significantly more IFN-γ than NK cells negative for CXCR3. Analyzing HSC-induced IFN-γ production in circulating CD56BrightCXCR3(+), CD56BrightCXCR3(−), CD56DimCXCR3(+), and CD56DimCXCR3(−) NK cells separately confirmed the sequential decrease in functional activity in these four subsets (Figure 2F).

Expression of NKG2D on CXCR3(+) and CXCR3(−) NK Cell Subsets

The activating NK cell receptor NKG2D has been shown to be critically involved in killing of hepatic stellate cells by NK cells. Thus, we next studied expression of this NK cell receptor in circulating CXCR3-expressing and CXCR3-negative NK cell subsets. Frequency of NKG2D(+) NK cells did not differ between the four studied NK cell subsets. However, we found CXCR3(+) NK cells to display a significantly higher NKG2D surface expression as compared to their CXCR3(−) counterpart (Figure 3A).

Thus, we next performed blocking experiments to confirm a functional role of NKG2D in NK cell-mediated killing of HSC. Indeed, we found that co-incubation with a NKG2D-specific blocking antibody significantly reduced NK cell degranulation following co-incubation with HSC in both CXCR3(+) and CXCR3(−)CD56Bright NK cells (Figure 3B). A role for NKG2D was furthermore supported by the fact that cytotoxic activity of CXCR3(+) and CXCR3(−) CD56Bright NK cells against HSC did not differ significantly when NKG2D was blocked with a specific antibody (Figure 3C).

CXCR3(+)CD56Bright NK Cells from HCV-positive Patients Show Impaired Activity Against Hepatic Stellate Cells and Accumulate in the Fibrotic Liver

Finally, we studied whether chronic HCV infection might affect phenotype and function of CXCR3-expressing NK cells.

Analyzing circulating NK cells obtained from HCV infected patients confirmed the dichotomous pattern of CXCR3 expression. However, chronic hepatitis C was associated with a significantly increased percentage of peripheral CXCR3(+)CD56Bright NK cells as compared to HCV(−) controls (Figure 4A).

Dys-regulated hepatic recruitment of CXCR3-expressing immunocompetent cells has been suggested as a potential mechanism involved in the observed association between levels of CXCR3 ligands and stages of HCV-induced liver fibrosis. Thus, we next studied intra-hepatic frequency of CXCR3(+)CD56Bright NK cells in patients showing different degrees of liver fibrosis. Given the strong anti-fibrotic potential of peripheral CXCR3(+)CD56Bright NK cells observed in healthy individuals we speculated that advanced stages of HCV-associated liver fibrosis may be associated with a decreased intra-hepatic frequency of this NK cell subset. Surprisingly, the opposite was true as we found a significantly higher frequency of CXCR3(+)CD56Bright NK cells in livers of patients with F3/4 fibrosis as compared to livers with less advanced fibrosis (Figure 3B).

To better understand this finding we next analyzed functional activity of NK cells against HSC in chronic HCV infection. Unlike

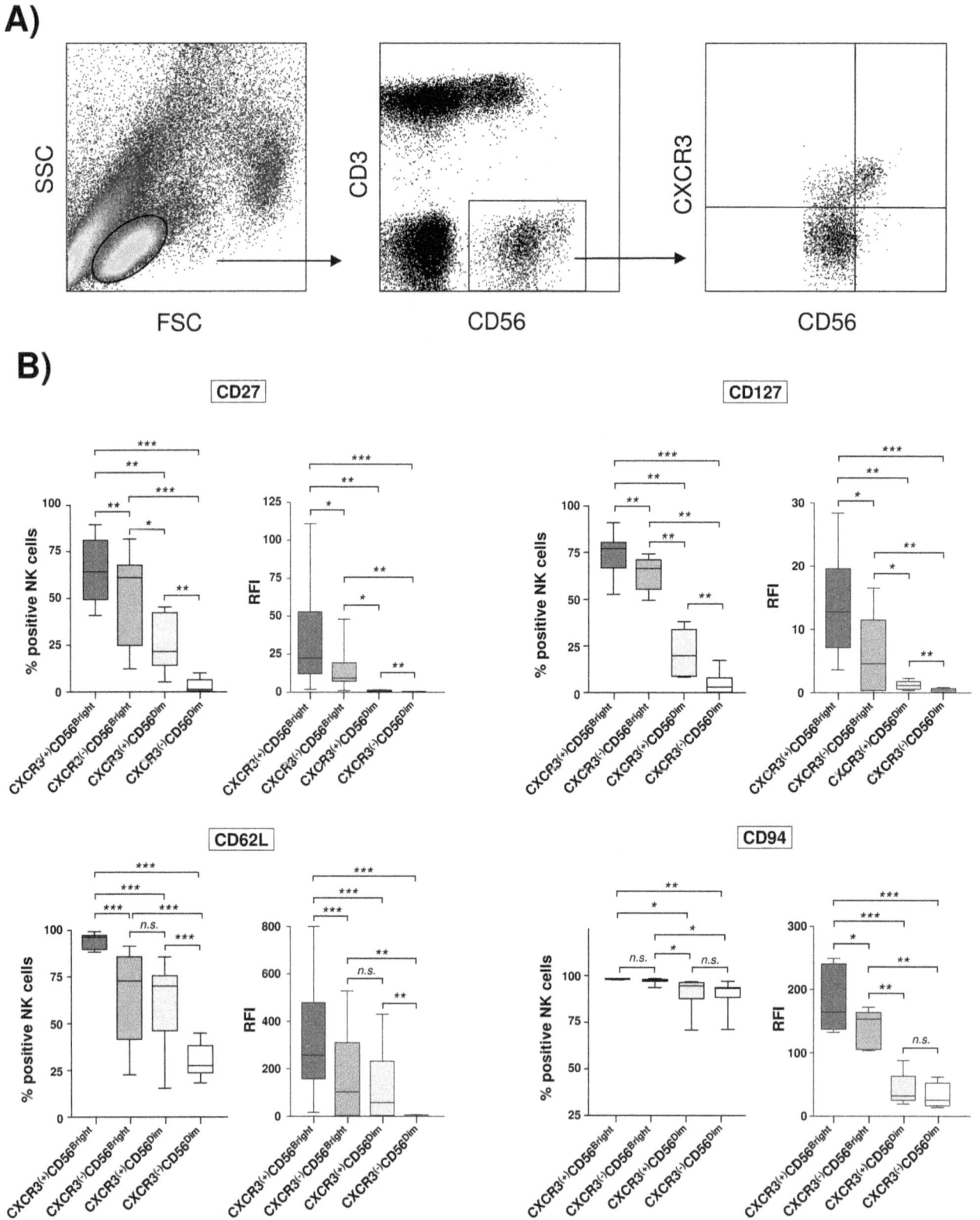

Figure 1. CXCR3 expression dissects phenotypically distinct NK cell subsets. Figure 1A: PBMCs in whole blood specimen were stained with anti-CD3, anti-CD56, and anti-CXCR3. CD3$^{(-)}$ CD56$^{(+)}$ NK cells were then gated for quantification of CXCR3 surface expression. Figure 1B: PBMCs from at least eight healthy donors were stained with anti-CD3, anti-CD56, and anti-CXCR3–conjugated mAb, as well as a mAb directed against the indicated maturation markers. CXCR3(+) and CXCR3(−) NK cell populations were then assessed for surface expression of the respective maturation marker. Results are given as box and whisker plots, with medians and 10th, 25th, 75th, and 90th percentiles. * indicates p<0.05; **indicates p<0.01; *** indicates p<0.001.

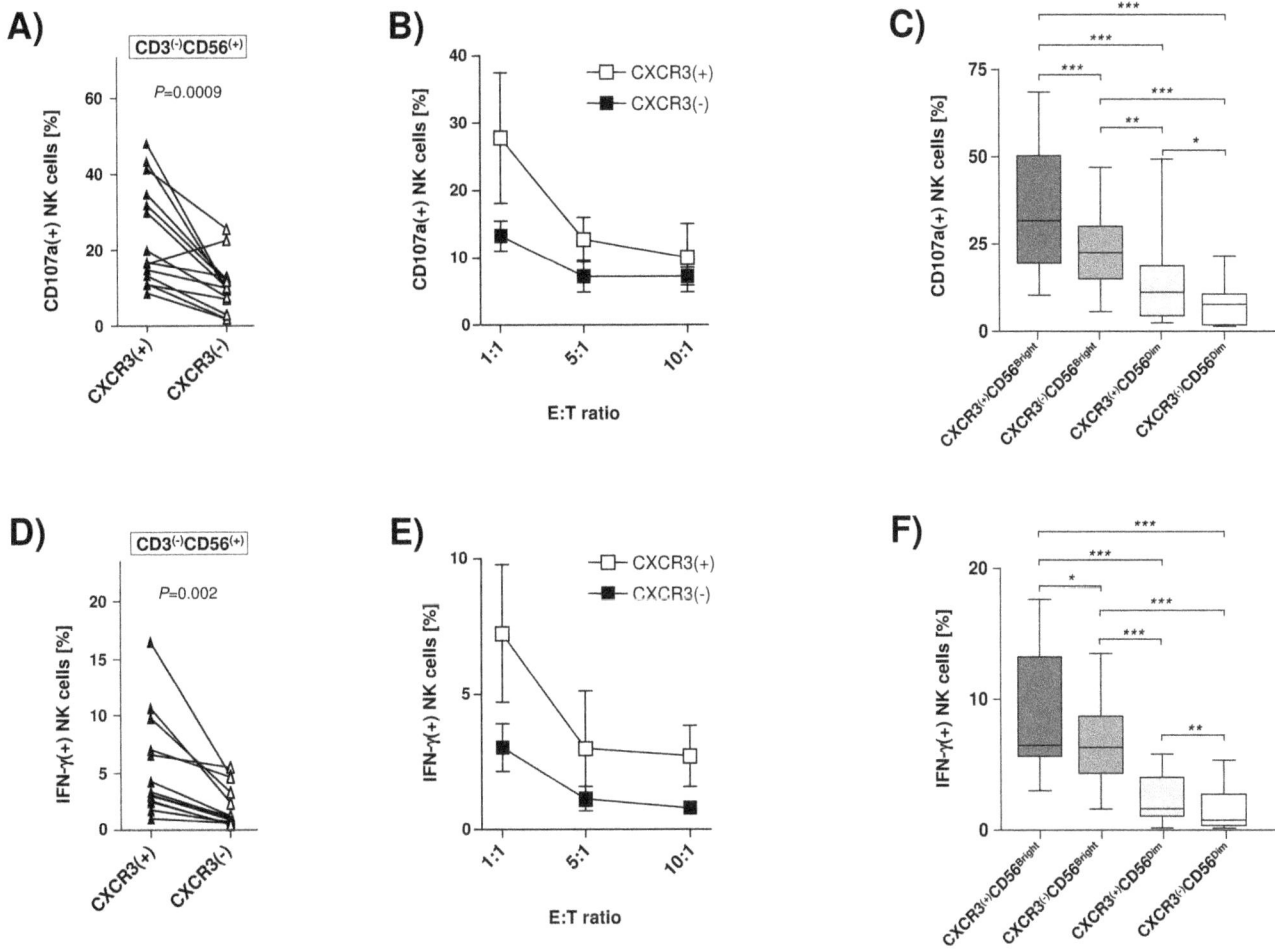

Figure 2. CXCR3(+)CD56Bright NK cells have strong anti-fibrotic potential. Figure 2A: Purified peripheral NK cells from healthy individuals (n = 14) were co-incubated with primary human hepatic stellate cells (E:T ratio 1:1) and then analyzed with respect to degranulation (CD107a) and expression of CXCR3 by flowcytometry. Figure 2B depicts NK cell degranulation following co-incubation with HSC at different effector : target (E:T) ratios as indicated (n = 5). Figure 2C shows CD107a expression of the four studied NK cell sub-populations obtained from healthy donors (n = 14) following co-incubation with primary hepatic stellate cells (E:T ratio 1:1). Figure 2D illustrates IFN-γ production of purified CXCR3(+) and CXCR3(−) NK cells obtained from HCV(-) individuals (n = 14) after co-culturing with primary HSC (E:T ratio 1:1). Figure 2E shows IFN-γ production of purified NK cells following co-incubation with hepatic stellate cells at different E:T ratios (n = 4). Figure 2F displays IFN-γ production of the four studied NK cell sub-populations isolated from healthy donors (n = 14) following co-incubation with primary hepatic stellate cells (E:T ratio 1:1).

natural killer cells obtained from healthy individuals we could not find any significant differences regarding HSC-induced degranulation and IFN-γ secretion between circulating CXCR3(+)CD56Bright and CXCR3(−)CD56Bright NK cell subsets in HCV-infected patients (Figure 5A). More importantly, peripheral CXCR3(+)CD56Bright NK cells obtained from HCV(+) patients exhibited significantly lower HSC-induced degranulation (p = 0.009) and IFN-γ production (p = 0.02) than CXCR3(+)CD56Bright NK cells from healthy controls (Figure 5B). Impaired cytotoxic activity was also found in the other NK cell subset. However, significantly decreased production of IFN-γ was a specific finding in the CXCR3(+)CD56Bright subset, suggesting that CXCR3(+)CD56Bright NK cells might represent a NK cell subset with dys-regulated anti-fibrotic potential in chronic hepatitis C. As a potential mechanism underlying this impaired functional activity we found chronic hepatitis C to be associated with a significantly decreased surface expression of NKG2D (Figure 5C).

Discussion

Infection with the hepatitis C virus often results in chronic liver disease and subsequent development of liver fibrosis/cirrhosis.

The exact mechanisms leading to liver injury are only partly understood. However, there is clear evidence indicating that activation of the immune response is a critical factor for the pathogenetic processes leading to progressive tissue injury and ultimately cirrhosis. Accordingly, liver cell damage has been shown to be associated with the presence of an intra-hepatic inflammatory infiltrate. On the other hand, there is increasing data suggesting that natural killer cells, a major component of the intra-hepatic lymphocyte pool, may mediate anti-fibrotic effects. In mouse models NK cells have been shown to exert anti-fibrotic activity by killing activated stellate cells. Moreover, impaired activity of murine NK cells has been associated with progressive liver fibrosis [14,15].

Hepatic recruitment of lymphocytes such as NK cells is regulated by chemokines and their respective receptors. Lymphocytes sense chemokine concentration gradients and move toward

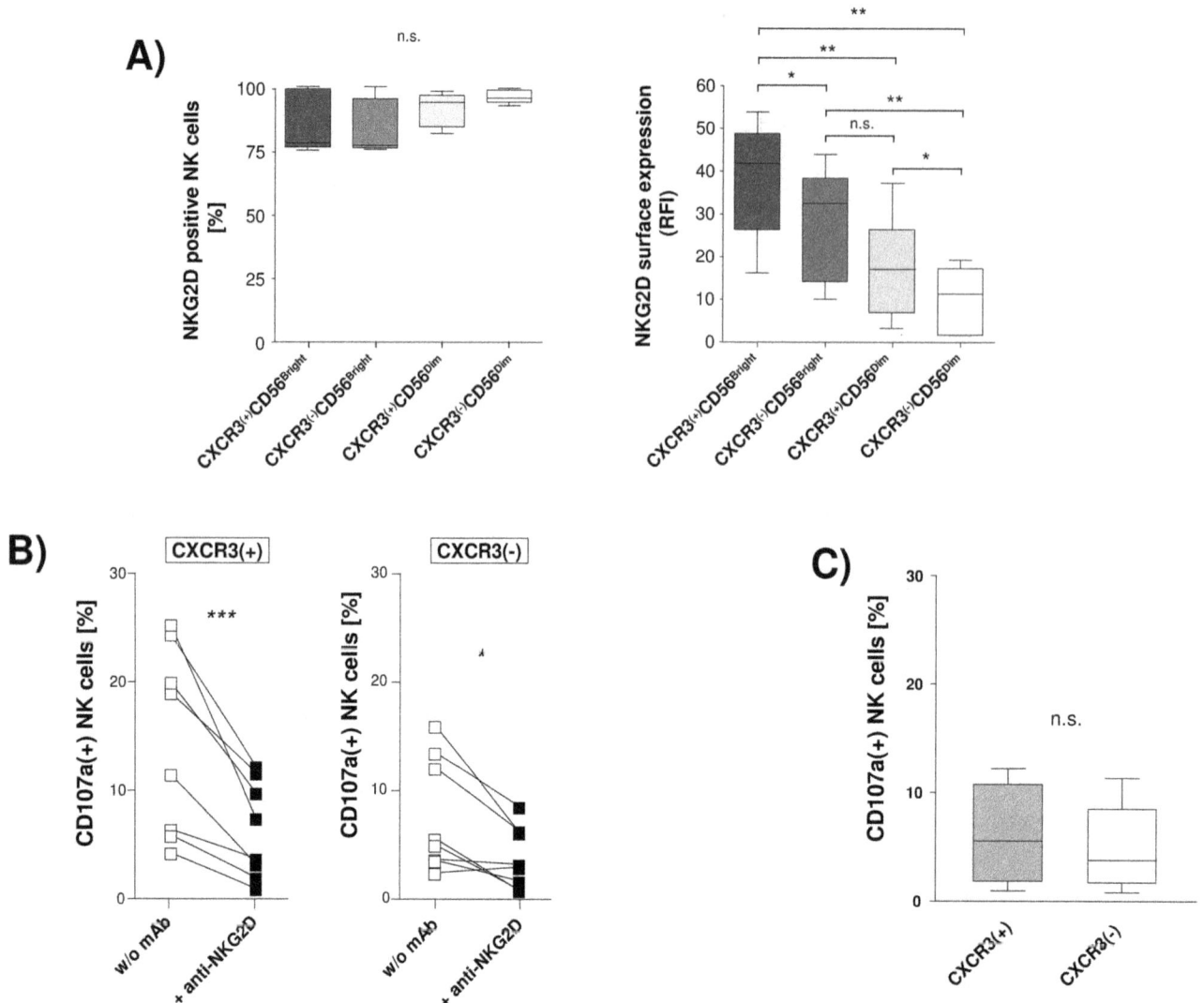

Figure 3. Role of NKG2D in anti-fibrotic activity of CXCR3-expressing NK cells. Figure 3A: Circulating NK cells obtained from HCV(-) individuals (n = 5) were analyzed for co-expression of NKG2D and CXCR3. The figure compares frequency of NKG2D-positive cells (left graph) as well as density of NKG2D surface expression (relative fluorescence intensity, RFI) (right graph) between the four studied NK cell subsets. Figure 3B shows the effect of NKG2D blockade on HSC-induced degranulation of CXCR3(+) and CXCR3(−) CD56Bright NK cell subsets obtained from healthy donors (n = 8). Figure 3C compares HSC-induced degranulation of CXCR3(+) and CXCR3(−) CD56Bright NK cell subsets (n = 8) following pre-incubation with anti-NKG2D. Results are given as box and whisker plots, with medians and 10th, 25th, 75th, and 90th percentiles. * indicates p<0.05; **indicates p<0.01; *** indicates p<0.001.

increasing concentrations. Thus, both differential chemokine secretion in the inflamed liver and selective expression of different chemokine receptors on distinct lymphocyte subsets regulate hepatic recruitment of lymphocytes [2]. Of note, recent data indicate that the chemokines receptor CXCR3 and its ligands, especially CXCL10 (IP-10) may play an important role in the regulation of HCV-associated liver fibrosis [5–8] by yet incompletely understood mechanisms. Given the observed anti-fibrotic potential of NK cells we speculated that CXCR3-mediated recruitment of functionally distinct NK cell subpopulation might play a role.

To clarify this issue, we first analyzed the *ex vivo* phenotypic characteristics of circulating CXCR3(+) and CXCR3(−) NK cells. CXCR3-expressing NK cells were found in both the CD56Dim and the CD56Bright subset although frequency of CXCR3(+) NK cells was higher among CD56Bright cells. More importantly,

comparing CD56BrightCXCR3(+), CD56BrightCXCR3(−), CD56DimCXCR3(+), and CD56DimCXCR3(−) NK cells separately we observed a progressive decrease in surface expression of the maturation markers CD27, CD62L, and CD127. In addition, the CXCR3(+) subset displayed significantly higher co-expression of the NK cell receptors NKG2A, NKG2C, and NKp44. Thus, our data suggest that expression of CXCR3 defines distinct NK cell subsets.

This concept was confirmed at the functional level, because in healthy controls CXCR3(+) and CXCR3(−) NK cell subsets differed significantly with respect to cytolytic activity and IFN-γ production after exposure to human hepatic stellate cells, with CD56BrightCXCR3(+) NK cells displaying the strongest activity against HSC. Activated HSC are considered to critically contribute to the establishment of hepatic fibrosis via excessive production of collagen. Thus, effective killing of HSC by

A)

B)

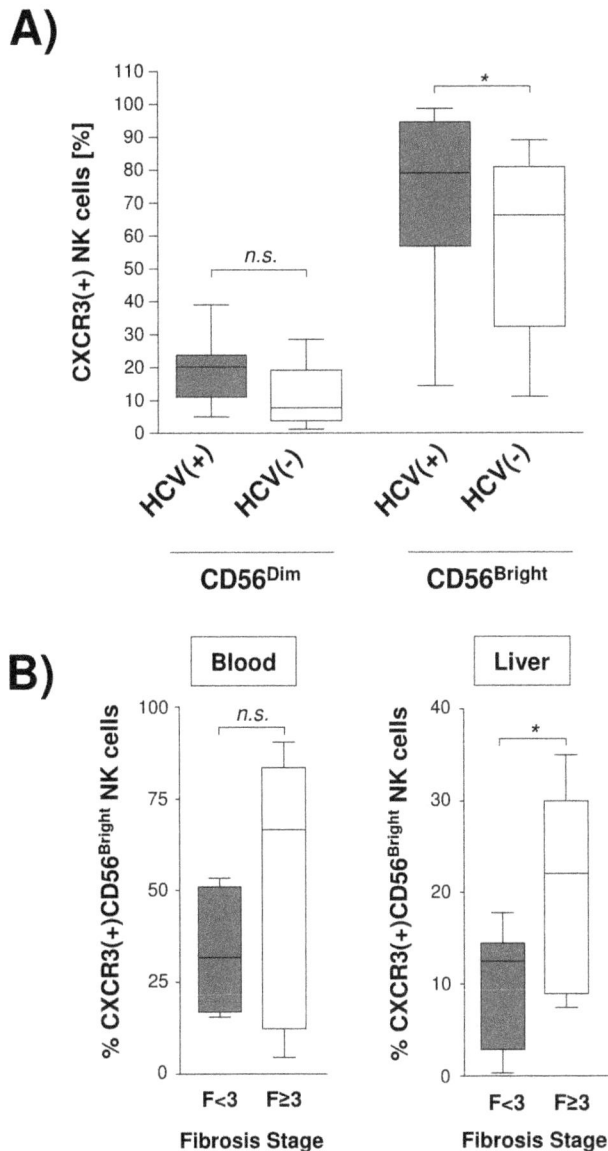

Figure 4. Frequency of CXCR3 expressing NK cells in chronic hepatitis C. Figure 4A compares frequency of peripheral CXCR3(+) NK cells in HCV infected (n = 14) and healthy individuals (n = 16). Figure 4B: Peripheral and liver-infiltrating NK cells from HCV-infected individuals were analyzed for expression of CXCR3 by flowcytometry Then frequency of circulating (left graph) and intra-hepatic (right graph) CXCR3(+)CD56Bright NK cells was compared between patients with progressive (F≥3; n = 6) and less advanced (F<3; n = 9) liver fibrosis. Results are given as box and whisker plots, with medians and 10th, 25th, 75th, and 90th percentiles. * indicates p<0.05.

CD56BrightCXCR3(+) NK cells suggests that this specific lymphocyte subset may play an important role in the regulation of HCV-associated liver fibrosis. However, in hepatitis C high levels of CXCR3 ligands have been associated with progressive liver cell damage and fibrosis [5–8]. Recently, these counterintuitive data could – at least in part – be explained by the identification of a chemokine antagonism in HCV infection which prevents CXCR3-mediated recruitment of immunocompetent cells into the liver thereby resulting in extra-hepatic accumulation of CXCR3-expressing cells [11]. Accordingly, we found chronic hepatitis C to be associated with a significantly increased

frequency of circulating CXCR3-expressing CD56Bright NK cells. However, we also observed a significantly increased frequency of CXCR3(+)CD56Bright NK cells in livers with advanced stages of fibrosis, suggesting that mechanism(s) other than dys-regulated hepatic migration may also play a role.

Indeed, our data indicate that hepatitis C may be associated with impaired activity of peripheral CXCR3(+) NK cells because we found that in HCV infected patients_specifically the CD56BrightCXCR3(+) subset displayed decreased degranulation and IFN-γ secretion in response to human HSC. Unfortunately, number of intra-hepatic NK cells in our study was insufficient to study activity of liver NK cells against HSC. Thus, it remains to be clarified whether intra-hepatic CXCR3-expressing NK cells also show dys-regulated activity against activated HSC or even exert pro-fibrotic effects.

The exact mechanisms responsible for this impaired functional activity of circulating CD56BrightCXCR3(+) NK cells in HCV infection remain incompletely understood but may involve altered surface expression of the NK cell receptor NKG2D. Mouse models indicate that NK cell killing of activated hepatic stellate cells is mediated via activating NK cell receptor NKG2D [14–16,20–24]. Accordingly, we found that blocking of NKG2D significantly reduced NK cell degranulation and IFN-γ secretion following co-incubation with HSC. Thus, our finding of decreased NKG2D surface expression in hepatitis C would be an intriguing explanation for our observation of impaired NK cell activity against HSC. However, the role of NKG2D in HCV infection is discussed controversially as some authors reported down-regulated expression of this NK cell receptor [25] whereas other studies found increased surface expression in hepatitis C [26,27]. In line with data presented by Sène and colleagues we found that differences in HCV(+) patients and healthy controls only affected expression levels of NKG2D, but not the frequency of NKG2D-positive cells [25].

However, reduced expression of NKG2D was not specific for the CXCR3(+)CD56Bright subset, indicating that other mechanisms may also play a role.

Taken together, we show that distinct NK cell subsets can be distinguished based on CXCR3 surface expression. Intra-hepatic accumulation of functionally impaired CD56BrightCXCR3(+) might be involved in the progression of HCV-induced liver fibrosis.

Methods

Patients

A total of 57 patients of Western European descent, all from the Bonn area in Germany, with chronic hepatitis C virus (HCV) infection were enrolled into this study (Table 1). None of these patients had histological evidence of liver cirrhosis and all were treatment naïve. As control we studied 27 healthy donors. Written informed consent was obtained from all patients. The study had been approved by the local ethics committee of the University of Bonn.

Flowcytometric Analysis. For FACS analysis the following antibodies were used: anti-CD3, anti-CD27, anti-CD56, anti-CD62L, anti-CD107a, anti-CD127 (BD Biosciences, Heidelberg, Germany); anti-CXCR3, anti-NKG2A, anti-NKG2C, anti-NKG2D, anti-NKp30, anti-NKp44, anti-NKp46, and anti-INF-γ (R&D Systems; Wiesbaden-Nordenstadt, Germany). After staining, cells were washed and analyzed on a FACSCalibur flowcytometer using the Flowjo 7.2.2 software package (Treestar, Ashland, USA).

A)

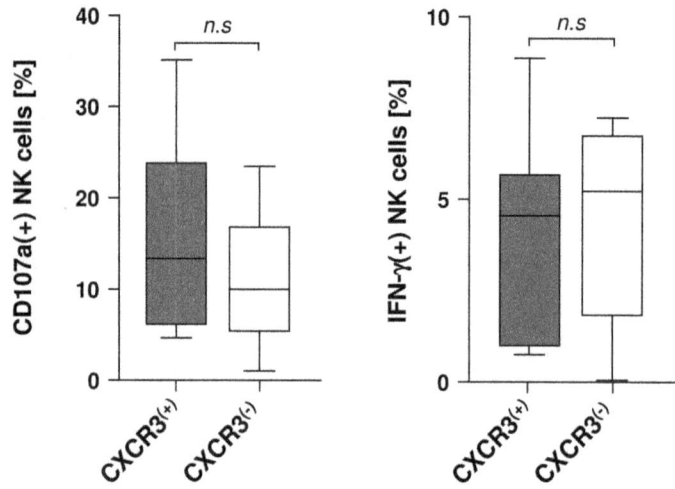

B)

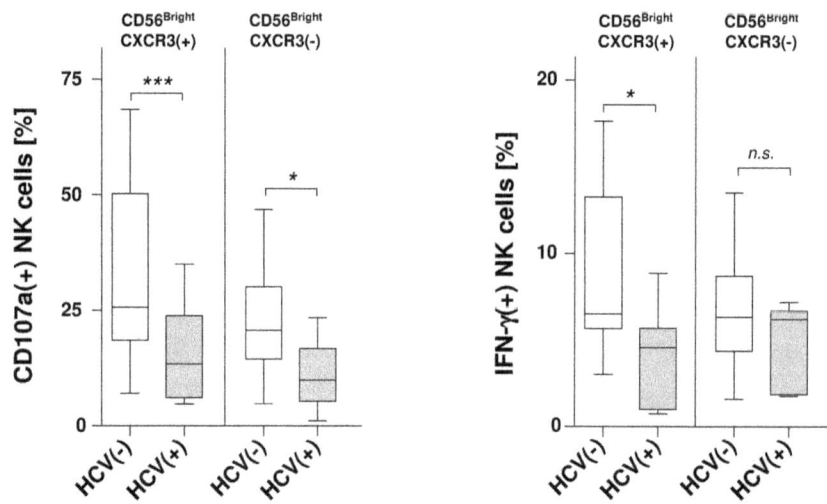

C)

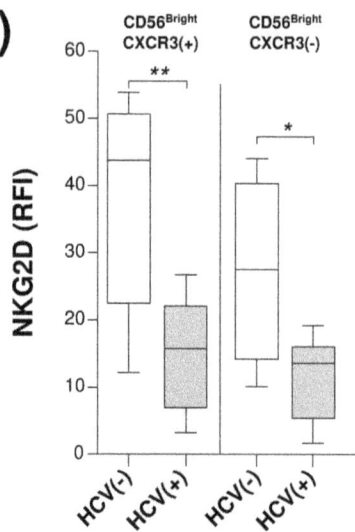

Figure 5. CXCR3(+)CD56Bright NK cells show impaired functional activity against HSC in chronic hepatitis C. Figure 5A: Circulating CXCR3(+) and CXCR3(−) CD56Bright NK cells from HCV(+) patients (n = 11) were co-incubated with primary human hepatic stellate cells and then assessed for degranulation (CD107a) as well as IFN-γ production by FACS analysis. Figure 5B compares HSC-induced degranulation and IFN-γ secretion between NK cell subsets obtained from healthy (n = 14) and HCV(+) (n = 11) donors. Figure 5C illustrates NKG2D surface expression on circulating CXCR3(+) and CXCR3(−) CD56Bright NK cells in hepatitis C (n = 7) in comparison to healthy controls (n = 4). Results are given as box and whisker plots, with medians and 10th, 25th, 75th, and 90th percentiles. * indicates p<0.05.

Cell Separation

NK cells were immunomagnetically separated from total PBMC by depletion of non-NK cells using EasySep Human NK Cell Enrichment Kit (StemCell Technologies, Grenoble, France). NK cells were cultured overnight for further experiments in RPMI1640 (PAA, Cölbe, Germany) supplemented with 25IU IL-2 (R&D Systems).

Purity of NK cells was >95% as determined by flowcytometric analysis.

Primary Human Hepatic Stellate Cells

Isolated primary activated human hepatic stellate cells (HSC; ScienCell, San Diego, CA, USA) [15-17] were cultured for 2–4 passages in defined Stellate Cell Medium (SteCM, ScienCell) supplemented with 2% fetal bovine serum, 5 ml stellate cell growth supplement, 10 U/ml penicillin and 10 µg/ml streptomycin (all ingredients obtained from ScienCell) at 37°C with 5% CO_2 and cryopreserved until further use.

Two days before HSC were used in an experiment the cells were thawed and cultured in SteCM medium. Then cells were harvested, washed, checked for viability using trypan blue, and then used in the respective experiments. Activated status of HSC was verified by immunofluorescence staining of α-smooth muscle actin.

IFN-γ Production

Isolated NK cells were co-cultured with HSC at 1:1 effector:target (E:T) ratio in 48-well round-bottom plates at 37°C for 5 h. Brefeldin A (10 µg/ml, Sigma-Aldrich) was added after 1hour of co-culture. Next, cells were harvested and washed in PBS. Finally,

cells were stained with anti-CXCR3-FITC, anti–CD56 APC, and anti-CD3 PerCP, fixed and permeabilized using Cytofix/Cytoperm (BD Biosciences), followed by intracellular staining with an anti–IFN-γ PE mAb and FACS analysis.

CD107a Degranulation Assay

Cytotoxic activity of NK cells was assessed by a CD107a degranulation assay as described before [18]. In brief, purified NK cells were co-incubated with HSC at 1:1 effector:target (E:T) ratio in the presence of CD107a mAb. After 1 h GolgiStop (BD Biosciences) was added and cells were cultured for an additional 3 h. Then, cells were stained, washed, and re-suspended in CellFix (BD Biosciences) followed by flowcytometric analysis.

Flow Cytometric Analysis of Cells in the Liver Specimens

Liver biopsy specimens for flowcytometric analysis of intra-hepatic cells were obtained from liver biopsies (n = 15) using 1.4 mm diameter disposable biopsy needles. Grading and staging of liver biopsies were performed according to the METAVIR score as part of the routine diagnostic work-up (F0: n = 5, F1: n = 1, F2: n = 3, F3: n = 4, F4: n = 2).

Fresh liver samples were washed twice in fresh medium and shaken gently to avoid blood contamination. Liver specimens were disrupted mechanically into small fragments in RPMI 1640 medium with 10% FCS using a forceps and scalpel. Then the fragments were homogenized on a cell strainer (BD Labware). The resulting cell suspension was washed and resuspended in RPMI 1640 medium. Intra-hepatic cells were then directly analyzed by flowcytometry.

Statistical Analysis

Statistical analyses were performed using GraphPad Prism Version 5.0a (GraphPad Software Inc, San Diego, CA) and the SPSS 17.0 (SPSS, Chicago, IL) statistical package. Mann–Whitney U tests were used to compare NK cell phenotype and cytolytic response between two independent groups. Wilcoxon tests were performed for individual comparison of the paired groups.

A 2-sided P value <0.05 was considered significant.

Acknowledgments

Disclaimer: The findings and opinion expressed herein belong to the authors and do not necessarily reflect the official views of the funder.

Parts of these data have been present at the 61st Annual Meeting of the American Association for the Study of the Liver (AASLD) 2010.

Author Contributions

Conceived and designed the experiments: ME TS US JN. Performed the experiments: ME AG BK CK PK BS. Analyzed the data: ME HDN TS US JN. Wrote the paper: ME JN US TS.

References

1. Butera D, Marukian S, Iwamaye AE, Hembrador E, Chambers TJ, et al. (2005) Plasma chemokine levels correlate with the outcome of antiviral therapy in patients with hepatitis C. Blood 106: 1175–1182.

Table 1. Patient Characteristics.

	HCV RNA(+)	healthy controls
Number	57	27
Female sex	16 (28.1%)	13 (48.1%)
Age (years)	46.95 (17–72)	29.1 (22–49)
Clinical data		
ALT U/L	96.2 (13–384)	n.a. [c]
γ-GT	142.9 (21–957)	n.a. [c]
HCV-Status		-
HCV Load (×10^6 copies/mL) [b]	5.2 (n.a. –23.3)	-
HCV-Genotypes:		
Genotype 1 [1a]	29 (50.9%)	-
Genotype 2 [1a]	3 (5.3%)	-
Genotype 3 [1a]	8 (14.0%)	-
Genotype 4 [1a]	4 (7.0%)	-
Undetermined Genotype [1a]	13 (22.8%)	-

[a] number of cases (number/total in %).
[b] mean (range).
[c] n.a. – not analyzed.

2. Lagging M, Romero AI, Westin J, Norkrans G, Dhillon AP, et al. (2006) IP-10 predicts viral response and therapeutic outcome in difficult-to-treat patients with HCV genotype 1 infection. Hepatology 44: 1617–1625.

3. Romero AI, Lagging M, Westin J, Dhillon AP, Dustin LB, et al. (2006) Interferon (IFN)-gamma-inducible protein-10: association with histological results, viral kinetics, and outcome during treatment with pegylated IFN-alpha 2a and ribavirin for chronic hepatitis C virus infection. J Infect Dis 194: 895–903.

4. Diago M, Castellano G, Garcia-Samaniego J, Perez C, Fernandez I, et al. (2006) Association of pretreatment serum interferon gamma inducible protein 10 levels with sustained virological response to peginterferon plus ribavirin therapy in genotype 1 infected patients with chronic hepatitis C. Gut 55: 374–379.

5. Harvey CE, Post JJ, Palladinetti P, Freeman AJ, Ffrench RA, et al. (2003) Expression of the chemokine IP-10 (CXCL10) by hepatocytes in chronic hepatitis C virus infection correlates with histological severity and lobular inflammation. J Leukoc Biol 74: 360–369.

6. Helbig KJ, Ruszkiewicz A, Semendric L, Harley HA, McColl SR, et al. (2004) Expression of the CXCR3 ligand I-TAC by hepatocytes in chronic hepatitis C and its correlation with hepatic inflammation. Hepatology 39: 1220–1229.

7. Zeremski M, Dimova R, Brown Q, Jacobson IM, Markatou M, et al. (2009) Peripheral CXCR3-associated chemokines as biomarkers of fibrosis in chronic hepatitis C virus infection. J Infect Dis 200: 1774–1780.

8. Zeremski M, Petrovic LM, Chiriboga L, Brown QB, Yee HT, et al. (2008) Intrahepatic levels of CXCR3-associated chemokines correlate with liver inflammation and fibrosis in chronic hepatitis C. Hepatology 48: 1440–1450.

9. Zeremski M, Dimova R, Astemborski J, Thomas DL, Talal AH (2011) CXCL9 and CXCL10 chemokines as predictors of liver fibrosis in a cohort of primarily African-American injection drug users with chronic hepatitis C. J Infect Dis 204: 832–836.

10. Tacke F, Zimmermann HW, Berres ML, Trautwein C, Wasmuth HE (2011) Serum chemokine receptor CXCR3 ligands are associated with progression, organ dysfunction and complications of chronic liver diseases. Liver Int 31: 840–849.

11. Casrouge A, Decalf J, Ahloulay M, Lababidi C, Mansour H, et al. (2011) Evidence for an antagonist form of the chemokine CXCL10 in patients chronically infected with HCV. J Clin Invest 121: 308–317.

12. Norris S, Collins C, Doherty DG, Smith F, McEntee G, et al. (1998) Resident human hepatic lymphocytes are phenotypically different from circulating lymphocytes. J Hepatol 28: 84–90.

13. Cruise MW, Lukens JR, Nguyen AP, Lassen MG, Waggoner SN, et al. (2006) Fas ligand is responsible for CXCR3 chemokine induction in CD4+ T cell-dependent liver damage. J Immunol 176: 6235–6244.

14. Radaeva S, Sun R, Jaruga B, Nguyen VT, Tian Z, et al. (2006) Natural killer cells ameliorate liver fibrosis by killing activated stellate cells in NKG2D-dependent and tumor necrosis factor-related apoptosis-inducing ligand-dependent manners. Gastroenterology 130: 435–452.

15. Melhem A, Muhanna N, Bishara A, Alvarez CE, Ilan Y, et al. (2006) Antifibrotic activity of NK cells in experimental liver injury through killing of activated HSC. J Hepatol 45: 60–71.

16. Jeong WI, Park O, Suh YG, Byun JS, Park SY, et al. (2011) Suppression of innate immunity (natural killer cell/interferon-gamma) in the advanced stages of liver fibrosis in mice. Hepatology 53: 1342–1351.

17. Morishima C, Paschal DM, Wang CC, Yoshihara CS, Wood BL, et al. (2006) Decreased NK cell frequency in chronic hepatitis C does not affect ex vivo cytolytic killing. Hepatology 43: 573–580.

18. Muhanna N, Abu Tair L, Doron S, Amer J, Azzeh M, et al. (2010) Amelioration of hepatic fibrosis by NK cell activation. Gut 60: 90–98.

19. Jeong WI, Gao B (2008) Innate immunity and alcoholic liver fibrosis. J Gastroenterol Hepatol 23 Suppl 1: S112–118.

20. Gao B, Radaeva S, Jeong WI (2007) Activation of natural killer cells inhibits liver fibrosis: a novel strategy to treat liver fibrosis. Expert Rev Gastroenterol Hepatol 1: 173–180.

21. Jeong WI, Park O, Gao B (2008) Abrogation of the antifibrotic effects of natural killer cells/interferon-gamma contributes to alcohol acceleration of liver fibrosis. Gastroenterology 134: 248–258.

22. Jeong WI, Park O, Radaeva S, Gao B (2006) STAT1 inhibits liver fibrosis in mice by inhibiting stellate cell proliferation and stimulating NK cell cytotoxicity. Hepatology 44: 1441–1451.

23. Muhanna N, Abu Tair L, Doron S, Amer J, Azzeh M, et al. (2011) Amelioration of hepatic fibrosis by NK cell activation. Gut 60: 90–98.

24. Radaeva S, Wang L, Radaev S, Jeong WI, Park O, et al. (2007) Retinoic acid signaling sensitizes hepatic stellate cells to NK cell killing via upregulation of NK cell activating ligand RAE1. Am J Physiol Gastrointest Liver Physiol 293: G809–816.

25. Sene D, Levasseur F, Abel M, Lambert M, Camous X, et al. (2010) Hepatitis C virus (HCV) evades NKG2D-dependent NK cell responses through NS5A-mediated imbalance of inflammatory cytokines. PLoS Pathog 6: e1001184.

26. Oliviero B, Varchetta S, Paudice E, Michelone G, Zaramella M, et al. (2009) Natural killer cell functional dichotomy in chronic hepatitis B and chronic hepatitis C virus infections. Gastroenterology 137: 1151–1160, 1160 e1151–1157.

27. Varchetta S, Oliviero B, Francesca Donato M, Agnelli F, Rigamonti C, et al. (2009) Prospective study of natural killer cell phenotype in recurrent hepatitis C virus infection following liver transplantation. J Hepatol 50: 314–322.

Discordance between Liver Biopsy and FibroScan® in Assessing Liver Fibrosis in Chronic Hepatitis B: Risk Factors and Influence of Necroinflammation

Seung Up Kim[1,2,5], **Ja Kyung Kim**[1,2,5], **Young Nyun Park**[3,4,5,6]*, **Kwang-Hyub Han**[1,2,5,6]*

1 Department of Internal Medicine, Yonsei University College of Medicine, Seoul, Korea, **2** Institute of Gastroenterology, Yonsei University College of Medicine, Seoul, Korea, **3** Department of Pathology, Yonsei University College of Medicine, Seoul, Korea, **4** Center for Chronic Metabolic Disease, Yonsei University College of Medicine, Seoul, Korea, **5** Liver Cirrhosis Clinical Research Center, Seoul, Korea, **6** Brain Korea 21 Project for Medical Science, Seoul, Korea

Abstract

Background: Few studies have investigated predictors of discordance between liver biopsy (LB) and liver stiffness measurement (LSM) using FibroScan®. We assessed predictors of discordance between LB and LSM in chronic hepatitis B (CHB) and investigated the effects of necroinflammatory activity.

Methods: In total, 150 patients (107 men, 43 women) were prospectively enrolled. Only LSM with ≥10 valid measurements was considered reliable. Liver fibrosis was evaluated using the Laennec system. LB specimens <15 mm in length were considered ineligible. Reference cutoff LSM values to determine discordance were calculated from our cohort (6.0 kPa for ≥F2, 7.5 kPa for ≥F3, and 9.4 kPa for F4).

Results: A discordance, defined as a discordance of at least two stages between LB and LSM, was identified in 21 (14.0%) patients. In multivariate analyses, fibrosis stages F3–4 and F4 showed independent negative associations with discordance (P = 0.002; hazard ratio [HR], 0.073; 95% confidence interval [CI], 0.014–0.390 for F3–4 and P = 0.014; HR, 0.067; 95% CI, 0.008–0.574 for F4). LSM values were not significantly different between maximal activity grades 1–2 and 3–4 in F1 and F2 fibrosis stages, whereas LSM values were significantly higher in maximal activity grade 3–4 than 1–2 in F3 and F4 fibrosis stage (median 8.6 vs. 11.3 kPa in F3, P = 0.049; median 11.9 vs. 19.2 kPa in F4, P = 0.009).

Conclusion: Advanced fibrosis stage (F3–4) or cirrhosis (F4) showed a negative correlation with discordance between LB and LSM in patients with CHB, and maximal activity grade 3–4 significantly influenced LSM values in F3 and F4.

Editor: Man-Fung Yuen, The University of Hong Kong, Hong Kong

Funding: This study was supported by the grant of the Good Health R & D Project from the Ministry of Health, Welfare and Family Affairs, Republic of Korea (A050021) and the National Research Foundation grant (R13-2002-054-03004-0) funded by the Korea government (MOST) (to YNP). The funders had no role in study design, data collection and analysis, decision to publish, or preparation of the manuscript.

Competing Interests: The authors have declared that no competing interests exist.

* E-mail: young0608@yuhs.ac (YNP); gihankhys@yuhs.ac (K-HH)

Introduction

Because the prognosis of and management strategies for patients with chronic liver diseases depend strongly on the severity of liver fibrosis, early detection of significant fibrosis is key [1]. To date, liver biopsy (LB) has been the gold standard for assessing liver fibrosis. However, its invasiveness, potential adverse events [2], sampling errors [3], and interpretational variability [4] have encouraged clinicians to seek more accurate and noninvasive tools for assessing liver fibrosis.

Recently, liver stiffness measurement (LSM) using FibroScan® was introduced as a noninvasive device to accurately assess liver fibrosis [5]. In view of the results achieved so far, LSM can help physicians decide treatment strategies, predict prognosis, and monitor disease progression or regression in patients with chronic liver disease. Despite the clinical usefulness of LSM, several confounding factors that can diminish the accuracy of LSM have been identified, such as necroinflammatory activity, reflected by a high alanine aminotransferase (ALT) level, cholestasis, or heart failure [6–12]. In addition to these extrinsic factors, LSM should satisfy the intrinsic prerequisites for preserving the validity of LSM: ≥10 valid measurements, a success rate ≥60%, and an interquartile range (IQR)/median LSM value among valid measurements (IQR/M) <0.3. However, because these criteria are not based on scientific evidence, several studies have tried to demonstrate the clinical relevance of these criteria by identifying factors that predict discordant results between LB and LSM in estimating liver fibrosis. Results from these studies have identified elevated ALT, high IQR/M, high body mass index (BMI), and fibrosis stage at the time of LB as predictors of discordance [13–15]. Although elevated ALT has been considered to be the single most important confounder on LSM, the effects of necroinflammatory activity, which is closely related to ALT level, on discordance between LB and LSM have not been determined.

Thus, in this study, we examined predictors of discordance between LB and LSM in patients with chronic hepatitis B

(CHB) and investigated the effects of necroinflammatory activity on LSM.

Methods

Patients

Between January 2007 and December 2009, 196 consecutive patients with CHB, defined by detectable hepatitis B virus surface antigen (HBsAg) for more than 6 months and positive hepatitis B virus (HBV) DNA by polymerase chain reaction assay, underwent both LB and LSM before starting antiviral treatment. Of them, 184 (93.9%) patients received LSMs on the same day as LB. The remaining LSMs were conducted at a median of 6 (range, 1–24) days before LB in 12 (6.1%) patients.

No patient had evidence of decompensated liver cirrhosis, such as a history of variceal bleeding, ascitic decompensation, hepatic encephalopathy, or Child-Pugh class B or C at the time of LB and LSM. Exclusions criteria were as follows: (1) previous antiviral treatment before LB, (2) evidence of liver cancer or another malignancy, (3) coinfection wtih hepatitis C virus, hepatitis D virus, or human immunodeficiency virus, (4) alcohol consumption in excess of 40 g/day for more than 5 years, (5) LB specimens shorter than 15 mm in length or unknown LB length, (6) right-sided heart failure, (7) LSM failure, or (8) unrelaible LSM (<10 valid measurments).

This study cohort includes a subset of a previous multicenter Korean study [14]. The study protocol was consistent with the ethical guidelines of the 1975 Declaration of Helsinki. Written informed consent was obtained from each participant or responsible family members after the possible complications of LB had been fully explained. This study was approved by the independent institutional review boards of Severance Hospital, Yonsei University College of Medicine.

Clinical data

Demographic details and BMI were collected. The following laboratory parameters were also collected from all the patients at the time of LSM; ALT, gamma-glutamyltranspeptidase (GGT), and platelet count. HBsAg was measured using standard enzyme-linked immunosorbent assays (Abbott Diagnostics, Abbott Park, IL, USA). The upper limit of normal (ULN) for ALT was defined as 40 IU/L.

Liver stiffness measurement

LSM was obtained according to the instructions provided by the manufacturer. Details of the technical background and examination procedure have been described previously [5,16–18]. The success rate was calculated as the number of valid measurements divided by the total number of measurements. Results are expressed in kilopascals (kPa). IQR was defined as an index of LSM intrinsic variability corresponding to the 25th and 75th percentiles intervals around the LSM result containing 50% of the valid measurements. The median value was considered representative of the elastic modulus of the liver. Only procedures with ≥10 validated measurements were considered reliable, regardless of success rate and IQR/M. The same experienced operator (>3,000 LSM examinations), blinded to LB results and the clinical data of the study population performed all LSM examinations.

Liver biopsy and histological evaluation

LB specimens were fixed in formalin and embedded in paraffin. Sections (4 μm) were stained with hematoxylin and eosin and Masson's trichrome. All liver tissue samples were evaluated by an experienced hepatopathologist (YN Park) who was blinded to the clinical data of study population, including LSM results. Liver fibrosis and necroinflammation were evaluated semiquantitatively according

to the Laennec system [19]. Fibrosis was scored in five grades at first: 0, no definite fibrosis, 1, minimal fibrosis (no septa or rare thin septum; may have portal expansion or mild sinusoidal fibrosis), 2, mild fibrosis (occasional thin septa), 3, moderate fibrosis (moderate thin septa; up to incomplete cirrhosis), and 4, liver cirrhosis. Then, liver cirrhosis was sub-classified into three groups: F4A, mild cirrhosis, definite or probable, 4B, moderate cirrhosis (at least two broad septa), and 4C, severe cirrhosis (at least one very broad septum or many minute nodules). The activity grade referred to the degree of necroinflammatory activity in the lobule and periportal area and was scored in five grades: A0, no activity, A1, minimal, A2, mild, A3, moderate, and A4, severe activity. Maximal activity grade was defined as the higher of the lobular and periportal activity. Steatosis in the liver specimen was graded on a four-point scale: S0 (insignificant, <5%), S1 (mild, 5–33%), S2 (moderate, 34–66%), and S3 (severe, ≥66% of hepatocytes with fat deposits) [20,21].

Statistical analysis

Patient characteristics are reported as means ± standard deviations, medians (ranges), or n (%), as appropriate. Continuous variables of patients with discordance and those without were compared with independent t-tests or Mann-Whitney U tests. The chi-squared or Fisher's exact test was used for categorical variables. A discordance was defined as a discordance of at least two stages between LB and LSM [13]. Cutoff LSM values for determining discordance were derived from our cohort, which maximized the sum of sensitivity (Se) and specificity (Sp). Positive and negative predictive value (PPV and NPV) was also computed. Spearman's analysis was used to investigate correlations between variables. Univariate and subsequent multivariate binary logistic regression analyses were performed to identify independent factors related to discordance between LB and LSM. Hazard ratios (HRs) and corresponding 95% confidence intervals (CIs) are also indicated. A two-sided P value of <0.05 was considered significant. All statistical analyses were performed with the SPSS software (ver. 12.0; SPSS Inc., Chicago, IL, USA).

Results

Baseline characteristics of the study population

After excluding 46 patients according to the predefined excludion criteria, 150 were included in the final analysis. Baseline characteristics of the excluded 46 patients including the percentage of discordance, were not significantly different from those of the remaining 150 patients (all P>0.05). The baseline characteristics of study population are listed in **Table 1**. The mean age, ALT level, and LSM values were 41.9 years, 74.1 IU/L, and 11.7 kPa, respectively. The proportions of patients with F2–4, F3–4, and F4 were 84.7% (n = 127), 56.0% (n = 84), and 45.3% (n = 68) and those of maximal A2–4, A3–4, and A4 were 88.0% (n = 132), 40.0% (n = 60), and 12.0% (n = 18), respectively. Among patients with cirrhosis (n = 68), 8 (11.8%), 44 (64.7%), and 16 (23.5%) patients showed F4A, F4B, and F4C, respectively.

Liver histology and corresponding LSM values

The median length of LB samples was 17 (range, 15–25) mm. The fibrosis stage and maximal activity grade are summarized in **Table 2**. Most patients (n = 126, 84.0%) showed no steatosis (S0) and only 1 (0.1%) patient with F1 fibrosis showed moderate steatosis (S2).

The median and range of LSM values according to maximal activity grade in each fibrosis stage are listed in **Table 2**. The median LSM values increased significantly as fibrosis stage increased (6.4 kPa for F1, 9.1 kPa for F2, 10.0 kPa for F3, and 12.0 kPa for F4; all P<0.05 between each fibrosis stage;

Table 1. Baseline characteristics.

	All patients	Patients with non-discordance	Patients with discordance	P value
	(n = 150)	(n = 129, 86.0%)	(n = 21, 14.0%)	
Age, years	41.9±14.2	43.1±13.4	34.3±16.7	0.008*
Male	107 (71.3)	93 (72.1)	14 (66.7)	0.610
BMI, kg/m²	23.2±2.8	23.1±2.7	23.8±3.5	0.321
Obesity (BMI ≥30 kg/m²)	4 (2.7)	2 (1.6)	2 (9.5)	0.094
Alanine aminotransferase, IU/L	74.1±98.3	72.9±103.1	81.6±62.3	0.707
Gamma glutamyltranspeptidase, IU/L	44.5±40.3	47.1±42.6	32.9±26.3	0.295
Platelet count, 10⁹/L	188±65	183±63	219±73	0.020*
Liver biopsy				
Fibrosis stage				
F2–4	127 (84.7)	113 (87.6)	14 (66.7)	0.055
F3–4	84 (56.0)	82 (63.6)	2 (9.5)	<0.001*
F4	68 (45.3)	67 (51.9)	1 (4.8)	<0.001*
Maximal activityᵃ				
A2–4	132 (88.0)	113 (87.6)	19 (90.5)	0.751
A3–4	60 (40.0)	49 (38.0)	11 (52.4)	0.236
A4	18 (12.0)	14 (10.9)	4 (19.0)	0.284
Lobular activity				
A2–4	125 (83.3)	106 (82.2)	19 (90.5)	0.530
A3–4	35 (23.3)	26 (20.2)	9 (42.9)	0.047*
A4	1 (0.7)	1 (0.8)	0	0.999
Periportal activity				
A2–4	118 (78.7)	100 (77.5)	18 (85.7)	0.568
A3–4	51 (34.0)	43 (33.3)	8 (38.1)	0.804
A4	18 (12.0)	14 (10.9)	4 (19.0)	0.284
Biopsy length, cm	17.9±2.2	18.0±2.2	17.1±2.0	0.125
LSM				
LSM value, kPa	11.7±7.3	11.7±7.7	11.3±3.2	0.659
Success rate, %	96.5±8.0	96.4±8.3	97.0±6.8	0.747
IQR/M, kPa	0.14±0.09	0.14±0.09	0.13±0.10	0.830
IQR/M >0.3	10 (6.7)	8 (6.2)	2 (9.5)	0.632

Variables are expressed as mean ± SD or n (%).
Maximal activityᵃ grade was defined as the higher one between lobular and periportal activity.
BMI, body mass index; LSM, liver stiffness measurement; kPa, kilopascal; IQR/M, interquartile range/median LSM value.
*P<0.05.

Figure 1(A)) and the median LSM values tended to increase as fibrosis stage and activity grade increased (**Figure S1**).

Histological sub-classification of cirrhosis also showed a significant increase in the median LSM values (8.5 kPa for F4A, 12.4 kPa for F4B, and 22.2 kPa for F4C; all P<0.05 among F4A, B, and C; **Figure 1(B)**) with no significant difference in ALT levels (median 32.5 (range, 19–70) IU/L for F4A. 42 (range, 12–112) IU/L for F4B, and 42.5 (range, 25–91) IU/L for F4C; all P>0.05).

Influence of necroinflammatory activity on LSM according to each fibrosis stage

LSM values between maximal activity grade 1–2 versus 3–4 were compared in each fibrosis stage (**Figure 2**). The median LSM values were not significantly different between maximal activity grade 1–2 and 3–4 in F1 and F2 fibrosis stage (P = 0.676 and 0.139, respectively), whereas those were significantly higher in maximal

activty grade 3–4 than 1–2 in F3 and F4 fibrosis stage (8.6 vs. 11.3 kPa in F3, P = 0.049; 11.9 vs. 19.2 kPa in F4, P = 0.009).

The ALT levels in F4 were 40.8±15.6 IU/L in the cases with maximal activity grade 1–2 and 60.7±23.3 IU/L in those with maximal activity grade 3–4, which were significantly different (P = 0.004). In contrast, the ALT levels in F1, F2, and F3 showed no significant difference between maximal activity grade 1–2 versus 3–4 (50.6±38.6 vs. 173.3±114.9 IU/L in F1, P = 0.121; 72.0±51.0 vs. 139.1±176.6 IU/L in F2, P = 0.224; 35.4±23.3 vs. 112.3±121.1 IU/L in F3, P = 0.146).

Correlations between variables

Among the study variables, the highest correlation was noted between ALT level and maximal activity grade (correlation coefficient, 0.497; P<0.001), followed by a correlation between ALT and age (correlation coefficient, −0.290; P<0.001) and

Table 2. Liver histology and corresponding LSM values (n = 150).

Fibrosis		Maximal activity		LSM (kPa)
Stage	n (%)	Grade	n	Median (range)
1	23 (15.3)	1	6	5.2 (3.7–8.7)
		2	13	5.4 (4.3–15.3)
		3	4	7.2 (6.0–8.7)
		4	-	-
2	43 (28.7)	1	-	-
		2	11	6.8 (4.6–11.0)
		3	21	7.8 (5.3–14.3)
		4	11	8.8 (5.0–17.1)
3	16 (10.7)	1	2	10.5 (10.0–11.0)
		2	7	8.3 (5.7–9.3)
		3	1	13.9
		4	6	11 (7.9–21.8)
4	68 (45.3)	1	10	9.1 (5.3–14.1)
		2	41	13.3 (7.6–34.3)
		3	16	18.2 (9.2–48.0)
		4	1	45.7

LSM, liver stiffness measurement; kPa, kilopascal.

another between ALT and gender (correlation coefficient, −0.170; $P = 0.038$).

Comparison between patients with non-discordance and those with discordance

Cutoff LSM values from our cohort were 6.0 kPa for ≥F2 (Se, 90.6%; Sp, 60.9%; PPV, 92.7%; NPV, 53.8%), 7.5 kPa for ≥F3 (Se, 96.4%; Sp, 57.6%; PPV, 74.3%; NPV, 92.7%), and 9.4 kPa for F4 (Se, 80.9%; Sp, 73.2%; PPV, 71.4%; NPV, 82.2%), giving a discordance between LSM and LB in 21 (14.0%) patients (**Table 3**). When we compared baseline characteristics between patients with non-discordance and those with discordance, age, platelet count, the proportion of F3–4 and F4, and the proportion of lobular activity grade 3–4 at the time of LB was significantly different from each other (all $P < 0.05$; **Table 1**). Although 10 (6.7%) patients with IQR/M>0.3 and one (0.7%) with a success rate <60% were identified, IQR/M and success rate were not selected as significant factors associated with discordance ($P = 0.830$ and $P = 0.747$, respectively).

Patients with discordance between LB and LSM

When we stratified these 21 patients with discordance into two groups (LB high group, defined as patients with higher fibrosis stage based on LB, and LSM high group, defined as those with higher fibrosis stage based on LSM), only 2 (9.5%) patients were stratified into the LB high group and 19 (90.5%) into the LSM high group. The distribution of fibrosis stages based on LB and LSM is indicated in **Table 3**.

The mean maximal activity grade and ALT levels of two patients with discordance in LB high group showed a trend to be lower than those of the 129 patients with non-discordance (1.5±0.7 vs. 2.4± 0.8, $P = 0.150$ and 25.0±12.7 vs. 72.9±103.1 IU/L, $P = 0.514$, respectively). The mean maximal activity grade of the 19 patients with discordance in the LSM high group was higher than the 129 patients with non-discordance with borderline statistical significance (2.7±0.9 vs. 2.4±0.8, $P = 0.074$), whereas ALT levels only showed a trend to be higher in the LSM high group than in the 129 patients with non-discordance (87.6±62.5 vs. 72.9±103.1 IU/L, $P = 0.547$).

Of the two cases in the LB high group, one was classified as F4A fibrosis stage, with a maximal activity grade of A, and the other was classified as stage F3, with a maximal activity of A2. The histology of the former patient with F4A showed a thin fibrous septa with minimal necroinflammatory activity (**Figure 3(A)**). Among the 19 cases in the LSM high group, 7 and 12 cases showed F1 and F2 fibrosis stage, respectively, and their maximal

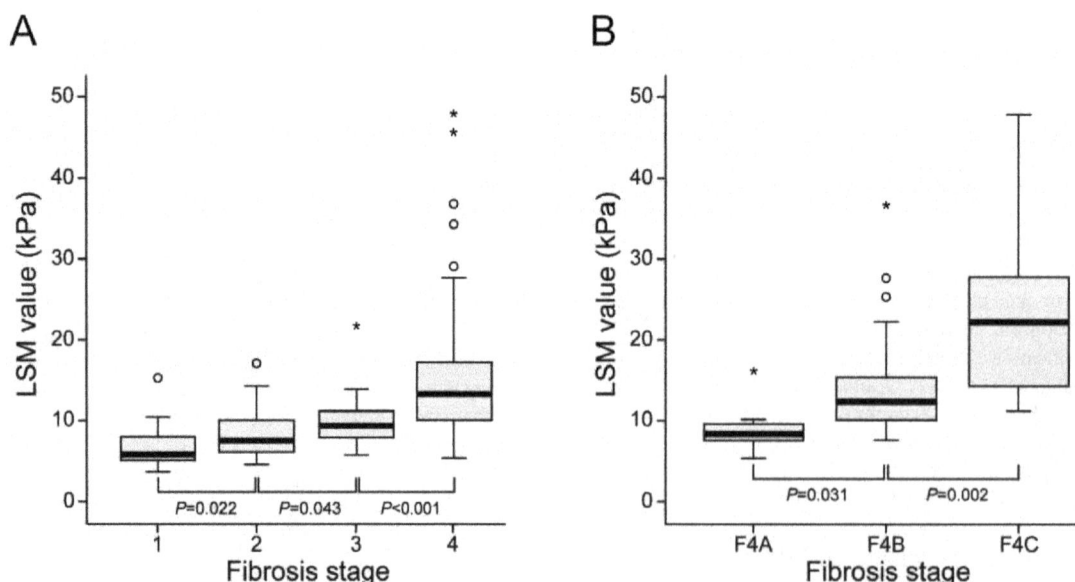

Figure 1. Box plots of LSM values according to fibrosis stage (A) and sub-classification of cirrhosis (B). Median LSM values increase significantly as fibrosis stage increases [6.4 kPa for F1 (range 3.7–15.3), 9.1 kPa for F2 (range 4.6–17.1), 10.0 kPa for F3 (range 5.7–21.8), and 12.0 kPa for F4 (range 5.3–48.0); all $P < 0.05$] and histologic sub-classification of cirrhosis also shows a significant increment in the median LSM values [8.5 kPa for F4A (range, 5.3–16.2), 12.4 kPa for F4B (range, 7.6–37.8), and 22.2 kPa for F4C (range, 11.2–48.0); all $P < 0.05$].

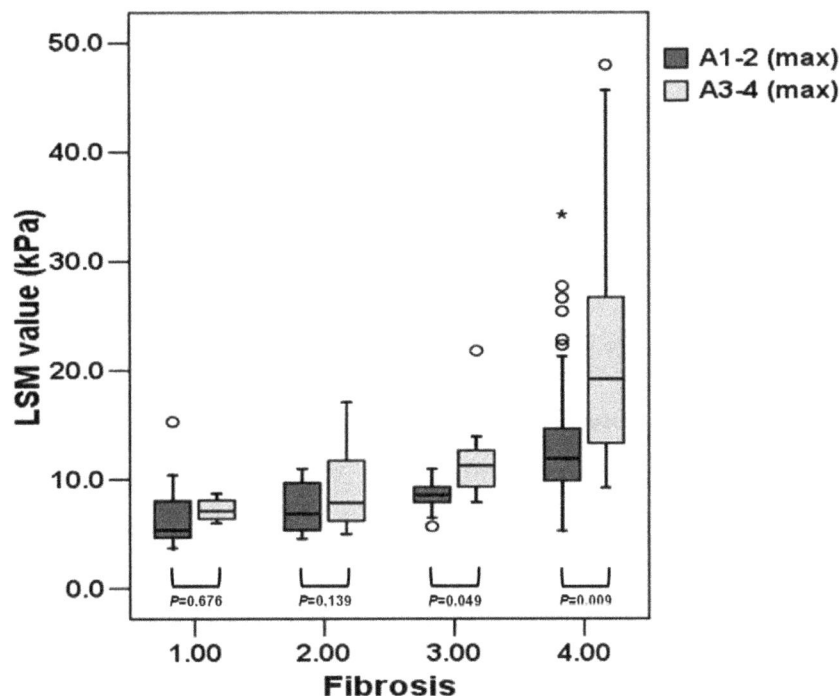

Figure 2. Distribution of LSM values according to fibrosis stage and maxiaml activity grade 1–2 vs. 3–4. The median LSM value was significantly higher in maxiaml activity grade 3–4 than 1–2 in F3 and F4 fibrosis stage (8.6 [range, 5.7–11.0] vs. 11.3 kPa [range, 7.9–21.8] in F3, P=0.049; 11.9 [range, 5.3–34.3] vs. 19.2 kPa [range, 9.2–48.0] in F4, P=0.009).

activity was A1–2 in 8, A3 in 8, and A4 in 3 cases, respectively. One histological example of the LSM high group showed periportal fibrosis with bridging necrosis (**Figure 3(B)**).

Independent predictors of discordance

In the multivariate binary logistic regression analysis, only F3–4 and F4 at the time of LB showed independent negative

Table 3. Distribution of fibrosis stage based on LB and LSM in patients with discordance (n = 21).

	LB high group[a]	LSM high group[b]
	(n = 2, 9.5%)	(n = 19, 90.5%)
Fibrosis stage		
F1	–	7
F2	–	12
F3	1	–
F4	1	–
LSM value, kPa		
F1 (<6.0 kPa)	2	–
F2 (≥6.0 kPa)	0	–
F3 (≥7.5 kPa)	–	4
F4 (≥9.4 kPa)	–	15

LB, liver biopsy; LSM, liver stiffness measurement; kPa, kilopascal.
A discordance was defined as a discordance of at least two stages between LB and LSM.
LB high group[a] was defined as patients with higher fibrosis stage based on LB.
LSM high group[b] was defined as patients with higher fibrosis stage based on LSM.

associations with discordance (P=0.002; HR, 0.073; 95% CI, 0.014–0.390 for F3–4 and P=0.014; HR, 0.067; 95% CI, 0.008–0.574 for F4). Given that IQR/M was demonstrated to be a significant predictor of discordance in previous studies [13,15], we adjusted F3–4 and F4 using IQR/M, although IQR/M was not a significant discriminating factor of discordance in our univariate analysis. However, IQR/M was not statistically significant (P=0.551 with F3–4 and P=0.495 with F4), whereas F3–4 and F4 at the time of LB remained significant independently (P=0.002; HR, 0.073, 95% CI, 0.014–0.387 for F3–4 and P=0.013; HR, 0.065; 95% CI, 0.008–0.559 for F4; **Table 4**).

Figure 4 showed the discordant rate according to F3–4 and F4. The estimated odds ratios of discordance, calculated by the chi-squared test, were 0.060 in patients with F3–4 (P<0.001; 95% CI, 0.013–0.271) and 0.046 in those with F4 (P<0.001; 95% CI, 0.006–0.355).

Discussion

Although LSM is an accurate method that evaluates the degree of liver fibrosis [5], many extrinsic factors have significant influences on LSM [6–10]. Additionally, LSM should satisfy the three intrinsic prerequisites of ≥10 valid measurements, success rate ≥60%, and IQR/M<0.3 to maintain the validity needed to reflect the real fibrotic state of liver [5]. However, these intrinsic prerequisites are only the manufacturer's recommendation.

As a result, several studies have investigated the influence of IQR/M on the accuracy of LSM [13–15]. Two studies with chronic hepatitis C (CHC) only [13] or mostly CHC [15] have proposed optimal cutoff IQR/M values of 0.21 and 0.17, respectively. In contrast, the other study with CHB did not identify IQR/M as a significant predictor of accuracy [14]. Indeed, in our study with CHB, IQR/M was not selected as a significant predictor of discordance. Reasons for this remain

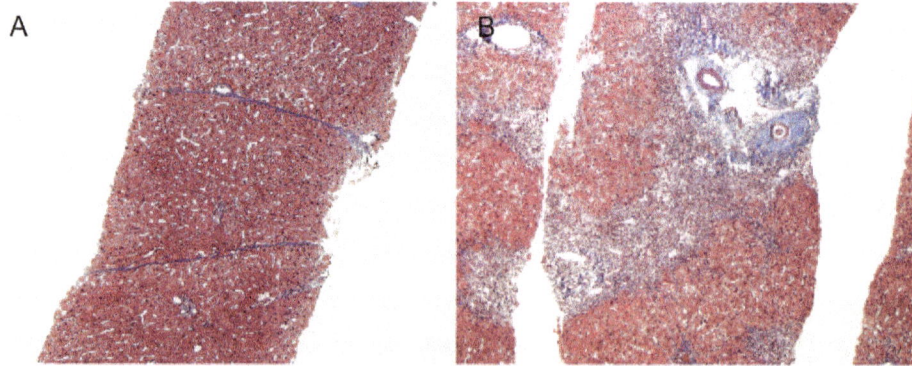

Figure 3. Histology of LB high group (A) and LSM high group (B) (Masson trichrome, original magnification ×100). (A) a patient in LB high group (F4A, maximal activity grade of A1, and ALT level of 34 IU/L) showed a thin fibrous septa and minimal necroinflammatory activity. (B) a patient in LSM high group (F2, maximal activity grade of A4, and ALT level of 168 IU/L) showed periportal fibrosis with bridging necrosis.

unclear although IQR/M in the previous CHB study [14] and ours (both mean IQR/M 0.14) was much lower than in CHC studies (0.23 [13] and 0.16 [15]) indicating that LSM performed more accurately. We believe that IQR/M may not be a sensitive marker to predict discordance in CHB because of the influence of inhomogeneous histological features or necroinflammation that overwhelm the influence of IQR/M on LSM [22]. Consistent with the literature [13–15], success rate was not a significant predictor of discordance in our study, which might mean that 'high quality,' reflected by lower IQR/M, does matter for the accurate interpretation of LSM, rather than a 'high percentage' of successful shots.

In addition to IQR/M, fibrosis stage (F0–2 vs. F3–4) and elevated ALT (>1.5–2× ULN) were proposed as significant extrinsic predictors of discordance [13–15]. However, controversy remains regarding fibrosis stage. Lucidarme et al. [13] concluded that advanced fibrosis (F3–4) was correlated with discordance, while Kim et al. [14] and Myers et al. [15] proposed minimal fibrosis (F0–2) as a significant predictor of discordance between LB and LSM. In our study, F3–4 and F4 showed a negative

correlation with discordance. The significantly lower rate of discordance in F4 may be explained by an unlimited upper cutoff LSM value for cirrhosis until 75 kPa in this study design. Accordingly, F3–4, which included a high proportion of F4 (80.9%), also showed a negative correlation with discordance. From these results, we suggest that a different predictor of discordance may be produced according to a different distribution of F4. Furthermore, this hypothesis may explain why ALT level was not selected as a significant predictor of discordance in our study with a higher prevalence of F3–4 (56.0%) than in a previous study (20.3%) that proposed ALT as a significant predictor of discordance [15]. This confounding effect of elevated ALT may have been attenuated in our study due to a higher proportion of F4, which is free to misdiagnosis due to LSM overestimation by elevated ALT, despite similar ALT levels between the two studies [mean 61 IU/L [15] vs. 74 IU/L in the present study].

Thus, the potentially masked influence of necroinflammation in F4, the consistent reports on the overestimating effects of elevated ALT, and the significant correlation between lobular activity grade 3–4 and discordance in our univariate analysis prompted us to

Table 4. Independent predictors of discordance between LSM and LB.

	Univariate	Multivariate			
	P value	P value (with F3–4)	P value (with F4)	Hazard ratio	95% confidence interval
Age	0.008*	0.906	0.640	-	-
Platelet count	0.020*	0.769	0.574	-	-
A3–4 (lobular)	0.047*	0.658	0.543	-	-
F3–4	<0.001*	0.002*	-	0.073	0.014–0.390
F4	<0.001*	-	0.014*	0.067	0.008–0.574
IQR/M adjusted					
Age	0.008*	0.851	0.596	-	-
Platelet count	0.020*	0.710	0.520	-	-
A3–4 (lobular)	0.047*	0.613	0.512	-	-
IQR/M	0.830	0.551	0.495	-	-
F3–4	<0.001*	0.002*	-	0.073	0.014–0.387
F4	<0.001*	-	0.013*	0.065	0.008–0.559

LSM, liver stiffness measurement; LB, liver biopsy; IQR/M, interquartile range/median value.
*P<0.05.

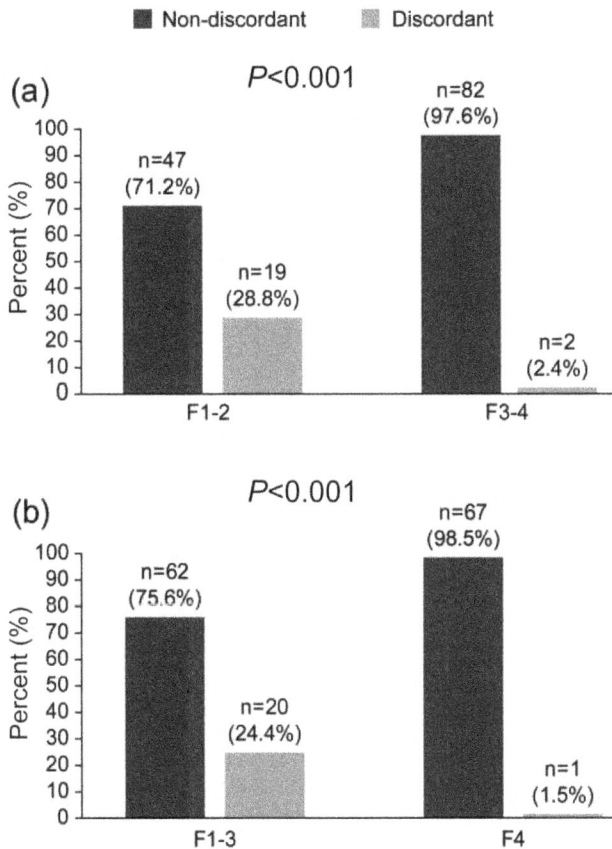

Figure 4. Percentage of patients with non-discordance and those with discordance in fibrosis stage F1–2 *vs.* F3–4 (A) and F1–3 *vs.* F4 (B). The estimated odds ratios of discordance were 0.060 in patients with F3–4 ($P<0.001$; 95% confidence interval [CI], 0.013–0.271) and 0.046 in those with F4 ($P<0.001$; 95% CI, 0.006–0.355).

'in the LSM high group, the clinical implications should be further investigated in future studies, considering the borderline statistical significance of high ALT ($P = 0.074$) and the small sample size of the LB high group. Indeed, clinical variables, such as ALT level, which showed the best correlation with necroinflammatory activity in our study, are needed to predict the discordance 'before LB,' because histological variables, such as fibrosis stage or activity grade, which are only available 'after LB' are not helpful for the prediction of the discordance between LB and LSM. Indeed, the concept of excluding subjects with high ALT to enhance the accuracy of LSM has already been proposed [17,25]. Although ALT was not a significant predictor, the optimal cutoff ALT level to predict discordance was 55 IU/L (data not shown). Furthermore, the mean ALTs of maximal activity grade 3–4 in F3 and F4 that raised LSM values significantly were 60.7 and 112.3 IU/L, respectively. Because the ALT cutoff seemed to be around 1.5–3× ULN in our study and 1.5–2× ULN in previous ones [14,15,26], ALT level ≤3× ULN may be optimal to enhance LSM performance.

Interestingly, LSM values showed a significant stepwise increment according to F4A, B, and C without a significant difference in ALT levels in our study, indicating that LSM can further stratify patients with cirrhosis. Thus, mild liver cirrhosis (F4A) might have a higher chance of being underestimated by LSM than moderate or severe cirrhosis (F4B or F4C), especially when necroinflammatory activity or ALT level is low. This could be a reason why one patient with F4A and A1 activity grade belonged to the LB high group. Although the histological sub-classification of cirrhosis is gaining clinical relevance [27], stratification of cirrhosis according to the Laennec system or LSM should be further validated via long-term follow-up studies using solid clinical end-points, such as liver-related death or development of hepatocellular carcinoma.

In conclusion, advanced fibrosis stage (F3–4) or cirrhosis (F4) showed a negative correlation with discordance between LB and LSM in patients with CHB, and maximal activity grade 3–4 significantly influenced LSM values in F3–4 and F4. Thus, future studies should investigate how to control for the clinical marker of ALT, which may bridge histological information to enhance the accuracy of LSM.

Acknowledgments

The authors are grateful to Dong-Su Jang, (Medical Illustrator, Medical Research Support Section, Yonsei University College of Medicine, Seoul, Korea) for his help with the figures.

Author Contributions

Conceived and designed the experiments: YNP KHH JKK. Analyzed the data: SUK. Contributed reagents/materials/analysis tools: SUK. Wrote the paper: SUK.

investigate further the effects of necroinflammatory activity grade on LSM. The maximal activity grade 3–4 significantly influenced LSM values in F3 and F4, but not in F1 or F2, which may be explained in several ways. First, the mean ALT level was not significantly different in A1–2 versus A3–4 in F1 and F2 in our cohort. Thus, the ALT effect could not be revealed. Second, extrinsic factors, such as liver congestion [7] and respiration [23] resulting in a change of portal flow concurrent with necroinflammation, may have influenced the performance of LSM when liver fibrosis was insufficient (≤F2) to be detected by LSM. These combined effects of several confounders might have concealed the effects of necroinflammation on LSM, consistent with a recent meta-analysis on LSM reporting the relatively lower performance of LSM to predict significant fibrosis (≥F2) [24].

Most patients (90.5%) with discordance were stratified into the LSM high group, indicating that LSM values were subject to overestimation due to necroinflammation or high ALT. Although statistical significance for necroinflammation and high ALT was not seen when we compared patients with non-discordance with those

References

1. Wright TL (2006) Introduction to chronic hepatitis B infection. Am J Gastroenterol 101(suppl 1): S1–6.
2. Bravo AA, Sheth SG, Chopra S (2001) Liver biopsy. N Engl J Med 344: 495–500.
3. Bedossa P, Darge're D, Paradis V (2003) Sampling variability of liver fibrosis in chronic hepatitis C. Hepatology 38: 1449–1457.
4. Rousselet MC, Michalak S, Dupré F, Croué A, Bedossa P, et al. (2005) Hepatitis Network 49. Sources of variability in histological scoring of chronic viral hepatitis. Hepatology 41: 257–264.
5. Sandrin L, Fourquet B, Hasquenoph JM, Yon S, Fournier C, et al. (2003) Transient elastography: a new noninvasive method for assessment of hepatic fibrosis. Ultrasound Med Biol 29: 1705–13.

6. Millonig G, Reimann FM, Friedrich S, Fonouni H, Mehrabi A, et al. (2008) Extrahepatic cholestasis increases liver stiffness (FibroScan) irrespective of fibrosis. Hepatology 48: 1718–1723.

7. Millonig G, Friedrich S, Adolf S, Fonouni H, Golriz M, et al. (2010) Liver stiffness is directly influenced by central venous pressure. J Hepatol 52: 206–210.

8. Kim SU, Han KH, Park JY, Ahn SH, Chung MJ, et al. (2009) Liver stiffness measurement using FibroScan is influenced by serum total bilirubin in acute hepatitis. Liver Int 29: 810–815.

9. Coco B, Oliveri F, Maina AM, Ciccorossi P, Sacco R, et al. (2007) Transient elastography: a new surrogate marker of liver fibrosis influenced by major changes of transaminases. J Viral Hepat 14: 360–369.

10. Arena U, Vizzutti F, Corti G, Ambu S, Stasi C, et al. (2008) Acute viral hepatitis increases liver stiffness values measured by transient elastography. Hepatology 47: 380–384.

11. Fung J, Lai CL, But D, Hsu A, Seto WK, et al. (2010) Reduction of liver stiffness following resolution of acute flares of chronic hepatitis B. Hepatol Int 4: 716–722.

12. Fung J, Lai CL, Cheng C, Wu R, Wong DK, et al. (2011) Mild-to-moderate elevation of alanine aminotransferase increases liver stiffness measurement by transient elastography in patients with chronic hepatitis B. Am J Gastroenterol 106: 492–496.

13. Lucidarme D, Foucher J, Le Bail B, Vergniol J, Castera L, et al. (2009) Factors of accuracy of transient elastography (fibroscan) for the diagnosis of liver fibrosis in chronic hepatitis C. Hepatology 49: 1083–1089.

14. Kim SU, Seo YS, Cheong JY, Kim MY, Kim JK, et al. (2010) Factors that affect the diagnostic accuracy of liver fibrosis measurement by Fibroscan in patients with chronic hepatitis B. Aliment Pharmacol Ther 32: 498–505.

15. Myers RP, Crotty P, Pomier-Layrargues G, Ma M, Urbanski SJ, et al. (2010) Prevalence, risk factors and causes of discordance in fibrosis staging by transient elastography and liver biopsy. Liver Int 30: 1471–1480.

16. Kim SU, Kim do Y, Park JY, Lee JH, Ahn SH, et al. (2010) How can we enhance the performance of liver stiffness measurement using FibroScan in diagnosing liver cirrhosis in patients with chronic hepatitis B? J Clin Gastroenterol 44: 66–71.

17. Kim SU, Kim YC, Choi JS, Kim KS, Choi GH, et al. (2010) Can preoperative diffusion-weighted MRI predict postoperative hepatic insufficiency after curative resection of HBV-related hepatocellular carcinoma? A pilot study. Magn Reson Imaging 28: 802–811.

18. Kim SU, Ahn SH, Park JY, Kim do Y, Chon CY, et al. (2008) Prediction of postoperative hepatic insufficiency by liver stiffness measurement (FibroScan®) before curative resection of hepatocellular carcinoma: a pilot study. Hepatol Int 2: 471–417.

19. Wanless IR, Sweeney G, Dhillon AP, Guido M, Piga A, et al. (2002) Lack of progressive hepatic fibrosis during long-term therapy with deferiprone in subjects with transfusion-dependent beta-thalassemia. Blood 100: 1566–1569.

20. Brunt EM, Janney CG, Di Bisceglie AM, Neuschwander-Tetri BA, Bacon BR (1999) Nonalcoholic steatohepatitis: a proposal for grading and staging the histological lesions. Am J Gastroenterol 94: 2467–2474.

21. Kim SU, Kim do Y, Ahn SH, Kim HM, Lee JM, et al. (2010) The impact of steatosis on liver stiffness measurement in patients with chronic hepatitis B. Hepatogastroenterology 57: 832–828.

22. Castera L, Forns X, Alberti A (2008) Non-invasive evaluation of liver fibrosis using transient elastography. J Hepatol 48: 835–847.

23. Yun MH, Seo YS, Kang HS, Lee KG, Kim JH, et al. (2010) The effect of the respiratory cycle on liver stiffness values as measured by transient elastography. J Viral Hepat 18: 631–636.

24. Friedrich-Rust M, Ong MF, Martens S, Sarrazin C, Bojunga J, et al. (2008) Performance of transient elastography for the staging of liver fibrosis: a meta-analysis. Gastroenterology 134: 960–974.

25. Chan HL, Wong GL, Choi PC, Chan AW, Chim AM, et al. (2009) Alanine aminotransferase-based algorithms of liver stiffness measurement by transient elastography (Fibroscan) for liver fibrosis in chronic hepatitis B. J Viral Hepat 16: 36–44.

26. Cho HJ, Seo YS, Lee KG, Hyun JJ, An H, et al. (2011) Serum aminotransferase levels instead of etiology affects the accuracy of transient elastography in chronic viral hepatitis patients. J Gastroenterol Hepatol 26: 492–500.

27. Kim MY, Cho MY, Baik SK, Park HJ, Jeon HK, et al. (2011) Histological subclassification of cirrhosis using the Laennec fibrosis scoring system correlates with clinical stage and grade of portal hypertension. J Hepatol 55: 1004–1009.

High Hepatitis B Surface Antigen Levels Predict Insignificant Fibrosis in Hepatitis B e Antigen Positive Chronic Hepatitis B

Wai-Kay Seto[1], Danny Ka-Ho Wong[1], James Fung[1], Philip P. C. Ip[2], John Chi-Hang Yuen[1], Ivan Fan-Ngai Hung[1], Ching-Lung Lai[1,3], Man-Fung Yuen[1,3]*

1 Department of Medicine, The University of Hong Kong, Queen Mary Hospital, Hong Kong, Hong Kong, 2 Department of Pathology, The University of Hong Kong, Queen Mary Hospital, Hong Kong, Hong Kong, 3 State Key Laboratory for Liver Research, University of Hong Kong, Queen Mary Hospital, Hong Kong, Hong Kong

Abstract

Introduction: There is no data on the relationship between hepatitis B surface antigen (HBsAg) levels and liver fibrosis in hepatitis B e antigen (HBeAg)-positive patients with chronic hepatitis B (CHB).

Methods: Serum HBsAg and HBV DNA levels in HBeAg-positive CHB patients with liver biopsies were analyzed. The upper limit of normal (ULN) of alanine aminotransferase (ALT) was 30 and 19 U/L for men and women respectively. Histologic assessment was based on Ishak fibrosis staging for fibrosis and Knodell histologic activity index (HAI) for necroinflammation.

Results: 140 patients (65% male, median age 32.7 years) were recruited. 56 (40%) had ALT $\leq 2 \times$ULN. 72 (51.4%) and 42 (30%) had fibrosis score ≤ 1 and necroinflammation grading ≤ 4 respectively. Patients with fibrosis score ≤ 1, when compared to patients with fibrosis score >1, had significantly higher median HBsAg levels (50,320 and 7,820 IU/mL respectively, p<0.001). Among patients with ALT $\leq 2 \times$ULN, serum HBsAg levels achieved an area under receiver operating characteristic curve of 0.869 in predicting fibrosis score ≤ 1. HBsAg levels did not accurately predict necroinflammation score. HBsAg $\geq 25,000$ IU/mL was independently associated with fibrosis score ≤ 1 (p = 0.025, odds ratio 9.042).Using this cut-off HBsAg level in patients with ALT $\leq 2 \times$ULN, positive and negative predictive values for predicting fibrosis score ≤ 1 were 92.7% and 60.0% respectively. HBV DNA levels had no association with liver histology.

Conclusion: Among HBeAg-positive patients with ALT $\leq 2 \times$ULN, high serum HBsAg levels can accurately predict fibrosis score ≤ 1, and could potentially influence decisions concerning treatment commencement and reduce the need for liver biopsy.

Editor: Heiner Wedemeyer, Hannover Medical School, Germany

Funding: The authors have no support or funding to report.

* E-mail: mfyuen@hkucc.hku.hk

Introduction

Chronic hepatitis B (CHB) is known for its highly variable disease course, ranging from an inactive carrier state to the development of clinical complications, including cirrhosis and hepatocellular carcinoma (HCC) [1]. CHB patients with repeated hepatitis flares were noted to have increased necroinflammation in liver histology, leading to increased fibrogenesis and subsequent disease progression [2].

Treatment guidelines by two international liver associations [3,4] recommend treatment commencement when serum alanine aminotransferase (ALT) is persistently >2×upper limit of normal (ULN) in hepatitis B e antigen (HBeAg)-positive patients. Guidelines from another international liver association recommend treatment when there is clinical evidence of significant liver fibrosis e.g. by using liver biopsy in patients with elevated ALT [5]. There is increasing evidence that patients with ALT $\leq 2 \times$ULN

could still eventually develop clinical complications [6]. HBeAg-positive patients with normal ALT are traditionally classified as in the immune tolerant phase of disease, with minimal histologic changes on liver biopsy [7]. However histologic studies of HBeAg-positive patients with "high normal" ALT have been shown to have significant fibrosis and necroinflammation [8,9]. In addition, the definition of "normal ALT" has also been re-evaluated. One study of 6835 healthy blood donors has suggested lowering the ULN of ALT to 30 U/L for men and 19 U/L for women [10]. A study from Asia involving 1105 potential liver donors also has similar recommendations [11]. Because of all these controversial issues, using ALT levels to classify patients for treatment initiation is suboptimal. Assessment of fibrosis is thus an important parameter in deciding treatment.

Given the invasive nature of liver biopsy, several non-invasive indices have been developed for the prediction of significant fibrosis in CHB [12,13,14]. These studies however are limited by their small sample sizes, the lack of large-scale external validation, and the use of serum markers not routinely available from standard laboratories. The use of predictive models established in chronic hepatitis C has also produced conflicting results [15,16]. Transient elastography is another method for assessing liver fibrosis [17]. However, it is often difficult to determine in obese patients, has reduced diagnostic accuracy with lower fibrosis scores, and is affected by even small degrees of ALT elevation, with 40–50% of patients still requiring other means of fibrosis assessment [17].

The quantification of hepatitis B surface antigen (HBsAg) levels has been recently advocated as a surrogate marker for intrahepatic closed covalently circular DNA (cccDNA) [18]. Recent evidence have shown serum HBsAg levels to be useful in identifying inactive CHB carriers [19], predicting subsequent HBsAg seroclearance [20,21,22], and predicting favorable outcomes with pegylated interferon therapy [23]. Serum HBsAg levels have been shown to be extremely high among HBeAg-positive patients with normal ALT [24,25], and it has been suggested high HBsAg levels could be supportive evidence of immune tolerance [26]. The aim of our study was to evaluate the use of serum HBsAg levels in assessing liver histology in HBeAg-positive CHB patients.

Methods

Ethics Statement

The present study was approved by the Institutional Review Board, the University of Hong Kong and West Cluster of Hospital Authority, Hong Kong. All patients had written consent prior to liver biopsy and study entry with all clinical investigation conducted according to the principles expressed by the Declaration of Helsinki.

Patients

The present study included treatment-naive HBeAg-positive CHB patients who were recruited for therapeutic drug trials between 1994 to 2008 in the Department of Medicine, the University of Hong Kong, Queen Mary Hospital. All patients were HBsAg-positive for at least 6 months before study entry. Other inclusion criteria included ALT <10×ULN and HBV DNA ≥20,000 IU/mL. Patients with concomitant liver diseases, including chronic hepatitis C or D infection, Wilson's disease, autoimmune hepatitis, primary biliary cirrhosis, significant intake of alcohol (30 grams per day for male, 20 grams per day for female) and decompensated liver disease were excluded.

Liver Biopsy

Two different biopsy needles were used. An 18G sheathed cutting needle (Temno Evolution, Cardinal Health, McGaw Park, IL) was used in 58 patients, while a 17G core aspiration needle (Hepafix, B. Braun Melsungen AG, Germany) was used for the remaining 82 patients. The biopsy lengths were 1.5 to 1.8 cm and 2 to 5 cm respectively. A single pathologist (initials PPCI), blinded to all biochemical, serologic and virologic parameters, was assigned to review all biopsy specimens. Biopsies were fixed, paraffin-embedded, and stained with hematoxylin and eosin for morphological evaluation and Masson's trichrome stain for assessment of fibrosis. Histologic staging of fibrosis and grading of necroinflammation was performed using the Ishak fibrosis score (range 0 to 6) [27] and Knodell histologic activity index (HAI) (range 0 to 18) [28] respectively. "Insignificant fibrosis" was defined as an Ishak fibrosis score of equal or less than 1. "Insignificant necroinflammation" was defined as a Knodell HAI score of equal or less than 4.

Laboratory Assays

Serum samples used for measurements were taken at the day of biopsy and stored at −20°C. Following recommendations of current treatment guidelines [3], the ULN of serum ALT was defined as 30 U/L for men and 19 U/L for women [10]. Serum HBsAg, HBeAg and antibody to the hepatitis B e antigen (anti-HBe) were measured using commercially available immunoassays (Abbott Laboratories, Chicago, IL). Serum HBV DNA levels were measured using Cobas Taqman assay (Roche Diagnostics, Branchburg, NJ), with a linear range of 20 to 1.98×10^8 IU/mL. Samples with HBV DNA levels higher than 1.98×10^8 IU/mL were diluted at 1:100 for retesting. Serum HBsAg titer was measured using the Elecsys HBsAg II assay (Roche Diagnostics, Gmbh, Mannheim), with a linear range of 0.05 to 52,000 IU/mL. Samples with HBsAg levels higher than 52,000 IU/mL were retested at a dilution of 1:100.

Statistical Analysis

All continuous variables are expressed in median (range). Statistical analyses were performed using SPSS version 18.0 (SPSS Inc, Chicago, Illinois). The Mann-Whitney U test was used for comparing continuous variables with a skewed distribution; Chi squared test was used for categorical variables. Correlation was performed using Spearman's bivariate correlation. The predictions of minimal histologic changes were first examined by the construction of corresponding receiver operating characteristic (ROC) curves, followed by the assessment of overall accuracy by areas under the curves (AUCs). The Youden Index, defined as the sensitivity plus the specificity minus one, was used to identify the optimal level of prediction. Multivariate logistic regression was used to identify factors independently associated with insignificant fibrosis. A two-sided p value of <0.05 was considered statistically significant.

Results

One hundred and forty HBeAg-positive patients were included in the present study. The baseline demographics are shown in Table 1. Three patients (2.1%) had histologic evidence of cirrhosis. Based on liver biochemistry, 17 (12.1%) were classified as immune tolerant with normal ALT; the remaining 123 (87.9%) were classified to be in immune clearance. There were no significant differences in age, gender, liver biochemistry and serum HBV DNA between the two groups of patients (Table 1, all p>0.05).

Median HBsAg levels for patients with normal ALT, ALT 1–2×ULN and ALT >2×ULN were 105,020 IU/mL (range: 13,490–319,800 IU/mL), 40,490 IU/mL (range: 257–286,300 IU/mL) and 9,362 IU/mL (range: 62–217,200 IU/mL) respectively (p<0.001). The distribution of HBsAg levels among patients stratified by ALT ≤2×ULN versus ALT >2×ULN is shown in Figure 1a. A significantly larger proportion of patients with ALT ≤2×ULN had serum HBsAg >25,000 IU/mL when compared to patients with ALT >2×ULN (73.2% versus 26.2%, p<0.001).

Serum HBsAg showed moderate correlation with serum HBV DNA levels (r=0.403, p<0.001), and moderate inverse correlation with ALT levels (r=−0.450, p<0.001).

Liver Histology

The distribution of fibrosis scores and necroinflammation gradings of all 140 patients stratified by ALT levels is shown in Figures 1b and 1c. Seventy-two (51.4%) and 42 (30%) patients had insignificant fibrosis and necroinflammation respectively. All immune tolerant patients with normal ALT (n = 17) had

High Hepatitis B Surface Antigen Levels Predict Insignificant Fibrosis in Hepatitis B e Antigen...

115

Table 1. Baseline characteristics of all 140 patients.

	All patients (n = 140)	ALT ≤2×ULN (n = 56)	ALT >2×ULN (n = 84)	p value*
Age	32.7 (16.6–60.1)	32.6 (16.6–55.0)	32.5 (18.0–60.1)	0.309
Number of male patients	91 (65.0%)	40 (71.4%)	51 (60.7%)	0.193
Albumin (U/L)	46 (37–54)	47 (39–52)	45 (37–54)	0.152
Bilirubin (umol/L)	10 (3–31)	9.5 (4–31)	10.5 (3–30)	0.088
ALT (U/L)	67.5 (14–175)	38 (14–60)	89 (46–175)	<0.001
HBV DNA (log IU/mL)	7.96 (4.41–12.4)	8.14 (4.83–11.9)	7.72 (4.41–12.4)	0.113
HBsAg (IU/mL)	17,680 (62–319,800)	52,535 (257–319,800)	9,362 (62–217,200)	<0.001

All continuous values expressed in median (range).
ALT, alanine aminotransferase; ULN, upper limit of normal; HBsAg, hepatitis B surface antigen.
ALT upper limit of normal: 30 U/L for men, 19 U/L for women.
*Comparison was between patients with ALT ≤2×ULN and ALT >2×ULN.

insignificant fibrosis. Among patients with ALT ≤2×ULN (n = 56), 44 (78.6%) had insignificant fibrosis, significantly more than among patients with ALT >2×ULN (33.3%, p<0.001). The proportion of patients with insignificant necroinflammation among the two patients groups was similar (33.9% and 27.4% respectively, p = 0.408). The type of biopsy needle used (i.e. the sheathed cutting needle versus the core aspiration needle) did not influence the degree of fibrosis and necroinflammation (p = 0.735 and 0.970 respectively). Serum HBsAg levels among all patients divided by their histologic scores and gradings are shown in Figures 2a and 2b. Patients with insignificant fibrosis had significantly higher median HBsAg levels (p<0.001). In the subgroup of 39 patients with ALT 1–2×ULN, median HBsAg levels were also significantly higher in those with insignificant fibrosis (51,400 IU/mL, range: 2,598 to 286,300 IU/mL) when compared to those with significant fibrosis (7,703 IU/mL, range 257 to 78,810 IU/mL) (p = 0.002). Comparing patients with insignificant necroinflammation and those with significant necroinflammation, median HBsAg levels showed no significant difference (p = 0.393).

Median serum HBV DNA levels showed no significant difference in patients with insignificant fibrosis compared to patients with significant fibrosis for the whole group (8.01 and 7.85 log IU/mL respectively, p = 0.794) and for the subgroup of patients with ALT ≤2×ULN (8.23 and 7.65 log IU/mL respectively, p = 0.318). There was also no significant difference in median HBV DNA levels among patients with insignificant necroinflammation versus significant necroinflammation for the whole group of patients (7.91 and 7.99 log IU/mL respectively, p = 0.897) and for the subgroup of patients with ALT ≤2×ULN (8.40 and 8.02 log IU/mL respectively, p = 0.095).

Serum HBsAg showed a moderate inverse correlation with fibrosis scores (r = −0.449, p<0.001). Serum HBsAg also had an inverse correlation with necroinflammation gradings, but with a lower correlation coefficient (r = −0.269, p = 0.001). Serum HBV DNA had no correlation with both fibrosis scores (r = −0.076, p = 0.373) and necroinflammation gradings (r = −0.042, p = 0.624).

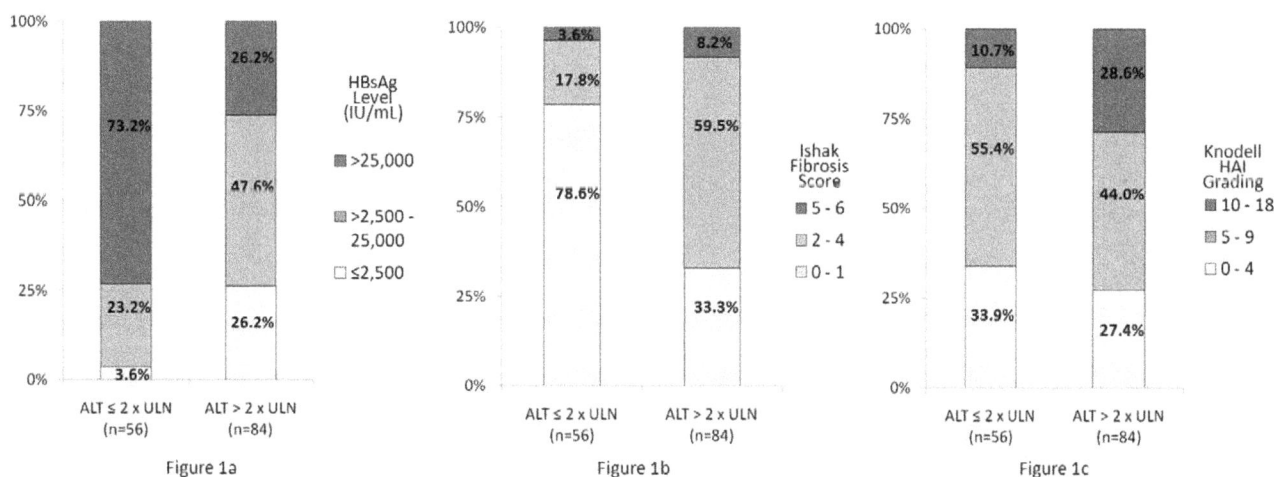

ALT, alanine aminotransferase; HAI, histologic activity index; HBsAg, hepatitis B surface antigen

Figure 1. Distribution of all patients stratified by ALT levels. HBsAg levels (Figure 1a), fibrosis scores (Figure 1b) and necroinflammation gradings (Figure 1c) of all patients are shown.

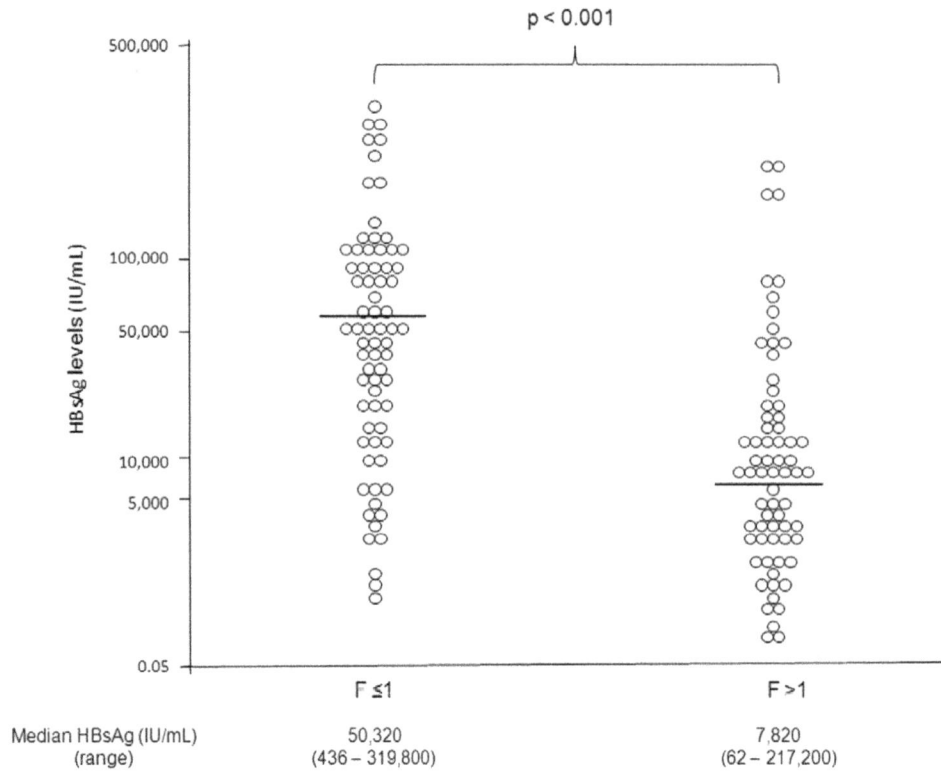

Figure 2a

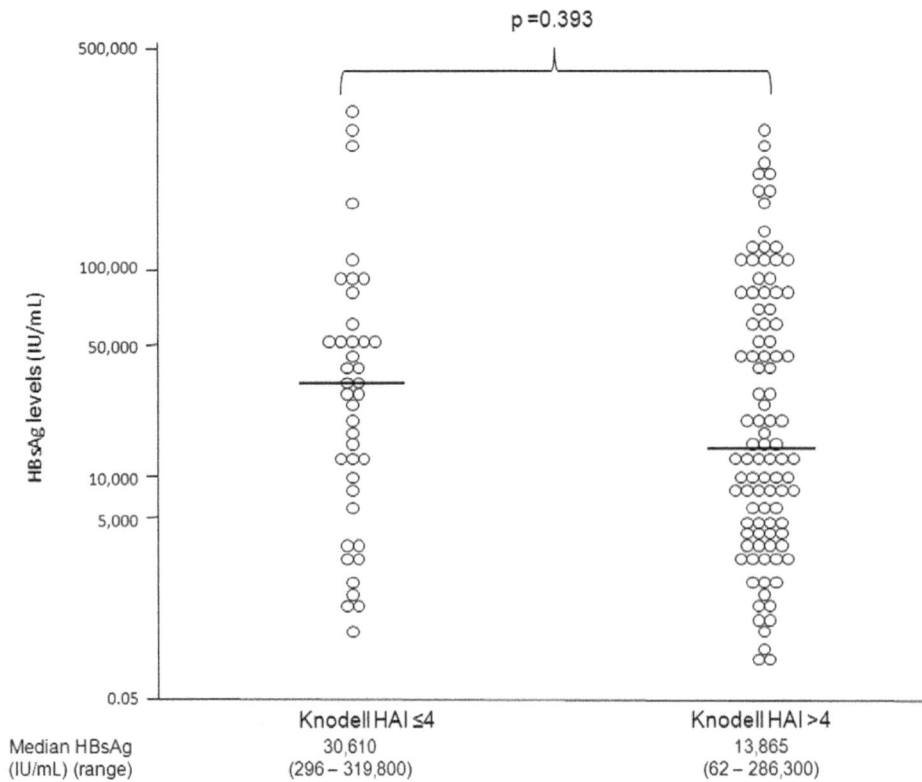

Figure 2b

HBsAg, hepatitis B surface antigen; F, Ishak fibrosis score, HAI, histologic activity index.
Insignificant fibrosis defined as F ≤1
Insignificant necroinflammation defined as Knodel HAI ≤4
Horizontal line denotes median HBsAg level

Figure 2. Distribution of serum HBsAg levels. Patients are stratified by fibrosis scores (Figure 2a) and necroinflammation gradings (Figure 2b).

Predictive Value of HBsAg for Minimal Histologic Changes

The ROC curves and the AUC values of serum HBsAg levels in predicting insignificant fibrosis and necroinflammation are depicted in Figure 3 and Table 2. Serum HBsAg levels produced a better AUC for insignificant fibrosis in patients with ALT ≤2×ULN (AUC 0.869) compared to the overall population (AUC 0.771). Serum HBsAg levels did not have any predictive value for insignificant necroinflammation (AUC 0.546 and 0.532 for all patients and patients with ALT ≤2×ULN respectively).

The sensitivity, specificity and predictive values of different HBsAg levels in predicting insignificant fibrosis among patients with ALT ≤2×ULN are shown in Table 3. Based on the Youden Index, the optimal level of serum HBsAg to predict insignificant fibrosis was ≥27,490 IU/mL (Youden index 0.697, sensitivity 86.4%, specificity 83.3%). Rounding off to the nearest five-thousandth level, serum HBsAg ≥25,000 IU/mL was able to predict insignificant fibrosis with a sensitivity of 86.4%, specificity of 75.0%, positive predictive value of 92.7% and negative predictive value of 60.0%. The 7.3% (3 out of 41) of patients with HBsAg ≥25,000 IU/mL but fibrosis score >1 had only stage 2 fibrosis. Serum HBsAg ≥100,000 IU/mL was 100% predictive of insignificant fibrosis.

Multivariate Analysis for Predicting Insignificant Fibrosis

Among patients with ALT ≤2×ULN, younger age (p<0.001), serum HBsAg ≥25,000 IU/mL (p<0.001) and lower serum ALT (p = 0.001) were associated with insignificant fibrosis by univariate analysis. The multivariate analysis of factors independently predictive of insignificant fibrosis is shown in Table 4. After adjusting for different clinical parameters, factors independently associated with insignificant fibrosis included serum HBsAg ≥25,000 IU/mL (p = 0.025, odds ratio 9.042, 95% confidence interval 1.325–61.716) and younger age (p = 0.030).

Discussion

An elevated ALT level classically differentiates immune clearance from immune tolerance in HBeAg-positive CHB. Nevertheless, studies have shown ALT to be an inaccurate marker of liver injury [7,9]. Although HBsAg staining patterns in liver histology [29] and antibody to the hepatitis B core antigen IgM titers [30] could assist in differentiating the two HBeAg-positive disease phases, the assessment of fibrosis remains an essential step in deciding treatment commencement [5]. Current non-invasive methods are unable to accurately identify patients with severe histologic abnormalities. Our present study showed serum HBsAg levels can play an important role in identifying HBeAg-positive patients with insignificant fibrosis and potentially reduce the need for liver biopsies. Although there had been preliminary analysis linking HBsAg levels with histologic severity [31], our study to our knowledge was the first to formally use liver histology as an outcome measure to assess the role of HBsAg titers in distinguishing insignificant and significant fibrosis.

The present study identified two serum HBsAg cut-off levels useful for predicting insignificant fibrosis among HBeAg-positive patients with ALT ≤2×ULN. Serum HBsAg ≥100,000 IU/mL was 100% predictive of insignificant fibrosis. Prior studies also found similarly high serum HBsAg levels in immune tolerant patients defined by normal ALT levels [24,25,32]. HBeAg-positive patients with HBsAg ≥100,000 are likely to have insignificant fibrosis even if ALT levels are minimally elevated.

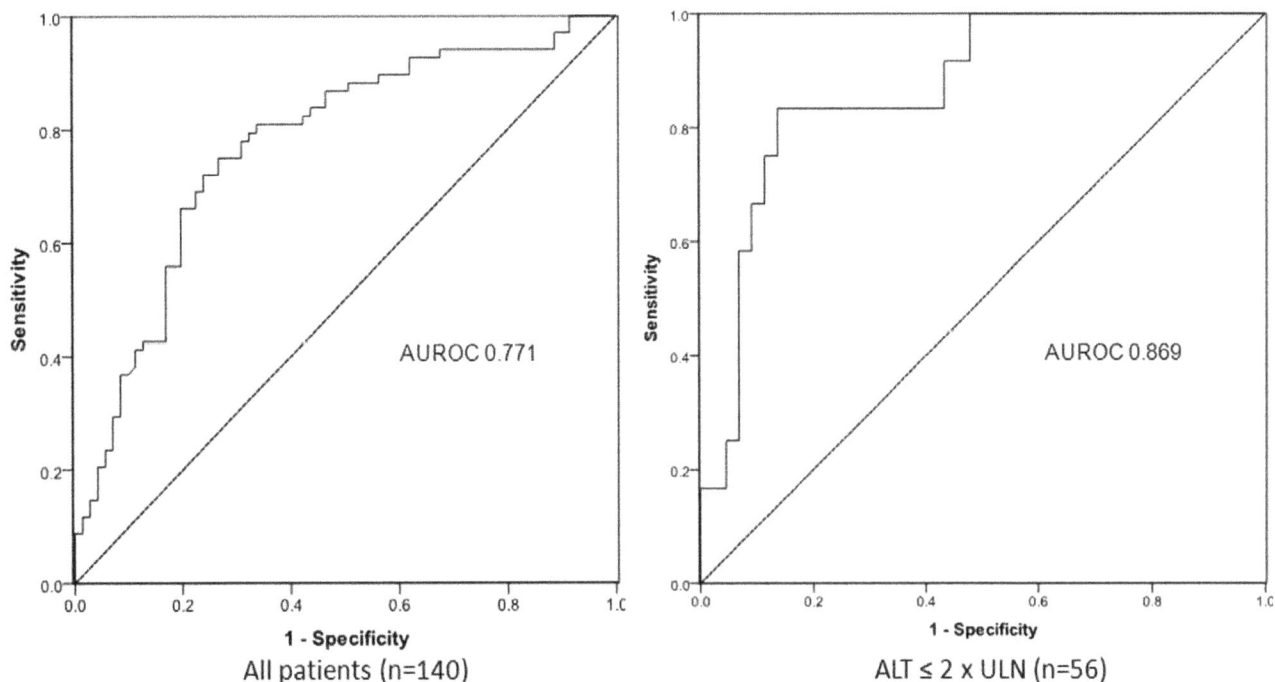

Figure 3. Receiver operating characteristic curves of serum HBsAg levels in predicting insignificant fibrosis (Ishak fibrosis score ≤1).

Table 2. Area under the receiver operating characteristic curve of serum HBsAg levels in predicting minor histologic changes.

		AUC	Standard Error	p value	95% CI
Insignificant fibrosis (F ≤1)	All patients (n = 140)	0.771	0.040	<0.001	0.692–0.851
	ALT ≤2×ULN (n = 56)	**0.869**	0.054	<0.001	0.763–0.976
Insignificant necroinflammation (Knodell HAI ≤4)	All patients (n = 140)	0.546	0.053	0.393	0.442–0.650
	ALT ≤×2 ULN (n = 56)	0.532	0.080	0.697	0.376–0.698

F, Ishak fibrosis score; HAI, histologic activity index; ALT, alanine aminotransferase; ULN, upper limit of normal; AUC, area under curve; CI, confidence interval.

The present study also found the optimal serum HBsAg cut-off level to predict insignificant fibrosis to be of ≥25,000 IU/mL. Among HBeAg-positive patients with ALT ≤2×ULN, serum HBsAg ≥25,000 IU/mL had a positive predictive value of 92.7% of predicting insignificant fibrosis. In addition, serum HBsAg ≥25,000 IU/mL was the best factor independently associated with insignificant fibrosis (p = 0.025, odds ratios 9.042). Our results suggest that HBeAg-positive patients with ALT ≤2×ULN and serum HBsAg ≥25,000 IU/mL can be observed without the need of liver biopsies. If serum HBsAg levels are below 25,000 IU/mL, other forms of assessment of fibrosis are necessary to decide for the commencement of therapy.

Our study failed to establish any association between serum HBV DNA levels and liver histology in HBeAg-positive patients. A possible explanation is that in these patients, the immune-mediated response during immune clearance may lead to fluctuating viremic levels with varying degrees of abnormalities in histology [33]. Several non-invasive predictive indices involving HBeAg-positive patients proposed in recent studies have also not included serum HBV DNA as a factor for prediction [13,14]. Serum HBV DNA levels are of greater predictive value in HBeAg-negative patients [34].

While the exact mechanism for the inverse relationship between the HBsAg levels and the degree of fibrosis remains to be examined, it may be related to the different stages of immune clearance. HBsAg is found extensively in immunohistochemical staining of liver histology in the immune tolerance phase [29]. With the transition from immune tolerance to early immune clearance, the immune system starts to increase its magnitude of immune control on the HBV. Serum HBsAg levels still remain high at the transition from immune tolerance to early immune clearance phase (ALT level may be at the high normal range) and it is to be expected that there will be minimal fibrosis because

immune mediated attack is still of low magnitude. Upon entering into a more full-blown stage of immune clearance with repeatedly greater immune mediated damage, more fibrosis develops, and viral control is achieved with decreasing HBsAg levels. HBsAg production could also be influenced by the development of preS/S mutants during immune clearance [35].

Intriguingly, high HBsAg levels are not always favorable in CHB, as shown by recent studies demonstrating high HBsAg levels to be associated with the development of HCC [36,37]. Hence, further longitudinal studies should be performed to examine the exact relationship between severity of fibrosis, disease progression and HBsAg levels by serial HBsAg measurement. Studies including non-Asian CHB patients would also be important, since such patients are infected later in life, with the classical immune tolerant phase absent or very short, and could well demonstrate different results.

Our study employed the lowered ULN for ALT (30 U/L for men, 19 U/L for women) as recommended by current treatment guidelines. Therefore, our cohort of patients with ALT ≤2×ULN accurately represents the HBeAg-positive population in which assessment of histologic severity is essential before deciding on treatment. In addition, the assay used for serum HBsAg measurement in our study has a broad dynamic range, minimizing the potential errors related to manual dilution in the measurement of high levels. Our study is limited by the lack of non-Asian CHB patients. In addition, HBV genotyping was not performed in our study, although prior studies have shown genotypes B and C, the two common genotypes in Hong Kong, have a similar risk of advanced fibrosis and histologic progression [38,39]. Future studies involving different CHB populations with different genotypes are required to validate our findings. The comparison of the predictive value of HBsAg levels (including for HBeAg-negative histology) with different non-invasive predictive indices

Table 3. Sensitivity, specificity and predictive values of different HBsAg levels for predicting insignificant fibrosis among patients with ALT ≤2×ULN (n = 56).

HBsAg (IU/mL)	Number of patients	Sensitivity	Specificity	PPV	NPV	LR+	LR−
≥10,000	45	90.9%	58.3%	*88.9%*	63.6%	2.18	0.16
≥25,000	41	86.4%	75.0%	*92.7%*	60.0%	3.46	0.18
≥50,000	32	68.2%	83.3%	*93.8%*	41.7%	4.08	0.38
≥75,000	24	52.3%	91.7%	*95.8%*	34.4%	6.30	0.52
≥100,000	16	36.4%	100%	*100%*	30.0%	–	0.64

Insignificant fibrosis defined as Ishak fibrosis score ≤1.
HBsAg, hepatitis B surface antigen; ALT, alanine aminotransferase; ULN, upper limit of normal; PPV, positive predictive value; NPV, negative predictive value, LR+, positive likelihood ratio; LR-, negative likelihood ratio.

Table 4. Multivariate analysis of factors independently associated with insignificant fibrosis among patients with ALT ≤2×ULN.

	p value	Odds ratio	95% Confidence Interval
HBsAg ≥25,000 IU/mL	*0.025*	*9.042*	1.325–61.716
Age (Years)	0.030	0.884	0.791–0.988
ALT (U/L)	0.078	0.936	0.869–1.007

Insignificant fibrosis defined as Ishak fibrosis score ≤1.
ALT, alanine aminotransferase; HBsAg, hepatitis B surface antigen.

(e.g. the asparate aminotransferase/platelet ratio index) and transient elastography are also needed. In additional, future clinical and cost-effectgive studies with larger cohorts, after the adjustment of HBV genotype, could consider fitting HBsAg levels and other available non-invasive markers as an algorithm for practical clinical usage.

In conclusion, serum HBsAg ≥25,000 IU/mL was independently associated with insignificant fibrosis. This level accurately predicted insignificant fibrosis in HBeAg-positive CHB patients with ALT ≤2×ULN (AUROC 0.869, positive predictive value 92.7%), the group of patients in which histologic evaluation is recommended. Measurement of serum HBsAg levels can thus assist treatment decisions among HBeAg-positive patients and potentially reduce the need for liver biopsies.

Author Contributions

Conceived and designed the experiments: WKS DKHW MFY. Performed the experiments: JF PPCI JCHY IFNH. Analyzed the data: WKS. Contributed reagents/materials/analysis tools: JF PPCI JCHY IFNH. Wrote the paper: WKS. Critical revision of manuscript: CLL MFY. Study supervision: MFY.

References

1. Lai CL, Yuen MF (2007) The natural history and treatment of chronic hepatitis B: a critical evaluation of standard treatment criteria and end points. Ann Intern Med 147: 58–61.
2. Rockey DC, Caldwell SH, Goodman ZD, Nelson RC, Smith AD (2009) Liver biopsy. Hepatology 49: 1017–1044.
3. Lok AS, McMahon BJ (2009) Chronic hepatitis B: update 2009. Hepatology 50: 661–662.
4. Liaw YF, Leung N, Kao JH, Piratvisuth T, Gane E, et al. (2008) Asian-Pacific consensus statement on the management of chronic hepatitis B: a 2008 update. Hepatol Int 2: 263–283.
5. European Association For The Study Of The L (2012) EASL Clinical Practice Guidelines: Management of chronic hepatitis B virus infection. J Hepatol 57: 167–185.
6. Yuen MF, Yuan HJ, Wong DK, Yuen JC, Wong WM, et al. (2005) Prognostic determinants for chronic hepatitis B in Asians: therapeutic implications. Gut 54: 1610–1614.
7. Andreani T, Serfaty L, Mohand D, Dernaika S, Wendum D, et al. (2007) Chronic hepatitis B virus carriers in the immunotolerant phase of infection: histologic findings and outcome. Clin Gastroenterol Hepatol 5: 636–641.
8. Kumar M, Sarin SK, Hissar S, Pande C, Sakhuja P, et al. (2008) Virologic and histologic features of chronic hepatitis B virus-infected asymptomatic patients with persistently normal ALT. Gastroenterology 134: 1376–1384.
9. Seto WK, Lai CL, Ip PP, Fung J, Wong DK, et al. (2012) A large population histology study showing the lack of association between ALT elevation and significant fibrosis in chronic hepatitis B. PLoS One 7: e32622.
10. Prati D, Taioli E, Zanella A, Della Torre E, Butelli S, et al. (2002) Updated definitions of healthy ranges for serum alanine aminotransferase levels. Ann Intern Med 137: 1–10.
11. Lee JK, Shim JH, Lee HC, Lee SH, Kim KM, et al. (2010) Estimation of the healthy upper limits for serum alanine aminotransferase in Asian populations with normal liver histology. Hepatology 51: 1577–1583.
12. Zeng MD, Lu LG, Mao YM, Qiu DK, Li JQ, et al. (2005) Prediction of significant fibrosis in HBeAg-positive patients with chronic hepatitis B by a noninvasive model. Hepatology 42: 1437–1445.
13. Fung J, Lai CL, Fong DY, Yuen JC, Wong DK, et al. (2008) Correlation of liver biochemistry with liver stiffness in chronic hepatitis B and development of a predictive model for liver fibrosis. Liver Int 28: 1408–1416.
14. Seto WK, Lee CF, Lai CL, Ip PP, Fong DY, et al. (2011) A new model using routinely available clinical parameters to predict significant liver fibrosis in chronic hepatitis B. PLoS One 6: e23077.
15. Myers RP, Tainturier MH, Ratziu V, Piton A, Thibault V, et al. (2003) Prediction of liver histological lesions with biochemical markers in patients with chronic hepatitis B. J Hepatol 39: 222–230.
16. Wai CT, Cheng CL, Wee A, Dan YY, Chan E, et al. (2006) Non-invasive models for predicting histology in patients with chronic hepatitis B. Liver Int 26: 666–672.
17. Fung J, Lai CL, Seto WK, Yuen MF (2011) The use of transient elastography in the management of chronic hepatitis B. Hepatol Int 5: 868–875.
18. Fung J, Lai CL, Yuen MF (2010) Hepatitis B virus DNA and hepatitis B surface antigen levels in chronic hepatitis B. Expert Rev Anti Infect Ther 8: 717–726.
19. Brunetto MR, Oliveri F, Colombatto P, Moriconi F, Ciccorossi P, et al. (2010) Hepatitis B surface antigen serum levels help to distinguish active from inactive hepatitis B virus genotype D carriers. Gastroenterology 139: 483–490.
20. Wiegand J, Wedemeyer H, Finger A, Heidrich B, Rosenau J, et al. (2008) A decline in hepatitis B virus surface antigen (hbsag) predicts clearance, but does not correlate with quantitative hbeag or HBV DNA levels. Antivir Ther 13: 547–554.
21. Tseng TC, Liu CJ, Su TH, Wang CC, Chen CL, et al. (2011) Serum hepatitis B surface antigen levels predict surface antigen loss in hepatitis B e antigen seroconverters. Gastroenterology 141: 517–525, 525 e511–512.
22. Seto WK, Wong DK, Fung J, Hung IF, Fong DY, et al. (2012) A large case-control study on the predictability of hepatitis B surface antigen (HBsAg) levels three years before HBsAg seroclearance. Hepatology.
23. Moucari R, Mackiewicz V, Lada O, Ripault MP, Castelnau C, et al. (2009) Early serum HBsAg drop: a strong predictor of sustained virological response to pegylated interferon alfa-2a in HBeAg-negative patients. Hepatology 49: 1151–1157.
24. Chan HL, Wong VW, Wong GL, Tse CH, Chan HY, et al. (2010) A longitudinal study on the natural history of serum hepatitis B surface antigen changes in chronic hepatitis B. Hepatology 52: 1232–1241.
25. Jaroszewicz J, Calle Serrano B, Wursthorn K, Deterding K, Schlue J, et al. (2010) Hepatitis B surface antigen (HBsAg) levels in the natural history of hepatitis B virus (HBV)-infection: a European perspective. J Hepatol 52: 514–522.
26. Chan HL, Thompson A, Martinot-Peignoux M, Piratvisuth T, Cornberg M, et al. (2011) Hepatitis B surface antigen quantification: why and how to use it in 2011 - a core group report. J Hepatol 55: 1121–1131.
27. Ishak K, Baptista A, Bianchi L, Callea F, De Groote J, et al. (1995) Histological grading and staging of chronic hepatitis. J Hepatol 22: 696–699.
28. Knodell RG, Ishak KG, Black WC, Chen TS, Craig R, et al. (1981) Formulation and application of a numerical scoring system for assessing histological activity in asymptomatic chronic active hepatitis. Hepatology 1: 431–435.
29. Mani H, Kleiner DE (2009) Liver biopsy findings in chronic hepatitis B. Hepatology 49: S61–71.
30. Colloredo G, Bellati G, Sonzogni A, Zavaglia C, Fracassetti O, et al. (1999) Semiquantitative assessment of IgM antibody to hepatitis B core antigen and prediction of the severity of chronic hepatitis B. J Viral Hepat 6: 429–434.
31. Martinot-Peignoux M, Carvalho-Filho R, Ferreira Netto Cardoso AC, Lapalus M, Lada O, et al. (2012) Significant genotype-specific association of hepatitis B surface antigen level and severity of liver disease in patients with chronic hepatitis B (abstract). J Hepatol 56: S211.
32. Nguyen T, Thompson AJ, Bowden S, Croagh C, Bell S, et al. (2010) Hepatitis B surface antigen levels during the natural history of chronic hepatitis B: a perspective on Asia. J Hepatol 52: 508–513.
33. Yuen MF, Ng IO, Fan ST, Yuan HJ, Wong DK, et al. (2004) Significance of HBV DNA levels in liver histology of HBeAg and Anti-HBe positive patients with chronic hepatitis B. Am J Gastroenterol 99: 2032–2037.
34. Yuen MF, Chow DH, Tsui K, Wong BC, Yuen JC, et al. (2005) Liver histology of Asian patients with chronic hepatitis B on prolonged lamivudine therapy. Aliment Pharmacol Ther 21: 841–849.

38. Sumi H, Yokosuka O, Seki N, Arai M, Imazeki F, et al. (2003) Influence of hepatitis B virus genotypes on the progression of chronic type B liver disease. Hepatology 37: 19–26.

35. Pollicino T, Amaddeo G, Restuccia A, Raffa G, Alibrandi A, et al. (2012) Impact of hepatitis B virus (HBV) preS/S genomic variability on HBV surface antigen and HBV DNA serum levels. Hepatology.

36. Chen CJ, Lee MH, Liu J, Batrla-Utermann R, Jen CL, et al. (2011) Quantitative serum levels of hepatitis B virus DNA and surface antigen are indepedent risk predictors of hepatocellular carcinoma (abstract). Hepatology 54: 881A.

37. Tseng TC, Liu CJ, Yang HC, Su TH, Wang CC, et al. (2012) High levels of hepatitis B surface antigen increase risk of hepatocellular carcinoma in patients with low HBV load. Gastroenterology 142: 1140–1149 e1143; quiz e1113–1144.

39. Yuen MF, Tanaka Y, Ng IO, Mizokami M, Yuen JC, et al. (2005) Hepatic necroinflammation and fibrosis in patients with genotypes Ba and C, core-promoter and precore mutations. J Viral Hepat 12: 513–518.

Quantification of Hepatic Iron Concentration in Chronic Viral Hepatitis: Usefulness of T2-weighted Single-Shot Spin-Echo Echo-Planar MR Imaging

Tatsuyuki Tonan[1][9], Kiminori Fujimoto[1,2][*][9], Aliya Qayyum[3], Takumi Kawaguchi[4], Atsushi Kawaguchi[5], Osamu Nakashima[6], Koji Okuda[7], Naofumi Hayabuchi[1], Michio Sata[8]

1 Department of Radiology, Kurume University School of Medicine, Kurume University Hospital, Kurume, Fukuoka, Japan, 2 Center for Diagnostic Imaging, Kurume University Hospital, Kurume, Fukuoka, Japan, 3 Department of Radiology and Biomedical Imaging, University of California San Francisco, San Francisco, California, United States of America, 4 Department of Digestive Disease Information & Research and Department of Internal Medicine, Kurume University School of Medicine, Kurume, Fukuoka, Japan, 5 Biostatics Center, Kurume University School of Medicine, Kurume, Fukuoka, Japan, 6 Department of Clinical Laboratory Medicine, Kurume University Hospital, Kurume, Fukuoka, Japan, 7 Department of Surgery, Department of Medicine, Kurume University School of Medicine, Kurume, Fukuoka, Japan, 8 Division of Gastroenterology, Department of Medicine, Kurume University School of Medicine, Kurume, Fukuoka, Japan

Abstract

Objective: To investigate the usefulness of single-shot spin-echo echo-planar imaging (SSEPI) sequence for quantifying mild degree of hepatic iron stores in patients with viral hepatitis.

Methods: This retrospective study included 34 patients with chronic viral hepatitis/cirrhosis who had undergone histological investigation and magnetic resonance imaging with T2-weighted gradient-recalled echo sequence (T2-GRE) and diffusion-weighted SSEPI sequence with b-factors of 0 s/mm^2 (T2-EPI), 500 s/mm^2 (DW-EPI-500), and 1000 s/mm^2 (DW-EPI-1000). The correlation between the liver-to-muscle signal intensity ratio, which was generated by regions of interest placed in the liver and paraspinous muscles of each sequence image, and the hepatic iron concentration (μmol/g dry liver), which was assessed by spectrophotometry, was analyzed by linear regression using a spline model. Akaike information criterion (AIC) was used to select the optimal model.

Results: Mean $\pm$ standard deviation of the hepatic iron concentration quantified by spectrophotometry was 24.6$\pm$16.4 (range, 5.5 to 83.2) μmol/g dry liver. DW-EPI correlated more closely with hepatic iron concentration than T2-GRE (R square values: 0.75 for T2-EPI, 0.69 for DW-EPI-500, 0.62 for DW-EPI-1000, and 0.61 for T2-GRE, respectively, all $P<0.0001$). Using the AIC, the regression model for T2-EPI generated by spline model was optimal because of lowest cross validation error.

Conclusion: T2-EPI was sensitive to hepatic iron, and might be a more useful sequence for quantifying mild degree of hepatic iron stores in patients with chronic viral hepatitis.

Editor: James Fung, The University of Hong Kong, Hong Kong

Funding: This study was partially supported by a Health and Labour Sciences Research Grants for Research on Hepatitis from the Ministry of Health, Labour and Welfare of Japan. No additional external funding received for this study. The funders had no role in study design, data collection and analysis, decision to publish, or preparation of the manuscript.

Competing Interests: The authors have declared that no competing interests exist.

* E-mail: kimichan@med.kurume-u.ac.jp

[9] These authors contributed equally to this work.

Introduction

Abnormalities of iron metabolism are frequently observed in patients with chronic liver diseases such as viral hepatitis, nonalcoholic fatty liver disease, and cirrhosis [1,2]. Iron excess, which increases oxidative stress via the formation of hydroxyl radicals and other highly reactive oxidizing molecules, leads to hepatotoxicity; it is related to the fibrogenesis and hepatocarcinogenesis associated with chronic viral hepatitis [1,3].

In recent years, several research groups have reported on the efficacy of iron reduction therapies by phlebotomy [4–10]. Yano et al. [6] reported that phlebotomy therapy contributed to improvement of biochemical markers in patients with hepatitis C virus

infection. Kato et al. [10] stated that phlebotomy therapy may potentially lower the risk of progression to hepatocellular carcinoma (HCC) in patients with hepatitis C virus infection. Therefore, precise quantification of hepatic iron overload might be beneficial for managing iron reduction therapy in patients with chronic viral hepatitis.

Assessment of body iron stores by measurement of serum ferritin concentration has poor specificity [11]. Liver biopsy, the most reliable method to measure hepatic iron stores, is an invasive procedure. Magnetic resonance imaging (MRI) is sensitive to hepatic iron because iron leads to a decline of MR signal due to T2-shortening effect related to paramagnetic properties. MRI has recently been recognized as a suitable noninvasive technique for quantifying hepatic iron overload [12]. Quantification of hepatic iron overload by MRI is useful in that it obviates the need for invasive liver biopsy and allows for repeat performance.

Generally, it is accepted that gradient-recalled echo (GRE) sequences are the most sensitive sequence to quantify mild degree of hepatic iron overload [13–20]. However, many studies evaluating GRE sequence with different echo-time and flip angle report variable results in the quantification of hepatic iron overload. Although the reproducibility of the technique and the quantification algorithm has been validated in various centers, these results are complicated.

Diffusion-weighted (DW) single-shot spin-echo echo-planar imaging (DW-EPI) has become a sequence used routinely in many institutions since the image quality was improved by recent technical progress such as parallel imaging and respiratory triggering [21–23]. In previous studies, it was reported that single-shot spin-echo EPI (SSEPI) sequence also had a high susceptibility effect [24,25].

We postulate that DW-EPI sequence might be superior to GRE sequence for quantifying mild degree of hepatic iron stores. To our knowledge, the investigation of hepatic iron overload by DW-EPI sequence has not been examined. The aim of this study was to investigate the usefulness of SSEPI sequence for quantifying mild degree of hepatic iron stores in patients with viral hepatitis.

Materials and Methods

Patients

The institutional review board (the Ethics Committee of Kurume University) approved this retrospective study (Approval No. 09112), which complied with the principles of the Declaration of Helsinki (2008 version). All included patients gave written informed consent to participate.

Our study was targeted at patients with viral chronic hepatitis/cirrhosis and HCC because such patients with chronic liver impairment may have increased liver iron and would have undergone both liver MR imaging and hepatic surgery.

We reviewed the patients who admitted use of both liver specimens and MR images before hepatic surgery at our institution between January 2007 and April 2008 and identified patients who met the following inclusion criteria: (a) patients had both chronic viral hepatitis/cirrhosis and HCC; (b) patients underwent abdominal MR imaging with T2-weighted GRE sequence and DW-EPI sequence with b-factors of 0 s/mm^2, 500 s/mm^2, and 1000 s/mm^2 (these sequences were part of our standard abdominal MR imaging protocol during this period); and (c) patients underwent an operation for HCC and received a histopathologic diagnosis of either chronic hepatitis or cirrhosis that was based on findings at surgical resection, performed within a month after MR imaging.

Forty-six patients fulfilled these criteria. Twelve of these 46 patients were excluded on the basis of the following reasons: (a) Available imaging data did not correspond to available histopathologic data because of interval surgery ($n = 5$), (b) MR studies were incomplete ($n = 3$), (c) an artifact was observed on MR images and precluded accurate measurement of signal intensity ($n = 1$), and (d) other causes of chronic liver disease such as alcoholic hepatitis ($n = 2$) and non-alcoholic steatohepatitis ($n = 1$). Thirty-four patients formed the final study group (21 men and thirteen women; median age, 65 years; range, 52–83 years). Histopathologic sampling of all patients included in the study was performed after MR imaging (median, 5 days; range, 1–30 days). The cause of chronic liver disease was hepatitis C virus infection (n = 26) or hepatitis B virus infection (n = 8). None of the patients had a

clinical diagnosis of hemochromatosis that was based on review of medical records.

Hepatic iron concentration and histological analysis

A partial hepatic resection was performed in all patients with HCC. For each patient, 50 mg of wet liver tissue was extracted from the surgically removed specimen by a MLS1200 MEGA microwave digestion system (Milestone General Co. Ltd., Kawasaki, Japan) for 1 min at 250 W, 1 min at 0 W, 5 min at 250 W, 5 min 400 W, and 5 min at 500 W. For determination of hepatic iron concentration (μmol/g dry liver), the resulting extracts were analyzed by spectrophotometry with a graphite atomic absorption camera (Polarized Zeeman Atomic Absorption Spectrophotometer, Hitachi, Ltd., Tokyo, Japan) and were converted to the units shown above [26].

For histological analysis, fibrosis stage and necroinflammation grade were evaluated semiquantitatively using the METAVIR scoring system [27]. Fibrosis stage graded on a scale of 0 to 4, as follows: F0 = no fibrosis; F1 = portal fibrosis without septa; F2 = portal fibrosis and few septa; F3 = numerous septa without cirrhosis; and F4 = cirrhosis. The necroinflammatory activity score was graded on a scale of 0 to 3, as follows: A0 = none; A1 = mild; A2 = moderate; A3 = severe. Distribution of steatosis was also retrospectively evaluated as the overall impression of the percentage of fat-containing hepatocytes on hematoxylin and eosin–stained specimens [28,29]. Steatosis grade was scored on a scale of 0 to 2, as follows: grade 0 = absence of steatosis; grade 1 = steatosis <5%; and grade 2 = steatosis ≥5%.

MRI technique and analysis

Within one month prior to surgery, MR imaging was performed at field strength of 1.5 T (Magnetom Symphony Advanced; Siemens, Erlangen, Germany) with use of a body phased-array surface coil. A series of DWIs and T2-weighted GRE sequence were obtained using parallel imaging with generalized auto calibrating partially parallel acquisition (GRAPPA) of acceleration factor 2 in all patients. DWI was performed in the transverse plane by respiratory-triggered combining SSEPI sequence with a chemical shift–selective pulse (CHESS). Any antiperistalsis drug was not used.

The imaging parameters for DW-EPI were as follows: repetition time (TR), 2000 msec; echo time (TE), 81 msec; directions of the motion-probing gradient, three orthogonal axes; gradient factor b values of 0 sec/mm^2 (T2-weighted SSEPI, hereafter T2-EPI), 500 sec/mm^2 (DW-EPI-500), and 1000 sec/mm^2 (DW-EPI-1000); 2170-Hz per pixel bandwidth; 350-mm field of view; 128×88 rectangular matrixes; 9-mm-thick sections; 1-mm intersection gap; six signals acquired; and acquisition time of approximately 1 minute 30 seconds.

T2-weighted GRE sequence (hereafter, T2-GRE) was performed in the transverse plane by fast low angle shot (FLASH) with one signal acquired during a 22-second breath hold. The imaging parameters for T2-GRE were as follows: TR, 246 msec; TE, 9.5 msec; flip angle (FA), 30°; 350-mm field of view; 9-mm-thick sections; 1-mm intersection gap; 16-number of sections; 256×192 matrix; and 130-Hz per pixel bandwidth.

Quantitative image analysis was conducted by measuring the signal intensities of the liver parenchyma and paraspinous muscles. Image analysis was performed by two independent radiologists using plug-in software developed in-house by one of the authors [30,31] (Figure 1). Five separate regions of interest (ROIs) were carefully placed manually in the anterior and posterior segments of the right hepatic lobe at the level of the porta hepatis (whenever possible) on each sequence; care was taken to avoid focal lesions, major vascular structures, and artifacts such as chemical shifts, magnetic susceptibility, and cardiac motion. Liver signal intensities were recorded as the mean values generated from the five measurements (total liver ROI area sampled, 500 mm^2). The procedure was repeated to measure muscle signal intensity by placing two separate ROIs on the right and left paraspinous muscles in the same slice section used to measure liver signal intensity; care was taken to avoid artifacts such as chemical shifts, magnetic susceptibility, and motion on each sequence.

Muscle signal intensities were recorded as the mean values generated from the two measurements (total muscle ROI area sampled, 200 mm^2). We calculated the liver-to-muscle signal intensity ratio (LMR) by dividing mean liver signal intensity by mean muscle signal intensity for each sequence [15].

Statistical analysis

A Bland-Altman plot was used to analyze the 95% limits of interobserver agreement for the LMR on each sequence [32]. The correlation of the LMR obtained by the two observers on each sequence was determined using the Pearson correlation coefficient (r).

The relationship between the LMR on each sequence and hepatic iron concentration was analyzed by means of scatter plots. These results were inspected for linearity and goodness of fit. The relationship between the LMR on each sequence and hepatic iron concentration was modeled by regression techniques using a spline model. Details of spline models are given in the next section.

To investigate effects of each LMR on hepatic iron concentration, we applied the linear models containing not only a main term but also knot terms which play a role as an inflection point. The

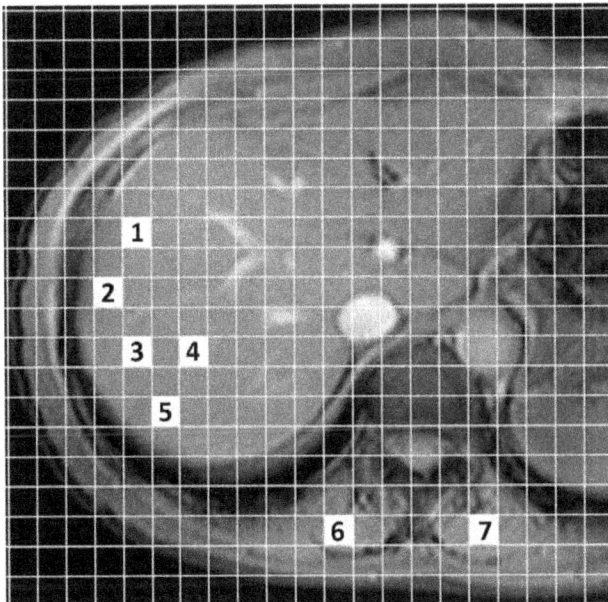

Figure 1. Illustration of the method used to measure regions of interest on an MR image. With use of computer software (developed in-house by the authors), two independent observers freely and easily selected a region of interest by clicking a mesh unit on the right hepatic lobe of an image while avoiding the large vessels, focal hepatic lesions, or artifacts. Seven regions of interest were chosen for liver parenchyma (1–5, total liver ROI area sampled, 500 mm^2) and paraspinous muscles (6 and 7, total muscle ROI area sampled, 200 mm^2) in the same slice section of each sequence.

Akaike information criterion (AIC) was used to evaluate these alternate models [33]. The number and location of knots were determined objectively with the minimum AIC among their prespecified candidates, which were 20, 40, 60, and 80 percentiles of each LMR. To evaluate the predictive accuracy, a leave one out cross validation (CV) error [34] was computed.

The Kruskal–Wallis test was used to determine significant differences in the LMR on each sequence among category classification in each histological finding (i.e. necroinflammation grade, fibrosis stage, and steatosis grade). All analyses were performed using SPSS statistical software (version 12.0 J; SPSS, Inc., Chicago, IL, USA). $P < 0.05$ was considered statistically significant.

Details of the spline models used in statistical analysis

Response and predictor variables are denoted by y and x, respectively. The general form of the univariate (first order) spline model is

$$y = \alpha + \beta x + \sum_{j=1}^{m} \gamma_j (x - r_j)_+ + \varepsilon \qquad (1)$$

where α, β, and γ_j ($j = 1, 2, \ldots, m$) are parameters to be estimated, $(z)_+ = \max(0, z)$, $r_1, r_2, \cdots, r_m$ are called knots which play a role as an inflection point, and ε is an error following a normal distribution with mean 0 and a constant variance. Note that in the case of $\gamma_1 = \gamma_2 = \cdots = \gamma_m = 0$ the model can be identified as a simple linear regression model. The parameters in the model (1) are estimated by an ordinary least squares method to minimize squared residuals Q in (2) from samples (x_i, y_i) ($i = 1, 2, \ldots, n$) from n patients.

$$Q = \sum_{i=1}^{n} \left(y_i - \alpha - \beta x_i - \sum_{j=1}^{m} \gamma_j (x_i - r_j)_+ \right)^2 \qquad (2)$$

To illustrate the interpretation of parameters in the spline model, we consider the model as with only one knot as in (3). This model contains two lines whose slope and intercept are changed at $x = r$.

$$y = \alpha + \beta x + \gamma (x - r)_+ + \varepsilon \qquad (3)$$

In the range $x \leq r$, the slope is β and the intercept is α. In the other range $x > r$, the slope is $\beta + \gamma$ and the intercept is $\alpha - \gamma r$. This modeling can be easily implemented by standard software such as SAS, SPSS, and R. Supposing that the data set has two columns corresponding to response (y) and predictor (x) variables, one can add the computed $(x - r)_+$ as the third column. Then, the multiple regression model can be applied with the response y and two predictors, x and $(x - r)_+$. If you want more knots, you can add the corresponding columns and predictors in the regression model.

The essential point in the use of this spline model is to select the number and location of knots. As used in this paper, one choice for candidates for knots is the quantiles for continuous variables taking into account the sample size. Once one specifies the candidates, the problem turns to the variable selection for predictor variables used in the multiple regression model, which can also be implemented by standard software. One effective method is to use information criteria such as AIC. This kind of modeling [35] is useful to investigate the flexible relationship between the response and predictor.

Results

Hepatic iron concentration and histological findings

Mean ± SD of the hepatic iron concentration quantified by spectrophotometry was 24.6±16.4 (range, 5.5 to 83.2) μmol/g dry liver. Histological necroinflammation grade was A1 in 21 patients and A2 in 13 patients. Fibrosis stage was F1 in 13 patients, F2 in 4 patients, F3 in 5 patients, and F4 (i.e. cirrhosis) in 12 patients. Steatosis grade was 0 in 14 patients, grade 1 in 11 patients, and grade 2 in 9 patients.

Interobserver agreement for the LMR on each sequence

There was no significant difference between measurements made by the two observers for the two parameters; the interclass Pearson correlation coefficients were 0.96 (95% confidence interval [CI]: 0.86, 1.00) for T2-GRE, 0.99 (95% CI: 0.92, 1.00) for T2-EPI, 0.97 (95% CI: 0.85, 1.00) for DW-EPI-500, and 0.98 (95% CI: 0.97, 1.00) for DW-EPI-1000; the mean difference (± standard deviation) was −0.0027±0.054 for T2-GRE, −0.0069± 0.052 for T2-EPI, 0.017±0.11 for DW-EPI-500, and 0.013±0.16 for DW-EPI-1000; and the coefficients of repeatability were 0.108 for T2-GRE, 0.105 for T2-EPI, 0.213 for DW-EPI-500, and 0.316 for DW-EPI-1000. Bland-Altman plots with 95% limits of

agreement for each sequence are shown in Figure 2. There was no proportional bias or fixed bias in each Bland-Altman plot for the two parameters.

Correlation between the LMR on each sequence and hepatic iron concentration

Figure 3 shows results for the line fit by the selected regression model. Created simple regression models to estimate the hepatic iron concentration in each sequence are as follows:

$$T2 - GRE : y = 103.7 - 85.7 \times LMR + 58.2 \times (LMR - 1.05)_+$$

$$T2 - EPI : y = 131.0 - 139.7 \times LMR + 106.5 \times (LMR - 0.73)_+ + 27.4 \times (LMR - 1.24)_+$$

$$DW - EPI - 500 : y = 80.2 - 51.8 \times LMR + 43.0 \times (LMR - 1.24)_+$$

$$DW - EPI - 1000 : y = 66.7 - 29.3 \times LMR + 25.7 \times (LMR - 1.76)_+$$

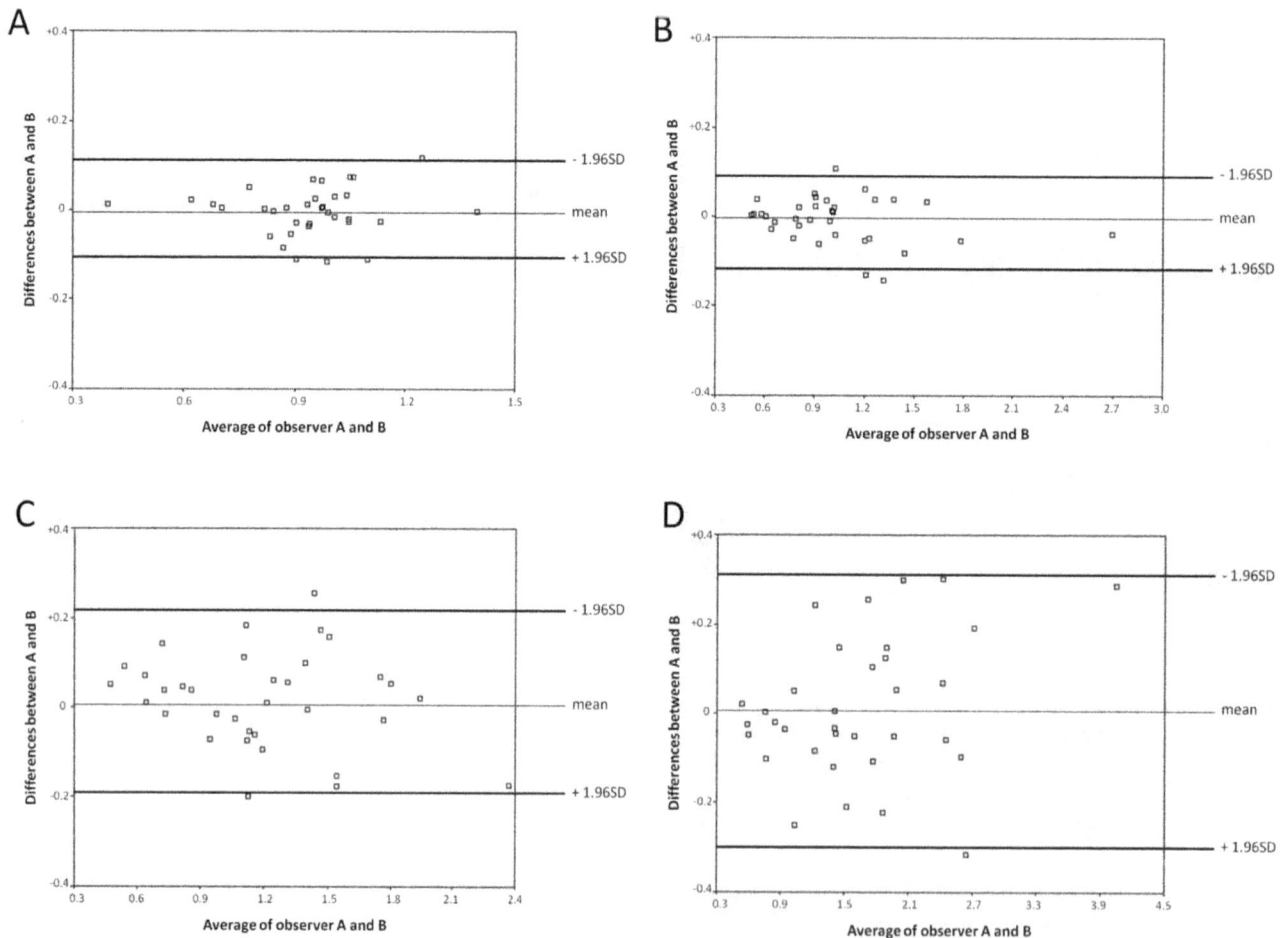

Figure 2. Bland-Altman plots for measurements of T2-GRE (A), T2-EPI (B), DW-EPI-500 (C), and DW-EPI-1000 (D) in liver parenchyma. Each Bland-Altman plots demonstrates good interobserver agreement and lack of proportional bias or fixed bias. The average of the measurements made by the two observers is plotted against the difference between the measurements made by the two observers. The thin lines represent the mean value of all differences between the two observers, and the thick lines represent the 95% limits of agreement. *SD* = standard deviation.

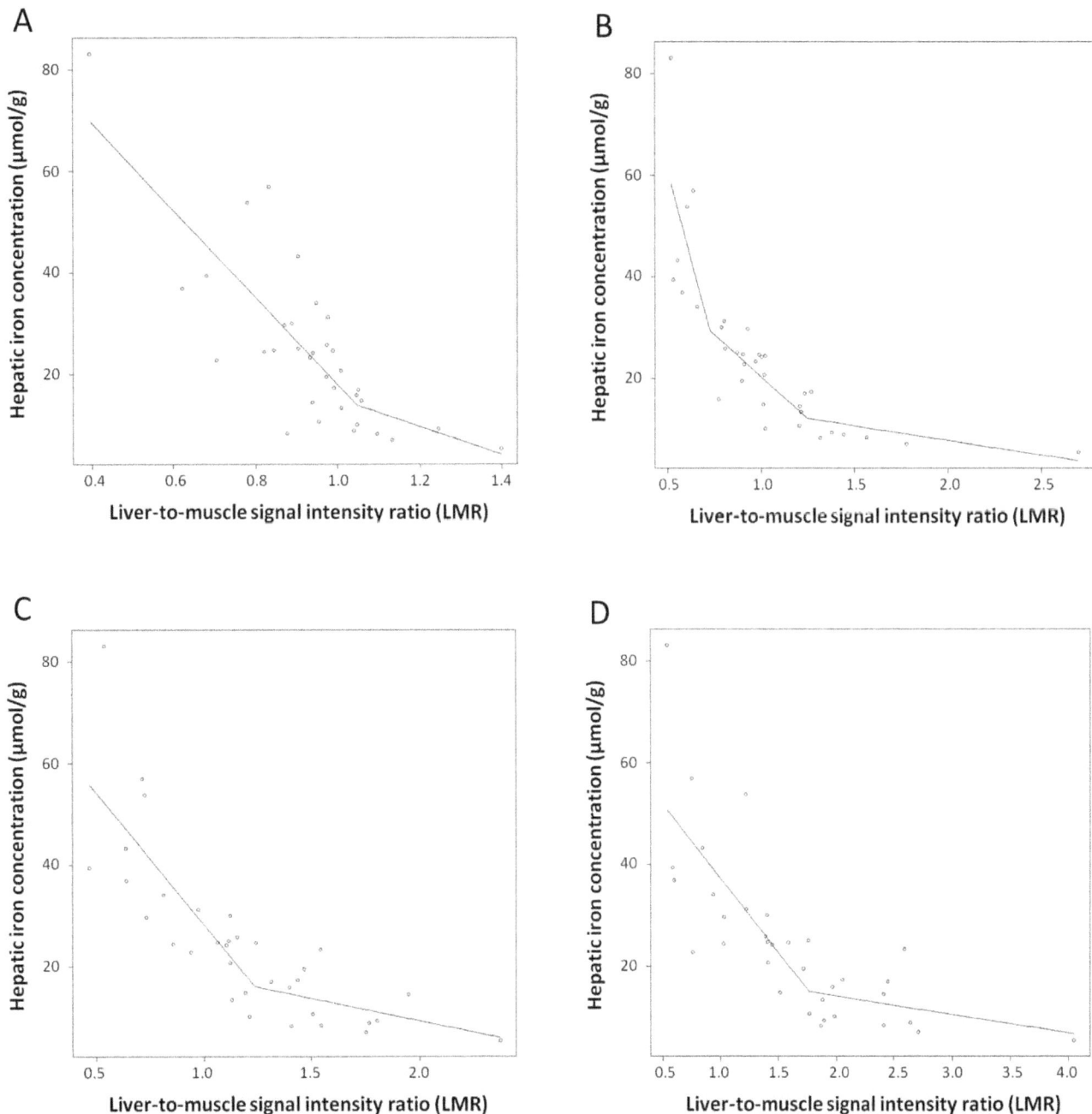

Figure 3. Scatter plots of LMR and hepatic iron concentration (μmol/g dry liver) on T2-GRE (A), T2-EPI (B), DW-EPI-500 (C), and DW-EPI-1000 (D). Correlation between LMR and hepatic iron concentration for linear regression with spline models are shown as solid lines on each sequence. The linear regression model [y = 131.0−139.7×LMR+106.5×(LMR−0.73)$_+$+27.4×(LMR−1.24)$_+$] on T2-EPI was optimal.

where LMR is the measurement value on each sequence (appendix).

The regression analyses showed an excellent overall negative correlation on each sequence. Particularly, T2-EPI correlated most closely with hepatic iron concentration. R square values on each sequence were as follows: 0.75 for T2-EPI, 0.69 for DW-EPI-500, 0.62 for DW-EPI-1000, and 0.61 for T2-GRE (F-test, $P<0.0001$, respectively).

Using the AIC, the linear regression model on T2-EPI [y = 131.0−139.7×LMR+106.5×(LMR−0.73)$_+$+27.4×(LMR−1.24)$_+$] was chosen as having the best fit, since it had the lowest CV error. The corresponding CV errors were as follows: 14161.3 for

T2-GRE, 11357.4 for T2-EPI, 12220.0 for DW-EPI-500, and 14376.2 for DW-EPI-1000.

Correlation between the LMR on each sequence and histological findings

No significant differences were found for the LMR on each sequence among category classification of histological findings (i.e. necroinflammation grade, fibrosis stage, and steatosis grade). P values (Kruskal-Wallis test) were as follows: (a) necroinflammation grade: $P=0.4$ for T2-GRE, $P=0.89$ for T2-EPI, $P=0.68$ for DW-EPI-500, and $P=0.6$ for DW-EPI-1000; (b) fibrosis stage: $P=0.39$

for T2-GRE, $P = 0.29$ for T2-EPI, $P = 0.19$ for DW-EPI-500, and $P = 0.38$ for DW-EPI-1000; (c) steatosis grade: $P = 0.75$ for T2-GRE, $P = 0.77$ for T2-EPI, $P = 0.69$ for DW-EPI-500, and $P = 0.95$ for DW-EPI-1000.

Discussion

In the present study, we found good correlation between DW-EPI and hepatic iron concentration in patients with chronic viral hepatitis, and also demonstrated that SSEPI sequence was more sensitive than T2-GRE sequence for quantifying small amount of hepatic iron overload; this is in concordance with prior studies reporting a high susceptibility effect with SSEPI sequence [24,25].

A lot of studies have evaluated the correlation between hepatic iron concentration and MRI measurements [13–20]. Particularly, GRE sequences, which are more sensitive to field heterogeneities than spin-echo sequences [15,16,18], were used for quantifying mild degree of hepatic iron stores in many studies. It was reported that the best means to evaluate mild degrees of hepatic iron overload was T2-GRE sequences with long TE (i.e. >15 ms) and with low FA (i.e. 20°–30°) [15,19]. Alternatively, Bonkovsky et al. [18] reported that GRE sequence with shortest TR and TE, which results in a short breath hold time, was useful to minimize motion artifact and other sources of noise. Results from studies of GRE sequence were variable in terms of quantification of hepatic iron overload [13–20].

The sensitivity to iron on T2-GRE sequences varies significantly with various different TE and FA [15]. Marked signal loss from proton dephasing will occur at longer TEs, and once signal intensity falls to the level of image noise, inaccuracies in signal intensity measurement can be expected [36]. From these points, in the routine examination, we employed the conventional TE which corresponds to second in-phase on T2-GRE sequence for quantifying mild degree of hepatic iron overload.

SSEPI sequences are very fast and have a high susceptibility effect, but suffer from limited image quality. This is mostly related to limited signal to noise ratio (SNR), especially at higher b-values, and limited spatial resolution, which constitute an obstacle for its widespread use in clinical practice [37]. However, techniques such as parallel imaging and pulse triggering improve image quality of SSEPI sequences by correcting magnetic field heterogeneity [21–23]. Recent data showed that respiratory triggering improved the image quality with SNR on SSEPI sequences. This method attempts to avoid motion artifacts prospectively by using respiratory signals to synchronize image acquisition with the patient's breathing cycle and by acquiring the imaging data during the relative quite end expiration phase [38–40].

In the present study, we employed SSEPI sequence with techniques such as parallel imaging and respiratory triggering. This sequence, which has the advantage of high susceptibility effects, was useful to assess mild degree of hepatic iron stores in patients with viral hepatitis. Of DW-EPIs, it was suggested that T2-EPI was the most suitable sequence because DW-EPI-500 and DW-EPI-1000 had loss of SNR caused by application of the motion-probing gradients pulse.

In patients with chronic viral hepatitis, steatosis is a common secondary phenomenon. Westphalen et al. [41] reported that iron stores in background liver complicated measurement of steatosis by opposed-phase MR imaging. Alternatively, a recent study reported that concomitant steatosis lowers the diagnostic performance of T2-GRE sequence and chemical shift imaging for quantifying mild degree of hepatic iron stores because intravoxel constructive and destructive interference between fat and water spins due to chemical shift effect of the second kind potentially affect the signal intensity measurements for T2-GRE sequence [36]. Therefore, it might be important to consider the influence of each factor in background liver tissue in the quantification of steatosis and iron stores using MR imaging.

On DW-EPI, we found no significant differences in LMR among histological steatosis grades. Use of fat saturation pulse (i.e., CHESS) on DW-EPIs could eliminate the influence of steatosis, which might support the better utility of this sequence for quantifying mild degree of hepatic iron stores. On the other hand, although previous studies reported that liver fibrosis decreased the diffusion signal [30,42,43], no significant differences were found in LMR on DW-EPIs among histological fibrosis stages, which suggest that influence of liver fibrosis to the signal of DW-EPIs was low as a result. The quantification of iron stores by DW-EPIs may have suffered potential influence by fibrosis, which might be one of the reasons that T2-EPI was most accurate sequence for quantifying mild degree of iron stores. Therefore, we recommend the T2-EPI with b values of 0 sec/mm^2, which is not affected to the diffusion signal, for quantifying mild degree of iron stores.

Several limitations of the present study warrant mention. First, the study was conducted retrospectively and sample size was small. Although a major effort was made to exclude sample bias, there was limited sample size for examination of liver iron concentration using spectrophotometry because of its retrospective nature. Second, all measurements for the LMR were obtained in the right lobe of the liver to avoid motion-related artifact. Because the pathologic specimens were obtained at surgery for an HCC, histologically sampled areas did not completely correspond to radiologically sampled areas. A prospective study with a substantially larger sample is needed to further validate our findings.

In conclusion, DW-EPI (especially, T2-weighted SSEPI) was sensitive to hepatic iron, and might be a more useful sequence for quantifying mild degree of hepatic iron stores in patients with chronic viral hepatitis.

Author Contributions

Conceived and designed the experiments: TT KF TK MS. Performed the experiments: TT KF TK ON. Analyzed the data: TT KF AK. Contributed reagents/materials/analysis tools: KF TK ON KO NH MS. Wrote the paper: TT KF AQ AK. Designed the software used in analysis: KF. Drafting the article or revising it critically for important intellectual content and final approval of the version to be published: TT KF AQ TK AK ON KO NH MS.

References

1. Bonkovsky HL, Banner BF, Rothman AL (1997) Iron and chronic viral hepatitis. Hepatology 25: 759–768.
2. Younossi ZM, Gramlich T, Bacon BR, Matteoni CA, Boparai N, et al. (1999) Hepatic iron and nonalcoholic fatty liver disease. Hepatology 30: 847–850.
3. Niederau C, Fischer R, Sonnenberg A, Stremmel W, Trampisch HJ, et al. (1985) Survival and causes of death in cirrhotic and in noncirrhotic patients with primary hemochromatosis. N Engl J Med 313: 1256–1262.
4. Hayashi H, Takikawa T, Nishimura N, Yano M, Isomura T, et al. (1994) Improvement of serum aminotransferase levels after phlebotomy in patients with chronic active hepatitis C and excess hepatic iron. Am J Gastroenterol 89: 986–988.
5. Di Bisceglie AM, Bonkovsky HL, Chopra S, Chopra S, Flamm S, et al. (2000) Iron reduction as an adjuvant to interferon therapy in patients with chronic hepatitis C who have previously not responded to interferon: a multicenter, prospective, randomized, controlled trial. Hepatology 32: 135–138.
6. Yano M, Hayashi H, Yoshioka K, Kohgo Y, Saito H, et al. (2004) A significant reduction in serum alanine aminotransferase levels after 3-month iron reduction

therapy for chronic hepatitis C: a multicenter, prospective, randomized, controlled trial in Japan. J Gastroenterol 39: 570–574.

7. Kawamura Y, Akuta N, Sezaki H, Hosaka T, Someya T, et al. (2005) Determinants of serum ALT normalization after phlebotomy in patients with chronic hepatitis C infection. J Gastroenterol 40: 901–906.

8. Sumida Y, Kanemasa K, Fukumoto K, Yoshida N, Sakai K (2007) Effects of dietary iron reduction versus phlebotomy in patients with chronic hepatitis C: results from a randomized, controlled trial on 40 Japanese patients. Intern Med 46: 637–642.

9. Yano M, Hayashi H, Wakusawa S, Sanae F, Takikawa T, et al. (2002) Long term effects of phlebotomy on biochemical and histological parameters of chronic hepatitis C. Am J Gastroenterol 97: 133–137.

10. Kato J, Kobune M, Nakamura T, Kuroiwa G, Takada K, et al. (2001) Normalization of elevated hepatic 8-hydroxy-2-deoxyguanousine levels in chronic hepatitis C patientsby phlebotomy and low iron diet. Cancer Res 61: 8697–8702.

11. Brissot P, Deugnier Y. Haemochromatosis In: McIntyre N, Benhamou JP, Bircher J, Rizzetto M, Rodes J, eds. Oxford textbook of clinical hepatology Oxford: Oxford University Press. pp 1379–1391.

12. Olthof AW, Sijens PE, Kreeftenberg HG, Kappert P, Irwan R, et al. (2007) Correlation between serum ferritin levels and liver iron concentration determined by MR imaging: impact of hematologic disease and inflammation. Magn Reson Imaging 25: 228–231.

13. Alústiza JM, Castiella A, De Juan MD, Emparanza JI, Artetxe J, et al. (2007) Iron overload in the liver diagnostic and quantification. Eur J Radiol 61: 499–506.

14. Alustiza JM, Artetxe J, Castiella A, Agirre C, Emparanza JI, et al. (2004) Gipuzkoa Hepatic Iron Concentration by MRI Study Group. MR quantification of hepatic iron concentration. Radiology 230: 179–404.

15. Gandon Y, Olivi'e D, Guyader D, Aubé C, Oberti F, et al. (2004) Non-invasive assessment of hepatic iron stores by MRI. Lancet 363: 357–362.

16. St Pierre TG, Clark PR, Chua-anusorn W, Fleming AJ, Jeffrey GP, et al. (2005) Noninvasive measurement and imaging of liver iron concentrations using proton magnetic resonance. Blood 105: 855–861.

17. Olthof AW, Sijens PE, Kreeftenberg HG, Kappert P, van der Jagt EJ, et al. (2009) Non-invasive liver iron concentration measurement by MRI:Comparison of two validated protocols. Eur J Radiol 71: 116–121.

18. Bonkovsky HL, Rubin RB, Cable EE, Davidoff A, Rijcken TH, et al. (1999) Hepatic iron concentration: noninvasive estimation by means of MR imaging techniques. Radiology 212: 227–234.

19. Gandon Y, Guyader D, Heautot JF, Reda MI, Yaouanq J, et al. (1994) Hemochromatosis: diagnosis and quantification of liver iron with gradient-echo MR imaging. Radiology 193: 533–538.

20. Kreeftenberg HG, Jr., Mooyaart EL, Huizenga JR, Sluiter WJ (2000) Quantification of liver iron concentration with magnetic resonance imaging by combining T1-, T2-weighted spin echo sequences and a gradient echo sequence. Neth J Med 56: 133–137.

21. Bammer R, Keeling SL, Augustin M, Pruessmann KP, Wolf R, et al. (2001) Improved diffusion weighted single-shot echo-planar imaging (EPI) in stroke using sensitivity encoding (SENSE). Magn Reson Med 46: 548–554.

22. Taouli B, Martin AJ, Qayyum A, Merriman RB, Vigneron D, et al. (2004) Parallel imaging and diffusion tensor imaging for diffusion weighted MRI of the liver: preliminary experience in healthy volunteers. AJR Am J Roentgenol 183: 677–680.

23. Murtz P, Flacke S, Traber F, van den Brink JS, Gieseke J, et al. (2002) Abdomen: diffusion-weighted MR imaging with pulse-triggered single-shot sequences. Radiology 224: 258–264.

24. Tanimoto A, Kuribayashi S (2006) Application of superparamagnetic iron oxide to imaging of hepatocellular carcinoma. Eur J Radiol 58: 200–216.

25. Coenegrachts K, Matos C, Ter Beek L, Metens T, Haspeslagh M, et al. (2009) Focal liver lesion detection and characterization: Comparison of non-contrast enhanced and SPIO-enhanced diffusion-weighted single-shot spin echo echo planar and turbo spin echo T2-weighted imaging. Eur J Radiol 72: 432–439.

26. Griesmann GE, Hartmann AC, Farris FF (2009) Concentrations and correlations for eight metals in human liver. Int J Environ Health Res 19: 231–238.

27. Ishak K, Baptista A, Bianchi L, Callea F, De Groote J, et al. (1995) Histological grading and staging of chronic hepatitis. J Hepatol 22: 696–699.

28. Kleiner DE, Brunt EM, Van Natta M, Behling C, Contos MJ, et al. (2005) ; Nonalcoholic Steatohepatitis Clinical Research Network. Design and validation of a histological scoring system for nonalcoholic fatty liver disease. Hepatology 41: 1313–1321.

29. Brunt EM, Janney CG, Di Bisceglie AM, Neuschwander-Tetri BA, Bacon BR (1999) Nonalcoholicsteatohepatitis: a proposal for grading and staging the histological lesions. Am JGastroenterol 94: 2467–2474.

30. Fujimoto K, Tonan T, Azuma S, Kage M, Nakashima O, et al. (2011) Evaluation of the mean and entropy of apparent diffusion coefficient values in chronic hepatitis C: Correlation with pathologic fibrosis stage and inflammatory activity grade. Radiology 258: 739–748.

31. Tonan T, Fujimoto K, Qayyum A, Azuma S, Ishibashi M, et al. (2011) Correlation of Kupffer cell function and hepatocyte function in chronic viral hepatitis evaluated with superparamagnetic iron oxide-enhanced magnetic resonance imaging and scintigraphy using technetium-99m-labelled galactosyl human serum albumin. Exp Ther Med 2: 607–613.

32. Bland JM, Altman DG (1986) Statistical methods for assessing agreement between two methods of clinical measurement. Lancet 1: 307–310.

33. Akaike H (1974) A new look at the statistical model identification. IEEE Trans Automatic Control 19: 716–723.

34. Stone M (1974) Cross-validatory choice and assessment of statistical predictions. Journal of Royal Statistical Society B 36: 111–147.

35. Kawaguchi A, Yonemoto K, Tanizaki Y, Kiyohara Y, Yanagawa T, et al. (2008) Application of functional ANOVA models for hazard regression to the Hisayama data. Stat Med 27: 3515–3527.

36. Lim RP, Tuvia K, Hajdu CH, Losada M, Gupta R, et al. (2010) Quantification of hepatic iron deposition in patients with liver disease: comparison of chemical shift imaging with single-echo T2*-weighted imaging. AJR Am J Roentgenol 194: 1288–1295.

37. Taouli B, Sandberg A, Stemmer A, Parikh T, Wong S, et al. (2009) Diffusion-weighted imaging of the liver: comparison of navigator triggered and breathhold acquisitions. J Magn Reson Imaging 30: 561–568.

38. Nasu K, Kuroki Y, Sekiguchi R, Nawano S (2006) The effect of simulta- neous use of respiratory triggering in diffusion weighted imaging of the liver. Magn Reson Med Sci 5: 129–136.

39. Gourtsoyianni S, Papanikolaou N, Yarmenitis S, Maris T, Karantanas A, et al. (2008) Respiratory gated diffusion weighted imaging of the liver: value of apparent diffusion coefficient measurements in the differentiation between most commonly encountered benign and malignant focal liver lesions. Eur Radiol 18: 486–492.

40. Asbach P, Klessen C, Kroencke TJ, Kluner C, Stemmer A, et al. (2005) Magnetic resonance cholangiopancreatography using a free-breathing T2-weighted turbo spin echo sequence with navigator-triggered prospective acquisition correction. Magn Reson Imaging 23: 939–945.

41. Westphalen AC, Qayyum A, Yeh BM, Merriman RB, Lee JA, et al. (2007) Liver fat: effect of hepatic iron deposition on evaluation with opposed-phase MR imaging. Radiology 242: 450–455.

42. Taouli B, Tolia AJ, Losada M, Babb JS, Chan ES, et al. (2007) Diffusionweighted MRI for quantifi cation of liver fibrosis: preliminary experience. AJR Am J Roentgenol 189(4): 799–806.

43. Taouli B, Chouli M, Martin AJ, Qayyum A, Coakley FV, et al. (2008) Chronic hepatitis:role of diffusion-weighted imaging and diffusion tensor imaging for the diagnosis of liver fibrosis and infl ammation . J Magn Reson Imaging 28(1): 89–95.

Immunization with a Recombinant Vaccinia Virus That Encodes Nonstructural Proteins of the Hepatitis C Virus Suppresses Viral Protein Levels in Mouse Liver

Satoshi Sekiguchi[1], Kiminori Kimura[2], Tomoko Chiyo[1], Takahiro Ohtsuki[1], Yoshimi Tobita[1], Yuko Tokunaga[1], Fumihiko Yasui[1], Kyoko Tsukiyama-Kohara[3], Takaji Wakita[4], Toshiyuki Tanaka[5], Masayuki Miyasaka[6], Kyosuke Mizuno[7], Yukiko Hayashi[8], Tsunekazu Hishima[8], Kouji Matsushima[9], Michinori Kohara[1]*

1 Department of Microbiology and Cell Biology, Tokyo Metropolitan Institute of Medical Science, Setagaya-ku, Tokyo, Japan, 2 Division of Hepatology, Tokyo Metropolitan Komagome Hospital, Bunkyo-ku, Tokyo, Japan, 3 Transboundary Animal Diseases Center, Joint Faculty of Veterinary Medicine, Kagoshima University, Korimoto, Kagoshima, Japan, 4 Department of Virology II, National Institute of Infectious Diseases, Shinjuku-ku, Tokyo, Japan, 5 Laboratory of Immunobiology, Department of Pharmacy, School of Pharmacy, Hyogo University of Health Sciences, Chuo-ku, Kobe, Japan, 6 Laboratory of Immunodynamics, Department of Microbiology and Immunology, Osaka University Graduate School of Medicine, Suita, Osaka, Japan, 7 Chemo-Sero-Therapeutic Research Institute, Okubo, Kumamoto, Japan, 8 Department of Pathology, Tokyo Metropolitan Komagome Hospital, Bunkyo-ku, Tokyo, Japan, 9 Department of Molecular Preventive Medicine, School of Medicine, University of Tokyo, Bunkyo-ku, Tokyo, Japan

Abstract

Chronic hepatitis C, which is caused by infection with the hepatitis C virus (HCV), is a global health problem. Using a mouse model of hepatitis C, we examined the therapeutic effects of a recombinant vaccinia virus (rVV) that encodes an HCV protein. We generated immunocompetent mice that each expressed multiple HCV proteins via a Cre/*loxP* switching system and established several distinct attenuated rVV strains. The HCV core protein was expressed consistently in the liver after polyinosinic acid–polycytidylic acid injection, and these mice showed chronic hepatitis C-related pathological findings (hepatocyte abnormalities, accumulation of glycogen, steatosis), liver fibrosis, and hepatocellular carcinoma. Immunization with one rVV strain (rVV-N25), which encoded nonstructural HCV proteins, suppressed serum inflammatory cytokine levels and alleviated the symptoms of pathological chronic hepatitis C within 7 days after injection. Furthermore, HCV protein levels in liver tissue also decreased in a CD4 and CD8 T-cell-dependent manner. Consistent with these results, we showed that rVV-N25 immunization induced a robust CD8 T-cell immune response that was specific to the HCV nonstructural protein 2. We also demonstrated that the onset of chronic hepatitis in CN2-29$^{(+/-)}$/MxCre$^{(+/-)}$ mice was mainly attributable to inflammatory cytokines, (tumor necrosis factor) TNF-α and (interleukin) IL-6. Thus, our generated mice model should be useful for further investigation of the immunological processes associated with persistent expression of HCV proteins because these mice had not developed immune tolerance to the HCV antigen. In addition, we propose that rVV-N25 could be developed as an effective therapeutic vaccine.

Editor: Naglaa H. Shoukry, University of Montreal, Canada

Funding: This study was supported by grants from the Ministry of Education, Culture, Sports, Science, and Technology of Japan; the Program for Promotion of Fundamental Studies in Health Sciences of the Pharmaceuticals and Medical Devices Agency of Japan; and the Ministry of Health, Labor, and Welfare of Japan. The funders had no role in study design, data collection and analysis, decision to publish, or preparation of the manuscript.

Competing Interests: The authors have declared that no competing interests exist.

* E-mail: kohara-mc@igakuken.or.jp

Introduction

Hepatitis C virus (HCV) is a major public health problem; approximately 170 million people are infected with HCV worldwide [1]. HCV causes persistent infections that can lead to chronic liver diseases such as chronic hepatitis, liver cirrhosis, and hepatocellular carcinoma (HCC) [2]. Antiviral drugs are not highly effective in individuals with a chronic infection; furthermore, an effective vaccine against HVC has not been developed. A convenient animal model of HCV infection will greatly facilitate the development of an effective HCV vaccine.

Transgenic mice that express HCV proteins have been generated to study HCV expression [3,4]; however, in each of these cases, the relevant transgenes is expressed during embryonic development; therefore, the transgenic mice become immunotolerant to the transgenic products, and consequently, the adult mice are not useful for investigations of the pathogenesis of chronic hepatitis C. To address this problem, we developed a system that can drive conditional expression of an HCV transgene; our system involves the Cre/*loxP* system and a recombinant adenovirus capable of expressing Cre recombinase [5,6]. Concerns have been expressed that an adenovirus and transient expression of HCV proteins could induce immune responses [5] and, therefore, obscure any evidence of the effect of the host immune responses on chronic liver pathology. Therefore, here, we used a Cre/*loxP* switching system to generate an immunocompetent mouse model of HCV protein expression; with this system, we could study the host immune responses against HCV proteins.

Folgori et al. (2006) reported effective vaccination of chimpanzees with an adenoviral vector and plasmid DNA encoding the HCV nonstructural region. This technique protected the liver tissues from acute hepatitis, which results when whole animals are challenged with virus [7]. However, this vaccine has not yet been shown to be effective against chronic HCV infection.

Here, we aimed to address how HCV expression causes chronic liver diseases and to provide new options for HCV vaccine development. Using LC16m8, a highly attenuated strain of vaccinia virus (VV), we generated three recombinant vaccinia viruses (rVVs) that each encoded one of three different HCV proteins and found that one recombinant virus (rVV-N25), which encoded nonstructural HCV proteins, resolved pathological chronic hepatitis C symptoms in the liver. We also found that immunization with rVV-N25 suppressed HCV core protein levels in the livers of transgenic mice; moreover, this suppression was mediated by CD4 and CD8 T cells, as has been previously reported [8].

Results

Generation of a Model of Persistent HCV Protein Expression

To produce adult mice that express an HCV transgene, we bred CN2-29 transgenic mice, which carry an HCV transgene, [5,6,9] with Mx1-Cre transgenic mice [10], which express Cre recombinase in response to interferon (IFN)-α or a chemical inducer of IFN-α, poly(I:C) (Figure 1A). Following poly(I:C) injection, the HCV transgene was rearranged, and HCV sequences were expressed in the livers of F1 progeny (CN2-29$^{(+/-)}$/MxCre$^{(+/-)}$ mice) within 7 days after poly(I:C) injection (Figure 1B).

To evaluate the characteristic features of these CN2-29$^{(+/-)}$/MxCre$^{(+/-)}$ mice, we analyzed serum alanine aminotransferase (ALT) and liver HCV core protein levels after poly(I:C) injection. As illustrated in Figure 1C, serum ALT levels increased and reached a peak at 24 h after the first poly(I:C) injection; this elevation appeared to be a direct result of the poly(I:C) treatment, which causes liver injury [11]. After this peak, serum ALT levels dropped continuously until day 4, and then ALT levels began to increase, as did HCV core protein levels. Thereafter, the HCV core protein was expressed consistently for at least 600 days.

Histological analysis showed HCV core protein expression in most hepatocytes of the transgenic mice; these mice showed evidence of lymphocytic infiltration that was caused by the HCV core proteins (Figure 1D and E). These observations, in addition to the modified histology activity index (HAI) scores, indicated that expression of HCV proteins caused chronic hepatitis in the CN2-29$^{(+/-)}$/MxCre$^{(+/-)}$ mice because a weak, though persistent, immune response followed an initial bout of acute hepatitis (Figure S1). Moreover, we observed a number of other pathological changes in these mice – including swelling of hepatocytes, abnormal architecture of liver-cell cords, abnormal accumulation of glycogen, steatosis, fibrosis, and HCC (Figures 1E and F, Table S1). Steatosis was mild in the younger mice (day 21) and became increasingly severe over time (days 120 and 180; Figure S2). Importantly, none of the pathological changes were observed in the CN2-29$^{(+/-)}$/MxCre$^{(-/-)}$ mice after poly(I:C) injection (Figure 1F).

Recombinant Vaccinia Virus Immunization in HCV Transgenic Mice

To determine whether activation of the host immune response caused the reduction with HCV protein levels in the livers of CN2-29$^{(+/-)}$/MxCre$^{(+/-)}$ mice, we used a highly attenuated VV strain, LC16m8, to generate three rVVs [12]. Each rVV encoded a different HCV protein; rVV-CN2 encoded mainly structural proteins, rVV-N25 encoded nonstructural proteins, and rVV-CN5 encoded the entire HCV protein region (Figure 2A). Because rVVs can express a variety of proteins and induce strong and long-term immunity, they have been evaluated as potential prophylactic vaccines [13].

We used western blots to confirm that each HCV protein was expressed in cell lines. Each of seven proteins – the core, E1, E2, NS3-4A, NS4B, NS5A, and NS5B – was recognized and labeled by a separate cognate antibody directed (Figure S3). To induce effective immune responses against HCV proteins in transgenic mice, we injected an rVV-HCV (rVV-CN2, rVV-CN5, or rVV-N25) or LC16m8 (as the control) intradermally into CN2-29$^{(+/-)}$/MxCre$^{(+/-)}$ mice 90 days after poly(I:C) injection (Figure 2B). Analysis of liver sections 7 days after immunization with rVV-N25 revealed dramatic improvement in a variety of pathological findings associated with chronic hepatitis – including piecemeal necrosis, hepatocyte swelling, abnormal architecture of liver-cell cords, abnormal accumulation of glycogen, and steatosis (Figures 2C–E). Collectively, these results demonstrated that only the rVV-N25 treatment resulted in histological changes indicative of improvement in the chronic hepatitis suffered by the transgenic mice.

To determine whether rVV-N25 treatment induced the same effect in other strains of HCV transgenic mice, we analyzed RzCN5-15$^{(+/-)}$/MxCre$^{(+/-)}$ mice, which express all HCV proteins; in these mice, chronic hepatitis was resolved within 28 days of immunization with rVV-N25. Taken together, these findings indicated that rVV-N25 had a dramatic therapeutic effect on both types of HCV transgenic mice (Figure S4).

Treatment with rVV-N25 Reduced the HCV Core Protein Levels in the Livers

To assess in detail the effects of rVV-HCV immunization on HCV protein clearance from the livers of CN2-29$^{(+/-)}$/MxCre$^{(+/-)}$ mice, we monitored the levels of HCV core protein in liver samples via ELISA. We found that within 28 days after immunization the HCV core protein levels were significantly lower in livers of rVV-N25-treated mice than in those of control mice (Figure 3A). Immunohistochemical analysis indicated that, within 28 days after immunization, levels of HCV core protein were substantially lower in the livers of CN2-29$^{(+/-)}$/MxCre$^{(+/-)}$ mice than in those of control mice (Figure 3B). Importantly, neither resolution of chronic hepatitis nor reduction in the HCV protein levels was observed in the mice treated with LC16m8, rVV-CN2, or rVV-CN5. These results indicated that HCV nonstructural proteins might be important for effects of therapeutic vaccines. In contrast, rVV-CN5 which encoded HCV structural and non-structural proteins did not show any significant effects. These results indicated that HCV structural proteins might have inhibited the therapeutic effects of the non-structural proteins. Therefore, it may be important to exclude the HCV structural proteins (aa 1–541) as antigenic proteins when developing therapeutic vaccines against chronic hepatitis C.

In addition, we measured serum ALT levels in CN2-29$^{(+/-)}$/MxCre$^{(+/-)}$ mice from all four treatment groups 28 days after rVV-HCV immunization. Serum ALT levels were not significant-

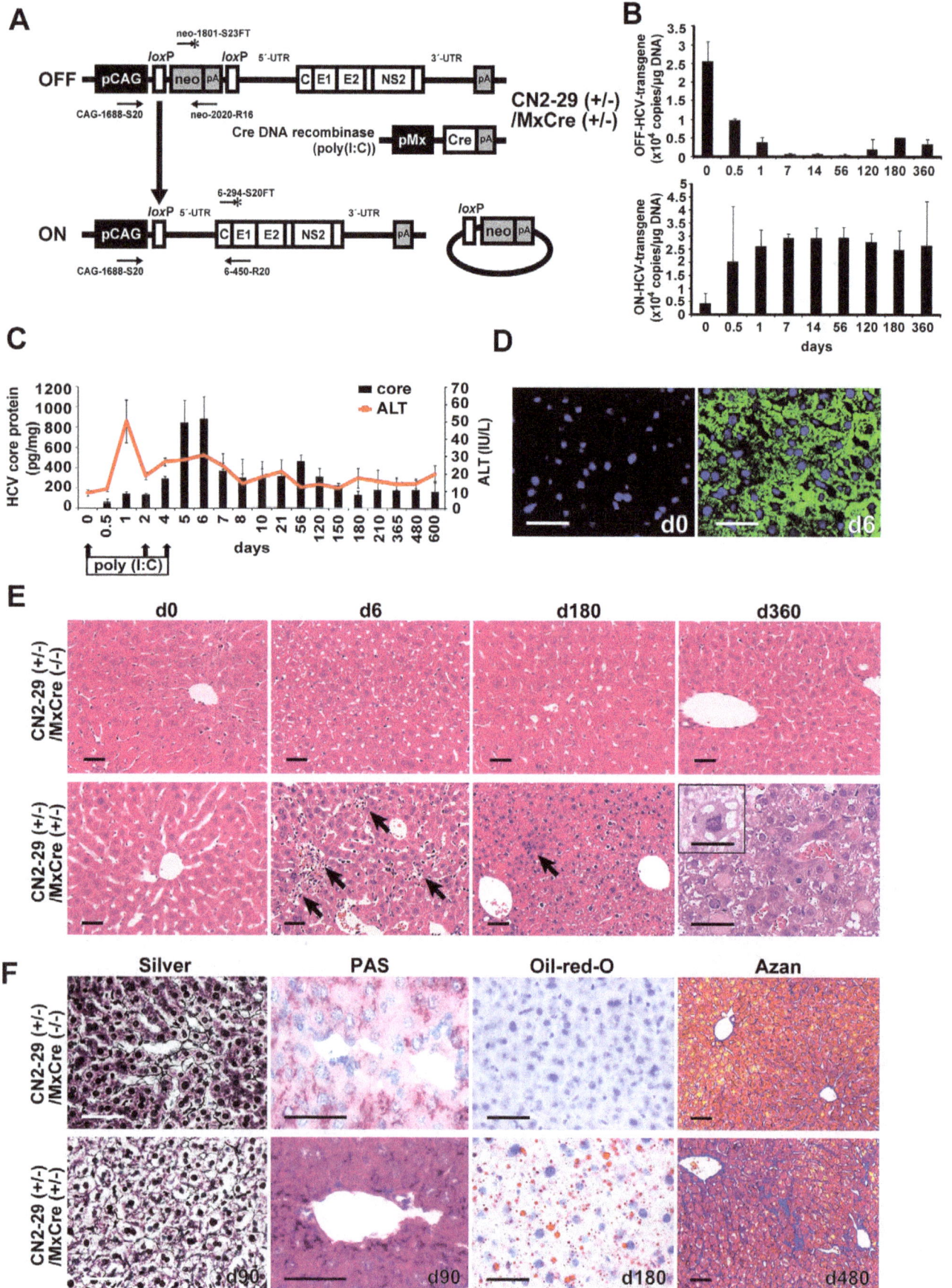

Figure 1. Pathogenesis in immunocompetent mice with persistent HCV expression. (**A**) Structure of CN2-29$^{(+/-)}$/MxCre$^{(+/-)}$ and the Cre-mediated activation of the transgene unit. R6CN2 HCV cDNA was cloned downstream of the CAG promoter, neomycin-resistant gene (*neo*), and poly A (pA) signal flanked by two *loxP* sequences. This cDNA contains the core, E1, E2, and NS2 regions. (**B**) Cre-mediated genomic DNA recombination. After poly(I:C) injection, genomic DNA was extracted from liver tissues and analyzed by quantitative RTD-PCR for Cre-mediated transgenic recombination. The transgene was almost fully recombined in transgenic mouse livers 7 days after the injection. In all cases, n = 3 mice per group. (**C**) HCV core protein expression was sustained for at least 600 days after poly(I:C) injection. (**D**) Immunohistochemical analysis revealed that most hepatocytes expressed the HCV core protein within 6 days after injection. (**E**) Liver sections from CN2-29$^{(+/-)}$/MxCre$^{(+/-)}$ mice after the poly(I:C) injection. Infiltrating lymphocytes (arrows) were observed on days 6 and 180; Hepatocellular carcinoma (HCC) was observed on day 360. In contrast, these pathological changes were not observed in CN2-29$^{(+/-)}$/MxCre$^{(-/-)}$ mice after the injection. The inset image shows abnormal mitosis in a tumor cell. (**F**) Hepatocyte swelling and abnormal architecture of liver-cell cords (silver staining), as well as abnormal glycogen accumulation (PAS staining) were observed on day 90 in CN2-29$^{(+/-)}$/MxCre$^{(+/-)}$ mice. We observed steatosis (oil-red-O staining) on day 180 and, subsequently, fibrosis (Azan staining) on day 480. The scale bars indicate 50 μm.

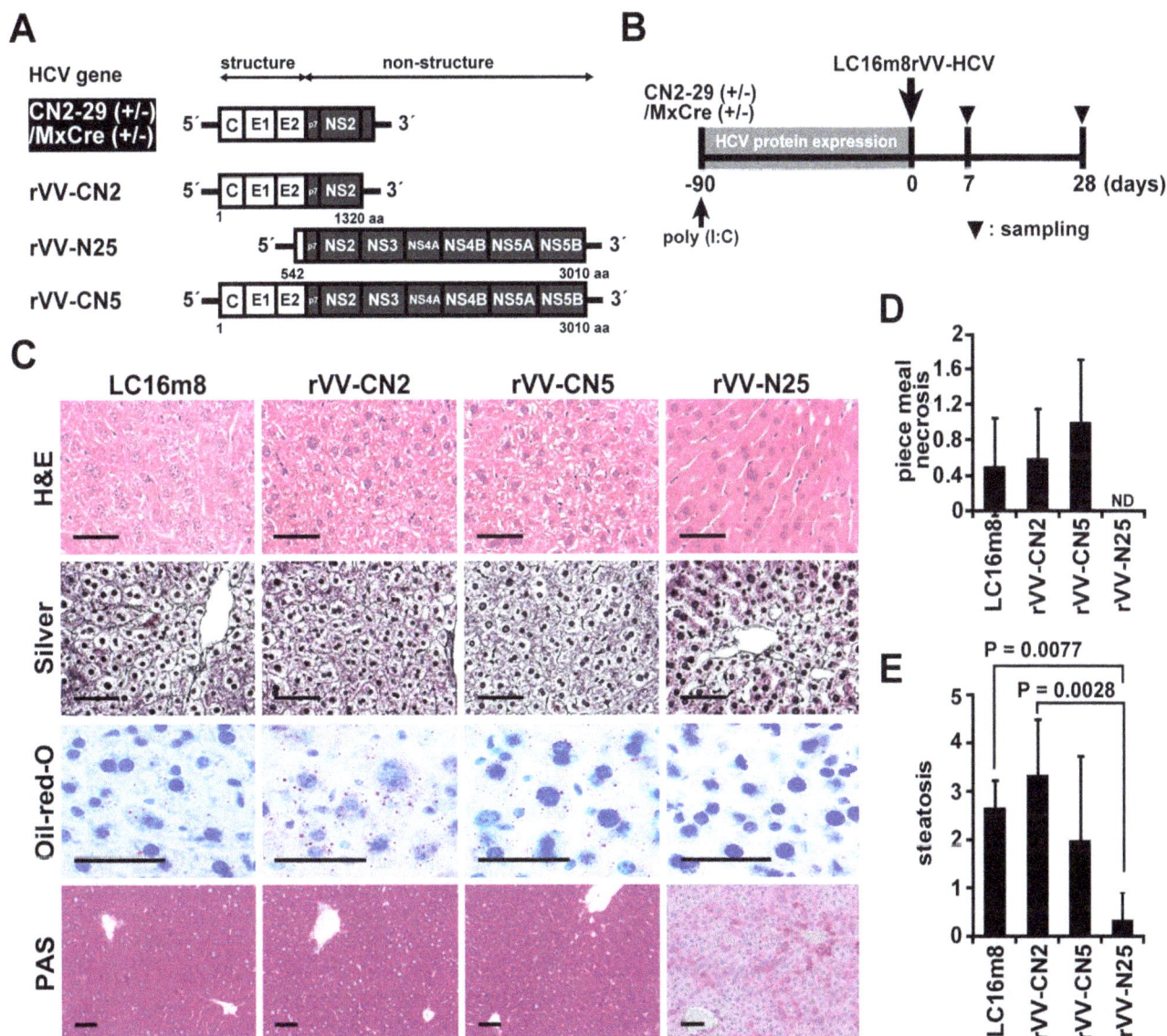

Figure 2. Effects of rVV-HCV treatment on the CN2-29$^{(+/-)}$/MxCre$^{(+/-)}$ mice. (**A**) HCV gene structure in the CN2-29$^{(+/-)}$/MxCre$^{(+/-)}$ mice and recombinant vaccinia viruses (rVV-HCV). MxCre/CN2-29 cDNA contains the core, E1, E2, and NS2 regions. The rVV-CN2 cDNA contains the core, E1, E2, and NS2 regions. The rVV-N25 cDNA contains the NS2, NS3, NS4A, NS4B, NS5A, and NS5B regions. The rVV-CN5 cDNA contains the entire HCV region. (**B**) Four groups of CN2-29$^{(+/-)}$/MxCre$^{(+/-)}$ mice were inoculated intradermally with rVV-CN2, rVV-N25, rVV-CN5, or LC16m8 90 days after the poly(I:C) injection. Blood, liver, and spleen tissue samples were collected 7 and 28 days after the inoculation. (**C**) Liver sections from the four groups of CN2-29$^{(+/-)}$/MxCre$^{(+/-)}$ mice 7 days after the inoculation. The sections were stained with H&E, silver, oil-red-O, or PAS. The scale bars indicate 50 μm. (**D**) Histological evaluation of piecemeal necrosis in the four groups of CN2-29$^{(+/-)}$/MxCre$^{(+/-)}$ mice 7 days after inoculation. (**E**) Histological evaluation of steatosis in the four groups of CN2-29$^{(+/-)}$/MxCre$^{(+/-)}$ mice 7 days after inoculation. Significant relationships are indicated by a P-value.

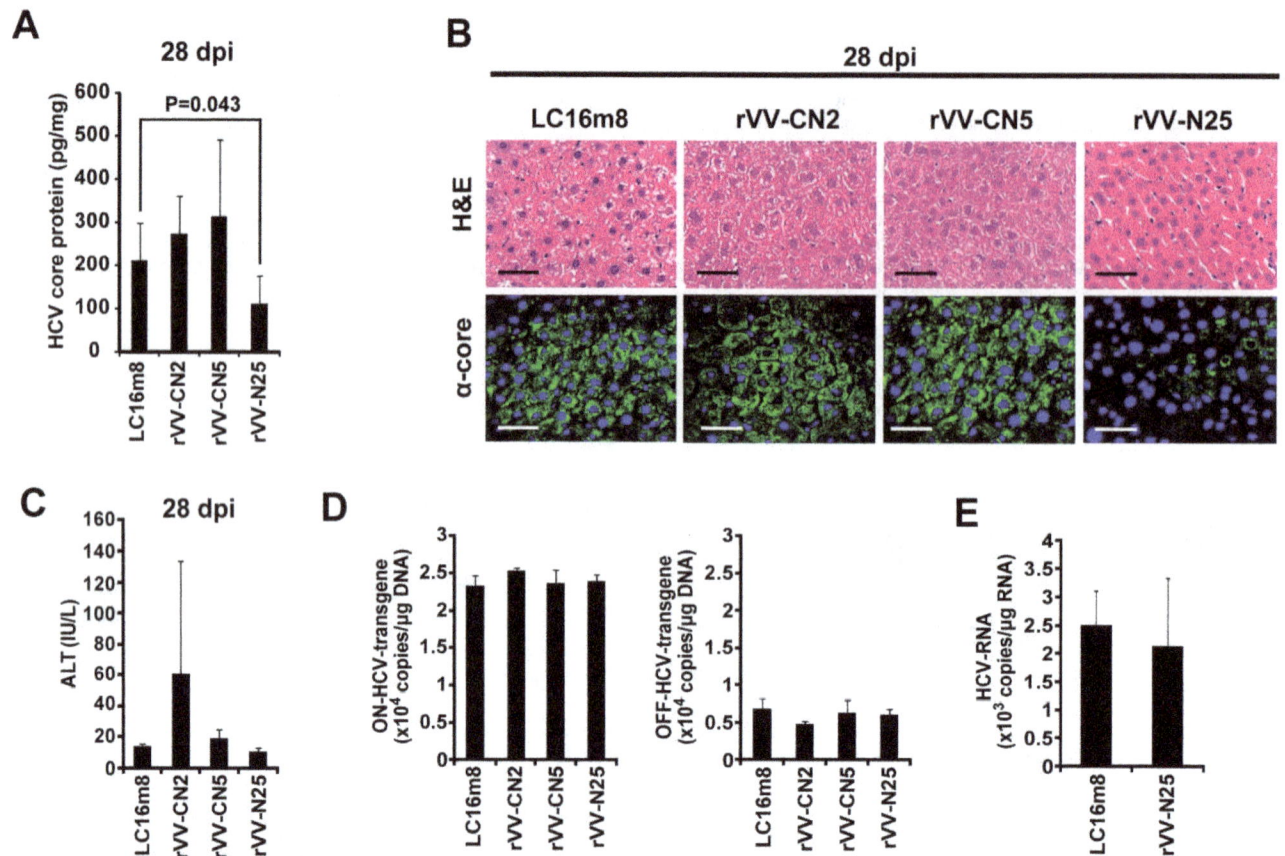

Figure 3. Effects of HCV core protein expression on the livers of CN2-29$^{(+/-)}$/MxCre$^{(+/-)}$ mice inoculated with rVV-HCV. (A) Expression of the HCV core protein in the four treatment groups of CN2-29$^{(+/-)}$/MxCre$^{(+/-)}$ mice 28 days after the inoculation. Significant relationships are indicated by a P-value. (B) H&E staining and immunohistochemical analysis for HCV core protein in the LC16m8-, rVV-CN2-, rVV-CN5-, or rVV-N25-treated CN2-29$^{(+/-)}$/MxCre$^{(+/-)}$ mice 28 days after the inoculation. Liver sections were stained with the anti-core monoclonal antibody. The scale bars indicate 50 μm. (C) Effects of HCV core protein expression on serum ALT levels in the four treatment groups of CN2-29$^{(+/-)}$/MxCre$^{(+/-)}$ mice 28 days after immunization. (D) Cre-mediated genomic DNA recombination in the four treatment groups 28 days after immunization. (E) Expression of HCV mRNA in the LC16m8- or rVV-N25-treated CN2-29$^{(+/-)}$/MxCre$^{(+/-)}$ mice 28 days after immunization. In all cases, n = 6 mice per group.

ly different in the rVV-N25-treated mice and control mice (Figure 3C); this finding indicated that rVV-N25 treatment did not cause liver injury and that the antiviral effect was independent of hepatocyte destruction.

We hypothesized that the reduction in the levels of HCV core protein in rVV-HCV-treated mice was not caused by cytolytic elimination of hepatocytes that expressed HCV proteins. To investigate this hypothesis, we conducted an RTD-PCR analysis of genomic DNA from liver samples of CN2-29$^{(+/-)}$/MxCre$^{(+/-)}$ mice. The recombined transgene was similar in rVV-N25-treated and control mice 28 days after immunization (Figure 3D). We also measured the expression of HCV mRNA in LC16m8-treated CN2-29$^{(+/-)}$/MxCre$^{(+/-)}$ mice with that in rVV-N25-treated CN2-29$^{(+/-)}$/MxCre$^{(+/-)}$ mice 28 days after immunization; the HCV mRNA levels did not differ between rVV-N25-treated CN2-29$^{(+/-)}$/MxCre$^{(+/-)}$ and control mice (Figure 3E). These results indicated that rVV-N25-induced suppression of HCV core protein expression could be controlled at a posttranscriptional level.

Role of CD4 and CD8 T cells in rVV-N25-treated Mice

Viral clearance is usually associated with CD4 and CD8 T-cell activity that is regulated by cytolytic or noncytolytic antiviral mechanism [14]. To determine whether CD4 or CD8 T-cell activity was required for the reduction in HCV core protein levels

in the livers of transgenic mice, we analyzed the core protein levels in CN2-29$^{(+/-)}$/MxCre$^{(+/-)}$ mice immunized with rVV-N25 in the absence of CD4 or CD8 T cells (Figure 4A). As expected, the mice lacking CD4 or CD8 T cells failed to show a reduction in HCV core protein levels (Figure 4B).

However, in mice lacking either CD4 or CD8 T-cells, the pathological changes associated with chronic hepatitis were resolved following rVV-N25 immunization, and the steatosis score of rVV-N25-treated mice was significantly lower than that of control mice (Figures 4C–E). These results indicated that CD4 and CD8 T cells were not responsible for the rVV-N25-induced amelioration of histological findings and that other inflammatory cell types may play an as-yet-unidentified role in the resolution of the pathological changes in these mice.

rVV-N25 Immunization Induced an NS2-specific Activated CD8 T cells Response

Because we found that HCV protein reduction in the liver required CD8 T cells, we tested whether HCV-specific CD8 T cells were present in splenocytes 28 days after immunization. To determine the functional reactivity of HCV-specific CD8$^+$ T cells, we performed a CD107a mobilization assay and intracellular IFN-γ staining. CN2-29 transgenic mice expressed the HCV structural protein and the NS2 region. However, rVV-N25 comprised only

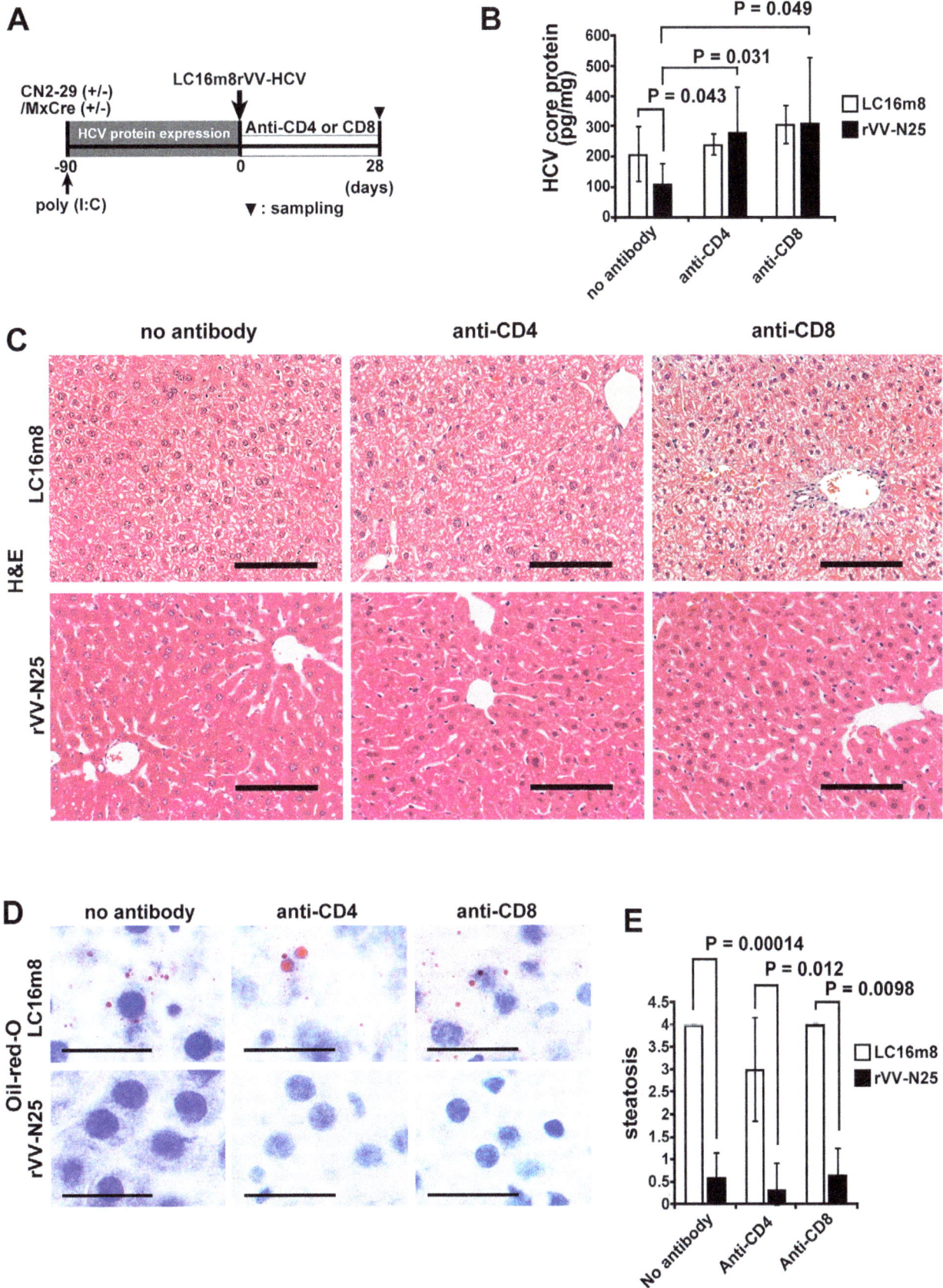

Figure 4. Role of CD4 and CD8 T cells in rVV-N25-treated mice. (**A**) Schematic diagram depicts depletion of CD4 and CD8 T cells via treatment with monoclonal antibodies. (**B**) Comparison of HCV core protein expression in control, CD4-depleted, and CD8-depleted mice 28 days after immunization with LC16m8 or rVV-N25. (**C, D**) Histological analysis of liver samples from CD4-depleted or CD8-depleted CN2-29$^{(+/-)}$/MxCre$^{(+/-)}$ mice

28 days after immunization with LC16m8 or rVV-N25. The scale bars indicate 100 μm (**C**) and 50 μm (**D**). (**E**) Histological evaluation of steatosis in liver samples from CD4-depleted or CD8-depleted CN2-29$^{(+/-)}$/MxCre$^{(+/-)}$ mice 28 days after immunization with LC16m8 or rVV-N25. Significant relationships are indicated by a P-value.

a HCV nonstructural protein. Thus, we focused on the role of the NS2 region as the target for CD8 T cells and generated EL-4 cell lines that expressed the NS2 antigen or the CN2 antigen.

Isolated splenocytes from immunized mice were co-cultured with EL-4CN2 or EL-4NS2 cell lines for 2 weeks and analyzed.

Cytolytic cell activation can be measured using CD107a, a marker of degranulation [15]. The ratio of CD8$^+$CD107a$^+$ cells to all CD8 T cells significantly increased in rVV-N25-treated splenocytes after co-culture with EL-4CN2 or EL-4NS2 ($P<0.05$), whereas splenocytes that had been treated with any other rVV were not detected (Figure 5A, B and C). These results indicated that rVV-N25 treatment increased the frequency of HCV NS2-specific activated CD8 T cells. Consistent with these results, the ratio of CD8$^+$IFN-γ^+ cells to all CD8 T cells for rVV-N25-treated mice was also significantly higher than that for mice treated with any other rVV ($P<0.05$). Taken together, these findings indicated that rVV-N25 induced an effective CD8 T-cell immune response and that NS2 is an important epitope for CD8 T cells.

rVV-N25 Immunization Suppressed Inflammatory Cytokines Production

To determine whether rVV-N25 treatment affected inflammatory cytokine production, we measured serum levels of inflammatory cytokines after rVV immunization. The serum levels of these inflammatory cytokines increased in the CN2-29$^{(+/-)}$/MxCre$^{(+/-)}$ mice (Figure 6A, Figure S5). Immunization with rVV-N25 affected serum levels of inflammatory cytokines in CN2-29$^{(+/-)}$/MxCre$^{(+/-)}$ mice and caused a return to the cytokine levels observed in wild-type untreated mice (Figure 6A). In wild-type mice, the cytokine levels remained unchanged after immunization (Figure 6A). These results indicated that inflammatory cytokines were responsible for liver pathogenesis in the transgenic mice.

To test the hypothesis that inflammatory cytokines were responsible for liver pathogenesis in CN2-29$^{(+/-)}$/MxCre$^{(+/-)}$ mice, we administered transgenic mouse serum intravenously into nontransgenic mice. We observed the development of chronic hepatitis in the nontransgenic mice within 7 days after the serum transfer (Figures 6B and C). This finding was consistent with the

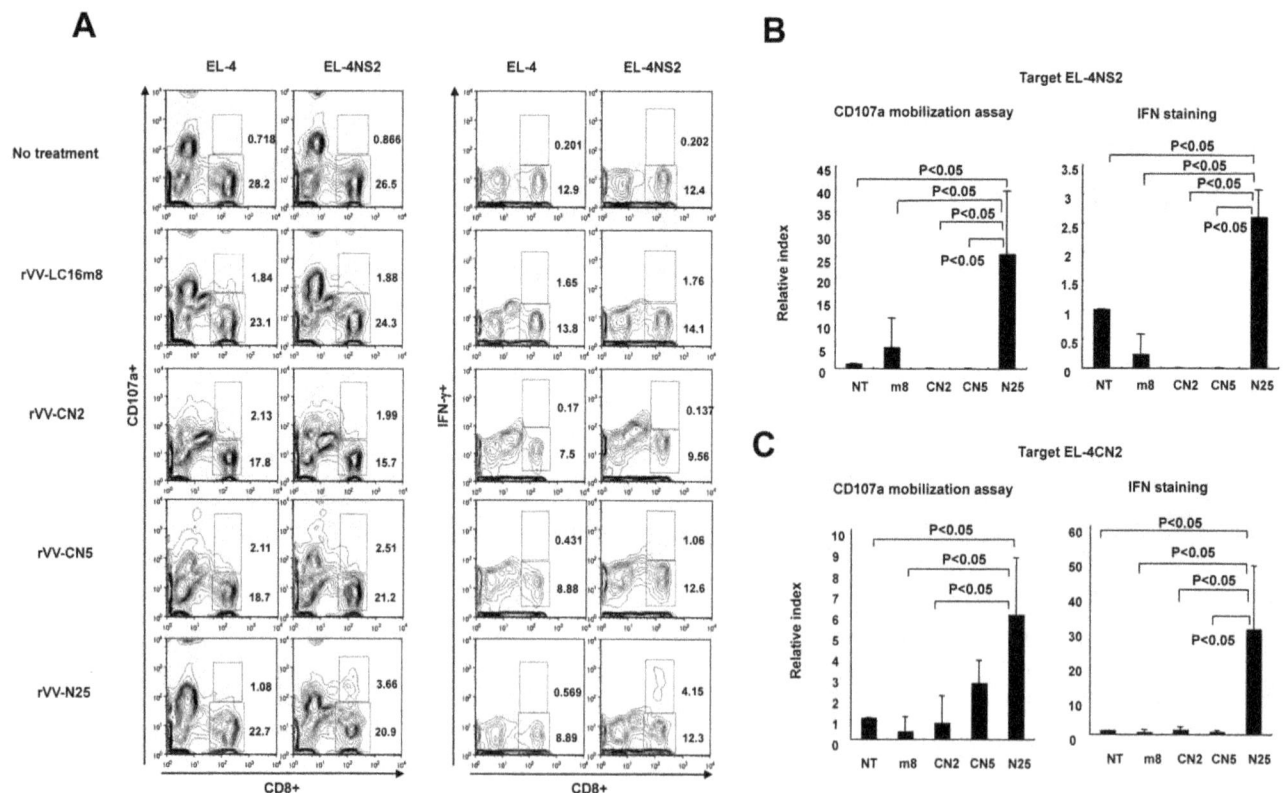

Figure 5. Immunization with rVV-N25 induced CD8 T-cell degranulation, a marker for cytotoxicity, and IFN-γ production. (A) The numbers represent the percentage of CD107a positive cells and negative cells (left two columns) and IFN-γ-positive cells and negative cells (right two columns). **(B, C)** The ratio of CD8$^+$IFN-γ^+ cells to all CD8 T cells for rVV-N25-treated mice was significantly higher than that for mice treated with any other rVV. Splenocytes (4 × 10^6 per well) were cultured with EL-4CN2 or EL-4NS2 cell lines in RPMI 1640 complete medium including 3% T-STIM^{TM} with ConA for 2 weeks. Harvested cells were incubated for 4 h with EL-4, EL-4CN2, or EL-4NS2 in combination with PE-labeled anti-CD107a mAb and monensin in RPMI 1640 complete medium with 50 IU/mL IL-2, according to the manufacturer's instruction. After incubation, cell suspensions were washed with PBS, and the cells were further stained with APC-labeled anti-IFN-γ mAb and Pacific blue-labeled anti-CD8 mAb. Harvested cells were stained with anti-CD107a-PE, anti-IFN-γ-APC, or anti-CD8-Pacific blue. Results that are representative of three independent experiments are shown. Significant relationships are indicated by P-value.

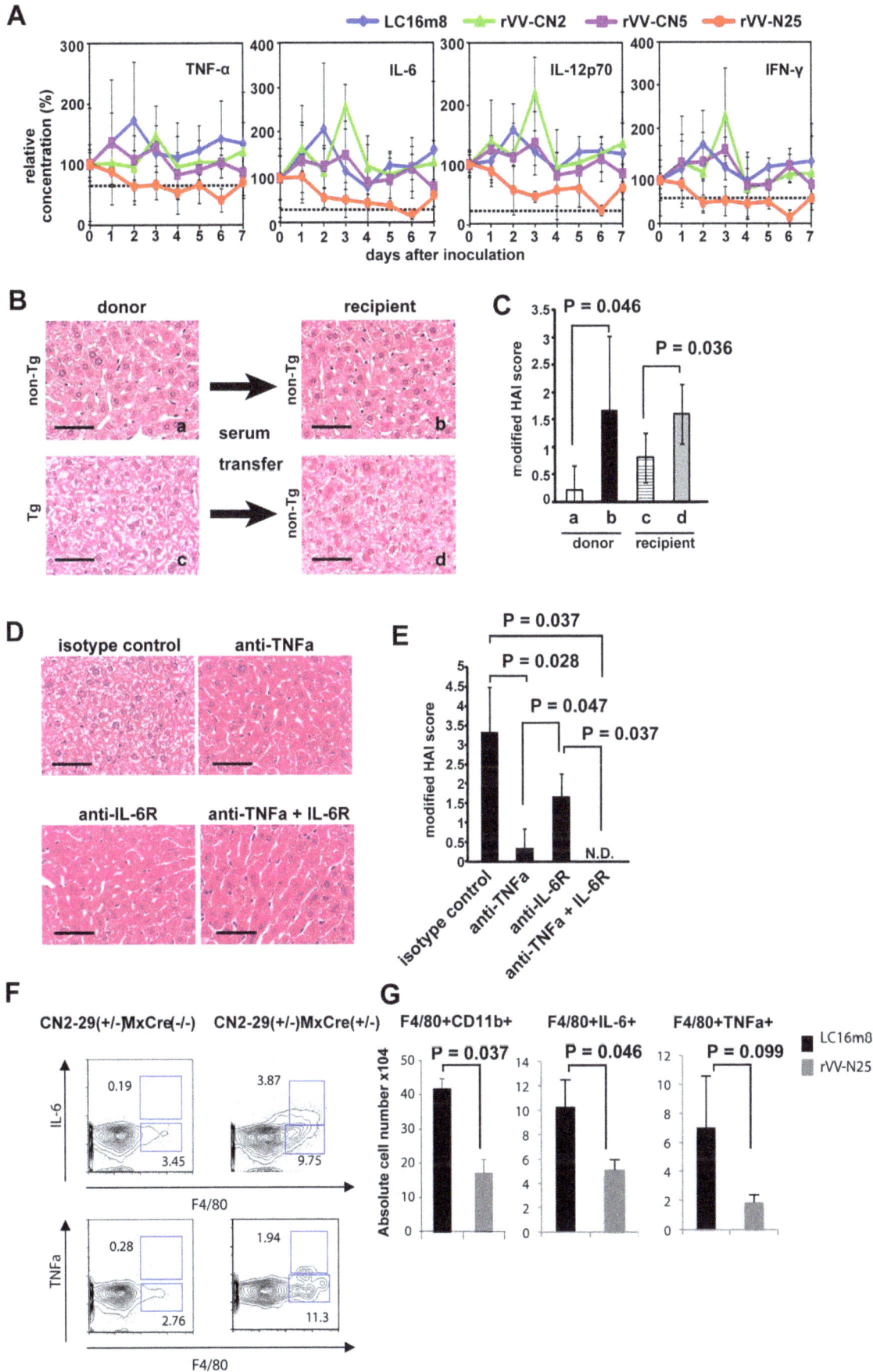

Figure 6. Immunization with rVV-N25 suppresses serum inflammatory cytokine levels. (**A**) Daily cytokine levels in the serum of CN2-29$^{(+/-)}$/MxCre$^{(+/-)}$ mice during the week following immunization with LC16m8, rVV-CN2, rVV-N25, or rVV-CN5. Values represent means ± SD (n = 3) and reflect the concentrations relative to those measured on day 0. The broken lines indicate the baseline data from wild-type mice. In all cases, n = 6 mice per group. (**B**) Liver sections from CN2-29$^{(+/-)}$/MxCre$^{(+/-)}$ and CN2-29$^{(+/-)}$/MxCre$^{(-/-)}$ mice. (**C**) Histology activity index (HAI) scores of liver samples taken from CN2-29$^{(+/-)}$/MxCre$^{(+/-)}$, or CN2-29$^{(+/-)}$/MxCre$^{(-/-)}$ mice. (**D**) Liver sections from CN2-29$^{(+/-)}$/MxCre$^{(+/-)}$ mice in which TNF-α was neutralized and the IL-6 receptor was blocked. The scale bars indicate 50 μm. (**E**) HAI scores of liver samples taken from CN2-29$^{(+/-)}$/MxCre$^{(+/-)}$ in which TNF-α was neutralized and the IL-6 receptor was blocked. Tg and non-Tg indicate CN2-29$^{(+/-)}$/MxCre$^{(+/-)}$ and CN2-29$^{(+/-)}$/MxCre$^{(-/-)}$, respectively. (**F**) Macrophages were the main producers of TNF-α and IL-6 in CN2-29$^{(+/-)}$/MxCre$^{(+/-)}$ mice following poly(I:C) injection. (**G**) Immunization with rVV-N25 reduced the number of macrophages in liver samples from CN2-29$^{(+/-)}$/MxCre$^{(+/-)}$ mice and suppressed TNF-α and IL-6 production from macrophages (Figure 6G). Significant relationships are indicated by a P-value.

hypothesis that inflammatory mediators played a key role in inducing hepatitis. Furthermore, to investigate whether TNF-α and IL-6 played particularly critical roles in the pathogenesis of chronic hepatitis in the transgenic mice, we neutralized TNF-α and blocked the IL-6 receptor in the livers of these mice. As expected, chronic hepatitis did not develop in these mice. (Figure 6D and E).

Next, to determine which cell population(s) produced TNF-α, IL-6, or both during continuous HCV expression in CN2-29$^{(+/-)}$/MxCre$^{(+/-)}$ mice, we isolated intrahepatic lymphocytes (IHLs) and labeled the macrophages (the F4/80$^+$ cells) with anti-TNF-α and anti-IL-6 antibodies using an intracellular cytokine detection method. Macrophages in CN2-29$^{(+/-)}$/MxCre$^{(-/-)}$ mice produced small amounts of TNF-α and IL-6, while those in CN2-29$^{(+/-)}$/MxCre$^{(+/-)}$ mice produced much larger amounts of these cytokines (Figure 6F).

Finally, we evaluated whether rVV-N25 treatment affected the number of macrophages, cytokine production by macrophages, or both; specifically, we isolated IHLs from CN2-29$^{(+/-)}$/MxCre$^{(+/-)}$ mice 7 days after immunization with rVV-N25 or with LC16m8. The percentage of macrophages (CD11b$^+$F4/80$^+$) among IHLs and IL-6 production from these macrophages were significantly lower in rVV-N25-treated mice than in control mice (Figure 6G). Though the percentage of TNF-α-producing macrophages was not significantly different in rVV-N25-treated and control mice (P = 0.099), rVV-N25 treatment appeared to suppress these macrophages. These results demonstrated that rVV-N25 had a suppressive effect on activated macrophages, and they indicated that this suppression ameliorated the histological indicators of chronic hepatitis.

Discussion

Various HCV transgenic mouse models have been developed and used to examine immune response to HCV expression and the effects of pathogenic HCV protein on hepatocytes [4,16,17]. However, these transgenic mice develop tolerance to the HCV protein; therefore, examining immune response to HCV protein has been difficult.

To overcome the problem of immune tolerance in mouse models of HCV expression, we developed an HCV model in mice that relies on conditional expression of the core, E1, E2, and NS2 proteins and the Cre/loxP switching system [5,6]; we showed that the injection of an Ad-Cre vector enhanced the frequency of HCV-specific activated CD8 T cells in the liver of these mice and caused liver injury. However, the Ad-Cre adenovirus vector alone causes acute hepatitis in wild-type mice. Nevertheless, the transgenic model was useful for evaluating interactions between the host immune system and viral protein (serum ALT level over 2,000 IU/L) [5]; HCV core protein levels were reduced and expression of this protein was transient (about 2 weeks). Therefore, this Ad-Cre-dependent model cannot be used to effectively investigate immune responses to chronic HCV hepatitis.

Here, we used poly (I:C)-induced expression of Cre recombinase to generate HCV transgenic mice in order to study the effect of HCV protein and confirmed that these mice developed chronic active hepatitis–including steatosis, lipid deposition, and hepatocellular carcinoma. These pathological findings in the transgenic mice were very similar to those in humans with chronic hepatitis C; therefore, this mouse model of HCV may be useful for analyzing the immune response to chronic hepatitis. However, experimental results obtained with this mouse model may not directly translate to clinical findings from patients with HCV infection because the expression of HCV proteins was not liver specific in these mice. Furthermore, poly(I:C) injection can activate innate immune responses and, consequently, might induce temporary liver injury [18]. Additionally, poly(I:C) injection has an adjuvant effect; specifically, it stimulates TLR3 signaling [19].

To evaluate whether poly(I:C) injection caused hepatitis in CN2-29$^{(+/-)}$/MxCre$^{(-/-)}$ mice, we examined serum ALT levels and liver histology following poly(I:C) injection. We found that, following poly(I:C) injection, serum ALT levels in CN2-29$^{(+/-)}$/MxCre$^{(-/-)}$ mice increased, reached a peak one day after injection, declined from day 1 to day 6, and were not elevated thereafter; this time-course indicated that poly(I:C) injection alone did not induced continuous liver injury (figure S6). Based on these findings, we believe that the effects of poly(I:C) injection in these mice did not confound our analysis of chronic hepatitis.

Immunization with rVV-N25 suppressed HCV protein levels in the liver, and this suppression was associated with ameliorated pathological chronic hepatitis findings (see Figure 3). Importantly, rVV-N25 treatment did not cause liver injury based on the serum ALT levels; therefore, this treatment was unlikely to have cytopathic effects on infected hepatocytes. These findings provided strong evidence that rVV-N25 treatment effectively halted the progression of chronic hepatitis. Immunization with plasmid DNA or with recombinant vaccinia virus can effectively induce cellular and humoral immune responses and exert a protective effect against challenge with HCV infection [20,21]. However, findings from these previous studies revealed HCV immunization of both uninfected, naïve animals and immune-tolerant animals induced a HCV-specific immune response. In the model describe here; the animals were immune competent for HCV; therefore, our findings provided further important evidence that rVV-N25 was effective in the treatment of chronic hepatitis.

In addition, we demonstrated that rVV-N25 treatment in the absence of CD4 and CD8 T cells had no effect on HCV clearance. This important observation indicated that rVV-N25-induced HCV clearance was mediated by CD4 and CD8 T cells. Many studies have shown that spontaneous viral clearance during acute HCV infection is characterized by a vigorous, broadly reactive CD4 and CD8 T-cell response. [8,22] HCV clearance and hepatocellular cytotoxicity are both mediated by CD8 antigen-specific (cytotoxic T lymphocyte) CTLs [23]. Consistent with these observations, rVV-N25 treatment effectively induced the accumulation of NS2-specific CD8 T cells, which express high levels of

CD107a and IFN-γin the spleen. Notably, even with rVV-N25 immunization, the frequency of activated CD8 T cells was very low, and a minimum of 2-weeks incubation was required to distinguish the difference between rVV treatments. Even if a small population of specific CD8+ T cells played a relevant role in the reduction of core protein, it is difficult to assert that the only NS2-specific CD8+ T cells were important to this reduction. However, based on the results presented in Figure 4B, we are able to conclude that at least CD8+ and/or CD4+ T cells were important to the reduction in HCV core protein. Therefore, to elucidate the mechanism of HCV protein clearance, further investigation of not only the other T cell epitopes but also other immunocompetent cells is required.

Interestingly, rVV-N25 treatment–but not the rVV-CN2 or rVV-CN5 treatment–efficiently induced a HCV-specific activated CD8 T cells response; this difference in efficacy could have one or more possible causes. The HCV structural proteins (core, E1, and E2 proteins) in the rVV-CN construct may cause the difference; Saito et al. reported that injection with plasmid constructs encoding the core protein induced a specific CTL response in BALB/c mice [24]. Reportedly, CTL activity against core or envelope protein is completely absent from transgenic mice immunized with a plasmid encoding the HCV structural proteins, but core-specific CTL activity is present in transgenic mice that were immunized with a plasmid encoding the HCV core [21]. In contrast, when recombinant vaccinia virus expressing different regions of the HCV polyprotein were injected into BALB/c mice, only the HCV core protein markedly suppressed vaccinia-specific CTL responses [25]. Thus, the HCV core protein may have an immunomodulatory function [26]. Based on these reports and our results, we hypothesize that the causes underlying the effectiveness of rVV-N25 treatment were as follows: 1) this rVV construct included the core and envelope proteins and 2) the core protein had an immune-suppressive effect on CTL induction. Therefore, we suggest that exclusion of the core and envelope antigen as immunogen is one important factor in HCV vaccine design.

Interestingly, immunization with rVV-N25 rapidly suppressed the inflammatory response; however, immunization with either of the other rVVs did not (see Figure 6A). This result indicated that rVV-N25 may modulate inflammation via innate immunity, as well as via acquired immunity. Reportedly, Toll-like receptor (TLR)-dependent recognition pathways play a role in the recognition of poxviruses [27]. TLR2 and TLR9 have also been implicated in the recognition of the vaccinia virus [28,29]. These findings indicate that TLR on dendritic cells may modulate the immunosuppressive effect of rVV-N25 in our model of HCV infection; however, further examination of this hypothesis is required. The finding that pathological symptoms in the HCV transgenic mice were completely blocked by intravenous injection of TNF-α and IL-6 neutralizing antibodies indicated that the progression of chronic hepatitis depended on inflammatory cytokines in serum, rather than the HCV protein levels in hepatocytes. Lymphocytes, macrophages, hepatocytes, and adipocytes each produce TNF-α and IL-6 [30,31], and HCV-infected patients have elevated levels of TNF-α and IL-6 [32,33]. Both cytokines also contribute to the maintenance of hepatosteatosis in mice fed a high-fat diet [34], and production of TNF-α and IL-6 is elevated in obese mice due to the low grade inflammatory response that is caused by lipid accumulation [35]. These findings indicate that both cytokines are responsible for HCV-triggered hepatosteatosis, and anti-cytokine neutralization is a potential treatment for chronic hepatitis if antiviral therapy is not successful.

The reduction of macrophages in number might be due to the induction of apoptosis by vaccinia virus *in vitro* infection as

previous reported [36]. To understand the mechanisms responsible for the reduction of the number of macrophage, we performed another experiment to confirm whether the macrophages were infected with vaccinia virus inoculation. However, based on PCR analyses; vaccinia virus DNA was not present in liver tissue that contained macrophages (Figure S7). Furthermore, apoptosis of macrophages was not detected in liver samples (Data not shown). Based on these results, it is unlikely that the reduction in the number of macrophages was due to apoptosis induced by vaccinia virus infection. Although rVV-N25 reduced the number of macrophage, precise mechanism is still unknown. Further examination to elucidate the mechanism is required.

In conclusion, our findings demonstrated that rVV-N25 is a promising candidate for an HCV vaccine therapy. Additionally, the findings of this study indicate that rVV-N25 immunization can be used for prevention of HCV infection and as an antiviral therapy against ongoing HCV infection.

Materials and Methods

Ethics Statement

All animal care and experimental procedures were performed according to the guidelines established by the Tokyo Metropolitan Institute of Medical Science Subcommittee on Laboratory Animal Care; these guidelines conform to the Fundamental Guidelines for Proper Conduct of Animal Experiment and Related Activities in Academic Research Institutions under the jurisdiction of the Ministry of Education, Culture, Sports, Science and Technology, Japan, 2006. All protocols were approved by the Committee on the Ethics of Animal Experiments of the Tokyo Metropolitan Institute of Medical Science (Permit Number: 11–078). All efforts were made to minimize the suffering of the animals.

Animals

R6CN2 HCV cDNA (nt 294–3435) [37] and full genomic HCV cDNA (nt 1–9611) [38,39] were cloned from a blood sample taken from a patient (#R6) with chronic active hepatitis (Text S1). The infectious titer of this blood sample has been previously reported [40]. R6CN2HCV and R6CN5HCV transgenic mice were bred with Mx1-Cre transgenic mice (purchased from Jackson Laboratory) to produce R6CN2HCV-MxCre and R6CN5HCV-MxCre transgenic mice, which were designated CN2-29$^{(+/-)}$/MxCre$^{(+/-)}$ and RzCN5-15$^{(+/-)}$/MxCre$^{(+/-)}$ mice, respectively. Cre expression in the livers of these mice was induced by intraperitoneal injection of polyinosinic acid–polycytidylic acid [poly(I:C)] (GE Healthcare UK Ltd., Buckinghamshire, England); 300 μL of a poly(I:C) solution (1 mg/mL in phosphate-buffered saline [PBS]) was injected three times at 48-h intervals. All animal care and experimental procedures were performed according to the guidelines established by the Tokyo Metropolitan Institute of Medical Science Subcommittee on Laboratory Animal Care.

Histology and Immunohistochemical Staining

Tissue samples were fixed in 4% paraformaldehyde in PBS, embedded in paraffin, sectioned (4-μm thickness), and stained with hematoxylin and eosin (H&E). Staining with periodic acid–Schiff stain, Azan stain, silver, or Oil-red-O was also performed to visualize glycogen degeneration, fibrillization, reticular fiber degeneration, or lipid degeneration, respectively.

For immunohistochemical staining, unfixed frozen liver sections were fixed in 4% paraformaldehyde for 10 min and then incubated with blocking buffer (1% bovine serum albumin in PBS) for 30 min at room temperature. Subsequently, the sections were incubated with biotinylated mouse anti-HCV core monoclonal antibody (5E3) for 2 h at room temperature. After being washed with PBS, the sections were incubated with streptavidin–Alexa Fluor 488 (Invitrogen). The nuclei were stained with 4',6-diamidino-2-phenylindole (DAPI). Fluorescence was observed using a confocal laser microscope (Laser scanning microscope 510, Carl Zeiss).

Generation of rVVs

The pBR322-based plasmid vector pBMSF7C contained the ATI/p7.5 hybrid promoter within the hemagglutinin gene region of the vaccinia virus, which was reconstructed from the pSFJ1-10 plasmid and pBM vector [41,42]. Separate full-length cDNAs encoding either the HCV structural protein, nonstructural protein, or all HCV proteins were cloned from HCV R6 strain (genotype 1b) RNA by RT-PCR. Each cDNA was inserted into a separate pBMSF7C vector downstream of the pBMSF7C ATI/p7.5 hybrid promoter; the final designation of each recombinant plasmid was pBMSF7C-CN2, pBMSF7C-N25, or pBMSF-CN5 (Figure 2). They were then transfected into primary rabbit kidney cells infected with LC16m8 (multiplicity of infection = 10). The virus–cell mixture was harvested 24 h after the initial transfection by scrapping; the mixture was then frozen at −80°C until use. The hemagglutinin-negative recombinant viruses were cloned as previously described [42] and named rVV-CN2, rVV-N25, or rVV-CN5. Insertion of the HCV protein genes into the LC16m8 genome was confirmed by direct PCR, and expression of each protein from the recombinant viruses was confirmed by western blot analysis. The titers of rVV-CN2, rVV-N25, and rVV-CN5 were determined using a standard plaque assay and RK13 cells.

Statistical Analysis

Data are shown as mean ± SD. Data were analyzed using the nonparametric Mann–Whitney or Kruskal–Wallis tests or ANOVA as appropriate; GraphPad Prism 5 for Macintosh (GraphPad) was used for all analyses. P values <0.05 were considered statistically significant.

Supporting Information

Figure S1   HAI score of liver samples taken from CN2-29$^{(+/-)}$/MxCre$^{(+/-)}$ mice.

Figure S2   Lipid degeneration in samples of liver taken from CN2-29$^{(+/-)}$/MxCre$^{(+/-)}$ mice.

Figure S3   HCV protein expression after infection of LC16m8, rVV-CN2, rVV-N25, or rVV-CN5 into HepG2 cells.

Figure S4   Effects of treatment with rVV-N25 in RzCN5-15$^{(+/-)}$/MxCre$^{(+/-)}$ mice.

Figure S5   Daily cytokine profiles of the serum from CN2-29$^{(+/-)}$/MxCre$^{(+/-)}$ mice during the week following inoculation with LC16m8, rVV-CN2, rVV-N25, or rVV-CN5.

Figure S6   The immune response following poly(I:C) injection in the acute phase.

Figure S7   Detection of vaccinia virus DNA in the skin, liver, and spleen after inoculation with attenuated vaccinia virus (Lister strain) or highly attenuated vaccinia virus (LC16m8 strain).

Table S1   Incidence of hepatocellular carcinoma in male and female transgenic mice at 360, 480, and 600 days after poly(I:C) injection.

Text S1   Supporting information including material and methods, and references.

Acknowledgments

We thank Dr. Fukashi Murai for supporting this study. We also thank Dr. Keiji Tanaka for providing the MxCre mice, Dr. Shigeo Koyasu for providing the GK1.5 (anti-CD4) and 53-6.72 (anti-CD8) monoclonal antibodies, and Dr Takashi Tokuhisa for helpful discussions.

Author Contributions

Performed the experiments: SS KK TC Y. Tobita TO FY Y. Tokunaga. Analyzed the data: SS KK TC MK. Contributed reagents/materials/analysis tools: KT-K TW TT MM K. Mizuno YH TH K. Matsushima. Wrote the paper: SS KK MK. Study concept and design: MK.

References

1. Lauer GM, Walker BD (2001) Hepatitis C virus infection. N Engl J Med 345: 41–52.
2. Alter MJ (1995) Epidemiology of hepatitis C in the West. Semin Liver Dis 15: 5–14.
3. Kawamura T, Furusaka A, Koziel MJ, Chung RT, Wang TC, et al. (1997) Transgenic expression of hepatitis C virus structural proteins in the mouse. Hepatology 25: 1014–1021.
4. Moriya K, Fujie H, Shintani Y, Yotsuyanagi H, Tsutsumi T, et al. (1998) The core protein of hepatitis C virus induces hepatocellular carcinoma in transgenic mice. Nat Med 4: 1065–1067.
5. Wakita T, Katsume A, Kato J, Taya C, Yonekawa H, et al. (2000) Possible role of cytotoxic T cells in acute liver injury in hepatitis C virus cDNA transgenic mice mediated by Cre/loxP system. J Med Virol 62: 308–317.
6. Wakita T, Taya C, Katsume A, Kato J, Yonekawa H, et al. (1998) Efficient conditional transgene expression in hepatitis C virus cDNA transgenic mice mediated by the Cre/loxP system. J Biol Chem 273: 9001–9006.
7. Folgori A, Capone S, Ruggeri L, Meola A, Sporeno E, et al. (2006) A T-cell HCV vaccine eliciting effective immunity against heterologous virus challenge in chimpanzees. Nat Med 12: 190–197.
8. Chisari FV, Ferrari C (1995) Hepatitis B virus immunopathology. Springer Semin Immunopathol 17: 261–281.
9. Machida K, Tsukiyama-Kohara K, Seike E, Tone S, Shibasaki F, et al. (2001) Inhibition of cytochrome c release in Fas-mediated signaling pathway in transgenic mice induced to express hepatitis C viral proteins. J Biol Chem 276: 12140–12146.
10. Kuhn R, Schwenk F, Aguet M, Rajewsky K (1995) Inducible gene targeting in mice. Science 269: 1427–1429.
11. Li K, Chen Z, Kato N, Gale M Jr, Lemon SM (2005) Distinct poly(I-C) and virus-activated signaling pathways leading to interferon-beta production in hepatocytes. J Biol Chem 280: 16739–16747.
12. Sugimoto M, Yamanouchi K (1994) Characteristics of an attenuated vaccinia virus strain, LC16m0, and its recombinant virus vaccines. Vaccine 12: 675–681.
13. Youn JW, Hu YW, Tricoche N, Pfahler W, Shata MT, et al. (2008) Evidence for protection against chronic hepatitis C virus infection in chimpanzees by immunization with replicating recombinant vaccinia virus. J Virol 82: 10896–10905.
14. Guidotti LG, Rochford R, Chung J, Shapiro M, Purcell R, et al. (1999) Viral clearance without destruction of infected cells during acute HBV infection. Science 284: 825–829.
15. Burkett MW, Shafer-Weaver KA, Strobl S, Baseler M, Malyguine A (2005) A novel flow cytometric assay for evaluating cell-mediated cytotoxicity. J Immunother 28: 396–402.

16. Pasquinelli C, Shoenberger JM, Chung J, Chang KM, Guidotti LG, et al. (1997) Hepatitis C virus core and E2 protein expression in transgenic mice. Hepatology 25: 719–727.

17. Lerat H, Honda M, Beard MR, Loesch K, Sun J, et al. (2002) Steatosis and liver cancer in transgenic mice expressing the structural and nonstructural proteins of hepatitis C virus. Gastroenterology 122: 352–365.

18. Lang KS, Georgiev P, Recher M, Navarini AA, Bergthaler A, et al. (2006) Immunoprivileged status of the liver is controlled by Toll-like receptor 3 signaling. The Journal of clinical investigation 116: 2456–2463.

19. Jasani B, Navabi H, Adams M (2009) Ampligen: a potential toll-like 3 receptor adjuvant for immunotherapy of cancer. Vaccine 27: 3401–3404.

20. Elmowalid GA, Qiao M, Jeong SH, Borg BB, Baumert TF, et al. (2007) Immunization with hepatitis C virus-like particles results in control of hepatitis C virus infection in chimpanzees. Proc Natl Acad Sci U S A 104: 8427–8432.

21. Satoi J, Murata K, Lechmann M, Manickan E, Zhang Z, et al. (2001) Genetic immunization of wild-type and hepatitis C virus transgenic mice reveals a hierarchy of cellular immune response and tolerance induction against hepatitis C virus structural proteins. J Virol 75: 12121–12127.

22. Crispe IN (2009) The liver as a lymphoid organ. Annu Rev Immunol 27: 147–163.

23. Chisari FV (2005) Unscrambling hepatitis C virus-host interactions. Nature 436: 930–932.

24. Saito T, Sherman GJ, Kurokohchi K, Guo ZP, Donets M, et al. (1997) Plasmid DNA-based immunization for hepatitis C virus structural proteins: immune responses in mice. Gastroenterology 112: 1321–1330.

25. Large MK, Kittlesen DJ, Hahn YS (1999) Suppression of host immune response by the core protein of hepatitis C virus: possible implications for hepatitis C virus persistence. Journal of immunology 162: 931–938.

26. Dustin LB, Rice CM (2007) Flying under the radar: the immunobiology of hepatitis C. Annu Rev Immunol 25: 71–99.

27. Bowie A, Kiss-Toth E, Symons JA, Smith GL, Dower SK, et al. (2000) A46R and A52R from vaccinia virus are antagonists of host IL-1 and toll-like receptor signaling. Proc Natl Acad Sci U S A 97: 10162–10167.

28. Zhu J, Martinez J, Huang X, Yang Y (2007) Innate immunity against vaccinia virus is mediated by TLR2 and requires TLR-independent production of IFN-beta. Blood 109: 619–625.

29. Samuelsson C, Hausmann J, Lauterbach H, Schmidt M, Akira S, et al. (2008) Survival of lethal poxvirus infection in mice depends on TLR9, and therapeutic vaccination provides protection. J Clin Invest 118: 1776–1784.

30. Sheikh MY, Choi J, Qadri I, Friedman JE, Sanyal AJ (2008) Hepatitis C virus infection: molecular pathways to metabolic syndrome. Hepatology 47: 2127–2133.

31. Tilg H, Moschen AR, Kaser A, Pines A, Dotan I (2008) Gut, inflammation and osteoporosis: basic and clinical concepts. Gut 57: 684–694.

32. Malaguarnera M, Di Fazio I, Laurino A, Ferlito L, Romano M, et al. (1997) Serum interleukin 6 concentrations in chronic hepatitis C patients before and after interferon-alpha treatment. Int J Clin Pharmacol Ther 35: 385–388.

33. Larrea E, Garcia N, Qian C, Civeira MP, Prieto J (1996) Tumor necrosis factor alpha gene expression and the response to interferon in chronic hepatitis C. Hepatology 23: 210–217.

34. Park EJ, Lee JH, Yu GY, He G, Ali SR, et al. (2010) Dietary and genetic obesity promote liver inflammation and tumorigenesis by enhancing IL-6 and TNF expression. Cell 140: 197–208.

35. Gregor MF, Hotamisligil GS (2011) Inflammatory mechanisms in obesity. Annu Rev Immunol 29: 415–445.

36. Humlova Z, Vokurka M, Esteban M, Melkova Z (2002) Vaccinia virus induces apoptosis of infected macrophages. The Journal of general virology 83: 2821–2832.

37. Choo QL, Kuo G, Weiner AJ, Overby LR, Bradley DW, et al. (1989) Isolation of a cDNA clone derived from a blood-borne non-A, non-B viral hepatitis genome. Science 244: 359–362.

38. Tsukiyama-Kohara K, Tone S, Maruyama I, Inoue K, Katsume A, et al. (2004) Activation of the CKI-CDK-Rb-E2F pathway in full genome hepatitis C virus-expressing cells. J Biol Chem 279: 14531–14541.

39. Nishimura T, Kohara M, Izumi K, Kasama Y, Hirata Y, et al. (2009) Hepatitis C virus impairs p53 via persistent overexpression of 3beta-hydroxysterol Delta24-reductase. J Biol Chem 284: 36442–36452.

40. Shimizu YK, Purcell RH, Yoshikura H (1993) Correlation between the infectivity of hepatitis C virus in vivo and its infectivity in vitro. Proc Natl Acad Sci U S A 90: 6037–6041.

41. Yasui F, Kai C, Kitabatake M, Inoue S, Yoneda M, et al. (2008) Prior immunization with severe acute respiratory syndrome (SARS)-associated coronavirus (SARS-CoV) nucleocapsid protein causes severe pneumonia in mice infected with SARS-CoV. J Immunol 181: 6337–6348.

42. Kitabatake M, Inoue S, Yasui F, Yokochi S, Arai M, et al. (2007) SARS-CoV spike protein-expressing recombinant vaccinia virus efficiently induces neutralizing antibodies in rabbits pre-immunized with vaccinia virus. Vaccine 25: 630–637.

Psychological Stress Exerts Effects on Pathogenesis of Hepatitis B via Type-1/Type-2 Cytokines Shift toward Type-2 Cytokine Response

YingLi He[1,4,ͽ], **Heng Gao**[2,ͽ], **XiaoMei Li**[3], **YingRen Zhao**[1,4]*

1 Department of Infectious Diseases, the First Affiliated Teaching Hospital, School of Medicine, Xi'an JiaoTong University, Xi'an, Shaanxi Province, China, **2** Xi'an Municipal Health College, Xi'an, Shaanxi Province, China, **3** Department of Psychology and Nursing, School of Medicine, Xi'an JiaoTong University, Xi'an, Shaanxi Province, China, **4** Institution of Hepatology, the First Affiliated Hospital of Xi'an JiaoTong University, Xi'an, Shaanxi Province, China

Abstract

Background: Psychological and physical stress has been demonstrated to have an impact on health through modulation of immune function. Despite high prevalence of stress among patients with hepatitis B virus (HBV) infection, little is known about whether and how stress exerts an effect on the course of hepatitis B.

Methods: Eighty patients with chronic hepatitis B(CHB) completed the Perceived Stress Scale-10(PSS-10) and State-Trait Anxiety Inventory(STAI). Fresh whole blood was subject to flow cytometry for lymphocytes count. Plasma samples frozen at $-80°C$ were thawed for cytokines, alanine aminotransferase (ALT), and virus load. These patients were grouped into high or low perceived stress, state anxiety and trait anxiety groups according to the scale score. Sociodemographic, disease-specific characteristics, lymphocytes count and cytokines were compared.

Results: Firstly, a negative association between ALT and stress (t = −4.308; p = .000), state anxiety (t = −3.085; p = .003) and trait anxiety (t = −4.925; p = .000) were found. As ALT is a surrogate marker of hepatocytes injury, and liver injury is a consequence of immune responses. Next, we tested the relationship between stress/anxiety and lymphocytes. No statistical significance were found with respect to counts of total T cells, CD4+ T cell, CD8+ T cell, NK cell, and B cell count between high and low stress group. Type-2 cytokine interleukin-10 (IL-10) level was significantly higher in high stress group relative to lower counterpart (t = 6.538; p = 0.000), and type-1 cytokine interferon-gamma (IFN-γ) level shown a decreased tendency in high stress group (t = −1.702; p = 0.093). Finally, INF-γ:IL-10 ratio displayed significant decrease in high perceived stress(t = −4.606; p = 0.000), state anxiety(t = −5.126; p = 0.000) and trait anxiety(t = −4.670; p = 0.000) groups relative to low counterparts.

Conclusion: Our data show stress is not related to the lymphocyte cells count in CHB patients, however, stress induces a shift in the type-1/type-2 cytokine balance towards a type-2 response, which implicated a role of psychological stress in the course of HBV related immune-pathogenesis.

Editor: Shawn Hayley, Carleton University, Canada

Funding: This study was supported by grants from the China National Natural Science Foundation (No. 30700712) and The Major National Science and Technology Projects for Infectious Diseases (11th and 12th Five Year, China) (No. 2008ZX10002-007, No. 2012ZX10002007). The funders had no role in study design, data collection and analysis, decision to publish, or preparation of the manuscript.

Competing Interests: The authors have declared that no competing interests exist.

* Email: zhaoyingren@mail.xjtu.edu.cn

ͽ These authors contributed equally to this work.

Introduction

An estimated 2 billion people worldwide are infected with the hepatitis B virus (HBV), and 350 million people are chronically infection[1]. HBV infection results in approximately 280 thousand deaths per year, caused by chronic hepatitis, cirrhosis, and hepatocellular carcinoma, which are associated with heavy psychological stress, enormous medical-care costs,and emotional and economic burden on those afflicted and/or their families[2]. HBV infection is a major life stressor, with up to 90% of those subjects reporting significant stress since the diagnosis of HBV infection[3]. Accumulating evidence has linked stress to the initiation, course and outcome of liver diseases[4]. Emotional stress, such as that induced by hypnotic of fear and anxiety, significantly decreased the hepatic blood flow. Moreover, the type I personality has been associated with the severity of chronic hepatitis C[5]. Stress has been reported to aggravate alpha-galactosylceramide induced hepatitis and carbon tetrachloride induced liver injury[6]. Recently, stress has been implicated in the hepatitis B antibody production in healthy participants[7], however little is known about the role of stress in the course of hepatitis B.

It has been reported that the stress is associated with a suppression of NK cell cytotoxicity[8], lymphocyte proliferation, and the production of IL-2 and IFN-γ, suggesting immunosuppression as a fundamental effect of stress. Moreover, recent data have suggested that dysregulation of type-1/type-2 cytokine balance may play a significant role in stress-associated immune alteration[9]. Type-1 and type-2 cytokines often have opposing actions thought to be critical in maintaining immunologic homeostasis. In the pathogenesis of hepatitis B, it is the host immune response targeting hepatocytes, but not HBV DNA itself, account for liver inflammation and injury. A considerable amount of data suggests that a switch from a predominantly type-1 cytokine-response pattern (e.g., relatively higher levels of IFN-γ) to a predominantly type-2 cell pattern (e.g., relatively higher IL-10) could impact on chronic hepatitis B progression[10–12]. Along these lines, we hypothesized that the stress involved in the immune alteration in the course of chronic hepatitis B. To test this, we investigated the association between psychological stress and hepatic inflammation and peripheral lymphocyte counts and circulating type-1 and type-2 cytokines in a series of 80 chronically ill hepatitis B patients.

Methods

Subjects

The study was approved by the Research Ethics Committee of the First Affiliated Hospital, Xian Jiaotong University, Shaanxi, China. All subjects signed a written informed consent. This study was performed with the participation of the Departments of Psychiatry, psychology, and Clinical Infectious Diseases between April 2006 and January 2010.

Patients with chronic hepatitis B with positivity for hepatitis B virus surface antigen (HBsAg) more than 6 months were recruited. Diagnoses of chronic hepatitis B were based on clinical, biochemical and virological findings. Criteria for recruitment were: 1) 20~50 years of age; 2) no cirrhosis by laboratory examination and ultrasonography; 3) AFP<20 ng/ml; 4) no psychosis; 5) no hypercortisolism; 6) no immunological disease and autoallergic disease or a history of illness associated with marked changes in the immune system; 7) no co-infection with other hepatitis virus and no alcoholic hepatitis; 8) without receiving interferon and other immunomodulators within the past one year. A series of 80 eligible patients were included in the study.

Assessment

All subjects signed a written informed consent. Besides the Stress and anxiety inventory, the subjects were asked to complete a questionnaire that included questions regarding age, sex, education level, Economic status, duration of disease. They subsequently provided disease history, underwent a physical examination, and had a small amount of blood drawn.

Peripheral blood T cell subset measurements were measured with flow cytometry, cell count were determined with 100 μl peripheral blood, using a three-color direct immunofluorescence method. In tube 1, CD3+CD4+ and CD3+CD8+ T cell analyzed with CD4/CD4/CD8 triple staining. In tube 2, B cell and natural killer cell was analyzed with CD16/CD19/CD3 triple staining on a CyFlow SL machine (PARTEC Company, Germany) using FloMax software, as described previously[13].

Plasma samples frozen at −80°C were thawed for cytokine, alanine aminotransferase, ALT, HBV DNA load and genotypes detection as described previously[14]. IL-10 and IFN gamma levels were assayed by using a Quantikine High Sensitivity Immunoassay kit (R & D Systems) according to kit instructions, and all samples from an individual were run in the same way.

Perceived stress

To obtain information about subjects' stress, we used the 10-item Perceived Stress scale (PSS): an instrument was designed to measure the degree to which situations in one's life are appraised as stressful. This scale assessed the amount of stress in one's life rather than in response to a specific stressor and has been used widely. This scale has good internal consistency ($\alpha = 0.80$–0.85) and test-retest reliability ($r = 0.73$–0.85) in Chinese people based on our data. Subjects rated each item from 0 (never) to 4(very often).

Anxiety

The State-Trait Anxiety Inventory (STAI) provided information on the degree of anxiety. The scales of both State anxiety and Trait anxiety consist of 20 self-report items, with each item running from 1 to 4, for a full score of 80 and a lower score reflecting a better psychological status.

Statistical analyses

In the present study, we dichotomized chronic hepatitis B subjects into high versus low perceived stress and anxiety score (n = 40/group) on the basis of a median split of the distribution of stress and anxiety score. Based on the scores obtained from these patients, subjects with perceived stress score ≥17 were assigned to the high stress group(P_H), while subjects with perceived stress score <17 were assigned to the low perceived stress(P_L); state anxiety ≥ 41 to the high state anxiety group(S_H), and <41 to the low state anxiety group(S_L); trait anxiety score ≥42 to the high trait anxiety(T_H), and <42 to the low trait anxiety(T_L).

Chi-square tests, Student-t test, as well as correlation analysis were used for comparing the difference between high and low perceived stress group, high and low state anxiety group and high and low trait anxiety group. SPSS 13.0 statistical software was used for statistical analysis. Reported p values were two-sided, and p values <0.05 were considered statistically significant.

Results

Perceived stress

The Perceived Stress Scale (PSS) is one of most widely used instruments to measure a global level of perceived stress in clinical and research settings[15]. It was reported that 10-item PSS be superior to 14-item PSS[16]. Since this is the first study designed to evaluate the stresses by using PSS-10 for patients with hepatitis B in Chinese population, the reliability of PSS-10 was assessed. The Cronnbach's alpha was 0.88 for the whole scale, the two-week test-retest reliability of PSS-10 was 0.72, suggesting PSS-10 is suitable for evaluating stress in Chinese hepatitis B patients.(During the preparation of this manuscript, the translated Chinese version of PSS-10, has been tested in Chinese policewomen with good internal consistency ($\alpha = 0.86$) and test-retest reliability ($r = 0.68$) [17].

Psychological stress lead to emotional reaction of anxiety when an individual perceive stress, therefore the extent of anxiety is associated with the stress level. The State-Trait Anxiety Inventory (STAI) provided information on the degree of anxiety. The scales of Table 1. Sociodemographic, disease-specific characteristics comparison between high and low perceived stress and anxiety patients with chronic hepatitis B.

Both state anxiety and trait anxiety consist of 20 self-report items, with each item running from 1 to 4, for a full score of 80 and a lower score reflecting a better psychological status. Higher scores are positively associated with higher levels of anxiety. To further test the validity of PSS-10, all the participants were encouraged to

Table 1. Sociodemographic, disease-specific characteristics comparison between high and low perceived stress and anxiety patients with chronic hepatitis B.

Variables[a]	P_H (n = 40)	P_L (n = 40)	p value	S_H (n = 40)	S_L (n = 40)	p value	T_H (n = 40)	T_L (n = 40)	p value
Gender(F/M)	8/32	10/30	0.79	8/32	10/30	0.79	10/30	8/32	0.79
Age, years	31.15 (8.85)	26.4 (6.01)	0.06	31.20 (8.21)	26.35 (6.85)	0.08	30.80 (8.41)	26.75 (6.88)	0.06
Education			0.005			0.050			0.043
<college	32	20		30	22		32	24	
≥college	8	20		10	18		8	16	
Marital			0.241			0.241			0.055
Married	28	24		28	24		28	20	
Single	12	16		12	16		12	20	
Economic status[b]			0.070			0.459			0.754
≥average	0	4		2	4		2	4	
common	12	16		10	18		14	14	
hard	26	20		28	18		24	22	
Disease duration[c]	8.25	7.80	0.080	6.75	9.30	0.06	7.15	8.90	0.100
mean(S.D.)	(6.3)	(5.8)		(5.8)	(6.08)		(5.89)	(6.1)	
ALT(U/L)	98.60	138.45	0.000	95.45	132.60	0.003	102.5	137.5	0.000
mean(S.D.)	(44.33)	(55.93)		(47.00)	(53.67)		(43.48)	(56.76)	
Virus Load[d]	6.38	6.24	0.18	6.31	6.32	0.28	6.37	6.27	0.26
mean(S.D.)	(1.1)	(1.13)		(1.1)	(1.1)		(1.2)	(1.1)	

[a]P_H, high stress group; P_L, low perceived stress; S_H, high state anxiety group; S_L, low state anxiety group; T_H, trait anxiety group; T_L, low trait anxiety; [b]Self reported economic status; [c]Years; [d]Log_{10}(copies/ml).

complete the STAI forms immediately after the completion of PSS-10. Consistency with the conception of psychological stress lead to emotional reaction of anxiety, we do found, a positive correlation between PSS-10 score and state anxiety (r = 0.811, p< 0.01), and trait anxiety (r = 0.782, p<0.01). These results also indicate that psychological stress is associated with mental health issues.

Sociodemographic comparison between high and low stress/anxiety patients

In China, most of these patients did not fullly covered by medical insurance, and hepatitis B virus infection has been link to substantial economic burden, stigmatization, and poor social support. As far as we know, this is the first study to test the stress of patients with hepatitis B in Chinese population. We want to know if there is association between perceived stress score and socio-demographic variable, clinical variable and virus replication variable. No significant difference was found(Table 1) between high and low stress/anxiety in sociodemographic (gender, age, marital state, and economic state, and disease duration.)

The knowledge of HBV related cirrhosis and hepatocelluar carcinoma and insufficient knowledge of the modes of transmission may results in isolation[3]. Consistently with this conception, in this study, the proportion of high stress scores patients was much higher in inadequate educated participants than well-educated subjects (61.5% vs 28.5%), while the proportion of well education was much lower in high stress group than that of the low stress group (20% vs 80%, chi-square 7.912, p = .009). A positive relationship between education and state anxiety (chi-square 3.516, p = .050), and trait anxiety (chi-square 3.810, p = .043) were also observed(Table 1).

Correlation between stress and liver inflammation

Next, we compared virus load, virus genotypes, and ALT between these two group. As shown in table 1, no differences were observed between high and low stree/anxiety group. However, a strong negative correlation(Figure. 1) between ALT and stress (t = − 4.308; p = .000), state anxiety (t = − 3.085; p = .003) and trait anxiety (t = − 4.925; p = .000) were found. ALT is a surrogate marker of hepatocytes injury. The HBV replication cycle is not directly cytotoxic toward hepatocytes. Much of the liver injury is thought to be a consequence of immune responses. Next, we analyzed the association between the subtypes of lymphocyte and the extent of stress/anxiety. The cell count of T cells (CD3+), T helper/inducer (CD3+CD4+), T suppressor/inducer (CD3+CD8+), NK (CD16+CD56+), B cells (CD19+) in those 80 patients enrolled are comparable with literature[18]. When we compared the cell count between low and high perceived stress group(-Table 2), no statistical significance were found with respect to counts of total T cells (t = −0.158; p = 0.875), CD4+ T cell (t = 0.648; p = 0.519), CD8+T cell (t = −1.810; p = 0.074), NK (t = −0.820; p = 0.414), and B cells (t = 0.11; p = 0.991). Similarly, no statistical significances were found between low and high state anxiety group, low and high trait anxiety in those subtypes of lymphocyte.

Studies suggest that the balance of cytokine production profiles may play a crucial role in determining the immune response in the liver. Th1 type cytokines (IFN-γ, TNF-α) are involved in immune activation and then the injury of HBV antigen expressed hepatocytes, while Th2 type cytokine productions (IL-10, IL-4) inhibit immune reaction and involved in the persistence of infection. In the current study we observed the level of IL-10 was significantly lower in chronic hepatitis B patients with minor stress than patients with major stress(t = 6.538; p = 0.000)(Fig-

ure. 2A). Since a close correlation between psychological stress and emotional reaction of anxiety was established in our previous data, the correlation between IL-10 and anxiety may be existence. Not surprisingly, IL-10 level was much lower in low state anxiety group (t = 5.821, p = 0.000) and low trait anxiety group (t = 6.238, p = 0.000), as compared with the higher counterpart. We also observed an increased tendency of Th1 cytokine IFN- γ level in high stress group than low stress group, but the statistical difference are not significant(t = 1.702; p = 0.093)(Figure. 2B). Similarity with those observations, no significant differences between low and high state anxiety group (t = 1.586, p = 0.121), and between low and high trait anxiety group (t = 1.711, p = 0.098).

The INF-γ:IL-10 ratio, reflecting the Th1/Th2 balance, has been implicated in psychological stress during an exam period[19]. Next, INF-γ: IL-10 ratio was calculated and then compared between high and low stress/anxiety groups. Consistent with our increased INF-γ and decreased IL-10 data in major stress/anxiety groups as shown above, the ratio displayed significantly increases in high perceived stress(t = 4.606; p = 0.000)(Figure. 2C), state anxiety(t = 5.126; p = 0.000) and trait anxiety(t = 4.670; p = 0.000) groups as compared with the low score groups.

Discussion

The PSS-10 is one of most widely used instruments to measure a global level of perceived stress in clinical and research settings and has been translated into many languages including Spanish[20], Arabic[21], Greek[22], Japanese[23],Korean[24]. At the beginning of the study, for the reason that this is the first study to employ the translated Chinese version of PSS-10 and STAI inventory scale to assess Chinese population, the reliability and validity were tested. The Cronnbach's alpha was 0.88 for the whole scale, the two-week test-retest reliability of PSS-10 was 0.72, suggesting the translated Chinese version of PSS-10 is suitable for evaluating stress in Chinese hepatitis B patients. The preliminary data were submitted to 13th International Congress on Infectious Diseases as a poster[25]. During the preparation of this manuscript, an independently translated Chinese version of PSS-10, has been tested in Chinese policewomen with comparable consistency and test-retest reliability[17].

Following the validation of the reliability of PSS-10, analysis was conducted in patients with CHB to found the relationship between stress/anxiety and sociodemographic and disease-specific characteristics. Data show stress/anxiety has no association with gender, age, marital state, economic state, disease duration, HBV virus load and HBV gene type. Positively relationship between stress and education was found, Moreover, a negative correlation between stress/anxiety and ALT were established. According to our knowledge, this is the first study discovered the relationship between stress/anxiety and ALT in patients with hepatitis B. The ALT reflects injury to hepatocytes[26]. It was well documented that it's the host immune response targeting infected hepatocytes, not the HBV replication itself in hepatocytes, led to liver injury[27–29]. To explorer the role of stress related immune alteration in the course of hepatitis B, we analyzed the stress/anxiety and immune cell count and cytokines, which account for the HBV related immunity response. However, no relationship was found between stress/anxiety and T cells, T helper/inducer, T suppressor/inducer, NK, and B cells count.

Among all the variables assessed, high circulating IL-10 levels was the only variable strongly associated with high stress/anxiety score, low IFN-γ levels was also observed in high stress/anxiety group, however the statistical differences was not significant. IL-10

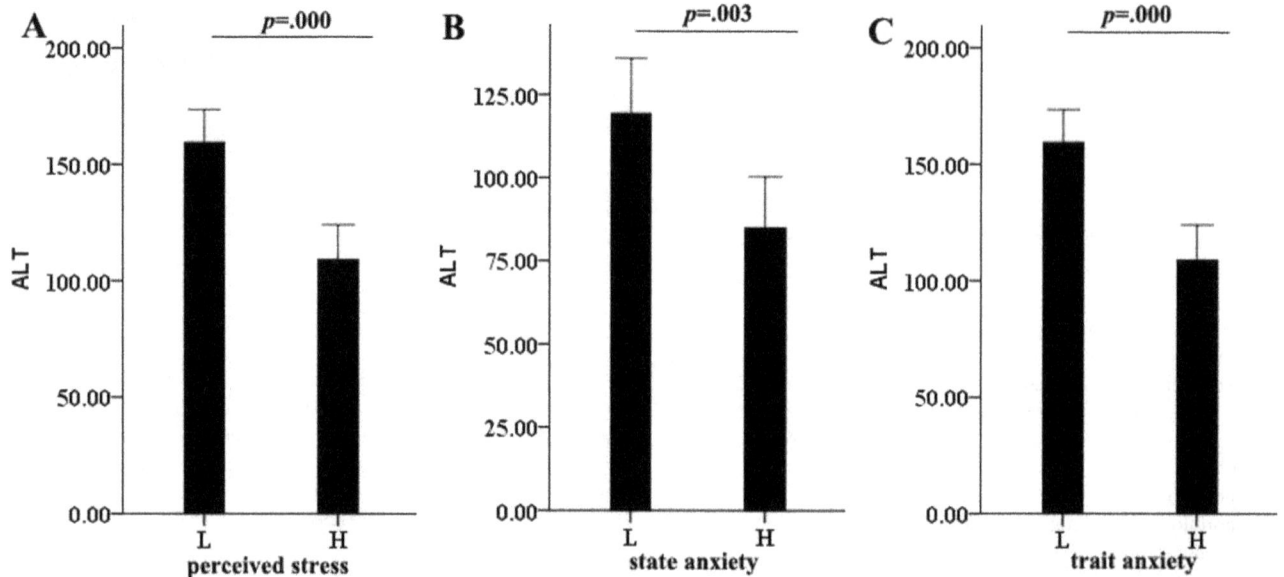

Figure 1. ALT level negatively associated with stress and anxiety. (A)Comparison of ALT between high and low perceived stress group; (B) Comparison of ALT between high and low state anxiety; (C) Comparison of ALT between high and low trait anxiety. *P* value was indicated.

and IFN-γ are important cytokines involved in chronic HBV infection, as level of IL-10 and IFN-γ associated greatly with course of chronic hepatitis B[30–32]. IL-10, a prototype of type-2 cytokine, is considered an anti-inflammatory cytokine and has inhibitory effect on immune response,whereas IFN-γ, a type-1 cytokine, is significantly increased in patients with acute hepatitis B, which would eventually eliminated viral from hepatocytes. Dysregulation of the Th1/Th2 cytokine production is thought to be involved in the pathogenesis of HBV related liver diseases. However, the reasons for the imbalance of Th1/Th2 cytokine still poorly studied in the progression of hepatitis B. Psychological distress has been shown to induce a shift in type-1/type-2 cytokine balance toward a type-2 responses through glucocorticoids and catecholamines. Consistently, we observed a higher IFN-γ/IL-10 ratio, indicating a shift toward a Th2 response, in high stress/anxiety group.

Stress has been reported to aggravate alpha-galactosylceramide induced hepatitis and carbon tetrachloride induced liver injury, however, out data shown stress linked to low ALT level. Thus, a discrepancy between our data and literature was observed. Firstly,

stressors are classified into acute, subchronic and chronic. The different duration of stress may elicit different neuroendocrine response and immune alteration. Acute stress may be associated with transient immune activation, while chronic stress seems consistently associated with immune suppression. Most of those studies, including alpha-galactosylceramide induced hepatitis and carbon tetrachloride induce liver injury in animal stress model, the duration of stress was just about weeks. In our study, the diseases duration was around 8 years. Consistent with the suppressive function of chronic stress on immunity, our *in vivo* data shown decreased liver inflammation and injury in high stress/anxiety subjects, as indicated by lower ALT level. Although ALT is a surrogated marker of liver inflammation in the context of hepatitis B and ALT has been widely clinically used, the golden diagnosis of liver inflammation is checking the necrosis of hepatocytes and infiltration of lymphocytes by liver biopsy, which call for further investigation. Secondly, consistent with the immune-suppressive notion of chronic stress, our data presented a markedly increased IL-10, a suppressive cytokine, and a decreased tendency of IFN-γ, an immune activation cytokine. Thirdly, ALT, a marker of liver

Table 2. Comparison of lymphocytes count and circulating cytokines between low and high perceived stress patients with hepatitis B.

	CHB with low stress	CHB with high stress	*p* value
CD3	1728 ±812	1605 ± 717	t = −0.158; p = 0.875
CD3/CD4	526±243	573 ± 194	t = 0.648; p = 0.519
CD3/CD8	519±223	489 ± 213	t = −1.810; p = 0.074
CD19	198±98	228 ± 148	t = 0.11; p = 0.991
CD16	217±103	197 ± 102	t = −0.820; p = 0.414
IFN-γ(pg/mL)	83.48±49.70	62.24±61.35	t = −1.702; p = 0.093
IL-10(pg/mL)	9.11±3.36	17.01±6.86	t = 6.538; p = 0.000
IFN-γ: IL-10	10.13±4.43	6.23±4.74	t = −4.606; p = 0.000

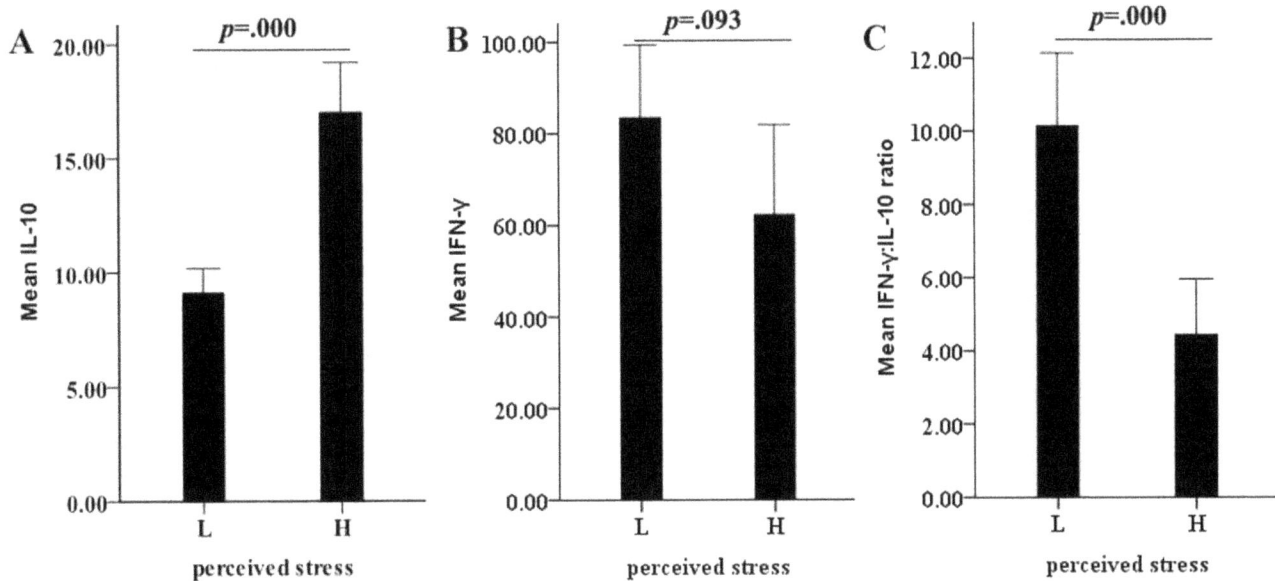

Figure 2. Shift of the type-1/type-2 cytokine balance towards a type-2 cytokine response in high perceived stress patients.
(A)Comparison of INF-γ between low and high perceived stress group; (B) Comparison of IL-10 between low and high perceived stress group; (C) Comparison of INF-γ:IL-10 ratio between low and high perceived stress group. *P* value was indicated.

inflammation, also an indicator of current immune competence, reflects the functional ability of body immunity system mounts a response to HB surface antigen and HB core antigen. It is reasonable that patients with major stress mount less extent of immune response relative to minor stress subjects. Finally, under the basic conception of deleterious effect of chronic stress on health, much attention has paid to the disease severity, while little paid to disease duration. Higher ALT level associated with earlier clearance of virus in both treatment naive patients and interferon treated patients, while lower or normal ALT level associated with persistent infection. In our study, profiles with low ALT, high IL-10, low IFN-γ and low IFN-γ:IL-10 ratio in major stress/anxiety patients is a typical characteristic of persistent infection, while the profiles with high ALT, low IL-10, high IFN-γ and high IFN-γ:IL-

10 ratio in minor stress/anxiety patients prone to immunity activation and maybe virus clearance.

To our knowledge, this is the first study to investigate the relation among stress, immunity and hepatitis B. Ours *in vivo* data support the model, at least in part, that alterations in IFN-γ:IL-10 ratio, particular the IL-10 level, secondary to increased psychological stress are involved in the persistent HBV infection.

Author Contributions

Conceived and designed the experiments: YRZ XML. Performed the experiments: YLH HG. Analyzed the data: YLH HG. Contributed reagents/materials/analysis tools: YLH HG YRZ XML. Wrote the paper: YLH. Statistical analysis: YLH.

References

1. Ioannou GN (2013) Chronic hepatitis B infection: a global disease requiring global strategies. Hepatology 58: 839–843.
2. Yang Y, Jin L, He YL, Wang K, Ma XH, et al. (2013) Hepatitis B virus infection in clustering of infection in families with unfavorable prognoses in northwest China. J Med Virol 85: 1893–1899.
3. Atesci FC, Cetin BC, Oguzhanoglu NK, Karadag F, Turgut H (2005) Psychiatric disorders and functioning in hepatitis B virus carriers. Psychosomatics 46: 142–147.
4. Vere CC, Streba CT, Streba LM, Ionescu AG, Sima F (2009) Psychosocial stress and liver disease status. World Journal Of Gastroenterology 15: 2980–2986.
5. Nagano J, Nagase S, Sudo N, Kubo C (2004) Psychosocial stress, personality, and the severity of chronic hepatitis C. Psychosomatics 45: 100–106.
6. Chida Y, Sudo N, Sonoda J, Sogawa H, Kubo C (2004) Electric foot shock stress-induced exacerbation of alpha-galactosylceramide-triggered apoptosis in mouse liver. Hepatology 39: 1131–1140.
7. Burns VE, Carroll D, Ring C, Harrison LK, Drayson M (2002) Stress, coping, and hepatitis B antibody status. Psychosomatic Medicine 64: 287–293.
8. Greeson JM, Hurwitz BE, Llabre MM, Schneiderman N, Penedo FJ, et al. (2008) Psychological distress, killer lymphocytes and disease severity in HIV/AIDS. Brain Behavior and Immunity 22: 901–911.
9. Palumbo ML, Canzobre MC, Pascuan CG, Rios H, Wald M, et al. (2010) Stress induced cognitive deficit is differentially modulated in BALB/c and C57Bl/6 mice Correlation with Th1/Th2 balance after stress exposure. Journal of Neuroimmunology 218: 12–20.
10. Lee M, Lee M, Lee SK, Son M, Cho SW, et al. (1999) Expression of Th1 and Th2 type cytokines responding to HBsAg and HBxAg in chronic hepatitis B patients. J Korean Med Sci 14: 175–181.
11. Szkaradkiewicz A, Jopek A, Wysocki J, Grzymislawski M, Malecka I, et al. (2003) HBcAg-specific cytokine production by CD4 T lymphocytes of children with acute and chronic hepatitis B. Virus Res 97: 127–133.
12. Luo GH, Wu JZ, Wu JL, Li GJ, Chen MW, et al. (2004) [Effects of cytokine in prognosis of chronic hepatitis B]. Zhonghua Gan Zang Bing Za Zhi12: 143–147.
13. Niu YH, Yin DL, Liu HL, Yi RT, Yang YC, et al. (2013) Restoring the Treg cell to Th17 cell ratio may alleviate HBV-related acute-on-chronic liver failure. World J Gastroenterol 19: 4146–4154.
14. Chen T, Wang J, Feng Y, Yan Z, Zhang T, et al. (2013) Dynamic changes of HBV markers and HBV DNA load in infants born to HBsAg(+) mothers: can positivity of HBsAg or HBV DNA at birth be an indicator for HBV infection of infants? BMC Infect Dis 13: 524.
15. Cohen S, Kamarck T, Mermelstein R (1983) A global measure of perceived stress. J Health Soc Behav 24: 385–396.
16. Lee EH (2012) Review of the Psychometric Evidence of the Perceived Stress Scale. Asian Nursing Research 6: 121–127.
17. Wang Z, Chen J, Boyd JE, Zhang H, Jia X, et al. (2011) Psychometric properties of the Chinese version of the Perceived Stress Scale in policewomen. PLoS One 6: e28610.
18. Cao W, Qiu ZF, Li TS (2011) Parallel decline of CD8+CD38+ lymphocytes and viremia in treated hepatitis B patients. World J Gastroenterol 17: 2191–2198.
19. Marshall GD Jr, Agarwal SK, Lloyd C, Cohen L, Henninger EM, et al. (1998) Cytokine dysregulation associated with exam stress in healthy medical students. Brain Behav Immun 12: 297–307.
20. Remor E (2006) Psychometric properties of a European Spanish version of the Perceived Stress Scale (PSS). Spanish Journal of Psychology 9: 86–93.

21. Chaaya M, Osman H, Naassan G, Mahfoud Z (2010) Validation of the Arabic version of the Cohen perceived stress scale (PSS-10) among pregnant and postpartum women. Bmc Psychiatry 10.

22. Andreou E, Alexopoulos EC, Lionis C, Varvogli L, Gnardellis C, et al. (2011) Perceived Stress Scale: Reliability and Validity Study in Greece. International Journal of Environmental Research and Public Health 8: 3287–3298.

23. Mimura C, Griffiths P (2004) A Japanese version of the perceived stress scale: translation and preliminary test. International Journal of Nursing Studies 41: 379–385.

24. Lee J, Shin C, Ko Y-H, Lim J, Han C (2012) Standardization of the Korean version of the Perceived Stress Scale. Asia-Pacific Psychiatry 4: 108–108.

25. YingLi H, Heng G, YingRen Z, Ke W (2008) Psychological Stress, Cortisol and Immune Status in Patients with Chronic Hepatitis B. International Journal of Infectious Diseases 12: E417–E418.

26. M'Kada H, Perazzo H, Munteanu M, Ngo Y, Ramanujam N, et al. (2012) Real time identification of drug-induced liver injury (DILI) through daily screening of ALT results: a prospective pilot cohort study. PLoS One 7: e42418.

27. Loggi E, Bihl FK, Cursaro C, Granieri C, Galli S, et al. (2013) Virus-specific immune response in HBeAg-negative chronic hepatitis B: relationship with clinical profile and HBsAg serum levels. PLoS One 8: e65327.

28. Pan LP, Zhang W, Zhang L, Wu XP, Zhu XL, et al. (2012) CD3Z genetic polymorphism in immune response to hepatitis B vaccination in two independent Chinese populations. PLoS One 7: e35303.

29. Arnaud N, Dabo S, Akazawa D, Fukasawa M, Shinkai-Ouchi F, et al. (2011) Hepatitis C virus reveals a novel early control in acute immune response. PLoS Pathog 7: e1002289.

30. Hyodo N, Tajimi M, Ugajin T, Nakamura I, Imawari M (2003) Frequencies of interferon-gamma and interleukin-10 secreting cells in peripheral blood mononuclear cells and liver infiltrating lymphocytes in chronic hepatitis B virus infection. Hepatol Res 27: 109–116.

31. Marinos G, Torre F, Chokshi S, Hussain M, Clarke BE, et al. (1995) Induction of T-helper cell response to hepatitis B core antigen in chronic hepatitis B: a major factor in activation of the host immune response to the hepatitis B virus. Hepatology 22: 1040–1049.

32. Rico MA, Quiroga JA, Subira D, Castanon S, Esteban JM, et al. (2001) Hepatitis B virus-specific T-cell proliferation and cytokine secretion in chronic hepatitis B e antibody-positive patients treated with ribavirin and interferon alpha. Hepatology 33: 295–300.

Predictability of Liver-Related Seromarkers for the Risk of Hepatocellular Carcinoma in Chronic Hepatitis B Patients

Yu-Ju Lin[1,2], Mei-Hsuan Lee[2,3], Hwai-I Yang[2,4,5], Chin-Lan Jen[2], San-Lin You[2], Li-Yu Wang[6], Sheng-Nan Lu[7], Jessica Liu[2], Chien-Jen Chen[2,8]*

1 Institute of Microbiology and Immunology, School of Life Sciences, National Yang-Ming University, Taipei, Taiwan, 2 Genomics Research Center, Academia Sinica, Taipei, Taiwan, 3 Institute of Clinical Medicine, National Yang-Ming University, Taipei, Taiwan, 4 Graduate Institute of Clinical Medical Science, College of Medicine, China Medical University, Taichung, Taiwan, 5 Molecular and Genomic Epidemiology Center, China Medical University Hospital, Taichung, Taiwan, 6 School of Medicine, MacKay Medical College, Taipei, Taiwan, 7 Department of Internal Medicine, Kaohsiung Chang-Gung Memorial Hospital, Kaohsiung, Taiwan, 8 Graduate Institute of Epidemiology and Preventive Medicine, College of Public Health, National Taiwan University, Taipei, Taiwan

Abstract

Background: Hepatitis B virus (HBV)-related hepatocellular carcinoma (HCC) is a major global health problem. A few risk calculators have been developed using mainly HBV seromarkers as predictors. However, serum HBV DNA level, HBV genotype, and mutants are not routinely checked in regular health examinations. This study aimed to assess the predictability of HCC risk in chronic hepatitis B patients, using a combination of liver-related seromarkers combined with or without HBV seromarkers.

Methods: A prospective cohort of 1,822 anti-HCV-seronegative chronic HBV carriers was included in this study. Liver-related seromarkers including aspartate aminotransferase (AST), alanine aminotransferase (ALT), alpha-fetoprotein (AFP), gamma-glutamyltransferase (GGT), total bilirubin, total protein, albumin, serum globulins, apolipoprotein A1, and apolipoprotein B were examined. Hazard ratios of HCC with 95% confidence intervals were estimated using Cox proportional hazards regression models. Regression coefficients of seromarkers significantly associated with HCC risk in multivariate analyses were used to create integer risk scores. The predictability of various risk models were assessed by area under receiver operating characteristic curves (AUROCs).

Results: During a median follow-up of 5.9 years, 48 newly-developed HCC cases were ascertained. Elevated serum levels of ALT ($\geq$28 U/L), AFP ($\geq$5 ng/mL), and GGT ($\geq$41 U/L), an increased AST/ALT ratio (AAR, $\geq$1), and lowered serum levels of albumin ($\leq$4.1 g/dL) and alpha-1 globulin ($\leq$0.2 g/dL) were significantly associated with an increased HCC risk ($P<0.05$) in multivariate analysis. The risk model incorporating age, gender, AAR, and serum levels of ALT, AFP, GGT, albumin, and alpha-1 globulin had an AUROC of 0.89 for predicting 6-year HCC incidence. The AUROC was 0.91 after the addition of HBV seromarkers into the model, and 0.83 for the model without liver-related seromarkers, with the exception of ALT.

Conclusion: Liver-related seromarkers may be combined into useful risk models for predicting HBV-related HCC risk.

Editor: Sang-Hoon Ahn, Yonsei University College of Medicine, Republic of Korea

Funding: Supported by research grants from Department of Health, Executive Yuan, Taipei, Taiwan; Bristol-Myers Squibb Co., USA; Academia Sinica, Taipei, Taiwan; and National Health Research Institutes (NHRI-EX98-9806PI), Chunan, Taiwan. The funders had no role in study design, data collection and analysis, decision to publish, or preparation of the manuscript.

Competing Interests: The funder, Bristol-Myers Squibb Co., supported the testing of serum levels of HBV DNA for this study. There are no patents, products in development or marketed products to declare.

* E-mail: chencj@gate.sinica.edu.tw

Introduction

Chronic hepatitis B virus (HBV) infection is one of the major causes of deaths from end-stage liver diseases. The lifetime risk (30–78 years of age) of developing cirrhosis and hepatocellular carcinoma (HCC) was estimated to be as high as 41.5% and 21.7%, respectively. [1] Chronic HBV infection accounts for around 50% of total HCC cases and virtually all childhood HCC cases. [2] Even though the prevalence of chronic HBV infection is gradually decreasing in most regions due to the implementation of HBV vaccination programs, it remains a serious public health problem worldwide. An updated statistic estimates that 240 million people are chronically infected with HBV in the world, with the highest burden lying in developing countries with inadequate medical resources such as sub-Saharan Africa and parts of Eastern Asia. [3].

A number of risk predictors for HBV-associated HCC have been identified in previous studies.[4–10] They include older age, male gender, family history of HCC, elevated serum level of alanine aminotransferase (ALT), alcohol drinking, cirrhosis status, hepatitis B e antigen (HBeAg) seropositivity, high HBV DNA viral load, HBV genotype C, and the HBV core promoter mutation. In addition, a few nomograms and risk scores have also been proposed in recent years to facilitate the identification of high-risk chronic hepatitis B patients for anti-viral treatment and screening of HCC. [11–14] Among the proposed risk models, serum HBV DNA level is an important HCC predictor. Continuous anti-viral treatment of patients with chronic hepatitis B has significantly reduced the subsequent development of hepatic decompensation and HCC. [15–17] Thus, prediction models may help chronic HBV carriers to be more conscious of the severity of their disease.

However, some HBV seromarkers included in previous risk calculators, such as HBV viral load, genotype, and mutants, are not routinely tested in regular health examinations. On the other hand, Liver-related seromarkers such as aspartate aminotransferase (AST), ALT, alpha-fetoprotein (AFP), total bilirubin, total protein, albumin, alpha-1 globulin, alpha-2 globulin, beta globulin, gamma globulin, gamma-glutamyltransferase (GGT), apolipoprotein A1 (apoA1), and apolipoprotein B (apoB) are frequently tested in clinical practice to assess liver injury, inflammation, fibrosis, and dysfunction. However, their capability to predict subsequent HCC risk has not been well assessed. [18,19].

This study aimed to assess the ability of liver-related seromarkers to predict HCC risk in chronic hepatitis B patients, both without, or in combination with HBV seromarkers. Several HCC risk prediction models with high validity were developed.

Methods

Study Participants

A sub-cohort derived from the R.E.V.E.A.L.-HBV Study was included in this analysis. The enrollment of the R.E.V.E.A.L.-HBV cohort has been described previously. [4,13,20] Briefly, it was a community-based cohort of participants seropositive for hepatitis B surface antigen (HBsAg) and seronegative for antibodies against hepatitis C virus (anti-HCV). Participants were enrolled from seven townships in Taiwan during 1991–1992 after obtaining each participant's informed consent. In addition to HBV seromarkers and serum ALT levels, a total of 12 liver-related seromarkers including AST, AFP, GGT, total bilirubin, total protein, albumin, alpha-1 globulin, alpha-2 globulin, beta globulin, gamma globulin, apoA1, and apoB were included in follow-up examination starting in July, 2002. The date each participant's first examination of liver-related seromarkers was defined as the entry date in this analysis. Only participants with complete seromarker data and without new HCV infections were included in this study. Furthermore, participants who developed HCC before or within 3 months after their first examination of liver-related seromarkers were excluded from this study. A total of 1,822 chronic HBV carriers (HBsAg-seropositive for more than 6 months) were included in this analysis (Figure 1).

Questionnaire Interview, Ascertainment of Cirrhosis, and Blood Collection

All participants were personally interviewed by well trained public health nurses using a structured questionnaire. Information on sociodemographic characteristics, dietary intake, habits of cigarette smoking and alcohol consumption, personal medical and surgical history, and family history of cancers and other major diseases was collected from each participant. Liver cirrhosis was diagnosed by high-resolution real-time ultrasound, based on a quantitative scoring system derived from the appearance of the liver surface, liver parenchymal texture, intrahepatic blood vessel size, and splenic size. All ultrasounds were performed and interpreted according to a standardized protocol. Computerized data linkage with National Health Insurance profiles in Taiwan was used to ensure the complete ascertainment of cirrhosis cases. [20] Cirrhosis status was defined as cirrhosis diagnosed before or at the time of each participant's first examination of liver-related seromarkers.

Laboratory Examinations

A 10-mL blood sample was collected from each participant during follow-up health examinations. Fractionated aliquots of serum samples were frozen at −70°C before tested. Serum samples were tested for a battery of 13 seromarkers including AST, ALT, AFP, total bilirubin, total protein, albumin, alpha-1 globulin, alpha-2 globulin, beta globulin, gamma globulin, GGT, apoA1, and apoB, in addition to HBV seromarkers such as serum HBV DNA level and HBeAg serostatus. AST, ALT, total bilirubin, total protein, GGT, apoA1, and apoB were tested by autoanalyzer (Toshiba TBA-200FR, Japan) with commercial reagents (Denka Seiken, Tokyo, Japan). AFP was measured by radioimmunoassay with the BRAHMS AFP KRYPTOR (Brahms France, Sartrouville, France). Albumin, alpha-1 globulin, alpha-2 globulin, beta globulin, and gamma globulin were analyzed using protein electrophoresis (Helena Lab., TX, USA).

Seromarkers of chronic HBV and HCV infection were examined using commercial kits: HBeAg and HBsAg by radioimmunoassay (Abbott Laboratories, North Chicago, IL), and anti-HCV by enzyme-linked immunoassay using second-generation test kits (Abbott Laboratories). Serum HBV DNA level was quantified using a polymerase chain reaction–based nucleic acid amplification test (Cobas Amplicor HBV monitor test kit; Roche Diagnostics, Indianapolis, IN) with a certified detection limit of 300 copies/mL.

Ascertainment of Newly-developed Hepatocellular Carcinoma

Every participant was tested by abdominal ultrasonography every 3–12 months. Suspected HCC cases identified in regular health examinations were referred for further examinations using liver biopsy, angiogram, or computed tomography. Newly-developed HCC cases were ascertained through computerized linkage with national cancer registration and death certification profiles. The diagnostic criteria included histopathological confirmation, two coincident imaging findings, or AFP levels ≥400 ng/mL plus one positive imaging finding. [21].

Statistical Analysis

All statistical analyses were performed with SAS version 9.2 (SAS Institute, Cary, NC). Hazard ratios (HR) with 95% confidence intervals (CI) were derived to assess associations between predictors and newly-developed HCC through Cox proportional hazards regression analyses after adjustment for age, gender, and residential township. All 13 seromarkers were dichotomized into binary data using either upper or lower quartiles of the seromarkers in all participants as the cut-off points. The cut-off point for the AST/ALT ratio (AAR) was defined as 1 according to a previous study. [22] During the derivation of risk models, only seromarkers significantly associated with newly-developed HCC in multivariate regression models were included. The correlations among predictors included in the

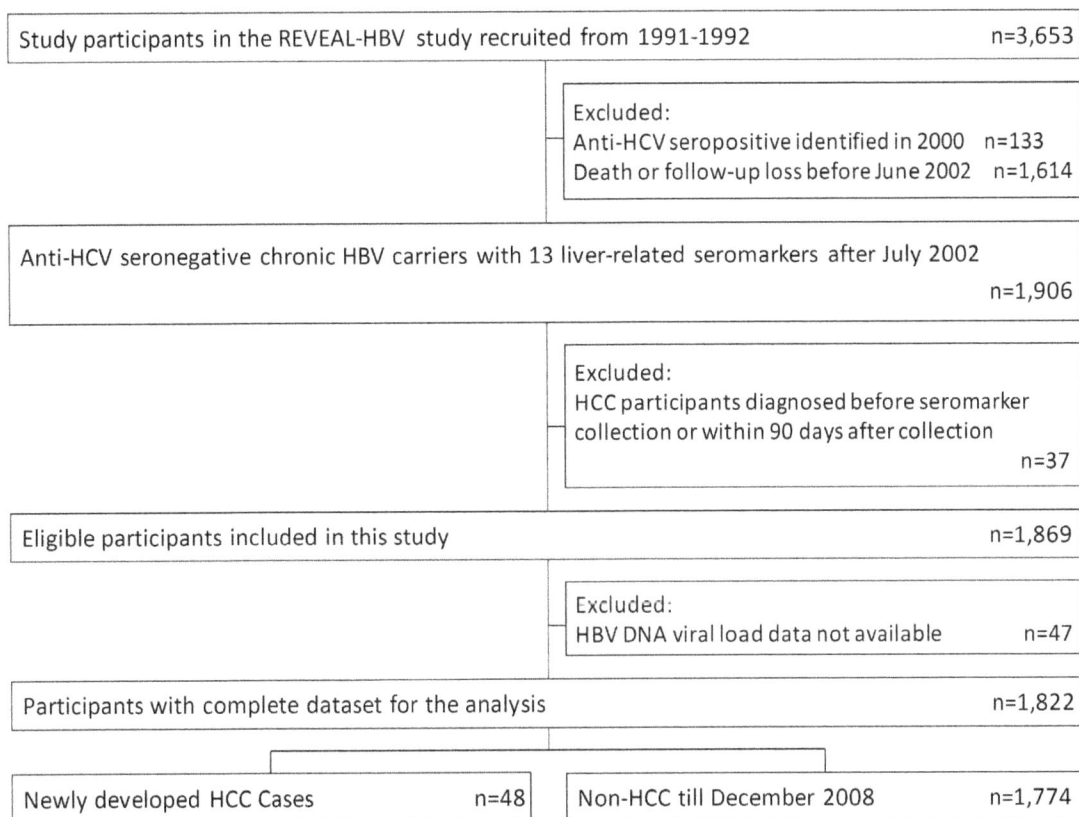

Figure 1. Flowchart of study participants selected from original REVEAL-HBV cohort and included in this analysis.

final scoring systems were evaluated by Pearson correlation coefficients.

The risk score for each 5-year increment in age was set as 1. Regression coefficients for other predictors included in the regression model were converted into integer scores by rounding the quotients of dividing each regression coefficient by the regression coefficient for each 5-year increment in age to the nearest integer. Sum scores were derived by adding the scores assigned to all risk predictors included in the specific model. The validity of risk models for the 6-year prediction of HCC risk was evaluated by using the area under the receiver operating characteristic curve (AUROC), the best Youden index (sensitivity+ specificity-1), the positive likelihood ratio [sensitivity/(1-specificity)], and the negative likelihood ratio [(1-sensitivity)/specificity] [23]. For evaluating and comparing the AUROCs of different prediction models, a nonparametric comparison of areas under correlated ROC curves was used. [24] The estimated 6-year cumulative incidence of HCC was calculated according to the following equation:

$$1 - S_0(t)^{\exp\left\{\left[\beta_{age}(42.5) + \beta_{age5y}(sum\ score)\right] - \sum_{i=1}^{p} \beta_i \bar{X}_i\right\}}$$

where $S_0(t)$ is the estimate of the average survival at 6 years, β_{age} is the regression coefficient of age, 42.5 is the age value we considered as the base, β_{age5y} is the regression coefficient for each 5-year increment in age, β_i is the regression coefficient for the ith covariate, and $\bar{X}_i$ is the mean level of the ith covariate. [13,14,25] The Student's t-test was used for comparing mean total scores between HCC and non-HCC groups among cirrhotic patients, and between

HCC participants with and without cirrhosis. The paired t-test was used for testing the stability of sum scores in model II.

Ethics Statement

This study was approved by the Institutional Review Board of the College of Public Health, National Taiwan University in Taipei, Taiwan.

Results

Risk Predictors of Hepatocellular Carcinoma

During the follow-up of 1,822 anti-HCV-seronegative chronic HBV carriers for a median period of 5.9 years (range, 0.3–6.5 years), 48 newly-developed HCC cases occurred. HCC incidence rates stratified by risk predictors including age, gender, cirrhosis status, HBV seromarkers of serum HBV DNA level and HBeAg serostatus, the 13 liver-related seromarkers, and AAR are shown in Table 1. A significantly increased HCC incidence was associated with older age, male gender, cirrhosis, serum HBV DNA levels >10,000 copies/mL, and HBeAg seropositivity. Elevated serum levels of AST, ALT, AFP, GGT, and gamma globulin, increased AAR, and lower serum levels of albumin and alpha-1 globulin were also significantly associated with increased HCC risk. In the multivariate analysis, 6 seromarkers including ALT, AAR, AFP, GGT, albumin, and alpha-1 globulin remained significantly associated with the risk of HCC, and were included in the models for the prediction of the 6-year risk of HCC. Serum levels of AST and gamma globulin were no longer significantly associated with HCC risk after adjustment for other HCC predictors in the multivariate analysis. Since ALT and AST were highly correlated with a Pearson correlation coefficient of 0.80, ALT and AST were included into separate multivariate regression analyses. However, AST was still not significantly associated with HCC risk after adjustment for other HCC predictors, even when both ALT and AAR were excluded. The correlations between AAR and ALT (or AST) were low, showing a Pearson correlation coefficient of -0.17 between AAR and ALT, and 0.23 between AAR and AST.

Risk Models Combining Different HCC Predictors

Three risk models combining different sets of HCC predictors with their assigned scores are shown in Table 2. Risk Model I was the "classical risk model" and included age, gender, serum ALT levels, and HBV seromarkers in the model. This set of predictors has been previously reported to have good validity in predicting the 3-, 5- and 10-year risk of HCC in patients with chronic hepatitis B. [14] Risk Model II included age, gender, and the liver-related seromarkers ALT, AAR, AFP, GGT, albumin, and alpha-1 globulin as predictors, but did not include HBV seromarkers. Risk Model III included HBV seromarkers in addition to the predictors included in Risk Model II. All predictors included in each model were statistically significant except gender. Considering that gender differences are usually observed in HBV-related HCC, it was still included in the three risk models with an assigned score of 1. The Pearson correlation coefficients among seromarkers included in the scoring models ranged from -0.34 to 0.29. Therefore, the effect of colinearity among these seromarkers was considered minimal.

Validity and AUROC of Three Risk Models

Figure 2 shows the ROC curves for predicting 6-year HCC risk using the total scores of the three risk models. Sum scores were derived by adding the scores assigned to all risk predictors included in each specific model. For example, when applying Risk Model III to a 62-years-old (score = 4) man (score = 1) with serum ALT levels of 90 U/L (score = 3), an AAR of 1.1 (score = 6), AFP of 3 ng/mL (score = 0), GGT of 29 U/L (score = 0), albumin of 4.7 g/dL (score = 0), and alpha-1 globulin of 0.3 g/dL (score = 0), as well as HBeAg-seronegative status with a serum HBV DNA level of 50,000 copies/mL (score = 3), the total score is 17.

The AUROC of Risk Model I was 0.83 for predicting 6-year HCC risk, which was consistent previous studies. [14] The best Youden index of Risk Model I was 0.50 for the 6-year prediction, while the positive likelihood ratio (LR+) and negative likelihood ratio (LR$-$) were 2.17 and 0.11, respectively. The AUROC, best Youden index, LR+, and LR$-$ were 0.89, 0.63, 10.38, and 0.33, respectively for Risk Model II, as well as 0.91, 0.68, 6.52 and 0.22, respectively for Risk Model III. When defining the cut-off point by using the highest Youden index, the best cut-off total scores were set as 6 for Model I, 22 for Model II, and 19 for Model III. The corresponding sensitivity and specificity according to these cut-offs were 0.93 and 0.57 for Model I; 0.70 and 0.93 for Model II; and 0.80 and 0.88 for Model III, respectively. The predictability of the three risk models was considered very good to excellent with significant improvements when comparing the AUROC of Risk Model I with the AUROCs of Risk Model II (P = 0.01) and Risk Model III (p<0.001).

As most of the predictors included in Risk Model II and Risk Model III were also seromarkers for cirrhosis, whether or not the risk models could differentiate HCC from cirrhosis was further assessed. The student's t-test was used for comparing the means of total scores between cirrhotic patients with or without HCC, and between HCC participants with or without cirrhosis. For Risk Model II, the mean (95% CI) sum score was 15.1 (14.1–16.2) for 135 cirrhotic patients without HCC, and 24.4 (22.0–26.8) for 27

cirrhotic patients with HCC. For Risk Model III, the mean (95% CI) sum score was 14.9 (13.9–15.9) for 135 cirrhotic patients without HCC and 24.0 (21.9–26.2) for 27 cirrhotic patients with HCC. The differences in means were statistically significant (P<0.001) between cirrhotic patients with or without HCC for both Risk Model II and III. However, the mean sum score was not significantly different between HCC patients with and without cirrhosis for either Risk Model II (P = 0.403) or Risk Model III (P = 0.300). This suggests that both Risk Models had good HCC risk predictability, regardless of cirrhosis status.

Since liver-related seromarkers may change over time, another set of seromarkers in blood samples collected on dates different from baseline was compared to that of blood samples collected and analyzed to derive the risk scores. Among the 1,822 participants, 1,543 had another blood sample collected at a later time point (mean time interval: 314 days, median time interval: 356 days). Comparing sum scores of ALT, AAR, AFP, GGT, albumin, and alpha-1 globulin from Risk Model II at the two time points, there was no significant difference in total score based on a paired t-test (P = 0.77). Similar results were found for HCC cases (n = 35, mean time interval: 229 days, median time interval: 184 days, P = 0.87) and non-HCC cases (n = 1,508, mean time interval: 316 days, median time interval: 356 days, P = 0.79), respectively.

Figure 3 shows the cumulative incidence of HCC for participants classified into three groups using their sum scores from each risk model. Cut-off points of sum scores were set as 8 and 12 for Risk Model I, 22 and 27 for Risk Model II, and 21 and 26 for Risk Model III, according to the best stratification of HCC cases into three approximately equal groups. There were striking differences in cumulative HCC incidence during follow-up between the three groups with high, medium, and low sum scores, suggesting that the three Risk Models had an excellent discriminating capability to triage chronic HBV carriers with regards to their 6-year risk of HCC.

Estimated HCC Incidence by Risk Model II and III

Table 3 shows the estimated 6-year cumulative HCC risk according to sum scores of Risk Model II and III. For Risk Model II, the estimated 6-year cumulative risk of HCC ranged from 0.01% for a total score of 0 to 96.71% for a total score of 34. For Risk Model III, the estimated 6-year cumulative risk of HCC ranged from 0.01% for a total score of 0 to 99.52% for a total score of 33. Both Risk Models had a wide range of estimated HCC risk, again suggesting their excellent discriminating capability.

Discussion

HBV-associated HCC remains a serious public health problem worldwide, especially in developing countries with lower income and inadequate medical resources. [26] In this study, we aimed to develop valid and easy-to-use HCC prediction models for chronic HBV carriers using liver-related seromarkers. In previous studies, various HBV seromarkers including serum HBV viral load, genotype, and mutants were used as predictors in HCC risk prediction models. [11–14] However, these seromarkers are not routinely tested in regular health examinations at most clinics. Therefore, we aimed to develop prediction models combining several liver-related seromarkers for HCC, even though we had already proposed a good prediction model (Risk Model I). In this study, we found that both models combining liver-related seromarkers with (Risk Model III) or without (Risk Model II) HBV seromarkers of serum HBV DNA level and HBeAg serostatus had good validity and discriminating capability to

Table 1. Incidence Rates and Adjusted Hazard Ratios of Developing Hepatocellular Carcinoma (HCC) by Risk Predictors in 1,822 Anti-HCV-Seronegative Chronic HBV Carriers.

Baseline Demographic or Characteristic[+]	Number (%) of Participants (n = 1,822)	Person-years of Follow-up (Total = 10,083)	Number of HCC cases (n = 48)	Incidence Rate per 100,000 Person-years	Adjusted Hazard Ratio* (95% confidence interval)	P-value
Age						
40–49	595 (32.7)	3,435	5	146	1.00	
50–59	540 (29.6)	3,039	12	395	2.70 (0.95–7.66)	0.062
60+	687 (37.7)	3,609	31	859	6.04 (2.35–15.55)	<0.001
Gender						
Female	407 (22.3)	2,235	6	268	1.00	
Male	1,415 (77.7)	7,848	42	535	2.62 (1.07–6.41)	0.035
Cirrhosis						
No	1,660 (91.1)	9,227	21	228	1.00	
Yes	162 (8.9)	856	27	3,154	12.55 (7.06–22.33)	<0.001
HBV seromarkers						
HBeAg negative and HBV DNA ≤10,000 copies/mL	1,251 (68.7)	7,024	12	171	1.00	
HBeAg negative and HBV DNA >10,000 copies/mL	448 (24.6)	2,404	19	790	5.99 (2.87–12.51)	<0.001
HBeAg positive	123 (6.8)	655	17	2,595	20.71 (9.64–44.50)	<0.001
Serum AST level						
<30 U/L	1,336 (73.3)	7,464	11	147	1.00	
≥30 U/L	486 (26.7)	2,619	37	1,413	9.56 (4.87–18.77)	<0.001
Serum ALT level						
<28 U/L	1,324 (72.7)	7,333	18	245	1.00	
≥28 U/L	498 (27.3)	2,750	30	1,091	5.83 (3.19–10.65)	<0.001
AAR						
<1	651 (35.7)	3,732	4	107	1.00	
≥1	1,171 (64.3)	6,351	44	693	5.78 (2.06–16.24)	0.001
Serum AFP level						
<5 ng/mL	1,390 (76.3)	7,814	15	192	1.00	
≥5 ng/mL	432 (23.7)	2,269	33	1,454	8.16 (4.42–15.07)	<0.001
Serum GGT level						
<41 U/L	1,353 (74.3)	7,600	14	184	1.00	
≥41 U/L	469 (25.7)	2,483	34	1,369	7.73 (4.09–14.60)	<0.001
Serum total bilirubin level						
<0.8 mg/dL	1,365 (74.9)	7,561	32	423	1.00	
≥0.8 mg/dL	457 (25.1)	2,522	16	634	1.39 (0.76–2.54)	0.285
Serum total protein level						
>7.1 g/dL	1,362 (74.8)	7,480	33	441	1.00	
≤7.1 g/dL	460 (25.3)	2,603	15	576	1.18 (0.64–2.18)	0.601
Serum albumin level						
>4.1 g/dL	1,330 (73.0)	7,302	21	288	1.00	
≤4.1 g/dL	492 (27.0)	2,781	27	971	3.11 (1.75–5.53)	<0.001
Serum alpha-1 globulin level						
>0.2 g/dL	1,219 (66.9)	6,701	23	343	1.00	
≤0.2 g/dL	603 (33.1)	3,382	25	739	2.20 (1.24–3.89)	0.007
Serum alpha-2 globulin level						
>0.6 g/dL	495 (27.2)	2,814	11	391	1.00	
≤0.6 g/dL	1,327 (72.8)	7,269	37	509	1.30 (0.66–2.55)	0.450

Table 1. Cont.

Baseline Demographic or Characteristic[+]	Number (%) of Participants (n = 1,822)	Person-years of Follow-up (Total = 10,083)	Number of HCC cases (n = 48)	Incidence Rate per 100,000 Person-years	Adjusted Hazard Ratio* (95% confidence interval)	P-value
Serum beta globulin level						
<1 g/dL	1,256 (68.9)	6,904	29	420	1.00	
≥1 g/dL	566 (31.1)	3,179	19	598	1.47 (0.82–2.63)	0.192
Serum gamma globulin level						
<1.4 g/dL	943 (51.8)	5,192	13	250	1.00	
≥1.4 g/dL	879 (48.2)	4,891	35	716	3.07 (1.62–5.81)	<0.001
Serum apolipoprotein A1 level						
<149 mg/dL	1,358 (74.5)	7,537	33	438	1.00	
≥149 mg/dL	464 (25.5)	2,546	15	589	1.64 (0.88–3.05)	0.116
Serum apolipoprotein B level						
>72 mg/dL	1,343 (73.7)	7,433	35	471	1.00	
≤72 mg/dL	479 (26.3)	2,650	13	491	1.17 (0.62–2.21)	0.636

+: Using the quartile of each seromarker as the cut-off point except AAR.
*: Age, gender, and study townships were included in Cox proportional hazards models.
Abbreviation: HCC, hepatocellular carcinoma; HBeAg, hepatitis B e antigen; Anti-HCV, antibodies against hepatitis C virus; HBV, hepatitis B virus; AST, aspartate aminotransferase; ALT, alanine aminotransferase; AAR, AST/ALT ratio; AFP, alpha-fetoprotein; GGT, gamma-glutamyltransferase.

differentiate chronic HBV carriers with variable risks of developing HCC.

All of the liver-related seromarkers we analyzed are associated with liver diseases such as fibrosis, cirrhosis, jaundice, and fatty liver. They may reflect the status of the liver, such as liver cells injury, inflammation, necroinflammation, or proliferation, at the time of examination. AAR has been suggested as a fibrosis marker. By analyzing these 13 liver-related seromarkers along with the AAR, we first tried to find out candidate predictors that had significant associations with HCC. Then, we further selected predictors according to the results of multivariate analysis and biological rationale. Finally, liver-related seromarkers included in the models were ALT, AAR, AFP, GGT, albumin, and alpha-1 globulin. All of them were significantly associated with HCC in multivariate analyses. Among the six predictors, ALT, AAR, AFP, GGT, and albumin are widely used. Although Alpha-1 globulin is not commonly used, it had an independent and significant association with HCC in this study, and is also available in clinical practice. In addition, both ALT and albumin have been found to be HCC predictors in chronic hepatitis B patients. [12–14] AFP is a well-known HCC seromarker, and AAR is a cirrhotic marker that may reflect progressive liver functional impairment if it equals 1 or higher. [22] Serum GGT mostly comes from liver; it has been found to be useful for the diagnosis of HCC in patients with low AFP levels or at a relatively early stage. [27] The deficiency of alpha-1-antitrypsin, the main (~90%) protein of the alpha-1 globulins, has been found to be associated with an increased risk for liver damage, cirrhosis and HCC. [28].

In the long natural history of chronic hepatitis B, risk predictors of HCC may change over time. Some HCC predictors are more appropriate for long-term prediction, while some are better short-term predictors. Usually, liver fibrosis and cirrhosis occur sequentially before the development of HCC in chronic hepatitis B patients. During the hepatopathogenic progression, however, various seromarkers are changing dynamically. These seromarkers may thus be categorized as long-term and short-term risk predictors. When the onset of HCC is closer, useful predictors

will shift from the long-term predictors, such as HBeAg serostatus and serum HBV DNA level, to the short-term predictors, which may be surrogate variables of severe fibrosis or even cirrhosis. Both ALT and GGT are inflammatory markers; AAR and albumin are associated with liver fibrosis; AFP is associated with liver cell proliferation; and decreased alpha-1 globulin proteins may either be a sign of alpha-1 antitrypsin deficiency related to the pathogenesis of HCC, or reflect the reduced production of required proteins due to impaired liver function. All are biomarkers that reflect the disease status of the liver, and may be referred to as short-term predictors. However, ALT is also a long-term predictor since it is related to the hosts immunoreactivity to HBV.

Thus, the importance of HBeAg serostatus and serum HBV DNA levels in the prediction of HCC risk may decrease when chronic hepatitis B progresses from the immune tolerance phase, through the immune clearance phase, to the residual phase. HBeAg serostatus and HBV DNA levels had less additional predictability for the short-term risk of HCC if seromarkers of liver necroinflammation and fibrosis/cirrhosis were also taken into consideration. As HBeAg serostatus and serum HBV DNA level are the most important long-term predictors of HCC, antiviral therapy to lower viral load has a very significant impact on the reduction of HCC risk, especially for those patients without severe fibrosis or cirrhosis. The efficacy of therapeutic intervention for hepatitis B has been assessed and proven. Although sustained HBV DNA suppression is rarely associated with HBV clearance, it results in reduced rates of liver complications, including HCC and the progression of cirrhosis. [17] Though the importance of HBeAg serostatus and serum HBV DNA level shows is minor for the 6-year prediction of HCC, they still provide useful information for the continued care of chronic hepatitis B patients. The findings of this study suggest that in addition to antiviral therapy to lower HBV viral loads, other interventions to reverse fibrosis and cirrhosis are also important for the reduction of HCC risk.

Besides HBV seromarkers, age, gender, and liver cirrhosis are usually considered as important predictors in HCC risk models.

Table 2. Multivariate-adjusted Hazard Ratios (HR), Regression Coefficients, and Assigned Scores for Hepatocellular Carcinoma Predictors in Three Risk Models.

Predictors		Hazard Ratio/Regression Coefficient/Assigned Score										
		Risk Model I				Risk Model II				Risk Model III			
		HR (95%CI)	β coefficient	Score	P-value	HR (95%CI)	β coefficient	Score	P-value	HR (95%CI)	β coefficient	Score	P-value
Age (5-year increments from 40 years old)		1.58 (1.35–1.86)	0.4601	1	<0.001	1.37 (1.16–1.61)	0.3110	1	<0.001	1.40 (1.18–1.66)	0.3355	1	<0.001
Gender	Female	1.00	Reference	0		1.00	Reference	0		1.00	Reference	0	
	Male	1.55 (0.65–3.71)	0.4372	1	0.317	1.59 (0.65–3.86)	0.4633	1	0.306	1.59 (0.64–3.96)	0.4634	1	0.320
ALT (U/L)	<28	1.00	Reference	0		1.00	Reference	0		1.00	Reference	0	
	≥28	3.06 (1.61–5.83)	1.1189	2	<0.001	4.65 (2.46–8.76)	1.5358	5	<0.001	2.68 (1.36–5.28)	0.9848	3	0.005
AAR	<1					1.00	Reference	0		1.00	Reference	0	
	≥1					9.04 (3.13–26.06)	2.2012	7	<0.001	7.19 (2.46–20.99)	1.9723	6	<0.001
AFP (ng/mL)	<5					1.00	Reference	0		1.00	Reference	0	
	≥5					4.71 (2.50–8.86)	1.5486	5	<0.001	3.65 (1.86–7.14)	1.2938	4	<0.001
GGT (U/L)	<41					1.00	Reference	0		1.00	Reference	0	
	≥41					3.50 (1.77–6.92)	1.2525	4	<0.001	3.44 (1.73–6.86)	1.2354	4	<0.001
Albumin (g/dL)	>4.1					1.00	Reference	0		1.00	Reference	0	
	≤4.1					3.13 (1.74–5.63)	1.1400	4	<0.001	2.54 (1.39–4.64)	0.9308	3	0.003
Alpha-1 globulin (g/dL)	>0.2					1.00	Reference	0		1.00	Reference	0	
	≤0.2					2.07 (1.15–3.72)	0.7266	2	0.015	1.94 (1.08–3.50)	0.6638	2	0.027
HBeAg negative and HBV DNA ≤10,000*		1.00	Reference	0						1.00	Reference	0	
HBeAg negative and HBV DNA >10,000*		4.11 (1.93–8.75)	1.4144	3						3.19 (1.46–6.98)	1.1608	3	0.004
HBeAg positive		14.50 (6.50–32.35)	2.6743	6						4.72 (1.99–11.19)	1.5524	5	<0.001

Abbreviation: HBeAg, hepatitis B e antigen; HBV, hepatitis B virus; ALT, alanine aminotransferase; AAR, aspartate aminotransferase/alanine aminotransferase ratio; AFP, alpha-fetoprotein; GGT, gamma-glutamyltransferase.
*: Serum HBV DNA level, copies per mL.

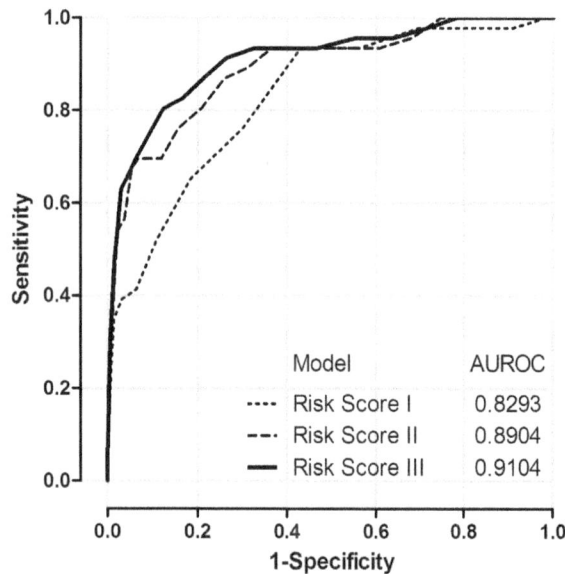

Figure 2. Receiver operating characteristic curves (ROCs) and areas under receiver operating characteristic curves (AUROCs). ROCs and AUROCs for the prediction of the 6-year incidence of hepatocellular carcinoma using sum scores of three risk models: The classical model (Risk Model I, dotted line), the model combining liver-related seromarkers without HBV seromarkers of HBeAg serostatus and serum HBV DNA level (Risk Model II, broken line), and the model combining liver-related seromarkers with HBV seromarkers (Risk Model III, solid line).

[11,12] Liver cirrhosis is a precursor to HCC. Each year, 2–8% of patients with HBV-related cirrhosis, either compensated cirrhosis or decompensated, may further develop HCC. [29] Cirrhosis status was not included as a predictor in our models because a confirmatory diagnosis of cirrhosis using liver biopsy was not feasible in a community-based cohort. Furthermore, most of the liver-related seromarkers used in our models are associated with liver stiffness and may be considered as surrogate biomarkers for cirrhosis. [30].

Since participants in this community-based prospective study were healthier than patients in hospital-based studies, most participants would be classified as "normal" for these liver-related seromarkers if current clinical cut-off points were applied. Therefore, in this study, the cut-off points of these seromarkers were set by their first or third quartiles instead of the normal limits routinely used in clinical practice, such as 40 U/L for ALT and 20 ng/mL for AFP. Indeed, the revised cut-off points of these seromarkers were found to be significantly associated with an increased risk of subsequent HCC. We used binary variables to reduce the influence of occasional fluctuations because the scoring was based on the dichotomous classification of "positive" or "negative" instead of exact measurements of liver-related seromarkers. In Risk Models I and III, serum HBV DNA level and HBeAg serostatus were combined to classify participants into three groups: 1) HBeAg-seronegatives with serum HBV DNA level ≤10,000 copies/mL, 2) HBeAg-seronegatives with serum HBV DNA level >10,000 copies/mL, and 3) HBeAg-seropositives, as almost all HBeAg-seropositives had very high serum levels of HBV DNA. The cut-off point of 10,000 copies/mL was used for serum HBV DNA levels according to our previous observation that serum HBV DNA levels seldom rebound again once they have spontaneously decreased ≤10,000 copies/mL. [1] The combina-

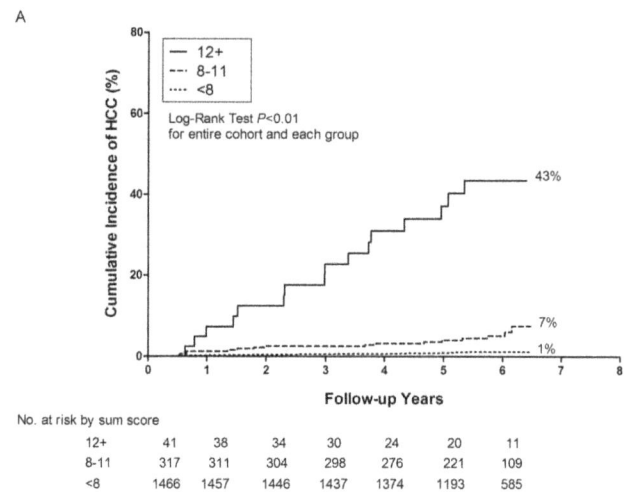

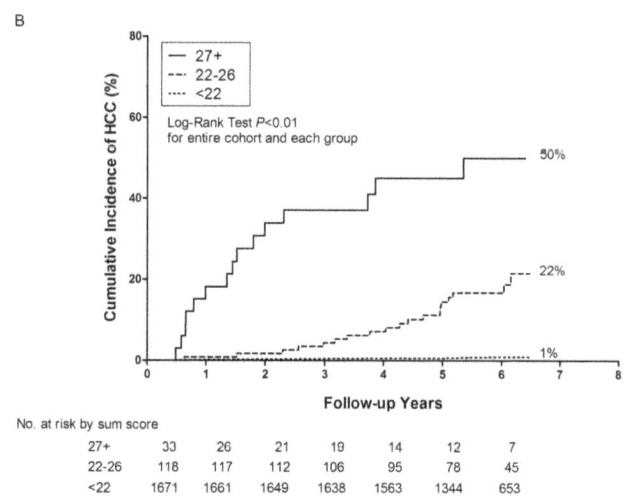

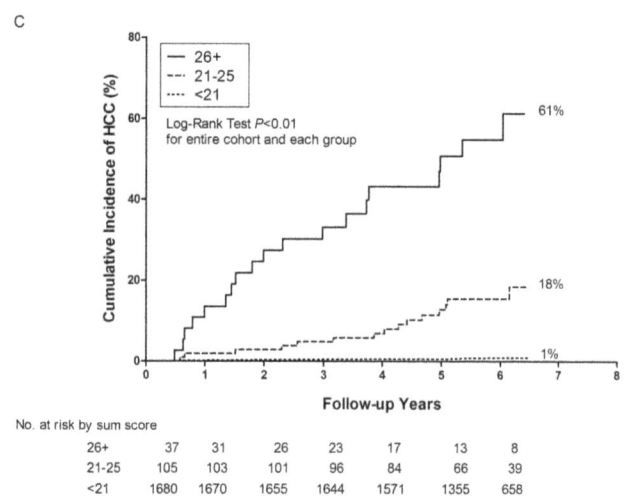

Figure 3. Cumulative incidence of hepatocellular carcinoma (HCC) by sum scores of each model at study entry. Classical model (Risk Model I, A), the model combining liver-related seromarkers without HBV seromarkers of HBeAg serostatus and serum HBV DNA level (Risk Model II, B), and the model combining liver-related seromarkers with HBV seromarkers (Risk Model III, C).

Table 3. Estimated 6-year Incidence of Hepatocellular Carcinoma Using Risk Models Combining Liver-related Seromarkers without (Model II) and with (Model III) HBV Seromarkers of HBeAg Serostatus and Serum HBV DNA Level.

Risk Model II		Risk Model III	
Sum Score	Estimate Risk (%)	Sum Score	Estimate Risk (%)
0	0.01	0	0.01
1	0.01	1	0.01
2	0.02	2	0.02
3	0.02	3	0.02
4	0.03	4	0.03
5	0.04	5	0.04
6	0.06	6	0.06
7	0.08	7	0.09
8	0.11	8	0.12
9	0.14	9	0.17
10	0.20	10	0.24
11	0.27	11	0.33
12	0.36	12	0.46
13	0.50	13	0.65
14	0.68	14	0.90
15	0.92	15	1.26
16	1.26	16	1.76
17	1.71	17	2.46
18	2.33	18	3.42
19	3.16	19	4.75
20	4.29	20	6.58
21	5.81	21	9.08
22	7.85	22	12.46
23	10.55	23	16.98
24	14.12	24	22.92
25	18.76	25	30.52
26	24.69	26	39.91
27	32.09	27	50.96
28	41.03	28	63.08
29	51.37	29	75.19
30	62.61	30	85.76
31	73.89	31	93.46
32	84.00	32	97.79
33	91.80	33	99.52
34	96.71		

tion of several seromarkers was considered adequate for deriving a stable risk estimation.

A specific aim of this study was to develop an evidence-based risk score to provide clinicians with the expected HCC risk for a patient infected with chronic hepatitis B. Developing such a score may help patient consultation and clinical management. The validity of the prediction models was evaluated using the AUROC as shown in Figure 2, and by assessing their discriminatory capability as shown in Figure 3. Furthermore, we provided an estimate of 6-year HCC risk according to total scores, which

makes it easy for clinicians to obtain a patient's 6-year risk of HCC and then give the patient clinical advice accordingly. Based on these findings, we suggest that chronic HBV carriers be tested for their liver-related seromarkers at their first clinical visit, and that our Risk Model II be used to calculate their probability of developing HCC in 6 years. Both HBeAg serostatus and serum HBV DNA level may be further tested to derive Risk Model III for the refinement of HCC risk prediction. Those who have high total scores should be further assessed for (1) whether or not they can be treated with antivirals or immune moderators to interrupt the progression of chronic hepatitis B to severe fibrosis, cirrhosis or even HCC; (2) how frequently they should be monitored by abdominal ultrasonography to detect HCC at a very early stage; and (3) what healthier lifestyles they should maintain.

There are some limitations to be considered if these risk models are to be applied to chronic HBV carriers in other populations. Firstly, almost all study participants were infected with HBV during early childhood and experienced the immune tolerance phase in this analysis. Whether or not the findings in this study may be applicable to patients infected in adulthood needs further elucidation. Secondly, participants enrolled in this study were middle aged adults. Therefore, the risk models may not apply to younger chronic HBV carriers. Thirdly, only seromarkers at study entry were included in this analysis, and whether seromarkers during follow-up are also important in risk prediction also deserves further elucidation. Lastly, all participants were infected with HBV genotype B and/or C, and whether or not the natural history of chronic HBV infection is the same for genotypes A, D or others also remains to be clarified.

In conclusion, we found that liver-related seromarkers may be combined to predict HCC risk of chronic hepatitis B patients, and two risk models incorporating liver-related seromarkers with and without HBV seromarkers were developed for the prediction of the 6-year risk of HCC. The models were found to have high validity and discriminating capability for the identification of high-risk groups for HCC. These risk models were accurate, inexpensive and easy-to-use. However, further external validation of the risk models is needed if they will be applied to chronic hepatitis B patients in different populations.

Acknowledgments

We thank the other members of the Risk Evaluation of Viral Load Elevation and Associated Liver Disease/Cancer-Hepatitis B Virus (R.E.V.E.A.L.-HBV) Study Group: C. Y. Hsieh, H.S. Lee, P. M. Yang, C. H. Chen, J. D. Chen, S. P. Huang, C. F. Jan (National Taiwan University Hospital); T. H. H. Chen (National Taiwan University); C. A. Sun (National Defense Medical Center); M. H. Wu (Taipei City Psychiatric Center); S. Y. Chen (Tzu Chi University); K. E. Chu (Shin Kong Wu Ho-Su Memorial Hospital); S. C. Ho, T. G. Lu (Huhsi Health Center, Penghu County); W. P. Wu, T. Y. Ou (Provincial Penghu Hospital); C. G. Lin (Sanchi Health Center, Taipei County); K. C. Shih (Provincial Chutung Hospital); W. S. Chung, C. Li (Provincial Potzu Hospital); C. C. Chen (Kaohsu Health Center, Pingtung County); W. C. How (Paihsa Health Center, Penghu County). Their efforts to complete the data collection are highly appreciated.

Author Contributions

Conceived and designed the experiments: YJL MHL HIY CLJ SLY LYW SNL JL CJC. Performed the experiments: YJL MHL HIY CLJ SLY LYW SNL JL CJC. Analyzed the data: YJL MHL HIY CLJ SLY LYW SNL JL CJC. Contributed reagents/materials/analysis tools: YJL MHL HIY CLJ SLY LYW SNL JL CJC. Wrote the paper: YJL MHL HIY CLJ SLY LYW SNL JL CJC.

References

1. Chen CJ, Yang HI (2011) Natural history of chronic hepatitis B REVEALed. J Gastroenterol Hepatol 26: 628–638.
2. El-Serag HB (2012) Epidemiology of viral hepatitis and hepatocellular carcinoma. Gastroenterology 142: 1264–1273 e1261.
3. Ott JJ, Stevens GA, Groeger J, Wiersma ST (2012) Global epidemiology of hepatitis B virus infection: new estimates of age-specific HBsAg seroprevalence and endemicity. Vaccine 30: 2212–2219.
4. Chen CJ, Yang HI, Su J, Jen CL, You SL, et al. (2006) Risk of hepatocellular carcinoma across a biological gradient of serum hepatitis B virus DNA level. JAMA 295: 65–73.
5. Morgan TR, Mandayam S, Jamal MM (2004) Alcohol and hepatocellular carcinoma. Gastroenterology 127: S87–96.
6. Fattovich G, Stroffolini T, Zagni I, Donato F (2004) Hepatocellular carcinoma in cirrhosis: incidence and risk factors. Gastroenterology 127: S35–50.
7. Yang HI, Lu SN, Liaw YF, You SL, Sun CA, et al. (2002) Hepatitis B e antigen and the risk of hepatocellular carcinoma. N Engl J Med 347: 168–174.
8. Chen CJ, Yang HI, Iloeje UH (2009) Hepatitis B virus DNA levels and outcomes in chronic hepatitis B. Hepatology 49: S72–84.
9. Chan HL, Hui AY, Wong ML, Tse AM, Hung LC, et al. (2004) Genotype C hepatitis B virus infection is associated with an increased risk of hepatocellular carcinoma. Gut 53: 1494–1498.
10. Kao JH, Chen PJ, Lai MY, Chen DS (2003) Basal core promoter mutations of hepatitis B virus increase the risk of hepatocellular carcinoma in hepatitis B carriers. Gastroenterology 124: 327–334.
11. Yuen MF, Tanaka Y, Fong DY, Fung J, Wong DK, et al. (2009) Independent risk factors and predictive score for the development of hepatocellular carcinoma in chronic hepatitis B. J Hepatol 50: 80–88.
12. Wong VW, Chan SL, Mo F, Chan TC, Loong HH, et al. (2010) Clinical scoring system to predict hepatocellular carcinoma in chronic hepatitis B carriers. J Clin Oncol 28: 1660–1665.
13. Yang HI, Sherman M, Su J, Chen PJ, Liaw YF, et al. (2010) Nomograms for risk of hepatocellular carcinoma in patients with chronic hepatitis B virus infection. J Clin Oncol 28: 2437–2444.
14. Yang HI, Yuen MF, Chan HL, Han KH, Chen PJ, et al. (2011) Risk estimation for hepatocellular carcinoma in chronic hepatitis B (REACH-B): development and validation of a predictive score. Lancet Oncol 12: 568–574.
15. Liaw YF, Sung JJ, Chow WC, Farrell G, Lee CZ, et al. (2004) Lamivudine for patients with chronic hepatitis B and advanced liver disease. N Engl J Med 351: 1521–1531.
16. Yuen MF, Seto WK, Chow DH, Tsui K, Wong DK, et al. (2007) Long-term lamivudine therapy reduces the risk of long-term complications of chronic hepatitis B infection even in patients without advanced disease. Antivir Ther 12: 1295–1303.
17. Aghemo A, Lampertico P, Colombo M (2012) Assessing long-term treatment efficacy in chronic hepatitis B and C: between evidence and common sense. J Hepatol 57: 1326–1335.
18. Imbert-Bismut F, Ratziu V, Pieroni L, Charlotte F, Benhamou Y, et al. (2001) Biochemical markers of liver fibrosis in patients with hepatitis C virus infection: a prospective study. Lancet 357: 1069–1075.
19. Baranova A, Lal P, Birerdinc A, Younossi ZM (2011) Non-invasive markers for hepatic fibrosis. BMC Gastroenterol 11: 91.
20. Iloeje UH, Yang HI, Su J, Jen CL, You SL, et al. (2006) Predicting cirrhosis risk based on the level of circulating hepatitis B viral load. Gastroenterology 130: 678–686.
21. Bruix J, Sherman M, Llovet JM, Beaugrand M, Lencioni R, et al. (2001) Clinical management of hepatocellular carcinoma. Conclusions of the Barcelona-2000 EASL conference. European Association for the Study of the Liver. J Hepatol 35: 421–430.
22. Giannini E, Risso D, Botta F, Chiarbonello B, Fasoli A, et al. (2003) Validity and clinical utility of the aspartate aminotransferase-alanine aminotransferase ratio in assessing disease severity and prognosis in patients with hepatitis C virus-related chronic liver disease. Arch Intern Med 163: 218–224.
23. Grimes DA, Schulz KF (2005) Refining clinical diagnosis with likelihood ratios. Lancet 365: 1500–1505.
24. DeLong ER, DeLong DM, Clarke-Pearson DL (1988) Comparing the areas under two or more correlated receiver operating characteristic curves: a nonparametric approach. Biometrics 44: 837–845.
25. Sullivan LM, Massaro JM, D'Agostino RB Sr. (2004) Presentation of multivariate data for clinical use: The Framingham Study risk score functions. Stat Med 23: 1631–1660.
26. Yang JD, Roberts LR (2010) Hepatocellular carcinoma: A global view. Nat Rev Gastroenterol Hepatol 7. 440–450.
27. Sawabu N, Nakagen M, Ozaki K, Wakabayashi T, Toya D, et al. (1983) Clinical evaluation of specific gamma-GTP isoenzyme in patients with hepatocellular carcinoma. Cancer 51: 327–331.
28. Eriksson S, Carlson J, Velez R (1986) Risk of cirrhosis and primary liver cancer in alpha 1-antitrypsin deficiency. N Engl J Med 314: 736–739.
29. Peng CY, Chien RN, Liaw YF (2012) Hepatitis B virus-related decompensated liver disease: Benefits of antiviral therapy. J Hepatol.
30. Fung J, Lai CL, Fong DY, Yuen JC, Wong DK, et al. (2008) Correlation of liver biochemistry with liver stiffness in chronic hepatitis B and development of a predictive model for liver fibrosis. Liver Int 28: 1408–1416.

Decreased Peripheral Natural Killer Cells Activity in the Immune Activated Stage of Chronic Hepatitis B

Yuan Li[1¤], Jiu-Jun Wang[1], Shan Gao[1], Qian Liu[1], Jia Bai[1], Xue-Qi Zhao[1], You-Hua Hao[2], Hong-Hui Ding[2], Fan Zhu[2], Dong-Liang Yang[2], Xi-Ping Zhao[1]*

1 Department of Infectious Diseases, Tongji Hospital, Tongji Medical College, Huazhong University of Science and Technology, Wuhan, P. R. China, 2 Division of Clinical Immunology, Tongji Hospital, Tongji Medical College, Huazhong University of Science and Technology, Wuhan, P. R. China

Abstract

Background & Aims: The natural course of chronic hepatitis B virus (HBV) infection is characterized by different immune responses, ranging from immune tolerant (IT) to immune activated (IA) stages. In our study, we investigated the natural killer (NK) cells activity in patients at different immunological stages of chronic HBV infection.

Methods: Blood samples obtained from 57 HBeAg positive patients with chronic hepatitis B (CHB), including 15 patients in the immune tolerant (IT) stage, 42 patients in the immune activated (IA) stage, and 18 healthy individuals (HI). The analyses included flow cytometry to detect NK cells, the determination of cytokine levels as well as of surface receptor expression and cytotoxicity.

Results: NK cells in peripheral blood were significantly lower in patients in the IA stage of CHB compared to HI (p<0.05). Patients in the IA stage of CHB had lower levels of NK cells activating receptor NKp30 and NKG2D expression, cytokine interferon-γ (IFN-γ) and tumor necrosis factor-α (TNF-α) production, as compared to patients in the IT stage and HI, respectively (p<0.05). Cytotoxicity of NK cells was lower in patients in the IA stage of CHB compared to patients in the IT stage and HI, respectively (p<0.05). The level of IFN-γ but not level of TNF-α and cytotoxicity of NK cells was inversely correlated with serum HBV load in patients with CHB. Peripheral NK cells activity did not correlate with ALT level.

Conclusion: NK cells activity was lower in CHB patients, especially in those in the IA stage.

Editor: Johan K. Sandberg, Karolinska Institutet, Sweden

Funding: This work was supported by grants from the National Science Fund of China (NSFC) (grant number 30771911), the National Key Basic Research Program of China (grant number 2009CB522502) and the National Science and Technology Major Project (grant numbers 2008ZX10002-014, 2008ZX10002-009, 2012ZX10002007-003). The funders had no role in study design, data collection and analysis, decision to publish, or preparation of the manuscript.

Competing Interests: The authors have declared that no competing interests exist.

* E-mail: xpzhao@tjh.tjmu.edu.cn

¤ Current address: Department of Liver Diseases, The First Affiliated Hospital of Guangxi University of Chinese Medicine, Nanning, P. R. China

Introduction

Hepatitis B virus (HBV) infection is a leading cause of liver diseases worldwide, especially in Asia and is associated with a wide spectrum of clinical manifestations, ranging from an asymptomatic course to active hepatitis B with progression to liver cirrhosis and hepatocellular carcinoma (HCC).

While HBV is not directly a cytopathic, the pathogenesis of HBV-related liver disease is immune mediated. The natural course of chronic HBV infection can present as different immunological stages, including immune tolerance and immune activation. The different immunological states of chronic HBV infection are associated with different levels of viral replication and inflammation as well as cellular immunity and humoral immunity [1]. The immune tolerant (IT) stage is characterized by HBeAg positivity, high levels of serum HBV DNA, normal serum alanine aminotransferase (ALT) levels and normal or minimally abnormal liver histology [2,3]. The HBV-specific immune response in the IT stage is very low or even absent. The immune activated (IA) stage is characterized by low levels of serum HBV DNA, elevated ALT levels, and active inflammation and even fibrosis in liver tissue [2,3]. In the IA stage, there is an HBV-specific immune response that is not strong enough, however, to result in HBV elimination.

Recently, the pathogenesis of innate immunity, including NK cell activity has been stressed in patients with viral hepatitis [4–7]. NK cells, which enriched markedly in liver and account for around one-third of total intrahepatic lymphocytes, are an important part of the innate immune system [8]. NK cells can not only directly kill virus-infected target cells without antigen-specific priming, but also regulate the adaptive immune response by producing cytokines such as IFN-γ and TNF-α, and thus take a central role in infection control [8]. Cross-talk of NK cells with CD8+ T cells strongly impact on the outcome of HBV infection. Early large amount of IFN-γ production by NK cells contribute to the initial control of infection and to allow timely development of an efficient adaptive immune response in self-limited acute HBV infection [9–11]. However, NK cells can negatively regulate specific antiviral immunity in chronic hepatitis B by directly killing HBV-specific CD8+ T cells which expressed TRAIL receptor, taking an important part in the failure of HBV elimination [12]. Besides, NK cells have important role in the pathogenesis of liver damage and inflammation through TRAIL- and Fas-mediated death [13,14]. The intensity and quality of NK cells function is determined by the precisely and dynamic coordinated balance of activating and inhibitory signals through their array receptors [15,16]. The activating receptors include NKp30, NKp46, NKG2C and NKG2D. NKp30 and NKp46 recognize MHC-independent ligands and transmit activating signals and induce NK cell cytotoxicity [15], while NKG2C and NKG2D recognize MHC-class I molecules. NKG2A, an inhibitory NK cells receptor, recognizes MHC-class I like molecules and transmits negative signals. NK cells activity is also regulated by cytokines microenvironment, with which the major immunosuppressive cytokines are TGF-β and IL-10 [17,18]. It had been reported that the frequency, subsets, surface receptors as well as the activity of NK cells had changed in patients infected with HBV as well as hepatitis C virus (HCV) [17,19–24], and the activity of NK ells altered after anti-viral treatment [25].

In this study, we analyzed NK cells activity in different immunological stages of chronic HBV infection. We found that NK cells activity is decreased in patients with chronic HBV infection, especially in patients in the IA stage. Unlike previous reports that NK cells function had dichotomy change in cytotoxicity and cytokine secretion [23,26,27], our study shown that both the cytotoxicity and secretion of cytokines were decreased, along with the decreased expression of activating receptors of NKp30 and NKG2D in NK cells in patients with chronic hepatitis B.

Results

PBMC subsets in patients with chronic HBV infection

CD3$^-$CD56$^+$ NK cells, CD4$^+$ T cells and CD8$^+$ T cells have all been shown to be involved in the antiviral immune response [30,31]. The frequency of these effector cells in patients with chronic HBV infection is summarized in Table 1. In patients with CHB in the IA stage, the frequency of NK cells was lower than that in HI (p<0.05). Non difference of NK cells frequency was observed between patients in the IA and IT stage, respectively. There were no obvious differences in the frequency of CD56dim and CD56bright NK cells between patients groups (data not shown). With respect to the frequency CD4$^+$ T cells and CD8$^+$ T cells there was no significant difference between the three study groups.

IFN-γ and TNF-α expression in NK cells

IFN-γ and TNF-α are pivotal functional cytokines for viral control and pathogenesis of hepatitis. After stimulated with PMA and ionomycin, IFN-γ and TNF-α expression in NK cells were

detected. We found that NK cells from subjects with chronic HBV infection had a reduced capacity to produce IFN-γ and TNF-α. As shown in Fig. 1, expression of IFN-γ as well as TNF-α was remarkable down regulated in NK cells from patients with CHB in the IA stage as compared to patients in the IT stage and HI, respectively (p<0.05).

NK cells cytotoxic activity

NK cells cytotoxicity was assessed by the analysis of different E:T ratios. The cytotoxic activity of NK cells gradually increased with increasing E:T ratios in the three study groups (Fig. 2A). As compared to HI, the cytotoxic activity of NK cells in patients with CHB was lower, especially in patients in the IA stage (p<0.05) (Fig. 2B).

Expression of NK cells surface receptors

We further analyzed NK cells receptors expression in the three study groups by flow cytometry (Fig. 3A). The receptors included the activating receptors NKp30, NKp46, NKG2D and NKG2C and the inhibitory receptor NKG2A. As illustrated in Fig. 3B, in patients with CHB in the IA stage the expression of the activating receptors NKp30 and NKG2D was down-regulated in peripheral NK cells compared to the patients in the IT stage and HI, respectively (p<0.05). No obvious difference of the expression of NKp46, NKG2C and NKG2A was observed in subjects in the three study groups.

Correlation of peripheral NK cells activity with serum HBV DNA or ALT level

NK cells exert their function through cytotoxicity and secretion of cytokines. The relationship of NK cells activity with HBV replication and liver damage was analyzed in the study. As shown in Fig. 4, in patients with CHB in the IA stage, there was no correlation between NK cell activity and the ALT level (Fig. 4A). The level of IFN-γ but not of TNF-α expressed by NK cells was inversely correlated to serum HBV load in subjects with chronic HBV infection (Fig. 4B). The relationship between IFN-γ and serum HBV load was seen only in IT stage when patients were grouped (Fig. 4C, 4D). No correlation was observed between NK cells cytotoxicity and serum HBV load.

Discussion

HBV infection can be roughly categorized in two stages: the IT and the IA stage, respectively, based on the serum HBV DNA level, serum ALT activity and the extent of liver damage. It is generally accepted that the HBV-specific immune response in the IT stage is lower than in the IA stage. Details regarding the innate immunity in the different stages of HBV infection are limited. NK cells,a major component of innate immune system, play a crucial role in the early clearance of HBV infection and the late developed adaptive immune response in CHB [32]. In this study we found that compared to health individuals, the frequency of peripheral NK cells was lower in patients with CHB in the IA stage. More important we demonstrated that the activity of NK cells, including cytotoxicity as well as IFN-γ and TNF-α production, was impaired in patients with CHB, especially in patients in the IA stage, and this functional impairment was companied with the phenotype changes of NK cells. Considering its significant role in anti-HBV infection, the reduced secretion of IFN-γ and TNF-α by NK cells, along with the decrease of its cytotoxicity which was shown in our study, might be associated with the chronicity of HBV infection.

It has been reported that the function of NK cells was dichotomy in chronic HBV and HCV infection [23,26], which

Table 1. Comparison of T lymphocyte subsets and NK cells (mean ± SEM).

groups	CD8$^+$ (%)	CD4$^+$ (%)	NK (%)
patients in IT stage	27.06±6.14	38.59±14.48	10.15±8.52
patients in IA stage	24.17±6.69	44.03±10.38	6.93±4.82*
HI subjects	26.96±5.47	44.10±4.57	11.56±6.85

Compared to HI,
*p<0.05.

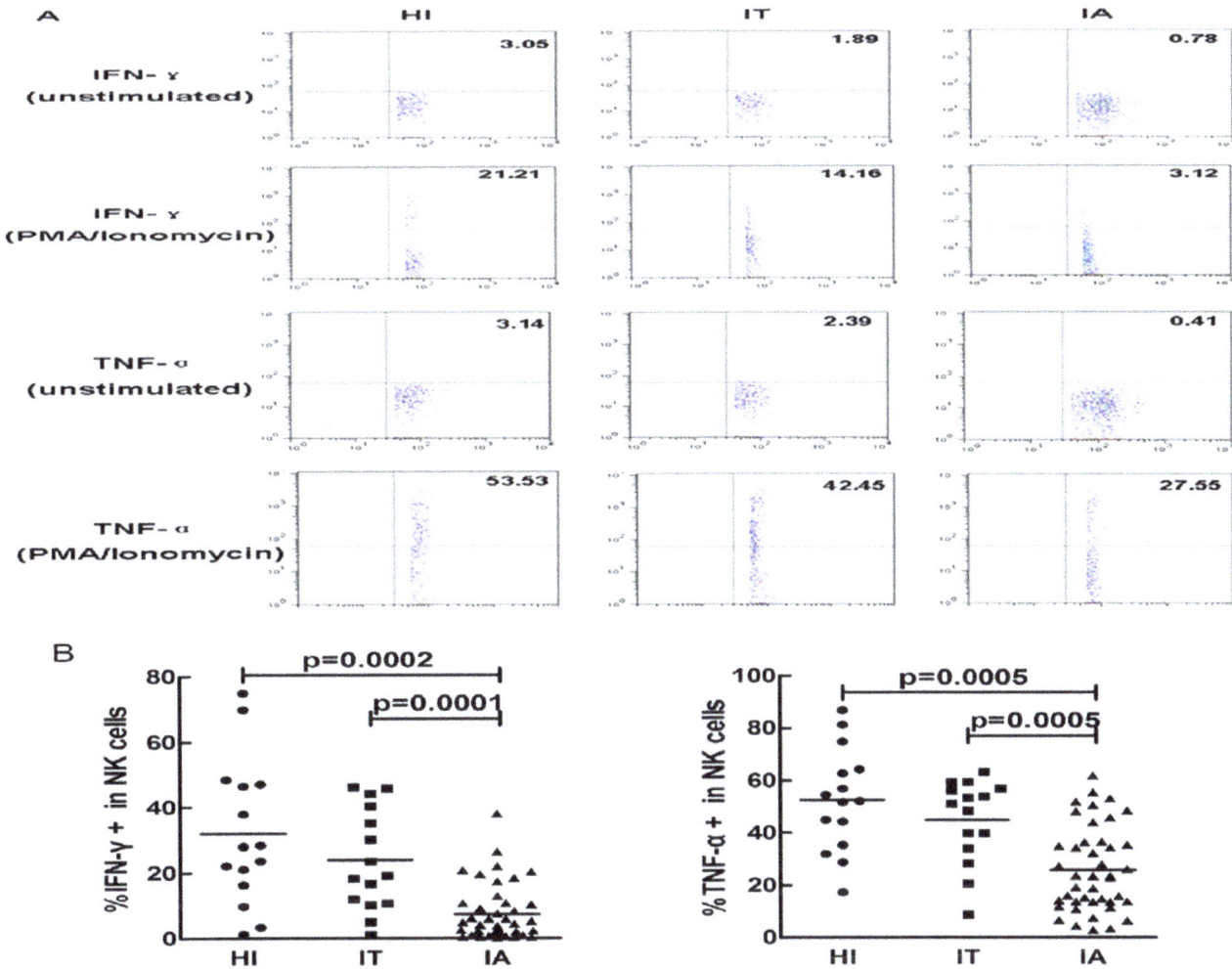

Figure 1. IFN-γ and TNF-α expression in peripheral NK cells. (A) The representative flow plots show IFN-γ and TNF-α expression including unstimulated controls and PMA/ionomycin stimulaton from the HI, IT and IA groups. (B) The percentage of peripheral NK cells expressing IFN-γ and TNF-α after stimulation with PMA/ionomycin in healthy individuals (HI) (circles), patients in the immune tolerant (IT) stage of CHB (squares) and patients in the immune activated (IA) stage of CHB (triangles) is shown. Each dot represents one individual. Horizontal lines represent the mean. The significance is calculated by the Mann-Whitney U test.

featuring in the conserved or enhanced cytolytic activity with the decreased cytokine production from NK cells. Zhang et al [24] also reported that NK cells from chronic hepatitis B patients had enhanced cytotoxicity but without the decrease of cytokine production. In contrast to these recent reports, our study shown that both the cytokine secretion and the cytolytic activity of NK cells were decreased in CHB patients, especially in patients in IA stage. The reason for this discrepancy is unknown, maybe partially due to the stimulation methods and target cells using in the cytotoxicity assay [33]. Indeed, as shown in the report from Oliviero and colleagues, the cytolytic activity of NK cells from CHB patients was significantly decreased when K562 cells was used as target cells while the cytotoxicity maintained when P815 target cells was used [23]. In our study, we also used K562 cells as the target cells for cytolytic assay. In this sense, our study had confirmed the results from Oliviero et al. Meanwhile, it was noteworthy to mention that there were also vigorous discrepancy reports of NK cells cytolytic activity in patients with chronic HCV infection [34–36]. The cytotoxicity of NK cells in CHB and CHC patients is thus needed to be further clarified. Methods used for stimulation of cytokine secretion by NK cells also might bring

some bias on the results. Though PMA/ionomycin-stimulation is more potent, it is not as physiological as cytokines such as IL 12 and IL 18 in NK cells activation. However, the trends for the change of cytokines secretion by NK cells were similar when NK cells were stimulated with different activators [9].

NK cells activity is thought to be maintained by the integrated signals from the inhibitory and activating receptors of NK cells. The functional impairrment might be due to the phenotype change of NK cells. In our study, NK cells from patients with CHB in the IA stage expressed significantly lower levels of activating receptors NKp30 and NKG2D compared to patients in the IT stage and HI, respectively (p<0.05). Decreased expression of NK cells activating receptors was observed in the study from Tjwa et al [26] but not from Zhang et al [24]. In previous reports, however, some studies shown that the phenotype of NK cells was not accordant with the functional change of NK cells [23,24,26]. In our study, we found that the reduced NKp30 and NKG2D expression of NK cells was well consistent with a decrease of cytotoxicity and cytokines production of NK cells in patients with CHB compared to HI.

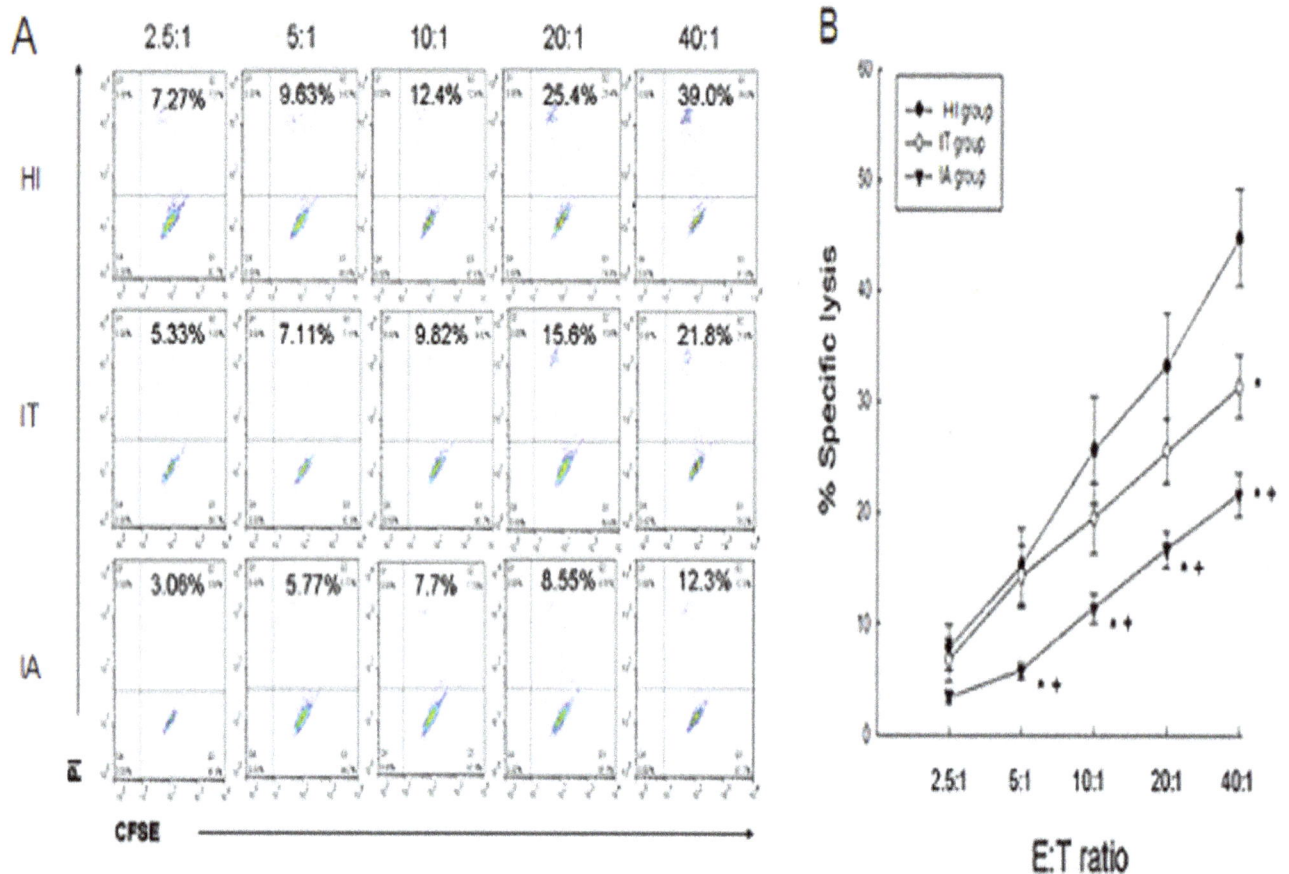

Figure 2. Cytotoxicity of peripheral NK cells. (A) Representative dot plots show K562 lysis by PBMCs from the three groups at different E:T ratios (2.5:1,5:1,10:1,20:1, and 40:1). (B) The cytotoxic activity of peripheral NK cells from the HI (n = 18), patients in the IT stage of CHB (n = 15), and patients in the IA stage of CHB (n = 42) at various E:T ratios. The mean and standard error are shown. Asterisk represents p<0.05 compared to HI. Crosses represent p<0.05 compared to patients in the IT stage of CHB.

Recently, Zhang et al [24] had investigated the activity of NK cells from patients with chronic hepatitis B in great detail. They found that NK cells from the IA stage CHB patients were phenotypic and functional activated which correlated with liver damage. In contrast, our study shown that NK cells from CHB patients was immunological tolerance both in function and in phenotype. Currently, it is hard to explain this obvious difference. The differences of patient's age, viral loads and ALT level might account to some extent for the discrepancy. All the IA patients in our study were e antigen positive. This is quite important because, compared to those IA patients with e negative, e antigen positive may indicate a relative earlier stage in immune activation. In view of the quite long process of the immune activation in CHB patients, it is understandable that the immune response including NK cells reaction might be quite different or maybe even opposite from the beginning to the end of the immune activation in chronic HBV infection. The longitudinal compared study of NK cells function in CHB patients from the beginning of the infection to viral clearance is needed to clarify this very important issue. Indeed, different levels of NK cell activity as well as HBV-specific CD4 and CD8 T cell reaction from the incubation to the clinical acute and the convalescent phase in self-limited acute HBV infection had been reported by Dunn et al [37] recently.

It is interesting to note that NK cells activity is much lower in patients in IA stage as compared to the IT stage. This phenomenon might be a reflection of the time required to mount an effective adaptive antiviral immune response. In the early stage of HBV infection, the first-line of defense is the relative strong innate immune response, including NK cells activity. With the development of adaptive immunity, the innate NK cells function is reduced. In line with this hypothesis, Sprengers et al found that the number of intrahepatic NK cells in IT stage was higher than that in IA stage of patients with CHB, while HBV-specific T cells increased in IA stage along with the decrease of viral loads [5]. The temporal relationship of NK cells activity with viral- specific adaptive immune reaction was demonstrated also in HIV infection [38]. Alternatively, the reduced NK cells activity in patients in the IA stage might be one of the mechanisms resulting in viral immune escape.

While NK cells activity was found to correlate with viral clearance in acute self-limited HBV infection in the chimpanzee model, in patients the correlation between NK cells activity and the level of HBV replication and liver damage is still controversial [24,26,39]. In this study, we found that NK cells expressed IFN-γ level, but not TNF-α level and NK cells cytotoxicity, was inversely correlated with HBV replication in CHB patients. Our study confirmed the important role of IFN-γ in HBV inhibition. Interestingly, the inverse relationship was observed only in the IT stage but not in the IA stage patients. However, we did not found positive relationship between NK cells activity and liver damage (as indicated by serum ALT level) in the IA stage patients. In this context it is not clear whether peripheral NK cells activity

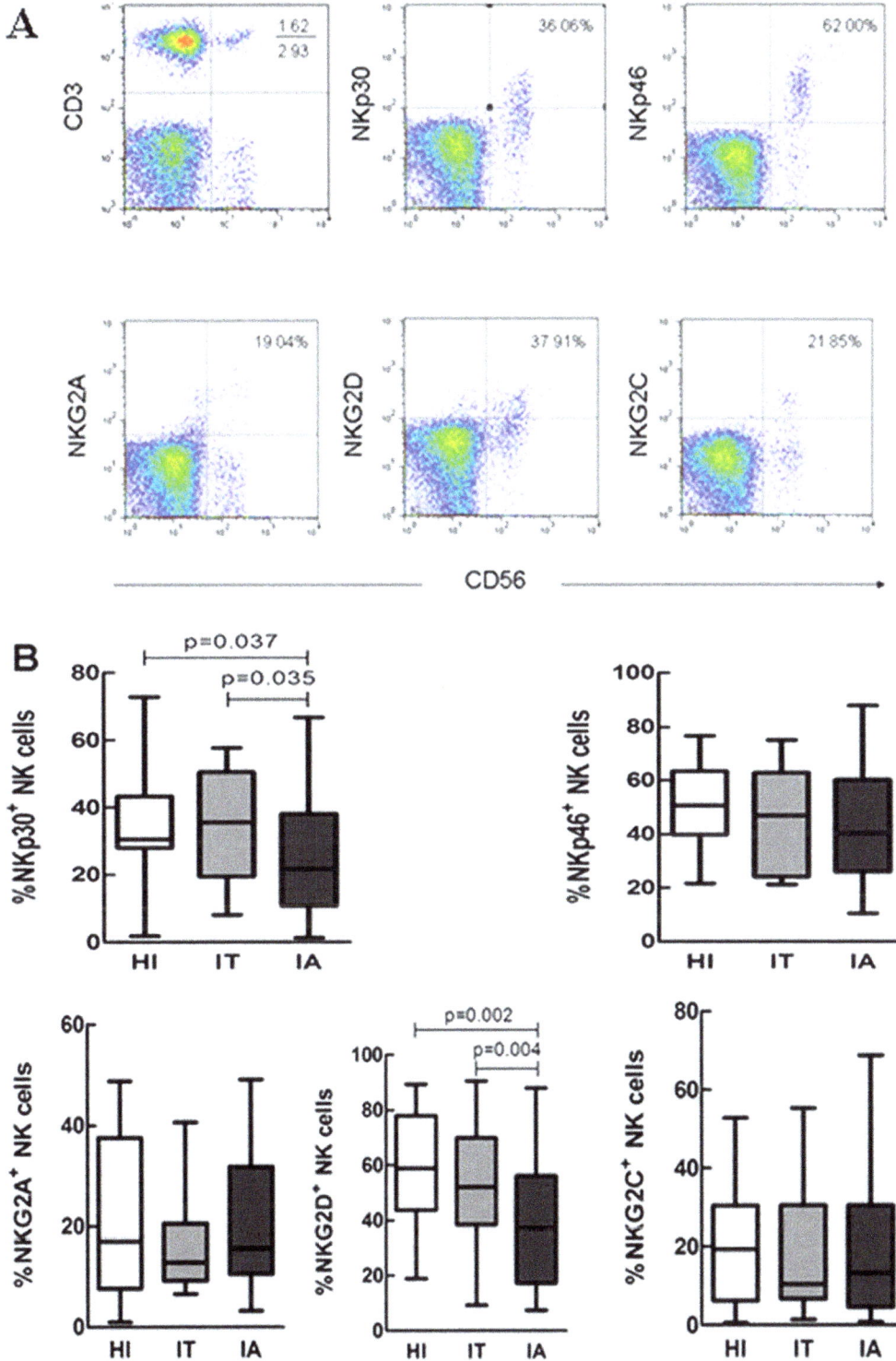

Figure 3. NK cell surface receptors expression in PBMC. (A) Representative dot plots of NK cells (CD3⁻CD56⁺) and their surface receptors (NKp30, NKp46, NKG2A, NKG2C, NKG2D) in PBMCs isolated from HBV-infected patients and HC are shown. (B) The percentage of NK cells expressing surface receptors in HI (n = 18), patients in the IT stage of CHB (n = 15), and patients in the IA stage of CHB (n = 42) is shown. The data are presented as boxplots showing medians (horizontal lines), upper and lower quartiles (boxes) and extreme values (whiskers). The significance is calculated by the Mann-Whitney U test.

reflects intrahepatic NK cells activity. Nevertheless, it is reasonable to assume that intrahepatic NK cell activity might correlate to liver damage. One can further assume that in patients with CHB the liver microenvironment has an important effect on immune effector cells, including NK cells, and thereby on HBV replication and the extent of liver damage.

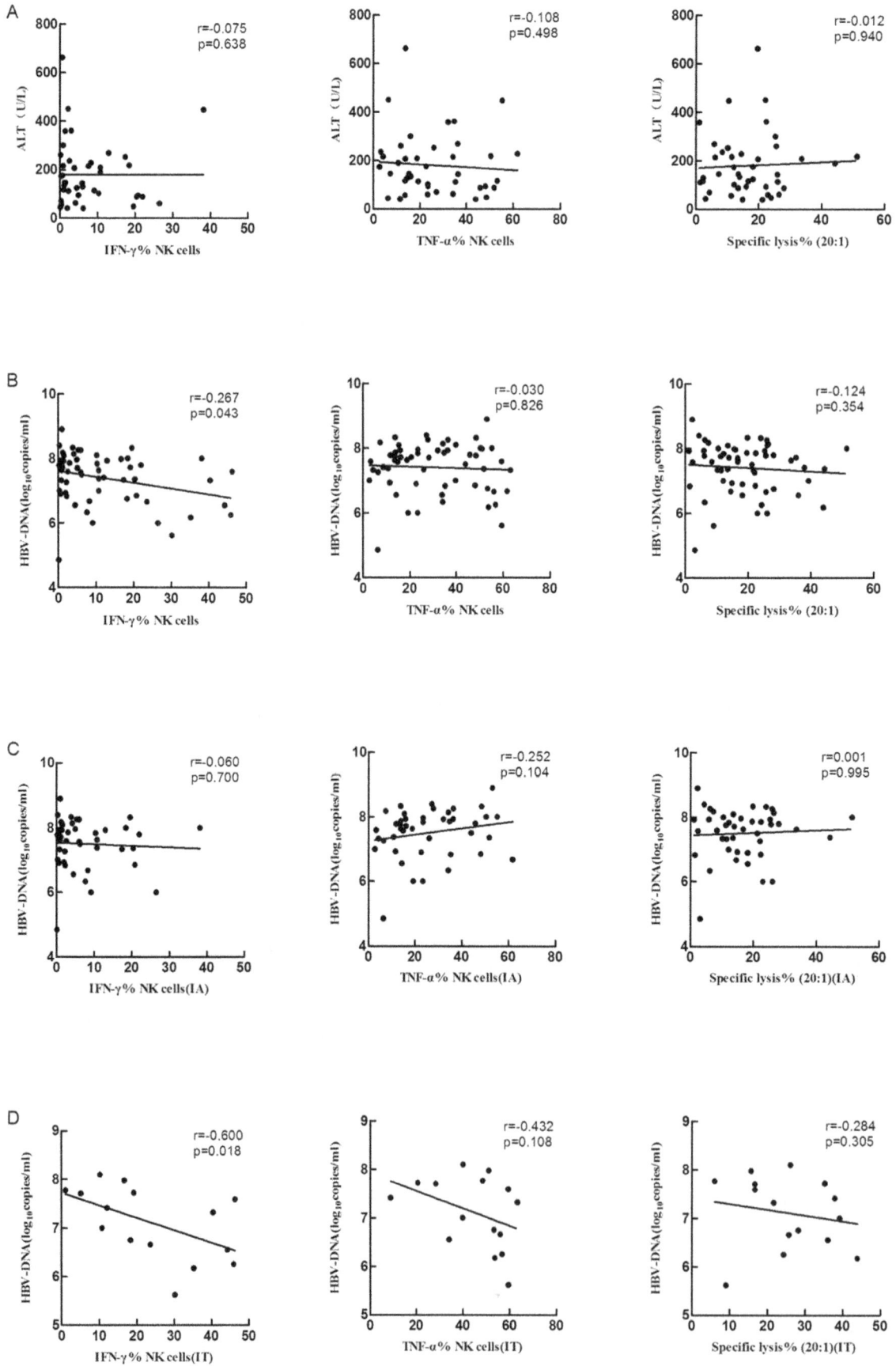

Figure 4. Relationship of NK cell activity with liver damage and HBV replication. Correlation between NK cells activity and ALT level in patients in the IA stage of CHB (A) and HBV replication in patients with CHB (B). Relationship of NK cell activity with HBV loads was further analyzed in IA stage (C) and in IT stage (D).

In conclusion, our study shown that NK cells, at least in this group of patients with chronic hepatitis B was immune tolerant, especially in patients at IA stage, which characterized by the reduced cytotoxicity, the down regulated expression of IFN-γ and TNF-α, along with the decreased expression of activating receptors of NKp30 and NKG2D. This immune tolerant status of NK cells might take important role in the pathogenesis of chronic HBV infection.

Materials and Methods

Ethics Statement

All subjects signed an informed consent form to participate in the study. Our study obtained approval from the ethics committee of Tongji Hospital, Tongji Medical College, Huazhong University of Science and Technology. We obtain informed consent from the next of kin, caretakers, or guardians on the behalf of the minors/children participants involved in our study. The consent was written.

Study Subjects

Overall, 57 patients with chronic HBV infection were recruited for the study and categorized according to the established criteria for viral hepatitis [28–29]. The immune tolerant (IT) stage was defined by high level HBV DNA in serum, HBeAg positivity and normal ALT levels. By contrast, the immune activated (IA) stage was defined by low level HBV DNA in serum and elevated ALT levels. All patients were negative for antibodies to hepatitis C virus, hepatitis D virus, human immunodeficiency virus, hepatitis A virus and hepatitis E virus. Further, the patients were not receiving immunosuppressive drugs during the last 6 months before recruitment and did not consume alcohol. Eighteen age and sex matched healthy individuals (HI) were enrolled as control group (Table 2). All subjects signed an informed consent form to participate in the study.

Serological test of liver function, HBV markers and HBV DNA

ALT activity in serum was measured with routine automated techniques (upper limit: 40 U/L). The HBV markers HBsAg, anti-HBs, HBeAg, anti-HBe, anti-HBc total, and anti-HBc IgM were determined by commercially available enzyme-linked immuno-sorbent assays. Serum HBV DNA was quantitated by real-time PCR (RT-PCR) using a commercially available kit (Shanghai KH Biology Co. Ltd.) and the Lightcycler PCR system FQD-33A, Bioer. The lower detection limit was 500 viral genome copies/ml.

Detection of lymphocyte subsets and NK cells surface receptors

Peripheral blood monouclear cells (PBMCs) were isolated from patients and healthy individuals, suspended in RPMI 1640 medium containing 2 mM/L L-glutamine and 10% fetal calf serum (Hyclone). Isolated PBMCs were stained with fluoro-chrome-conjugated antibodies to CD3-PerCP/cy5.5, CD56-FITC, CD8-FITC and CD4-FITC (Biolegend, San Diego, CA). NK cells surface receptors were stained with fluorochrome-conjugated antibodies to NKp46-PE, NKG2A-PE, NKp30-APC, NKG2C-APC, NKG2D-APC and isotype matched controls (Biolegend, San Diego, CA). Stained PBMC were isolated using a FACS Calibur flow cytometer (Becton Dickinson, USA) and analyzed by FlowJo analysis software (Treestar, Ashland, OR).

Intracellular cytokine staining

After stimulation with 20 ng/ml phorbol myristate acetate (PMA) (Sigma, USA) plus 1 µg/ml ionomycin (Sigma) for 1 hour at 37°C in 5% CO_2, cells were cultured for 4 hours in the presence of 2 µM/L monensin (Sigma). Then, cells were stained with fluorochrome-conjugated antibodies to CD3-PerCP/cy5.5, CD56-FITC, CD8-FITC and CD4-FITC (Biolegend, San Diego, CA) at 4°C in the dark. Cells were then fixed and permeabilized, followed by intracellular staining for IFN-γ-PE, TNF-α-PE and isotype matched controls (Biolegend, San Diego, CA) at 4°C in the dark. Finally, cells were detected by flow cytometry.

Cytotoxicity assay

K562 cells were labeled with 3 µM/L carboxyfluorescein diacetate succinimidyl ester (CFSE) (Molecular Probes, Eugene, OR). PBMCs were subsequently incubated with the CFSE-labeled K562 cells at effector to target (E:T) ratios of 2.5:1, 5:1, 10:1, 20:1, and 40:1 and incubated for the 4 hours at 37°C in 5% CO_2. Then, 100 µg/mL propidium iodide (PI) (BD Bioscience, San Jose, CA) was added to identify dead cells. The target cells alone were used as controls. The percentage lysis was calculated as: [(experimental release (%)−spontaneous release (%))/(1−spontaneous release (%))]×100.

Statistical analysis

All data were analyzed with SPSS 13.0 for Windows (SPSS, Inc., Chicago, IL). Comparisons between various individuals were performed with the Mann-Whitney U test. Correlations between variables were calculated with the Spearman rank correlation test. P values<0.05 were considered significant.

Table 2. Characteristics of study subjects.

	HI subjects (n = 18)	patients in IT stage (n = 15)	patients in IA stage (n = 42)
Age, yrs (mean±SEM)	25.35±9.65	28.27±8.93	30.82±10.58
Gender (Female:male)	10:8	8:7	8:34
ALT IU/L (mean±SEM)	20.50±1.50	22.20±7.12	199.85±192.93
HBV DNA log$_{10}$ copies/ml (mean±SEM)	na	7.58±0.21	6.62±0.18

na = not applicable.

Acknowledgments

The authors thank Prof. Dr. Hubert E. Blum for helpful discussions and support in the preparation of manuscript. Thanks also go to all individuals for their participation in this study.

References

1. Lok AS, McMahon BJ (2001) Practice guidelines committee, American Association for the Study of Liver Diseases. Chronic hepatitis B. Hepatology 34:1225–1241.
2. Rehermann B, Nascimbeni M (2005) Immunology of hepatitis B virus and hepatitis C virus infection. Nat Rev Immunol 5:215–229.
3. Ganem D, Prince AM (2004) Hepatitis B virus infection—natural history and clinical consequences. N Engl J Med 350:1118–1129.
4. Tian Z, Chen Y, Gao B (2013) Natural killer cells in liver disease. Hepatology 57:1564–1662.
5. Sprengers D, van der Molen RG, Kusters JG, Hansen B, Niesters HG, et al. (2006) Different composition of intrahepatic lymphocytes in the immune-tolerance and immune-clearance phase of chronic hepatitis B. J Med Virol 78:561–568.
6. Zou Z, Xu D, Li B, Xin S, Zhang Z, et al. (2009) Compartmentalization and its implication for peripheral immunologically-competent cells to the liver in patients with HBV-related acute-on-chronic liver failure. Hepatol Res 39:1198–1207.
7. Rehermann B (2013)Pathogenesis of chronic viral hepatitis: differential roles of T cells and NK cells. Nat Med 19:859–68.
8. Mondelli MU, Varchetta S, Oliviero B (2010) Natural killer cells in viral hepatitis: facts and controversies. Eur J Clin Invest 40:851–863.
9. Zhao J, Li Y, Jin L, Zhang S, Fan R, et al. (2012) Natural killer cells are characterized by the concomitantly increased interferon-γ and cytotoxicity in acute resolved hepatitis B patients. PLoS One 7:e49135.
10. Webster GJ, Reignat S, Maini MK, Whalley SA, Ogg GS, et al. (2000) Incubation phase of acute hepatitis B in man: dynamic of cellular immune mechanisms. Hepatology 32:1117–1124.
11. Fisicaro P, Valdatta C, Boni C, Massari M, Mori C, et al. (2009) Early kinetics of innate and adaptive immune responses during hepatitis B virus infection. Gut 58:974–982.
12. Peppa D, Gill US, Reynolds G, Easom NJ, Pallett LJ, et al. (2013) Up-regulation of a death receptor renders antiviral T cells susceptible to NK cell-mediated deletion. J Exp Med 210:99–114.
13. Dunn C, Brunetto M, Reynolds G, Christophides T, Kennedy PT, et al. (2007) Cytokines induced during chronic hepatitis B virus infection promote a pathway for NK cell-mediated liver damage. J Exp Med 204:667–680.
14. Zou Y, Chen T, Han M, Wang H, Yan W, et al. (2010) Increased killing of liver NK cells by Fas/Fas ligand and NKG2D/NKG2D ligand contributes to hepatocyte necrosis in virus-induced liver failure. J Immunol 184:466–475.
15. Lanier LL (2001) On guard-activating NK cell receptors. Nat Immunol 2:23–27.
16. Iwaszko M, Bogunia-Kubik K (2011) Clinical significance of the HLA-E and CD94/NKG2 interaction. Arch Immunol Ther Exp (Warsz) 59:353–367.
17. Peppa D, Micco L, Javaid A, Kennedy PT, Schurich A, et al. (2010) Blockade of immunosuppressive cytokines restores NK cell antiviral function in chronic hepatitis B virus infection. PLoS Pathog 6:e1001227.
18. Sun C, Fu B, Gao Y, Liao X, Sun R, et al. (2012) TGF-β1 down-regulation of NKG2D/DAP10 and 2B4/SAP expression on human NK cells contributes to HBV persistence. PLoS Pathog 8:e1002594.
19. Golden-Mason L, Madrigal-Estebas L, McGrath E, Conroy MJ, Ryan EJ, et al. (2008) Altered natural killer cell subset distributions in resolved and persistent hepatitis C virus infection following single source exposure. Gut 57:1121–1128.
20. Zarife MA, Reis EA, Carmo TM, Lopes GB, Brandão EC, et al. (2009) Increased frequency of CD56 (bright) NK-cells, CD3-CDl6+CD56-NK-cells and activated CD4+T-cells or B-cells in parallel with CD4+CD25 high T-cells control potentially viremia in blood donors with HCV. J Med Virol 81:49–59.
21. Mantegani P, Tambussi G, Galli L, Din CT, Lazzarin A, et al. (2010) Perturbation of the natural killer cell compartment during primary human immunodeficiency virus l infection primarily involving the CD56(bright) subset. Immunology 129:220–233.
22. Tseng CT, Klimpel GR (2002) Binding of the hepatitis C virus envelope protein E2 to CD8l inhibits natural killer cell functions. J Exp Med 195:43–49.
23. Oliviero B, Varchetta S, Paudice E, Michelone G, Zaramella M, et al. (2009) Natural killer cell functional dichotomy in chronic hepatitis B and chronic hepatitis C virus infections. Gastroenterology 137:1151–1160.
24. Zhang Z, Zhang S, Zou Z, Shi J, Zhao J, et al. (2011) Hypercytolytic activity of hepatic natural killer cells correlates with liver injury in chronic hepatitis B patients. Hepatology 53:73–85.
25. Zhao PW, Jia FY, Shan YX, Ji HF, Feng JY, et al. (2013) Downregulation and altered function of natural killer cells in hepatitis B virus patients treated with entecavir. Clin Exp Pharmacol Physiol 40:190–196.
26. Tjwa ET, van Oord GW, Hegmans JP, Janssen HL, Woltman AM (2011) Viral load reduction improves activation and function of natural killer cells in patients with chronic hepatitis B. J Hepatol 54:209–218.
27. Mondelli MU, Oliviero B, Mele D, Mantovani S, Gazzabin C, et al. (2012) Natural killer cell functional dichotomy: a feature of chronic viral hepatitis? Front Immunol 3:351.
28. Lai CL, Yuen MF (2007) The natural history of chronic hepatitis B. J Viral Hepatol 14:6–10.
29. Lok AS, McMahon BJ (2007) Chronic hepatitis B. Hepatology 45:507–539.
30. Kakimi K, Guidotti LG, Koezuka Y, Chisari FV (2000) Natural killer T cell activation inhibits hepatitis B virus replication in vivo. J Exp Med 192:921–930.
31. Webster GJ, Reignat S, Brown D, Ogg GS, Jones L, et al. (2004) Longitudinal analysis of CD8+ T cells specific for structural and nonstructural hepatitis B virus proteins in patients with chronic hepatitis B: Implications for immunotherapy. J Virol 78:5707–5719.
32. Vivier E, Tomasello E, Baratin M, Walzer T, Ugolini S (2008) Functions of natural killer cells. Nat Immunol 9:503–510.
33. Rehermann B, Naoumov NV (2007) Immunological techniques in viral hepatitis. J Hepatol 46:508–520.
34. Nattermann J, Feldmann G, Ahlenstiel G, Langhans B, Sauerbruch T, et al. (2006) Surface expression and cytolytic function of natural killer cell receptors is altered in chronic hepatitis C. Gut 55: 869–877.
35. Meier UC, Owen RE, Taylor E, Worth A, Naoumov N, et al. (2005) Shared alterations in NK cell frequency, phenotype, and function in chronic human immunodeficiency virus and hepatitis C virus infections. J Virol 79:12365–12374.
36. Morishima C, Paschal DM, Wang CC, Yoshihara CS, Wood BL, et al. (2006) Decreased NK cell frequency in chronic hepatitis C does not affect ex vivo cytolytic killing. Hepatology 43:573–580.
37. Dunn C, Peppa D, Khanna P, Nebbia G, Jones M, et al. (2009) Temporal analysis of early immune responses in patients with acute hepatitis B virus infection. Gastroenterology 137:1289–1300.
38. Alter G, Teigen N, Ahern R, Streeck H, Meier A, et al. (2007) Evolution of innate and adaptive effector cell functions during acute HIV-1 infection. J Infect Dis 195:1452–1460.
39. Guidotti LG, Rochford R, Chung J, Shapiro M, Purcell R, et al. (1999) Viral clearance without destruction of infected cells during acute HBV infection. Science 284:825–829.

Author Contributions

Conceived and designed the experiments: YL JJW XPZ. Performed the experiments: YL JJW SG QL JB XQZ HHD FZ. Analyzed the data: YL XPZ. Contributed reagents/materials/analysis tools: YHH FZ DLY. Wrote the paper: YL XPZ.

Regulatory Phenotype, PD-1 and TLR3 Expression in T Cells and Monocytes from HCV Patients Undergoing Antiviral Therapy: A Randomized Clinical Trial

Shan-shan Su[1], Huan He[1], Ling-bo Kong[1], Yu-guo Zhang[1], Su-xian Zhao[1], Rong-qi Wang[1], Huan-wei Zheng[2], Dian-xing Sun[3], Yue-min Nan[1]*, Jun Yu[4]

1 Department of Traditional and Western Medical Hepatology, Third Hospital of Hebei Medical University, Shijiazhuang, China, 2 Department of Infectious Disease, The Fifth Hospital of Shijiazhuang City, Shijiazhuang, China, 3 Department of Liver Disease, Bethune International Peace Hospital, Shijiazhuang, China, 4 Institute of Digestive Disease and Department of Medicine and Therapeutics, State Key Laboratory of Digestive Disease, Li Ka Shing Institute of Health Sciences, The Chinese University of Hong Kong, Hong Kong, China

Abstract

Background & Aims: The cellular immunity has a profound impact on the status of hepatitis C virus (HCV) infection. However, the response of cellular immunity on the virological response In patients with antiviral treatment remains largely unclear. We aimed to clarify the response of peripheral T cells and monocytes in chronic hepatitis C patients with antiviral treatment.

Methods: Patients with chronic hepatitis C were treated either with interferon alpha-2b plus ribavirin (n = 37) or with pegylated interferon alpha-2a plus ribavirin (n = 33) for up to 24 weeks. Frequencies of peripheral regulatory T-cells (Tregs), programmed death-1 (PD-1) expressing CD4+ T-cells or CD8+ T-cells and toll-like receptor (TLR) 3 expressing CD14+ monocytes were evaluated by flow cytometry in patients at baseline, 12 and 24 weeks following treatment and in 20 healthy controls.

Results: Frequencies of Tregs, PD-1 and TLR3 expressing cells were higher in patients than those in control subjects ($P < 0.05$). Patients with complete early virological response (cEVR) showed lower Tregs, PD-1 expressing CD4+ or CD8+ T-cells than those without cEVR at 12 weeks ($P < 0.05$). Patients with low TLR3 expressing CD14+ monocytes at baseline had a high rate of cEVR ($P < 0.05$).

Conclusions: Low peripheral TLR3 expressing CD14+ monocytes at baseline could serve as a predictor for cEVR of antiviral therapy in chronic HCV-infected patients. The cEVR rates were significantly increased in the patients with reduced circulating Tregs, PD-1 expressing CD4+ or CD8+ T-cells.

Editor: T. Mark Doherty, Glaxo Smith Kline, Denmark

Funding: This study was supported by the Key Program for Science and Technology Development of Hebei Province named Study on Prevention and Control of Viral Hepatitis (10276102D). The funders had no role in study design, data collection and analysis, decision to publish, or preparation of the manuscript.

Competing Interests: The authors have declared that no competing interests exist.

* E-mail: nanyuemin@163.com

Introduction

Hepatitis C virus (HCV) infection is a growing public health problem, with roughly 3% of the population infected worldwide [1,2]. Interferon alpha (IFNα) in combination with ribavirin (RBV) remains a gold standard treatment for chronic HCV infection. However, approximately one-half of chronic hepatitis C genotype 1 patients fail to achieve viral clearance [3]. Thus, it is important to identify the factors that may be valuable in improving antiviral strategy and treatment response.

Both innate and adaptive immunity have a profound impact on status of HCV infection. Impairment of host immunity, especially HCV-specific cellular immune response, may lead to chronic infection [4,5]. Regulatory T-cells (Tregs) have been shown to be increased in the peripheral blood of patients with chronic HCV infection and can suppress the proliferation of HCV-specific cytotoxic T lymphocytes, which may affect the antiviral treatment response [6–8]. Programmed cell death-1 (PD-1), expressing in activated T cells, B cells and monocytes, plays an essential role in regulation of adaptive immune responses [9]. Virus-specific CD8+ T cell response generated during acute HCV infection can be gradually exhausted in settings of persistent virus infections by the high expression of PD-1 [10–13]. Studies have shown that toll-like receptors (TLRs) can detect the presence of HCV infection through recognition of viral pathogen-associated molecular patterns (PAMPs) and control activation of the adaptive immune responses by inducing dendritic cell maturation [14,15]. In human monocytes, TLR3 is localized in intracellular endosomal compartments and the agonist of TLR3 represents an attractive target for pursuing the HCV clearance [16]. However, up to now, the effects of Tregs, PD-1 expressing CD4$^+$ T-cells or CD8$^+$ T-cells and TLR3 expressing CD14$^+$ monocytes on virological response in patients treated with IFNα plus RBV remains poorly understood. In this study, we aimed to clarify the role of Tregs, PD-1 and TLR3 in treatment response by assessing the baseline levels and dynamic changes of these immune mediators in patients receiving the combined antiviral treatment.

Patients and Methods

Ethics Statement

The protocol for this trial and supporting CONSORT checklist are available as supporting information; see Checklist S1 and Protocol S1. This was a randomized parallel-group study conducted in Shijiazhuang, China. The study protocol conformed to the guidelines of the 1975 Declaration of Helsinki and was approved by the ethics committees of Third Hospital of Hebei Medical University, Shijiazhuang, China, and all patients provided written informed consent. The registration number was ChiCTR-TNRC-10001090.

Subjects

A total of 70 patients chronically infected with HCV were recruited from Third Hospital of Hebei Medical University, the Fifth Hospital of Shijiazhuang City and Bethune International Peace Hospital (Shijiazhuang, China). The complete date range for patient recruitment and follow-up was from January 2011 to October 2012. HCV infection was diagnosed on the basis of the serum positive antibodies to HCV and the presence of HCV RNA in the plasma. Eligible patients were ≥18 years of age. Subjects meeting with the following criteria were excluded: presence of decompensated cirrhosis, co-infection with human immunodeficiency virus (HIV), hepatitis A, B or D virus, other causes of chronic liver disease or co-morbidities precluding interferon

therapy. Twenty age and gender matched healthy subjects were used as controls. Peripheral blood was collected from all of the healthy controls and chronic hepatitis C patients at baseline, 12 and 24 weeks after treatment.

HCV Antibodies Tests

The serum antibodies to HCV were detected by enzyme linked immunosorbent assay (ELISA) with a commercial detection kit (Livzon diagnostics INC, Zhuhai, China).

Quantitative Detection of HCV RNA

HCV RNA load was determined using qualitative reverse transcriptase polymerase chain reaction (RT-PCR) assay (Cobas Taqman HCV Test, Roche Diagnostics, Indianapolis, IN) and the low limit quantification was 15 IU/ml.

Biochemical Assays

Serum alanine aminotransferase (ALT) and aspartate aminotransferase (AST) were detected by an Olympus AU5400 automatic chemical analyzer.

HCV Genotyping

The HCV genotypes were identified using the HCV genotyping oligochip (Tianjin Third Central Hospital, China) [17].

Treatments and Assessments of Virological Responses

Participants were randomly assigned following simple randomization procedures. Eligible subjects were randomly divided into 2 groups: IFNα-2b plus RBV (IFNα-2b/RBV) group (n = 37), patients underwent therapy of recombinant IFNα-2b (300 million units for body weight<60 kg and 500 million units for body weight≥60 kg, on alternate days) (Beijing Kawin Technology Share-holding Co, Ltd. China) plus weight-based RBV (13–15 mg/kg·d) (Zhejiang Chengyi pharmaceuticals Co, Ltd. China); PegIFNα-2a plus RBV (PegIFNα-2a/RBV) group (n = 33), patients received PegIFNα-2a (135 μg/week for body weight< 60 kg and 180 μg/week for body weight≥60 kg, subcutaneously) (Pegasys, Roche, Basel, Switzerland) plus weight-based RBV (13–15 mg/kg·d) (Fig. 1). Responses to the treatment were assessed by detecting plasma HCV RNA levels at baseline, 12 and 24 weeks after the treatment. Standard definitions of responses were used to evaluate the therapeutic effect [18]. Complete early virological response (cEVR) was defined as undetectable plasma HCV RNA at 12 weeks after treatment. Full details of the trial protocol can be found in the Supplementary Appendix, available with the full text of this article at www.chictr.org/cn/.

Flow Cytometry Assay for Tregs, PD-1 Expressing T-cells and TLR3 Expressing CD14$^+$ Monocytes

Fluorescent dye conjugated antibodies consisted of cell surface monoclonal antibodies CD4-fluorescein isothiocyanate (FITC), CD8-peridinin-chlorophyll-protein complex (PerCP)-Cy5.5, PD-1-phycoerythrin (PE), CD25-PE and CD14-FITC (all from BD Biosciences, San Jose, CA), and intracellular monoclonal antibodies FoxP3-Alexa Flour 647 (BD Biosciences) and TLR3-PE (from eBioscience, San Diego, CA). All appropriate isotype controls were obtained from BD Biosciences. Intracellular staining of FoxP3 was performed according to the manufacturer's staining kit (BD Biosciences) instructions. Cell surface antigens to identify the PD-1 expression on CD4$^+$ or CD8$^+$ T-cells were detected with CD4-FITC, CD8-PerCP-Cy5.5 and PD-1-PE. To detect intracellular TLR3 expression in monocytes, cells were stained with surface antibodies CD14-FITC, fixed, permeabilized using FACS^{TM}

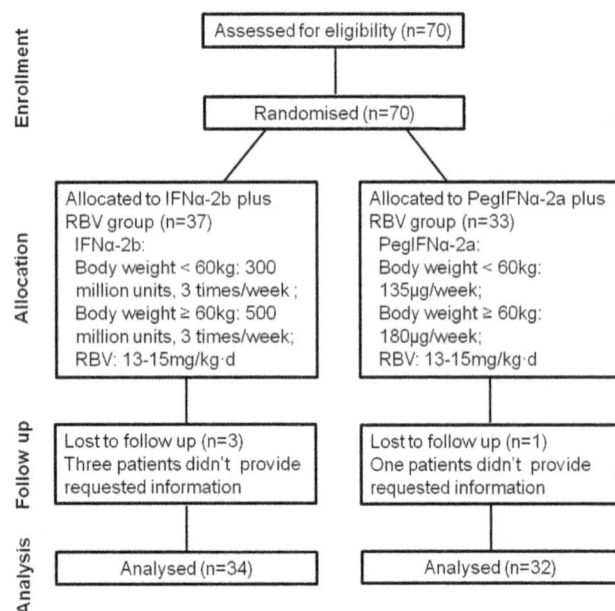

Figure 1. Flow diagram of the progress through the phases of the parallel randomised trial of two groups.

Table 1. Baseline Characteristics of the Subjects.

Parameter	IFNα-2b/RBV (n = 37)	PegIFNα/RBV (n = 33)	P-value
Gender (M/F)	16/21	16/17	0.660
Age, mean±SD	47.7±12.1	48.5±13.7	0.767
Body mass index (kg/m^2), mean±SD	23.3±2.9	23.4±2.7	0.938
ALT (IU/L), median (range)	68.5 (15–259)	66.6 (10–191)	0.457
AST (IU/L), median (range)	56.4 (17–189)	53.6 (15–228)	0.452
HCV RNA (IU/ml), median (range)	5.4×10^5 (403–6.0×10^8)	7.6×10^5 (1220–2.8×10^7)	0.723
Possible route of contamination			
Transfusion, n (%)	23 (62.2)	24 (72.7)	0.348
Previous surgery, n (%)	4 (10.8)	3 (9.1)	0.811
Stomatologic treatments, n (%)	1 (2.7)	1 (3.0)	0.935
Others or unknown, n (%)	9 (24.3)	5 (15.2)	0.338
HCV genotypes (1b/2a)	30/5	31/1	0.110

Abbreviations: IFN: Interferon; RBV: Ribavirin; ALT: Alanine transaminase; AST: Aspartate transaminase.

permeabilizing solution 2 (BD Biosciences) and incubated with TLR3-PE.

At least 100,000 cells were acquired on FACS CantoII (Becton Dickinson, San Jose, CA) and analyzed using Cellquest software. For data analyses, an initial lymphocyte gate was set based on side scatter (SSC)/forward scatter (FSC) and additional gates introduced as required. Results were present as the percentage of positively stained cells within the gated population.

Statistics Analysis

The statistical power calculation was performed based on predictive significance of cEVR to sustained virological response

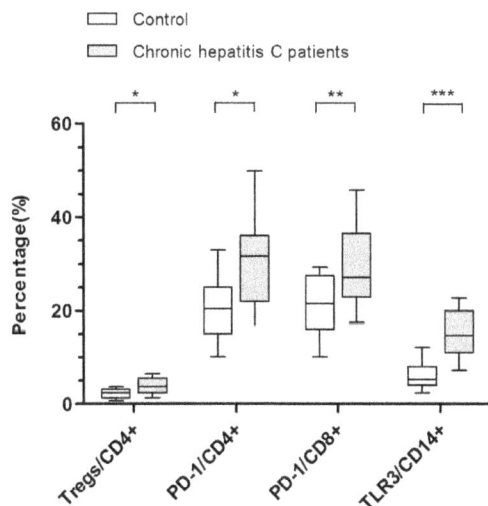

Figure 2. Proportions of Tregs, PD-1 expressing CD4$^+$ T-cells or CD8$^+$ T-cells and TLR3 expressing CD14$^+$ monocytes. Boxes represent the interquartile range and horizontal lines inside each box represent the median. The vertical lines from the ends of each box encompass the extreme data points. Proportions of Tregs, PD-1 expressing CD4$^+$ T-cells or CD8$^+$ T-cells and TLR3 expressing CD14$^+$ monocytes were measured by flow cytometry and data were presented by percentage. P-values were determined by Mann-Whitney test. *P< 0.05, **P<0.01, ***P<0.001.

(SVR) achievement. The target sample size gave 95% power at the 5% significance level to detect a difference of 58% in SVR rates (82.2% vs 24.2%) between the cEVR and non-cEVE patients according to the outcome of our completed clinical trial. Categorical data were expressed as numbers or proportions of subjects with the specific features. The chi-square test was used to compare categorical data. Continuous variables not normally distributed were summarized as medians and ranges, and Nonparametric Mann-Whitney U test was used to compare the differences between two groups. Kruskal-Wallis H test was used for comparison of differences between three groups and further comparisons between any two groups within these multiple groups were conducted using Nemenyi method. A mixed-effects model analysis of variance was applied to evaluate the time and group effects as well as the time by group interaction. If the overall P-value was significant, we used a step-down test based on the Bonferroni correction method to determine pairwise differences. Correlations between the variables were calculated using Spearman rank order correlations. Multivariate logistic regression analysis was performed to identify independent predictors of cEVR. All P-values were two-tailed, and were considered significant when lower than 0.05. Data were analyzed using SPSS 16.0 software package (v. 16.0; SPSS Inc., Chicago, IL).

Results

Patient Characteristics

At baseline, there were no significant differences between IFNα-2b/RBV and PegIFNα-2a/RBV treatment groups for the demographic and clinical characteristics, including gender, age, body mass index, serum ALT, AST, HCV RNA levels, percentages of different contaminated ways and HCV genotypes (Table 1). The age and gender between chronic hepatitis C patients and healthy controls were also no significant difference (data not shown).

Among 70 patients, 61 (87.1%, 61/70) of them were infected with HCV genotype 1b and 6 (8.6%, 6/70) patients were infected with HCV genotype 2a. The HCV genotype data were missing in 3 (4.3%, 3/70) patients.

A

B

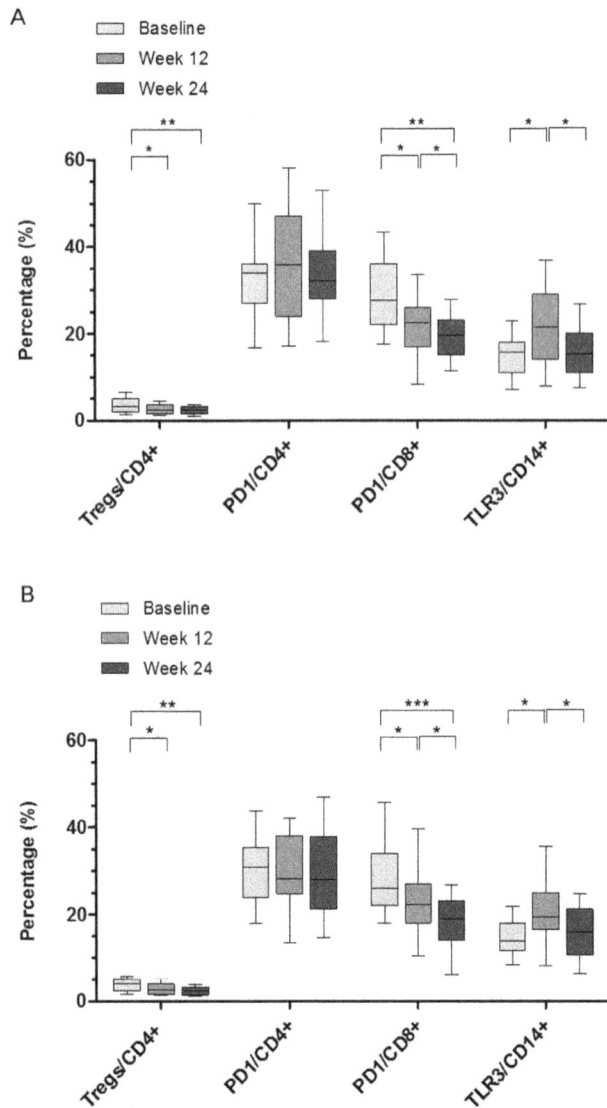

Figure 3. Proportions of Tregs, PD-1 expressing CD4$^+$ T-cells or CD8$^+$ T-cells and TLR3 expressing CD14$^+$ monocytes in patients treated with (A) IFNα-2b/RBV or (B) PegIFNα-2a/RBV. Boxes represent the interquartile range and horizontal lines inside each box represent the median. The vertical lines from the ends of each box encompass the extreme data points. Proportions of Tregs, PD-1 expressing CD4$^+$ T-cells or CD8$^+$ T-cells and TLR3 expressing CD14$^+$ monocytes were measured by flow cytometry and data were presented by percentage. P-values were determined by Kruskal-Wallis H test and Nemenyi test. *$P<0.05$, **$P<0.01$, ***$P<0.001$.

Treatment Responses

As 4 cases who didn't provide requested information at 12 weeks after treatment were missing, 66 subjects were included in the efficacy analysis for cEVR assessment (34 patients treated with IFNα-2b/RBV and 32 cases with PegIFNα-2a/RBV). Among 34 patients treated with IFNα-2b/RBV, 25 (73.5%, 25/34) achieved cEVR, and 25 (78.1%, 25/32) underwent PegIFNα-2a/RBV treatment achieved cEVR. There was no significant difference in the cEVR incidences between the two groups ($P=0.663$).

We evaluated the potential relationship between HCV genotypes and early response patterns (cEVR or non-cEVR). Among 66 subjects included in the efficacy analysis for cEVR assessment

(60 patients infected with HCV genotype 1b and 6 cases with HCV genotype 2a), 45 (75.0%, 45/60) patients with HCV genotype 1b infection achieved cEVR, while 5 (83.3%, 5/6) patients infected with HCV genotype 2a achieved cEVR.

Tregs and Virological Response

The effect of different types of interferon combined with RBV on peripheral CD4$^+$CD25$^+$FoxP3$^+$ Tregs proportion in CD4$^+$ T-cells was assessed. The Tregs frequency was higher in chronic hepatitis C patients than that in the controls ($P=0.031$) (Fig. 2), which was significantly decreased at 12 weeks after treatment with IFNα-2b/RBV ($P=0.015$) (Fig. 3A) or PegIFNα-2a/RBV ($P=0.034$) (Fig. 3B). No further change was observed at 24 weeks compared with 12 weeks following treatment. With respect to the Tregs levels, no significant difference was observed between IFNα-2b/RBV and PegIFNα-2a/RBV groups in any time point ($P>0.05$). A representative flow cytometry dot plot of Tregs proportion in CD4$^+$ T-cells was shown in Fig. 4A and 4B.

As compared with the baselines, the Tregs frequency was significantly decreased at 12, 24 weeks in cEVR patients ($P<0.001$) and at 24 weeks in non-cEVR cases ($P=0.001$ and $P=0.015$, respectively) after treatment with IFNα-2b/RBV or PegIFNα-2a/RBV (Fig. 5A and 5B). Futhermore, Tregs frequency was significantly lower in cEVR patients than that in non-cEVR cases after 12 weeks of medication ($P<0.001$ and $P=0.015$, respectively) (Fig. 5C and 5D), whereas no significant difference in the proportion was found at baseline and 24 weeks after therapy (Fig. 5C and 5D).

PD-1 Expressing CD4$^+$ Or CD8$^+$ T-cells and Virological Response

PD-1 expression on T-cell subsets was determined by the percentage of PD-1 positive cells. The PD-1 expressing CD4$^+$ T-cells ($P=0.012$) or CD8$^+$ T-cells ($P=0.004$) were significantly higher in chronic hepatitis C patients than those in healthy controls at baseline (Fig. 2). Compared with its baseline level, PD-1 expressing CD8$^+$ T-cells was decreased after 12 weeks of therapy in patients received IFNα-2b/RBV ($P=0.035$) or PegIFNα-2a/RBV ($P=0.015$), and further reduced at 24 weeks after treatment compared with its 12 weeks level ($P=0.034$ and $P=0.029$, respectively) (Fig. 3A and 3B). However, the PD-1 expressing CD4$^+$ T-cells did not show significant change after antiviral treatment. In addition, there was no significant difference of the PD-1 expressing CD4$^+$ T-cells or CD8$^+$ T-cells between IFNα-2b/RBV and PegIFNα-2a/RBV groups in any parallel time point ($P>0.05$). A representative flow cytometry dot plot of PD-1 expressing CD4$^+$ or CD8$^+$ T-cells was shown in Fig. 6A and 6B.

By analyzing the relationship between PD-1 level and virological response, compared with the baseline levels, PD-1 expressing CD4$^+$ T-cells were markedly decreased after 12 weeks of therapy with IFNα-2b/RBV ($P=0.004$) or PegIFNα-2a/RBV ($P<0.001$) in cEVR patients, but it did not show significant change in non-cEVR cases (Fig. 5A and 5B). As respect to PD-1 expressing CD8$^+$ T-cells, we found that it's frequency was significantly decreased at 12, 24 weeks in cEVR patients ($P<0.001$) and at 24 weeks in non-cEVR cases ($P=0.009$ and $P=0.006$, respectively) after treatment with IFNα-2b/RBV or PegIFNα-2a/RBV (Fig. 5A and 5B). Compared with non-cEVR patients, frequencies of PD-1 expressing CD4$^+$ ($P=0.005$ and $P=0.002$, respectively) in two treatment groups and PD-1 expressing CD8$^+$ T-cells ($P=0.001$) in IFNα-2b/RBV treated group were significantly lower in patients who achieved cEVR after 12 weeks of therapy (Fig. 5C and 5D), though no differences were seen at baseline and 24 weeks after treatment (Fig. 5C and 5D).

A

B

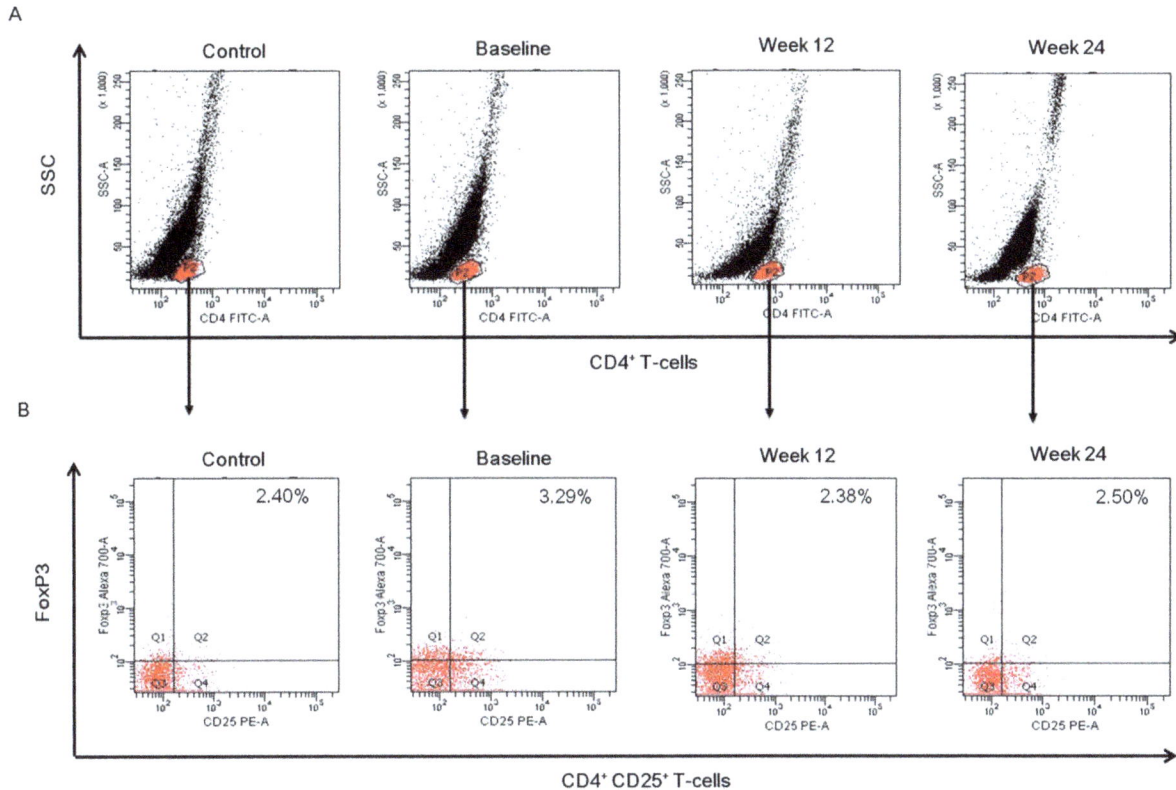

Figure 4. Representative dot plots of Tregs frequencies in peripheral CD4⁺ T-cells in healthy controls and chronic HCV-infected patients. (A) CD4⁺ lymphocytes were gated by positive staining of CD4 and side scatter (SSC). (B) Dot plots illustrating CD4⁺CD25⁺FoxP3⁺ Tregs in CD4⁺ cells. Cells were stained with monoclonal antibodies to CD4, CD25 and FoxP3. The lymphocyte subpopulation was selected on the basis of forward scatter (FSC) and SSC from peripheral blood cells. The percentage of positive cells is indicated in the upper right region.

TLR3 Expressing CD14⁺ Monocytes and Virological Response

TLR3 expressing CD14⁺ monocytes, determined by the percentage of TLR3 positive cells, were higher in chronic hepatitis C patients than those in healthy controls ($P<0.001$) (Fig. 2), and further increased after 12 weeks of treatment ($P=0.033$ and $P=0.018$, respectively), but returned to baseline level at 24 weeks in the two treatment groups (Fig. 3A and 3B). No significant difference was presented in TLR3 expressing CD14⁺ monocytes between IFNα-2b/RBV and PegIFNα-2a/RBV groups in any parallel time point ($P>0.05$). A representative flow cytometry dot plot of TLR3 expressing CD14⁺ monocytes was shown in Fig. 7A and 7B.

TLR3 expressing CD14⁺ monocytes were significantly increased after 12 weeks of treatment ($P<0.001$), and restored close to the baseline levels at 24 weeks in cEVR patients of the two treatment groups, but this changes were not significant in non-cEVR cases (Fig. 5A and 5B). Notably, the baseline TLR3 expressing CD14⁺ monocytes were significantly lower in patients achieved cEVR than those with non-cEVR ($P=0.009$ and $P=0.011$, respectively) (Fig. 5C and 5D), whereas there was no relationship between TLR3 expressing CD14⁺ monocytes and virological response at 12 and 24 weeks after treatment in the two groups (Fig. 5C and 5D).

Predict Factors of Treatment Response

Variables that may be related to treatment response were assessed by multivariate logistic regression analysis, including baseline laboratory parameters, consisting of Tregs, PD-1 expressing CD4⁺ T-cells or CD8⁺ T-cells, TLR3 expressing CD14⁺ monocytes, serum viral load, ALT and AST, as well as the use of interferon types. It was found that low proportion of baseline TLR3 expressing CD14⁺ monocytes was a single predictor of cEVR in chronic hepatitis C patients with antiviral treatment [odds ratio (OR) $=2.11$, 95% confidence intervals (CI) (1.15–3.88), $P=0.023$].

Lack of Association of Tregs, PD-1 and TLR3 with HCV Genotype, Viral Load, ALT and AST

Relationships of the baseline levels and the dynamic changes during treatment of Tregs, PD-1 expressing CD4⁺ T-cells or CD8⁺ T-cells and TLR3 expressing CD14⁺ monocytes with HCV genotypes were analyzed. No difference was found between HCV genotype 1b and 2a infected patients at each time point (data not shown). Moreover, there was no correlation of Tregs, PD-1 expressing CD4⁺ T-cells or CD8⁺ T-cells and TLR3 expressing CD14⁺ monocytes with baseline HCV load, ALT and AST levels as well (data not shown).

Discussion

Patients who achieved cEVR have the best chance of achieving SVR [19,20]. In our study, the cEVR rates were 73.5% and 78.1% in patients treated with IFNα-2b/RBV and PegIFNα-2a/RBV, respectively. The results were better than others reported on the early pivotal clinical trials, in which only 50%–66% patients infected with HCV achieved cEVR [21–23]. The reasons for this

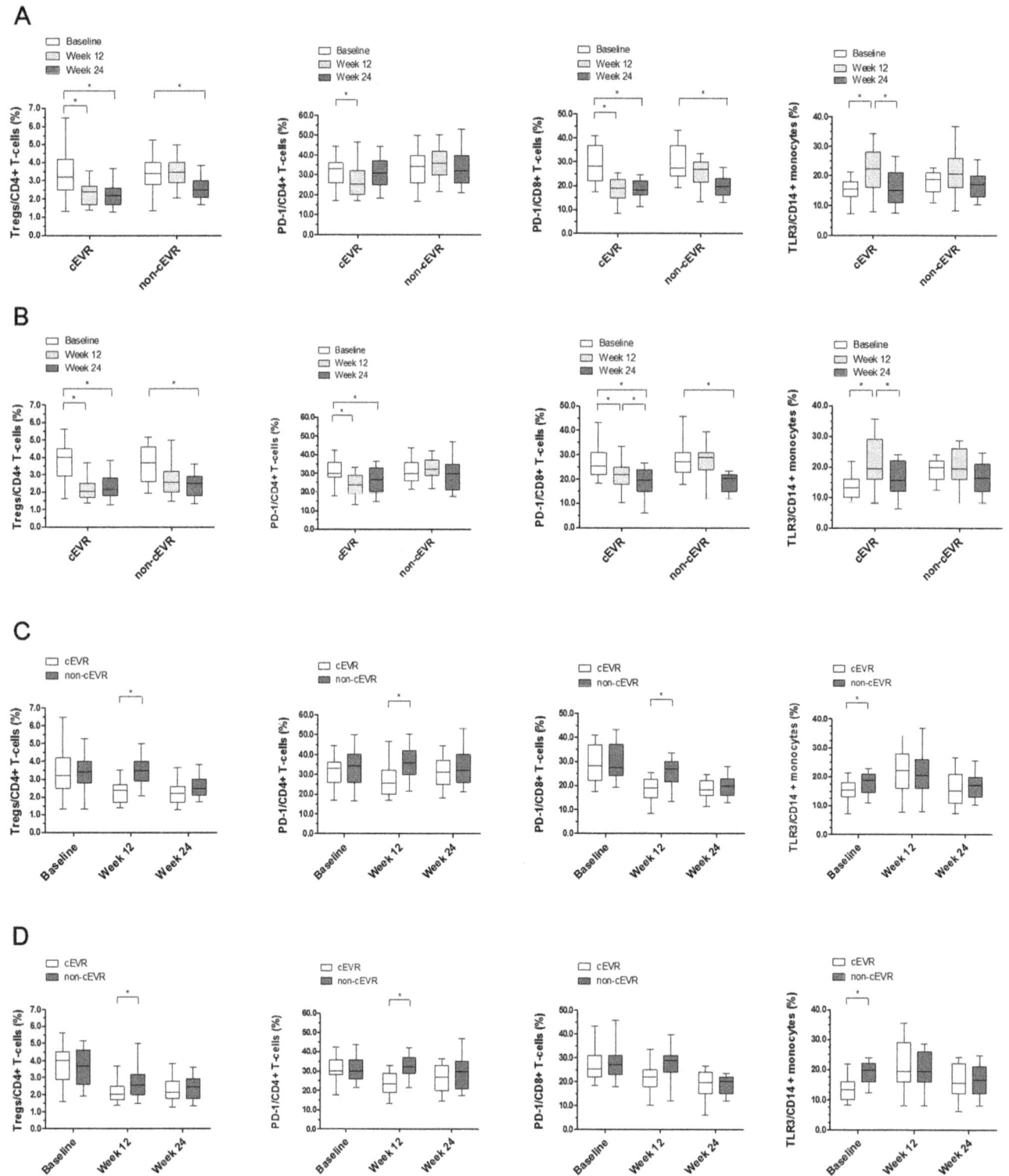

Figure 5. Proportions of Tregs, PD-1 expressing CD4+ T-cells or CD8+ T-cells and TLR3 expressing CD14+ monocytes at three time points treated with (A) IFNα-2b/RBV or (B) PegIFNα-2a/RBV and in cEVR or non-cEVR patients treated with (C) IFNα-2b/RBV or (D) PegIFNα-2a/RBV. Boxes represent the interquartile range and horizontal lines inside each box represent the median. The vertical lines from the ends of each box encompass the extreme data points. Proportions of Tregs, PD-1 expressing CD4+ T-cells or CD8+ T-cells and TLR3 expressing CD14+ monocytes were measured by flow cytometry and data were presented by percentage. *P*-values were determined by mixed model and Bonferroni correction method. *$P<0.0167$.

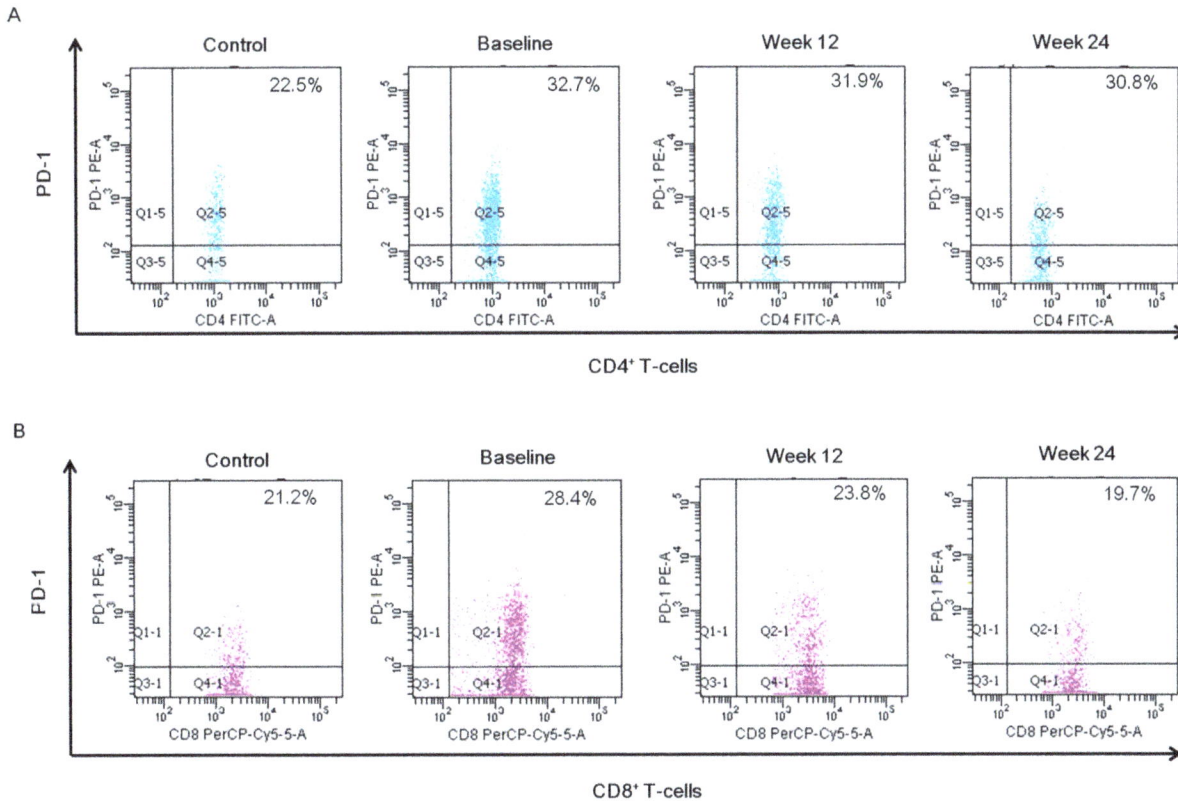

Figure 6. Representative dot plots of PD-1 expressing CD4$^+$ T-cells or CD8$^+$ T-cells in healthy controls and chronic HCV-infected patients. (A) Dot plots illustrating PD-1 expressing CD4$^+$ cells and (B) CD8$^+$ cells. Cells were stained with monoclonal antibodies to CD4, CD8 and PD-1. The lymphocyte subpopulation was selected on the basis of forward scatter (FSC) and side scatter (SSC) from peripheral blood cells. CD4$^+$ or CD8$^+$ lymphocytes were gated by positive staining of CD4 or CD8 and SSC. The percentage of positive cells is indicated in the upper right region.

disparity might arise from host IL-28B genetic variation (rs12979860 CC genotype) [24] and low body weight in Chinese population which were associated with interferon sensitivity and treatment-induced viral clearance.

A favorable treatment response includes a strong cellular immune response against HCV antigens [25,26]. To seek the role of cellular immune response in chronic hepatitis C patients with antiviral treatment, we investigated the dynamic changes of peripheral Tregs, PD-1 expressing T-cells and TLR3 expressing CD14$^+$ monocytes in the patients. In the present study, proportions of Tregs and PD-1 expressing CD4$^+$ T-cells or CD8$^+$ T-cells were significantly increased in the patients at baseline as compared with the controls, indicating that the impaired cellular immune function might contribute to chronic HCV infection. It was reported that HCV infection had a high propensity to develop persistent viremia and was associated with ineffective viral-specific CD4$^+$ and CD8$^+$ T-cells responses [27,28]. The cause of T-cells failure might relate to up-regulation of CD4$^+$CD25$^+$FoxP3$^+$ Tregs [6] and PD-1 expressions [11,13,29–32] which inhibited HCV-specific CD4$^+$ and CD8$^+$ T-cells function.

Feld et al. [33] has suggested that the immune-modulatory activity of interferon and ribavirin therapy may be associated with enhancing T effector cells response to HCV, thus, the impaired cellular immunity by persistent HCV infection might be partially restored by interferon and ribavirin administration. In our study, there was a significant decrease of Tregs and PD-1 expressing CD8$^+$ T-cells in chronic hepatitis C patients at 12 weeks after treatment compared with their baseline levels, indicating that

IFN/RBV treatment could restore HCV-specific T-cells response by reducing circulating CD4$^+$CD25$^+$FoxP3$^+$ Tregs and PD-1 expressing CD8$^+$ T-cells. Furthermore, the decrease proportions of Tregs and PD-1 expressing CD4$^+$ T-cells or CD8$^+$ T-cells were more obvious in cEVR patients than those in non-cEVR cases. According to Thimme et al. [34,35], T cell exhaustion contributed to the failure of about half of HCV-specific CD8$^+$ T cell responses and the antiviral efficacy of HCV-specific CD8$^+$ T cells was linked to surface expression of PD-1. Other studies had also reported that PD-1 was up-regulated on total CD4$^+$ and CD8$^+$ T cells in patients with chronic infection compared with normal subjects, and antiviral therapy that led to sustained elimination of circulating HCV RNA was associated with down-regulation of PD-1 on a wide range of cells [36,37]. Besides PD-1 modulation, activation of Tregs also involved in impairment of HCV-specific T effector cells. Langhans's study proposed that antiviral therapy is likely to shift the functional balance in the immune system between Tregs and T effector cells towards more efficacious effector responses in chronic hepatitis C patients. Our finding was in accordance with Langhans report [38], which indicated that interferon combined with ribavirin therapy could enhance proliferation of T effector cells as well as inhibit functions of Tregs, thus, reverses Treg-mediated suppression of T effector cells in chronic hepatitis C.

Treatment with IFNα-2b/RBV or PegIFNα-2a/RBV for 12 weeks, the frequencies of circulating Tregs and PD-1 expressing CD4$^+$ in two groups or PD-1 expressing CD8$^+$ T-cells in IFNα-2b/RBV group in patients who achieved cEVR were significantly lower than those in patients without cEVR. For

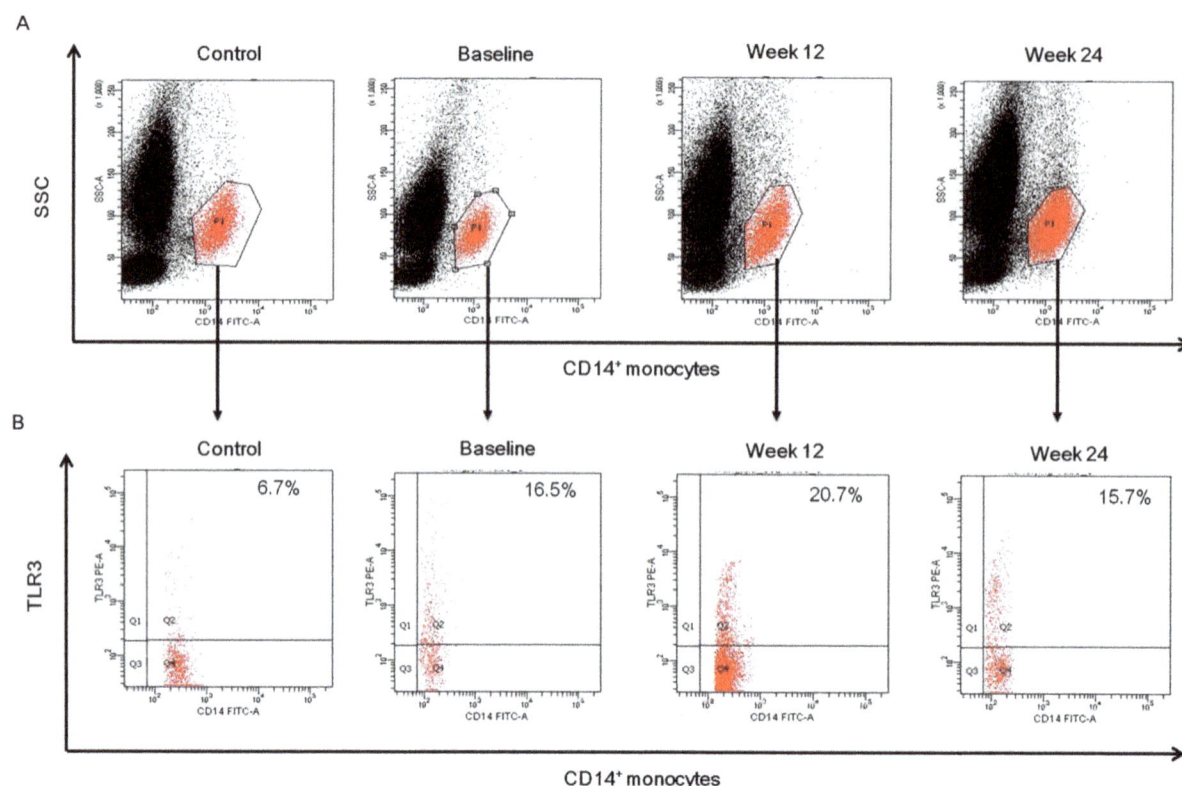

Figure 7. Representative dot plots of TLR3 expressing CD14$^+$ monocytes in healthy controls and chronic HCV-infected patients. (A) CD14$^+$ monocytes were gated by positive staining of CD14 and side scatter (SSC). (B) Dot plots illustrating TLR3 expressing CD14$^+$ cells. Cells were stained with monoclonal antibodies to CD14 and TLR3. The percentage of positive cells is indicated in the upper right region.

PegIFNα-2a/RBV treated group, the frequencies of PD-1 expressing CD8$^+$ was also lower in cEVR patients, but the P value was higher than 0.0167, perhaps on account of small sample size. Therefore, we speculated that Tregs and PD-1 could inhibit the responder cells population and function, which correlated with the risk of developing non-response. In contrast, patients who showed relatively abrogated capacity of Tregs and PD-1 might achieve cEVR and recover from HCV infection. This demonstrated that the suppression of Tregs and PD-1 might correlate with cEVR as it could generate an effective immune response and which provide a possible therapeutic target for immune modulation. However, whether the decrease in the frequency of Tregs and PD-1 expressing CD4$^+$ or CD8$^+$ T-cells were the necessary causes of cEVR warranted further investigation. No significant differences of the Tregs and PD-1 expressing CD4$^+$ T-cells or CD8$^+$ T-cells were found between IFNα-2b/RBV and PegIFNα-2a/RBV treated groups at any parallel time either from cEVR or non-cEVR, indicating that the immunomodulatory effects of IFNα-2b and PegIFNα-2a were comparable.

Activation of TLRs can induce both innate and adaptive immunity [39]. TLR3 signaling is induced by double-stranded (ds) RNA, a molecular signature of viruses, and is mediated by the TIR domain-containing adaptor-inducing IFN-β (TRIF) adaptor molecule. Thus, TLR3 plays an important role in the host response to viral infections [40]. The innate immune response activated through recognition of viral PAMPs by TLR3 leads to IFN-β induction, which in turn increases the interferon stimulated genes (ISGs) expression. Thus far, TLR3 expression in peripheral blood has not been well analyzed in chronic hepatitis C patients under antiviral treatment. Monocytes in peripheral blood were

identified as the cells responding to TLRs stimulation [41]. In present study, we found that the level of TLR3 expressing CD14$^+$ monocytes was elevated in chronic hepatitis C patients and further increased at 12 weeks, but returned to baseline level at 24 weeks after treatment with IFNα-2b/RBV or PegIFNα-2a/RBV. This change was more significant in cEVR patients than that in non-cEVR ones. This suggested that the anti-HCV treatment could increase TLR3 expressing CD14$^+$ monocytes to enhance antiviral activity at early stage of treatment and restore the cell number and function to baseline level as HCV was cleared. An important finding coming from our TLR3 analysis was that lower peripheral TLR3 expressing CD14$^+$ monocytes at baseline was an independent predictor for cEVR. In keeping with our findings, Hashad et al. [22] and Yuki et al. [23] found that pretreatment up-regulation of hepatic TLR3 expression was a predictive factor for non-respond. HCV infection could activate monocytes via TLRs pathway and elevate the expression of TLR3 as our study found, but pre-existing monocytes activation was a factor mediating reduced responses to TLR3 stimulation [42]. Thus, infection of monocytes by HCV may account for a defective response to HCV infection. Furthermore, the endogenous IFN system activation in the liver before treatment not only was ineffective in HCV clearance but also hampered further response to exogenous IFN plus RBV [37]. These reasons might explain why the level of TLR3 expressing CD14$^+$ monocytes was lower in cEVR patients than that in non-cEVR ones, but further and expanded investigations were needed to clarify the underlying mechanisms. Therefore, the baseline level of peripheral TLR3 expressing CD14$^+$ monocytes might serve as a predictor of response to antiviral therapy and have a substantial impact on treatment decision-making.

Conclusions

In summary, the present study suggested that low peripheral TLR3 expressing CD14$^+$ monocytes at baseline was a novel predictor for early virological response of antiviral therapy in chronic HCV-infected patients. The patients treated with interferon plus ribavirin could achieve completely early virological response through the modulation of peripheral CD4$^+$CD25$^+$FoxP3$^+$ regulatory T-cells, PD-1 expressing CD4$^+$ or CD8$^+$ T-cells and TLR3 expressing CD14$^+$ monocytes.

Supporting Information

Checklist S1   CONSORT 2010 checklist information to report the randomized parallel-group study. The study process, reported sections and topics, checklist item numbers, content and described sections in this manuscript were described.

Protocol S1   Study protocol in English. Study design and exclusion criteria for this study was presented in English in this protocol.

Protocol S2   Study protocol in Chinese. Study design and exclusion criteria for this study was presented in Chinese in this protocol.

Acknowledgments

We are grateful to all subjects who generously provided blood samples for this study. A special thanks to Prof. Qing-bao Tian, Ms. Ying-jun Bei and Mrs. Xue-min Niu for their precious help in the statistic analysis of this manuscript.

Author Contributions

Conceived and designed the experiments: YN HZ DS. Performed the experiments: SS HH LK YZ SZ RW. Analyzed the data: YN HZ DS. Wrote the paper: SS YN JY.

References

1. Hadigan C, Kottilil S (2011) Hepatitis C virus infection and co-infection with human immunodeficiency virus: challenges and advancements in management. JAMA 306: 294–301.
2. Munir S, Saleem S, Idrees M, Tariq A, Butt S, et al. (2010) Hepatitis C treatment: current and future perspectives. Virol J 7: 296.
3. Shepard CW, Finelli L, Alter MJ (2005) Global epidemiology of hepatitis C virus infection. Lancet Infect Dis 5: 558–567.
4. Marukian S, Jones CT, Andrus L, Evans MJ, Ritola KD, et al. (2008) Cell culture-produced hepatitis C virus does not infect peripheral blood mononuclear cells. Hepatology 48: 1843–1850.
5. Shiina M, Rehermann B (2008) Cell culture-produced hepatitis C virus impairs plasma cytoid dendritic cell function. Hepatology 47: 385–395.
6. Zheng Y, Rudensky AY (2007) Foxp3 in control of the regulatory T cell lineage. Nat Immunol 8: 457–462.
7. Speletas M, Argentou N, Germanidis G, Vasiliadis T, Mantzoukis K, et al. (2011) Foxp3 expression in liver correlates with the degree but not the cause of inflammation. Mediators Inflamm 827565: 1–9.
8. Tseng KC, Ho YC, Hsieh YH, Lai NS, Wen ZH, et al. (2012) Elevated frequency and function of regulatory T cells in patients with active chronic hepatitis C. J Gastroenterol 47: 823–833.
9. Sarikonda G, von Herrath MG (2011) Immunosuppressive mechanisms during viral infectious diseases. Methods Mol Biol 677: 431–447.
10. Nakamoto N, Cho H, Shaked A, Olthoff K, Valiga ME, et al. (2009) Synergistic reversal of intrahepatic HCV-specific CD8 T cell exhaustion by combined PD-1/CTLA-4 blockade. PLoS Pathog 5: e1000313.
11. Nakamoto N, Kaplan DE, Coleclough J, Li Y, Valiga ME, et al. (2008) Functional restoration of HCV-specific CD8 T cells by PD-1 blockade is defined by PD-1 expression and compartmentalization. Gastroenterology 134: 1927–1937.
12. Urbani S, Amadei B, Tola D, Pedrazzi G, Sacchelli L, et al. (2008) Restoration of HCV-specific T cell functions by PD-1/PD-L1 blockade in HCV infection: effect of viremia levels and antiviral treatment. J Hepatol 48: 548–558.
13. Missale G, Pilli M, Zerbini A, Penna A, Ravanetti L, et al. (2012) Lack of full CD8 functional restoration after antiviral treatment for acute and chronic hepatitis C virus infection. Gut 61: 1076–1084.
14. Pasare C, Medzhitov R (2003) Toll pathway-dependent blockade of CD4$^+$CD25$^+$ T cell-mediated suppression by dendritic cells. Science 299: 1033–1036.
15. Hackl D, Loschko J, Sparwasser T, Reindl W, Krug AB (2011) Activation of dendritic cells via TLR7 reduces Foxp3 expression and suppressive function in induced Tregs. Eur J Immunol 41: 1334–1343.
16. Thomas A, Laxton C, Rodman J, Myangar N, Horscroft N, et al. (2007) Investigating Toll-like receptor agonists for potential to treat hepatitis C virus infection. Antimicrob Agents Chemother 51: 2969–2978.
17. Gao YT, Chen RY, Song WQ, Chen CB, Qi ZL, et al. (2004) Prepare and clinical application of HCV genotyping oligochip. Chin J Lab Med 27: 690–693.
18. Ghany MG, Nelson DR, Strader DB, Thomas DL, Seeff LB; American Association for Study of Liver Diseases. (2011) An update on treatment of genotype 1 chronic hepatitis C virus infection: 2011 practice guideline by the American Association for the Study of Liver Diseases. Hepatology 54: 1433–1444.
19. Chung HJ, Lee JW, Kim YS, Lee JI (2013) Prediction of sustained virologic response based on week 4 and week 12 response in hepatitis C virus genotype 1 patients treated with peginterferon and ribavirin: assessment in a favorable IL28B allele-prevalent area. Intervirology 56: 178–183.
20. Huang CF, Yang JF, Huang JF, Dai CY, Chiu CF, et al. (2010) Early identification of achieving a sustained virological response in chronic hepatitis C patients without a rapid virological response. J Gastroenterol Hepatol 25: 758–765.
21. Rodriguez-Torres M, Sulkowski MS, Chung RT, Hamzeh FM, Jensen DM (2010) Factors associated with rapid and early virologic response to peginterferon alfa-2a/ribavirin treatment in HCV genotype 1 patients representative of the general chronic hepatitis C population. J Viral Hepat 17: 139–147.
22. Hashad DI, Salem PE, Abdallah DM (2011) Toll like receptor 3 expression as a novel predictor of response to treatment in chronic hepatitis C virus patients. Scand J Clin Lab Invest 71: 641–646.
23. Yuki N, Matsumoto S, Kato M, Yamaguchi T (2010) Hepatic Toll-Like Receptor 3 expression in chronic hepatitis C genotype 1 correlates with treatment response to peginterferon plus ribavirin. J Viral Hepat 17: 130–138.
24. Liao XW, Ling Y, Li XH, Han Y, Zhang SY, et al. (2011) Association of genetic variation in IL28B with hepatitis C treatment-induced viral clearance in the Chinese Han population. Antivir Ther 16: 141–147.
25. Kamal SM, Fehr J, Roesler B, Peters T, Rasenack JW (2002) Peginterferon alone or with ribavirin enhances HCV-specific CD4 T-helper 1 responses in patients with chronic hepatitis C. Gastroenterology 123: 1070–1083.
26. Fitzmaurice K, Klenerman P (2008) Cellular immunity and acute hepatitis C infection. Curr Pharm Des 14: 1666–1677.
27. Bowen DG, Walker CM (2005) Adaptive immune responses in acute and chronic hepatitis C virus infection. Nature 436: 946–952.
28. Frebel H, Richter K, Oxenius A (2010) How chronic viral infections impact on antigen-specific T-cell responses. Eur J Immunol 40: 654–663.
29. Yao S, Wang S, Zhu Y, Luo L, Zhu G, et al. (2009) PD-1 on dendritic cells impedes innate immunity against bacterial infection. Blood 113: 5811–5818.
30. Golden-Mason L, Palmer B, Klarquist J, Mengshol JA, Castelblanco N, et al. (2007) Upregulation of PD-1 expression on circulating and intrahepatic hepatitis C virus-specific CD8$^+$ T cells associated with reversible immune dysfunction. J Virol 81: 9249–9258.
31. Rutebemberwa A, Ray SC, Astemborski J, Levine J, Liu L, et al. (2008) High-programmed death-1 levels on hepatitis C virus-specific T cells during acute infection are associated with viral persistence and require preservation of cognate antigen during chronic infection. J Immunol 181: 8215–8225.
32. Shen T, Zheng J, Liang H, Xu C, Chen X, et al. (2011) Characteristics and PD-1 expression of peripheral CD4$^+$CD127^{lo}CD25^{hi}FoxP3$^+$ Treg cells in chronic HCV infected-patients. Virol J 8: 279.
33. Feld JJ, Hoofnagle JH (2005) Mechanism of action of interferon and ribavirin in treatment of hepatitis C. Nature 436: 967–972.
34. Bengsch B, Seigel B, Ruhl M, Timm J, Kuntz M, et al. (2010) Coexpression of PD-1, 2B4, CD160 and KLRG1 on exhausted HCV-specific CD8$^+$ T cells is linked to antigen recognition and T cell differentiation. PLoS Pathog 6: e1000947.
35. Seigel B, Bengsch B, Lohmann V, Bartenschlager R, Blum HE, et al. (2013) Factors that determine the antiviral efficacy of HCV-specific CD8(+) T cells ex vivo. Gastroenterology 144: 426–436.
36. Raziorrouh B, Ulsenheimer A, Schraut W, Heeg M, Kurktschiev P, et al. (2011) Inhibitory molecules that regulate expansion and restoration of HCV-specific CD4$^+$ T cells in patients with chronic infection. Gastroenterology 141: 1422–1431.

37. Golden-Mason L, Klarquist J, Wahed AS, Rosen HR (2008) Cutting edge: programmed death-1 expression is increased on immunocytes in chronic hepatitis C virus and predicts failure of response to antiviral therapy: race-dependent differences. J Immunol 180: 3637–3641.

38. Langhans B, Nischalke HD, Arndt S, Braunschweiger I, Nattermann J, et al. (2012) Ribavirin exerts differential effects on functions of Cd4⁺ Th1, Th2, and regulatory T cell clones in hepatitis C. PLoS One 7: e42094.

39. Gay NJ, Gangloff M (2007) Structure and function of Toll receptors and their ligands. Annu Rev Biochem 76: 141–165.

40. Schroder M, Bowie AG (2005) TLR3 in antiviral immunity: key player or bystander? Trends Immunol 26: 462–468.

41. Villacres MC, Literat O, DeGiacomo M, Du W, Frederick T, et al. (2008) Defective response to Toll-like receptor 3 and 4 ligands by activated monocytes in chronic hepatitis C virus infection. J Viral Hepat 15: 137–144.

42. Sarasin-Filipowicz M, Oakeley EJ, Duong FH, Christen V, Terracciano L, et al. (2008) Interferon signaling and treatment outcome in chronic hepatitis C. Proc Natl Acad Sci USA 105: 7034–7039.

Serum GP73, a Marker for Evaluating Progression in Patients with Chronic HBV Infections

Hongshan Wei[1][*][9]**, Boan Li**[2][9]**, Renwen Zhang**[1]**, Xiaohua Hao**[1]**, Yubo Huang**[1]**, Yong Qiao**[1]**, Jun Hou**[2]**, Xin Li**[1]**, Xingwang Li**[1]

1 Beijing Ditan Hospital, Capital Medical University, Chaoyang District, Beijing, China, **2** Center of Lab test, 302 Military Hospital, Beijing, China

Abstract

This study was designed to investigate the role of serum GP73 for diagnosing significant fibrosis in patients with chronic hepatitis B virus (HBV) infections. Two populations were enrollment. All subjects were patients with chronic HBV infections. First population included 761 patients, who received liver stiffness measurement; the second population included 633 patients, who undertaken liver biopsy, in which 472 patients with nearly normal ALT. All patients received serum GP73 test. The effect of GP73 recombinant protein to HepG2 cells and LX2 cells were observed *in vitro*. Results showed that serum GP73 concentration is correlated with liver stiffness (r = 0.601). The area under ROC curve is 0.76. The sensitivity and specificity of GP73 for significant fibrosis (≥F2) diagnosis were 62.81%, 80.05% respectively (cut off: 76.6 ng/ml). Serum GP73 concentration was significantly correlated with the grading of fibrosis (r = 0.32, and 0.35, in 633 and 472 patients, respectively.) GP73 had a striking performance for diagnosing S2 in patients with chronic HBV infections. In 472 patients with nearly normal ALT, the sensitivity and specificity of GP73 for S2 diagnosis were 62.5% and 80.0% respectively, where the cut-off was set at 82 ng/ml. GP73 recombinant protein may prompt LX2 cells proliferation at the concentration 10–100 ng/ml. The present results indicated that GP73 may be a marker for diagnosing significant fibrosis in patients with chronic HBV infections, and may be a new contributor to fibrogensis.

Editor: Sang-Hoon Ahn, Yonsei University College of Medicine, Republic of Korea

Funding: Supported by grant from the National Natural Science Foundation of China (No.30872243; No.81071411) to Prof. HW; and grant from the Fund of Capital Clinical Investigation (No.111107058811068) to Prof. BL. The funders had no role in study design, data collection and analysis, decision to publish, or preparation of the manuscript.

Competing Interests: The authous have declared than no competing interests exist.

* E-mail: drwei@ccmu.edu.cn

9 These authors contributed equally to this work.

Introduction

Hepatic fibrosis, the common response associated with almost of all chronic hepatitis B virus (HBV) infection, ultimately leads to cirrhosis [1]. With great advancements in the antiviral therapy used for the treatment of chronic virus hepatitis, the accurate assessment of liver fibrosis is a vital need for successful individualized management. Current guidelines recommend antiviral therapy in chronic hepatitis B patients with significant fibrosis (≥2), whether or not ALT is abnormal [2]. Moreover, the significant fibrosis correlated strongly with poor clinical outcomes, compared with mild fibrosis [3]. Lack of accurate, reproducible and easily applied methods for fibrosis assessment is the major limitation in the clinical management. The current 'gold standard' for liver fibrosis detection is liver biopsy [4]. Liver biopsy can provide physicians useful clinical information, such as appropriate time to start antiviral therapy, predicting the response to treatment, assessing the natural course of hepatitis, and estimating prognosis of hepatitis. Although accuracy in detailed fibrosis classification may provide by liver biopsy; however, this method does has innate limits, such as invasive, sampling error and sample size effect, which limits its application. Consequently, the highly specific set of biomarkers for fibrosis grading always pursue by professionals.

In the past two decades, a number of markers in combination with clinical risk factors are used to evaluate fibrosis grade, such as FibroMeter, FibroTest, etc [5,6], all being used for diagnosing significant fibrosis. In fact, the combination of several biomarker for evaluating fibrosis grading were better prognosis predictors than histological staging [7,8]. Those methods have one common point, i.e., consisting of several serum marker and mathematical model used to calculate fibrosis index. Since all of those non-invasive models have moderate accuracy for determining significant fibrosis, new biomarkers for the diagnosis of significant fibrosis are still in strong demand by clinicians.

Recently, a novel Golgi protein, GP73, was used to diagnosing hepatocelullar carcinoma [9]. This protein initially reported by Kladney RD, et al [10], and they also found that GP73 expression is increased in cultured cells by viruses infection [10], Subsequently, several investigations demonstrated that GP73 protein is overexpressed in a variety of acute and chronic liver diseases [11], and serum concentration correlated with progression of chronic liver disease [12,13]. However, the relationship between serum GP73 concentration and staging or grading of chronic liver disease is still a pendent question. The present study was designed to evaluate the serum GP73 for diagnosing significant fibrosis and liver cirrhosis.

Table 1. Patient's clinical characteristic.

Parameter	Description	
Group	FibroScan (761)	liver biopsy (633)
Sex/age		
Male	492 (39.48±12.32 yrs)	440(36.11±10.72 yrs)
Female	269 (40.62±13.76 yrs)	193(34.07±10.37 yrs)*
Clinical diagnosis		
Chronic hepatitis	649 (85.28%)	582(91.94%)
Liver cirrhsis	112 (14.72%)	51(8.06%)
Comorbidity		
Diabetes	48(6.31%)	17(2.69%)
Hypertension	11(1.45%)	7(1.11%)
Coronary heart disease	4(0.53%)	2(0.32%)
HBeAg		
Positive	436(57.29%)	397(62.72%)
Negative	325(42.71%)	236(37.28%)
HBV DNA		
< 2 log	68(8.94%)	36(5.69%)
≥ 2 log	693(91.06%)	597(94.31%)
BMI (Kg/m^2)		
Male(mean ± S.D.)	22.60±5.12	24.26±6.67
Female(mean ± S.D.)	20.73±4.93*	21.33±3.91*
Total bilirubin (μmol/L)	22.79±38.0	21.30±37.54
Albumin (g/L)	43.36±6.11	42.86±6.06
Prothrombin time (s)	12.88±2.20	12.71±9.35

*Compared with male group, p<0.05.
Since without any patients with ascites, no related information was showed.

Materials and Methods

Study design

This study registered at ChiCTR.org (No.DDT-11001397) Oct, 2010, and included two populations. First population consisted of 761 patients with chronic hepatitis B, who were received liver stiffness measurement; second populations involved 633 patients with chronic HBV infections, in which 472 patients with nearly normal ALT (<80 U/L). Patients in second populations were received liver biopsy and pathological examination. All patients consecutively admitted to two centers (Beijing Ditan Hospital and 302 Military Hospital), between Aug. 2010 and Mar.2012. The study was approved by the Institutional Review Board of the Beijing Ditan Hospital, Capital Medical University. For group enrollment, liver stiffness measurement or liver biopsy were based on clinical requirement. Before initiating drug therapy, the serum samples were collected, and stored at −70°C.

Biochemical analysis

The liver function tests including serum albumin, total bilirubin (TB), and alanine aminotransferase (ALT) were measured using a Roche Hitachi 717 chemistry analyzer at the central laboratory of Beijing Ditan hospital. Quantitative determination of GP73 in serum was performed using commercially available enzyme-linked immunosorbent assay (ELISA)

(Hotgen Biotech Inc., Beijing, China), according to the manufacturer's protocol.

Transient elastography measurement

Liver stiffness was measured with a FibroScan® device (FibroScan®, Philips, France), based on manufacturer's protocol. Results were expressed in kilopascals (kPa). Ten successful acquisitions were performed for each patient, and the median value was calculated by the device. The cut-off point of liver stiffness score for significant fibrosis, and liver cirrhosis referenced to the previous report [14,15] i.e. 8.8 kPa(F2), for significant fibrosis, 16.9 kPa for liver cirrhosis.

Liver biopsy and Immunohistochemistry

Liver biopsies were obtained using 16G disposable needles (Hepafix, Germany). Fibrosis staging was considered reliable when the liver specimen length was ≥1.5 cm or the portal tract number ≥10. Liver specimens were stained with Masson trichrome and interpreted by two highly experienced liver pathologists. Liver fibrosis was scored on a 0–4 scale according to the METAVIR scoring system [16]. For GP73 staining, 3–5 μm formalin-fixed, paraffin-embedded samples were dewaxed and rehydrated. After slides incubating in 3% hydrogen peroxide, sections were incubated with GP73 antibody (HotGen Biotech, Beijing, China) overnight at 4°C; HRP-labeling anti-rabbit (Boster Bio., Wuhan, China) were used as secondary antibodies. 3,3′-Diaminobenzidine (DAB) Substrate Chromogen System (Dako) and was employed in the detection procedure. Images were acquired on an Olympus E520 (Tokyo, Japan) microscope.

Cell culture and proliferation assay

Hepatoma cell line (HepG2) was reserved in our laboratory. Hepatic stellate cell line (LX2) was conferred by Prof. Cheng (Institute of Infectious Disease, Capital Medical University). LX2 cells line is a widely used hepatic stellate cell in the fibrosis investigation [17]. HepG2 and LX2 cells were cultured at 37°C in a humidified atmosphere containing 5% CO_2 in Eagle's minimum essential medium supplemented with10% fetal bovine serum. The ultimate concentration of GP73 recombinant protein added in supernatant was 1.0, 10.0, 20.0, 50.0, and 100.0 ng/ml respectively. After 48 hours coculturing, cell proliferation was evaluated with OD value, which was detected by CCK8 assay kit (Dojindo, Kumamoto, Japan), based on manufacture's protocol.

Western blot

Western blot was performed with standard protocol. Briefly, after cells cocultured with GP73 recombinant protein 48 hours, whole-cell extracts were prepared in assay buffer containing a protease inhibitor cocktail. Protein assays were performed using a BCA Protein assay kit (Pierce/Thermo Scientific, USA) according to the manufacturer's instructions. Total protein was electrophoresed in SDS–PAGE gels, and transferred to nitrocellulose membranes and then blocked with 5% milk in PBS, pH 7.4 with 0.05% Tween-20, incubated with collagen I or collagen III polyclonal antibody (Santa Cruz, USA) and anti-rabbit secondary antibody conjugated to horseradish peroxidase (Santa Cruz., USA). GP73 was detected by chemiluminescence.

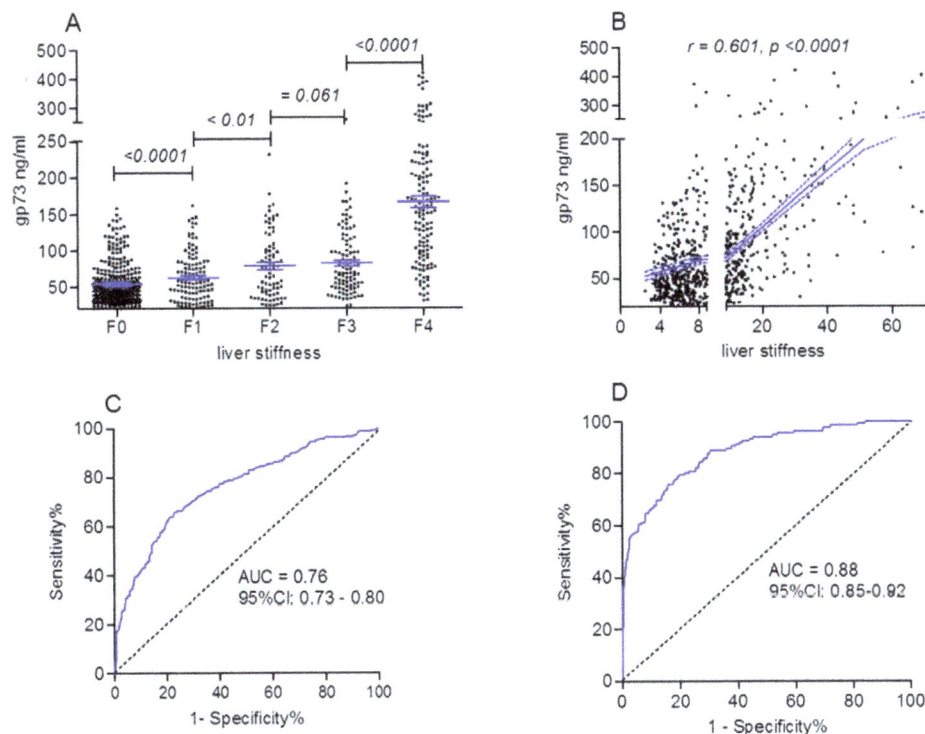

Figure 1. Serum GP73 concentration was correlated with liver stiffness (761 patients). A: Different GP73 levels were observed in patients with different groups of liver stiffness. B: serum GP73 concentration was correlated with liver stiffness. C and D: the ROC analysis of GP73 was performed on diagnosis of significant fibrosis and liver cirrhosis. The numbers after symbols "<"or " =" are p value.

Statistical analysis

Statistical analysis was performed using GraphPad Prism 5.0. Student t test was used to compare the difference of serum GP73 concentrations between different patients groups (mild and significant fibrosis group). Correlation between serum GP73 concentration and liver stiffness scores were calculated using Pearson's correlation coefficient (r). Data were expressed as mean ± SEM. P-values <0.05 were considered to be statistically significant. With liver stiffness value (FibroScan) or biopsy as the "gold standard", the diagnostic performance of GP73 was evaluated by performing the Area under the ROC curve (AUROC) with 95% confidence interval (CI). For adjusting other confounders (Sex, Age, ALT, Total Bilirubin, Albumin, Platelet), we performed multivariate ordinal logistic regression analysis by SPSS 16.0.

Results

Patient's characteristics

From Aug. 2010 to Mar 2012, 761 patients received liver stiffness measurements; 633 patients received liver biopsy, in which 472 patients with nearly normal ALT. Those patients consecutively admitted into Beijing Ditan Hospital, Capital Medical University and 302 Military Hospital. The demological materials of two populations were showed in table 1.

Serum GP73 concentration significantly correlated with hepatic stiffness

Based on more recently report, the diagnostic thresholds of liver stiffness in discriminating fibrosis stages ≥ F1, ≥ F2, ≥ F3 and = F4 were 7.1 kPa, 8.8 kPa, 10.7 kPa, and 16.9 kPa, respectively.

Based on data of liver stiffness, 57.95% (441/761) patients had mild fibrosis (324 patients with very mild fibrosis; 117 patients with F1 grade). 42.05% (320/761) patients were significant or severe fibrosis (F2:79, F3:105, F4:136). Obviously, more cirrhotic patients were confirmed with liver stiffness than initially clinician's diagnosis (Fig. 1A, Table 2).

To ascertain the correlation between serum GP73 concentration and liver stiffness, we firstly performed correlated analysis. Results showed that serum GP73 concentration is correlated with the value of liver stiffness (Correlation coefficient $r = 0.601$, p<0.0001). (Fig. 1B) Serum GP73 concentrations were significantly different between patients with different fibrotic group, except for F3 group (Fig. 1A). The important is that GP73 levels in patients of F2 group (78.46±45.35 ng/ml) is significantly higher than those of in patients of F1 group (62.54±34.31 ng/ml, p<0.01). This result suggested that GP73 concentration may be a marker for differentiating significant fibrosis (≥ F2) with mild fibrosis (<F2). The other interesting result is, for most cirrhotic patients, serum GP73 concentrations were especially higher than patients in F2 or F3 group. Despite serum GP73 concentration in patients of F3 group (81.90±44.51 ng/ml) were higher than those of patients in F2 group (78.46±45.35 ng/ml), this difference is no significant.

To clarify the optimal cut-off value of GP73 in diagnosing significant fibrosis (≥F2) in patients with chronic hepatitis B, we performed receiver operator characteristic (ROC) curve analysis. ROC curve analyses showed that the sensitivity and specificity of GP73 for significant fibrosis diagnosis were 62.81% (95% CI: 57.26%–68.12%), 80.05% (95% CI: 80.05%–83.68%) respectively, where the cut-off value was set at 76.6 ng/ml. The area under ROC curve is 0.76 (95% CI:

Table 2. Serum GP73 concentration related with liver stiffness (FibroScan), ALT, Fibrosis grading, and serum HBV DNA.

Parameter	N	GP73(ng/mL)	
		Mean ± SD	95%CI
Liver stiffness[a]			
< F1	324	53.70±28.84	50.55–56.85
F1	117	62.54±34.31	56.27–68.60
F2	79	78.46±45.35	68.30–88.61
F3	105	91.90±44.51	73.28–90.51
F4	136	166.0±87.39	151.2–180.8
Fibrosis grading[b]			
0.5	48	56.75±38.33	45.62–67.88
1.0	232	60.37±40.07	55.19–65.55
1.5	35	72.03±37.75	59.06–84.99
2.0	57	80.03±59.48	64.25–95.81
2.5	26	93.80±49.04	73.99–113.6
3.0	40	92.28±69.69	68.10–120.7
3.5	18	94.40±52.88	68.10–120.7
4.0	16	458.1±119.1	94.67–221.6
ALT(U/L)[c]			
≤ 40	274	71.90±55.28	65.33–78.48
< 80	197	72.52±53.07	65.08–79.98
80–200	93	88.35±77.53	72.38–104.3
> 200	69	137.0±89.25	115.5–158.4
HBV DNA(log10 IU/ml)[b]			
negative	25	49.13±17.39	41.95–56.31
< 4	99	65.00+41.52	56.72–73.29
≥ 4	106	91.88±88.7*	74.79–109.0
≥ 6	194	81.93±63.81	72.89–90.96
≥ 8	48	83.08±58.15	66.20–99.97

[a]. 761 patients received liver stiffness measurements; [b]. 472 patients with nearly normal ALT; [c]. 633 patients with chronic hepatitis B infections; * P<0.05 Compared with patients with HBV DNA less than 4 Log.

0.73–0.80). The positive predictive value (PPV), the negative predictive value (NPV), and acuuracy were 74.73%, 67.69, and 72.01%, respectively. If the diagnostic cut-off value was set at 135.4 ng/ml, the sensitivity and specificity of GP73 for diagnosing liver cirrhosis (F4) were 60.29% (95% CI: 51.55%–68.58%), 94.01% (95% CI: 91.84%–95.75%) respectively. The area under ROC curve is 0.88 (95%CI: 0.85–0.92). (Fig. 1.C, D). The PPV, the NPV, and acuuracy were 91.68%, 60.29%, and 86.07%, respectively.

Sensitivity and specificity of GP73 for diagnosis significant fibrosis

Serum GP73 concentration was significantly correlated with the grading of fibrosis (correlation coefficient r = 0.32, and 0.35, in 633 patients with chronic hepatitis B, and in which 472 patients with nearly normal ALT, respectively.) (Fig. 2.A, B). The mean GP73 concentration increased with liver grading aggravation, but significantly statistical differences only observed in several groups (Table 2; Fig. 2C).

To characterize GP73 as a new diagnostic tissue marker of significant fibrosis (≥S2), or moderate/severe inflammation (≥G2), we conducted a ROC analysis. The results showed that GP73 had a striking performance for diagnosing S2 or G2 in patients with chronic HBV infections. In patients with nearly normal ALT, the sensitivity and specificity of GP73 for S2 diagnosis were 62.5% (95%CI: 56.26–68.45%) and 80.0% (75.9–83.68%) respectively, where the cut-off was set at 82 ng/ml (Fig. 2D); The PPV, NPV, and diagnosing accuracy were 87.76%, 67.98%, and 80.29%, respectively. For G2 diagnosis, the sensitivity and specificity were 53.2% (95% CI: 47.35–58.95%) and 80.21(75.89–84.05%) respectively, the cut-off was 85 ng/ml (Fig. 2, E). The PPV, NPV, and diagnosing accuracy were 73.11%, 54.78%, and 68.64%, respectively. If the cut-off was set at 138.4 ng/ml for cirrhosis (S 3.5–4) diagnosis, the sensitivity and specificity were 38.24% (22.17–56.44%) and 90.18% (87.00–92.80%) respectively (Fig. 2.F). The PPV, NPV, and diagnosing accuracy were 94.95%, 23.21%, and 86.44%, respectively.

Which factors related with serum GP73 levels?

Multivariate ordinal logistic regression analysis was performed to adjust other potential confounders (Sex, Age, ALT, total bilirubin, albumin, Platelet). The results showed that serum GP73 was an independent risk factor of liver fibrogenesis in CHB patients with nearly normal ALT. The relative risk was increased 1.106 with the serum GP73 increasing 10 ng/mL. The results were showed in table 3. To explore the causes of GP73 increasing in serum, we further performed a Pearson's correlation analysis on several biomarkers, which reflected virus replication, hepatocytes injury, and other liver functions. As Fig. 3A and 3B showed, that ALT, total bilirubin (Tbil) were positively correlated with serum GP73 concentration. The correlation coefficient r were 0.25, 0.18, respectively (Fig. 3, B, F). The interesting data was that ALT seemed not significantly correlated with GP73 concentration in 472 patients with nearly normal ALT (r = 0.014, p = 0.76), by contraries, the total of 633 patients was (r = 0.25, p = 0.0003) (Fig. 3B, Table 2). Similarly, although HBV DNA was not correlated with serum GP73 concentration (r = 0.01, p = 0.89), the serum GP73 concentration of patients with HBV DNA above 4log was significantly higher than those of patients with HBV DNA below 4 log (p = 0.007) (Fig. 3C and 3D; Table 2). The other interesting result was that patient's GP73 levels were negatively correlated with their ALB levels (Fig. 3E).

To further validate GP73 expression in liver tissue with different fibrotic gradings, we observed character of GP73 staining in different biopsy sample. Immunohistochemical analysis showed that GP73 positive cells mainly scattered in parenchymal cells, but several non parenchymal cells also positive staining (Fig. 4). This result was consistent with Iftikhar R, et al. [12], report. Compared with mild fibrotic tissue, GP73 was strongly expressed in significant or severe fibrotic liver tissue.

Serum GP73 may be a contributor to liver fibrosis

To investigate the effect of GP73 to hepatocytes or hepatic stellate cells, we used different concentration of GP73 recombinant protein (1.0, 10.0, 20.0, 50.0, and 100.0 ng/ml) coculturing with HepG2 cells, or LX2 cells. The result showed that GP73 may obviously prompt proliferation of LX2 cells (Talbe.4; Fig. 5.A), but without any effect on HepG2 cells in vitro (data not show). With concentration of GP73 recombinant protein increasing (from 10 ng/mL to 80 ng/mL), the OD values of cultured LX2 cells also increased (Fig. 5A). The results suggested

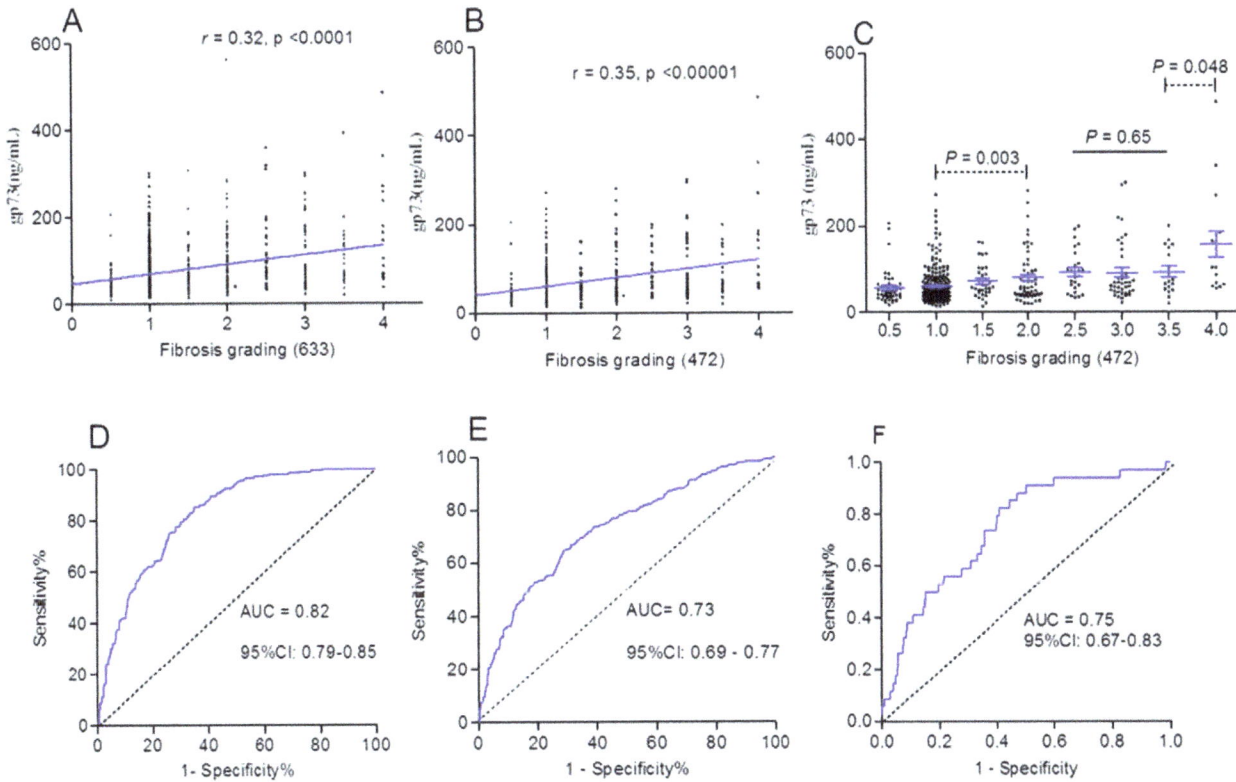

Figure 2. Serum GP73 was correlated with grading of patients. A: serum GP73 was correlated with grading of 633 patients. B and C: serum GP73 was correlated with grading of 472 patients with nearly normal ALT. D, E, F: ROC analysis of GP73 was performed on diagnosing S2(D), G2(E), and cirrhosis (F) respectively.

Table 3. The Multivariate ordinal logistic regression analysis for the factors assocaited with Fibrogenesis.

Parameter	b	stb	Wald χ^2 P		OR	95%CI for OR	
						Lower	Upper
Fibrosis grading							
4	0.25	0.88	0.08	0.771	-	-	-
3.5	1.22	0.86	2.02	0.155	-	-	-
3	2.21	0.86	6.62	0.010	-	-	-
2.5	2.64	0.86	9.39	0.002	-	-	-
2	3.37	0.87	15.17	<.0001	-	-	-
1.5	3.73	0.87	18.41	<.0001	-	-	-
1	6.59	0.91	52.65	<.0001	-	-	-
0.5	8.00	0.95	70.86	<.0001	-	-	-
GP73 (per 10 ng/mL)	0.01	0.00	30.62	<.0001	1.010	1.007	1.014
ALB (per 10 g/L)	−0.08	0.02	18.03	<.0001	0.927	0.895	0.960
PLT (per 10 ×109/L)	−0.01	0.00	30.87	<.0001	0.992	0.990	0.995

Note: Adjusted the factors including Sex, Age, ALT, total bilirubin, albumin, and platelet.

that GP73 recombinant protein may prompt LX2 cells proliferation *in vitro*. After cocultured 48 hours, the collagen III expression in LX2 cells was increased, but the collagen I was not (Fig. 5.B). We speculated that GP73 might regulate hepatic stellated cells by autocrine, since LX2 also expressed GP73 *in vitro* (Fig. 5C).

Discussion

The ultimate aim of fibrosis grading is provided clinicians with accurate information for treatment decision and prognosis judgment. Identifying significant fibrosis is also one of critical factors for treatment decision, especially for patients with mild abnormal ALT [18]. Avoided or reduced times of liver biopsy, but obtained pathological information from liver tissue, is always pursued by clinicians. Multi-marker combination can provide more accurate information about fibrosis [19], but result in increasing the patient's expenditure and clinician's working load. Based on our present data, GP73 might be a useful single marker for diagnosing significant fibrosis and cirrhosis in patients with chronic HBV infections.

The first question is why serum GP73 concentration correlated with liver stiffness? Based on recently reports, serum GP73 concentration related with progression of chronic liver diseases [13,20]. Different with other HCC marker, increased serum GP73 is related to hepatic impairment and chronic fibrosis [21,20]. In patients with Wilson disease, serum GP73 levels were associated with liver inflammation, fibrosis, and dysplasia, rather than copper overload [22]. More importantly, other experimental research showed that hepatic stellate cells

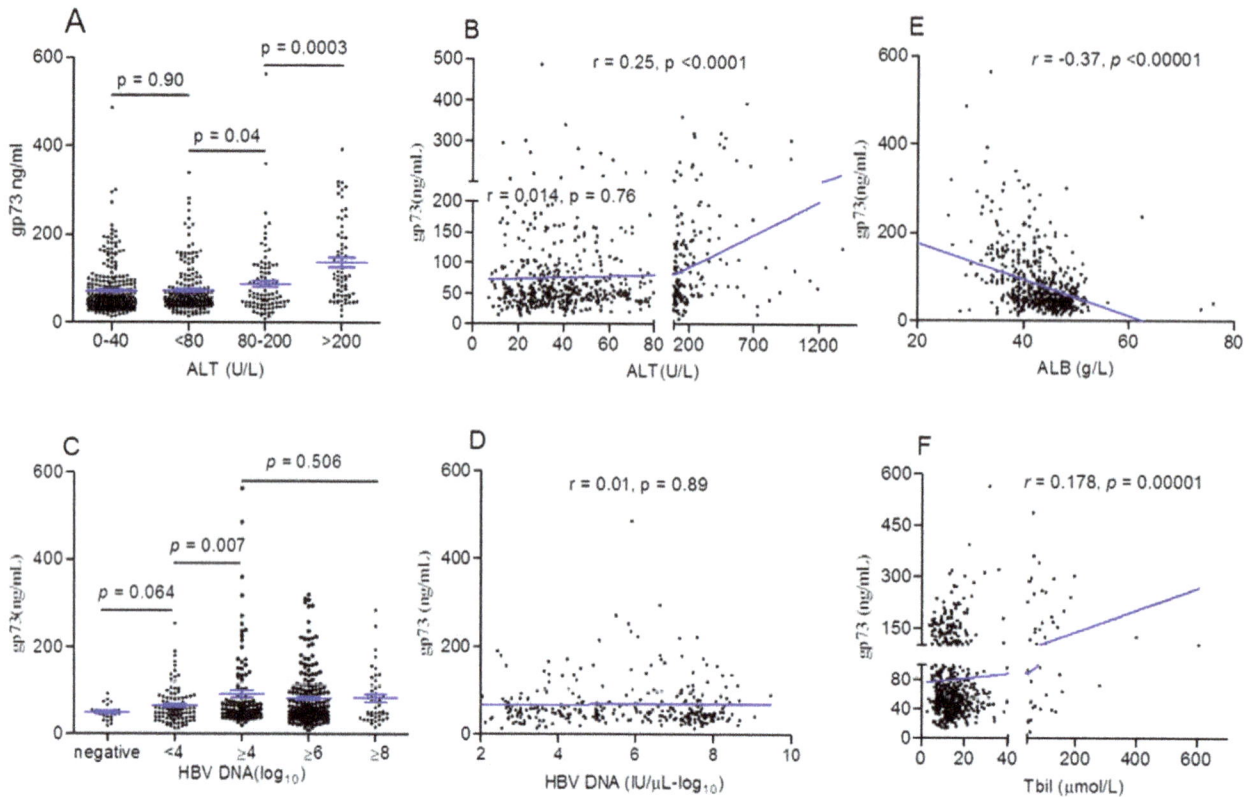

Figure 3. Serum GP73 concentration was related with levels of different biochemical marker. A and B: serum GP73 concentration was correlated with ALT in patients with ALT ≥ 80 U/L, but nearly normal ALT was not. Although different HBV DNA levels had their different GP73 concentration (C), the correlation was not significant (D). Sample number may be one of most important causes. GP73 were also correlated with total bilirubin (F), especially, significantly correlated with serum ALB negatively (E).

are also expressed GP73 [23]. This result consistent with our data, and indicated that more hepatic stellate cells activation, more significant fibrosis, and resulting in serum GP73 more increasing.

Strict adherence to practice guidelines of chronic hepatitis B, will make a number of patients with nearly normal ALT lost opportunities of receiving antiviral therapy. In fact, recommended

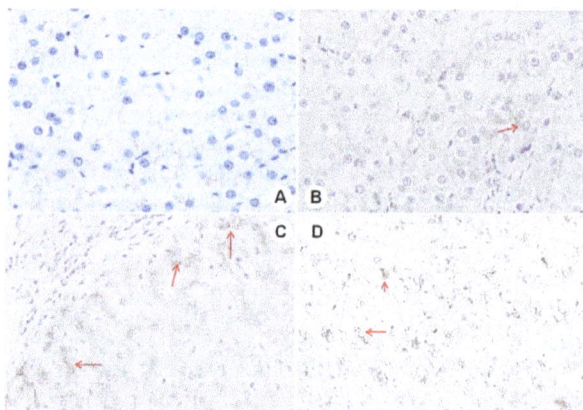

Figure 4. GP73 were stained in different liver tissue. GP73 was stained in brown. Arrow indicated positive cells. A: mild fibrosis (S1); B: significant fibrosis (S2); C: severe fibrosis (S3–4); D: cirrhosis (S4).

ALT thresholds may not absolutely reflect disease activity or degree of fibrosis [24]. More importantly, significant fibrosis (≥F2, or S2), or moderate hepatocytes injury (G2) are markers for beginning antiviral therapy in patients with chronic hepatitis B, based on present guideline [25]. Compared with other multi-parameter prediction models for grading fibrosis, GP73 is a single marker, which can be analysis with general enzyme-linked immunosorbent method. This new marker may be conveniently used in clinical practice, especially in developing countries for differentiating significant fibrosis with mild fibrosis in patients with chronic hepatitis B.

Liver stiffness is believed one of best non-invasive methods for evaluation liver fibrosis stage and disease progression. However, one question is what optimal cut-off value being chosen for fibrosis grading. Because numerous investigations provided different cut-off value for liver fibrosis classification, it was difficult to select optimal grading standard [26]. Based on recently reports, different research team presented different cut-off value for diagnosing significant fibrosis. Guha IN, et al [27], Stabinski L. et al [28], and Fung J, et al [29], presented 8.8 kPa, 9.3 kPa, 8.1 kPa respectively as optimal cut-off value for diagnosing significant fibrosis (≥F2). Since too higher cut-off value may be to lower the diagnostic sensitivity, we selected the relatively higher cut-off value, 8.8 kPa, for diagnosing significant fibrosis, in order to increase diagnostic specificity and accuracy. Difference of body constitution between east and west countries is other factor in our consideration, because liver stiffness variation in different populations [30]. Based on

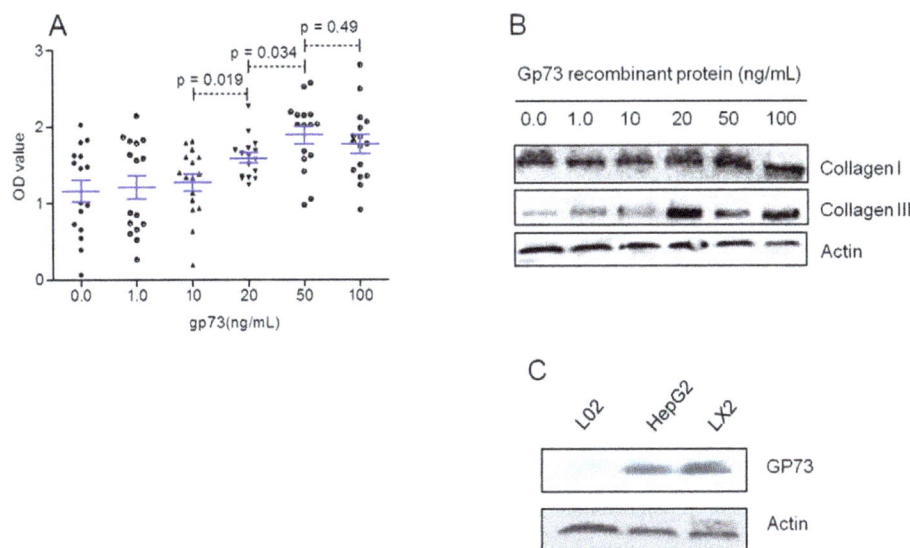

Figure 5. Gp73 recombinant protein prompted LX2 cells proliferation. A: when the concentration of GP73 recombinant protein was above 20 ng/ml, the LX2 proliferation was prompted. B: GP73 recombinant protein up-regulated collagen III expression, but collagen I was not. C: GP73 expression evaluated in different cells *in vitro*.

our present results, significant statistical differences only observed in several groups, although serum GP73 concentrations increasing with fibrosis progression. We speculated that these phenomena may be, at least in part, result in numbers of sample.

Based on data of stiffness measurement, setting 76.6 ng/ml as cut-off value may be appropriate for significant fibrosis diagnosis in chronic hepatitis B population. The impressive finding of this study was a obvious difference in GP73 concentration in patients with different fibrotic grading, especially in patients with nearly normal ALT (Table 2). According to results of liver biopsy, 80.21 ng/ml and 85 ng/ml, may effectively differentiate significant fibrosis (S2) or moderate injury (G2) from mild fibrosis or injury respectively. Integrating all abovementioned results, we proposed that 85 ng/ml may be an appropriate cut-off value for diagnosing significant fibrosis of moderate/severe hepatocytes injury from patients with chronic HBV infections. If the cut-off

value was set at 135 ng/ml, GP73 was also a potent marker for diagnosing liver cirrhosis.

Although GP73 (tr/tr) mice (with a severe truncation of the GP73 C-terminus) developed marked abnormity in liver, the role of GP73 in liver disease is still unknown [31]. The other interesting result is that GP73 may be not only a fibrosis marker, but also a contributor to fibrogenesis in patients with chronic HBV infections. Since unexplained high GP73 serum concentration was observed in patients with chronic HBV infection, this suggested that soluble GP73 may be playing a role in disease progression. This histological information indicated that non parenchymal cells may be another source of serum GP73. The present interpretation to serum GP73 levels is that HBV replication might increase GP73 secretion, and inflammation might result in GP73 releasing from hepatocytes. The molecular mechanism of GP73 mediating hepatic stellate cells proliferation needed to further elucidated. The main defects of our study is that patients received liver biopsy did not perform liver stiffness measurement, or *vice versa*, since most patients was willing to undertake FinroScan test, rather than liver biopsy. In fact, only thirteen patients received liver biopsy and liver stiffness measurements. We did not perform analysis to those patients separately.

In summary, GP73 may be a useful marker for liver fibrosis grading, especially for diagnosing significant fibrosis and cirrhosis in patients with chronic HBV infections.

Table 4. Effects of gp73 recombinant protein on LX2 cells.

GP73 recombinant Protein (ng/ml)	N	OD value	
		Mean ± SD	95%CI
0.0	16	1.17±0.58	0.86–1.48
1.0	16	1.22±0.61	0.90–1.54
10.0	16	1.27±0.44	1.04–1.51
20.0	16	1.59±0.27	1.45–1.73
50.0	16	1.89±0.46	1.64–2.13
100.0	16	1.77±0.48	1.52–2.03

Acknowledgments

We thank Dr. Gang Wan f or some statistical help.

Author Contributions

Conceived and designed the experiments: HW BL. Performed the experiments: RZ XH YH YQ. Analyzed the data: HW JH Xin Li. Contributed reagents/materials/analysis tools: HW Xingwang Li BL. Wrote the paper: HW.

References

1. Teixeira-Clerc F, Julien B, Grenard P, Tran Van Nhieu J, Deveaux V, Li L, et al. (2006) CB1 cannabinoid receptor antagonism: a new strategy for the treatment of liver fibrosis. Nat Med 12: 671–696.
2. Tong MJ, Hsien C, Hsu L, Sun HE, Blatt LM (2008) Treatment recommendations for chronic hepatitis B: an evaluation of current guidelines based on a natural history study in the United States. Hepatology 48: 1070–1078.
3. Hoefs JC, Shiffman ML, Goodman ZD, Kleiner DE, Dienstag JL, et al. (2011) Rate of progression of hepatic fibrosis in patients with chronic hepatitis C: results from the HALT-C Trial. Gastroenterology 141: 900-908.e1–2.
4. Callewaert N, Van Vlierberghe H, Van Hecke A, Laroy W, Delanghe J, et al. (2004) Noninvasive diagnosis of liver cirrhosis using DNA sequencer-based total serum protein glycomics. Nat Med 10: 429–434.
5. Munteanu M, Imbert-Bismut F, Messous D, Morra R, Thabut D, et al. (2008) Reproducibility of non-invasive fibrosis biomarkers, FibroMeter and FibroTest, could be improved by respecting the analytical standardizations. Clin Biochem 41: 1113–1114.
6. Imbert-Bismut F, Ratziu V, Pieroni L, Charlotte F, Benhamou Y, et al. (2001) Biochemical markers of liver fibrosis in patients with hepatitis C virus infection: a prospective study. Lancet 357: 1069–1075.
7. Mayo MJ, Parkes J, Adams-Huet B, Combes B, Mills AS, et al. (2008) Prediction of clinical outcomes in primary biliary cirrhosis by serum enhanced liver fibrosis assay. Hepatology 48: 1549–1557.
8. Naveau S, Gaudé G, Asnacios A, Agostini H, Abella A, et al. (2009) Diagnostic and prognostic values of noninvasive biomarkers of fibrosis in patients with alcoholic liver disease. Hepatology 49: 97–105.
9. Riener MO, Stenner F, Liewen H, Soll C, Breitenstein S, et al. (2009) Golgi phosphoprotein 2 (GOLPH2) expression in liver tumors and its value as a serum marker in hepatocellular carcinomas. Hepatology 49: 1602–1609.
10. Kladney RD, Bulla GA, Guo L, Mason AL, Tollefson AE, et al. (2000) GP73, a novel Golgi-localized protein upregulated by viral infection. Gene 249: 53–65.
11. Liu X, Wan X, Li Z, Lin C, Zhan Y, et al. (2011) Golgi protein 73(GP73), a useful serum marker in liver diseases. Clin Chem Lab Med 49: 1311–1316.
12. Iftikhar R, Kladney RD, Havlioglu N, Schmitt-Gräff A, Gusmirovic I, et al. (2004) Disease- and cell-specific expression of GP73 in human liver disease. Am J Gastroenterol 99: 1087–1095.
13. Sun Y, Yang H, Mao Y, Xu H, Zhang J, et al. (2011) Increased Golgi protein 73 expression in hepatocellular carcinoma tissue correlates with tumor aggression but not survival. J Gastroenterol Hepatol 26: 1207–1212.
14. Castera L, Forns X, Alberti A (2008) Non-invasive evaluation of liver fibrosis using transient elastography. J Hepatol 48: 835–847.
15. Corpechot C, Carrat F, Poujol-Robert A, Gaouar F, Wendum D, et al. (2012) Noninvasive elastography-based assessment of liver fibrosis progressionand prognosis in primary biliary cirrhosis. Hepatology 56(1): 198–208.
16. Bedossa P, Poynard T (1996) An algorithm for the grading of activity in chronic hepatitis C. The METAVIR Cooperative Study Group. Hepatology 24: 289–293.
17. Cao Q, Mak KM, Lieber CS (2007) Leptin represses matrix metalloproteinase-1 gene expression in LX2 human hepatic stellate cells. J Hepatol 46(1): 124–33.
18. Alberti A, Caporaso N (2011) HBV therapy: guidelines and open issues. Dig Liver Dis 43 Suppl 1: S57–63.
19. Adams LA, George J, Bugianesi E, Rossi E, De Boer WB, et al. (2011) Complex non-invasive fibrosis models are more accurate than simple models in non-alcoholic fatty liver disease. J Gastroenterol Hepato 26 (10): 1536–1543.
20. Tian L, Wang Y, Xu D, Gui J, Jia X, et al. (2011) Serological AFP/golgi protein 73 could be a new diagnostic parameter of hepatic diseases. Int J Cancer 129(8): 1923–1931.
21. Gu Y, Chen W, Zhao Y, Chen L, Peng T (2009) Quantitative analysis of elevated serum Golgi protein-73 expression in patients with liver diseases. Ann Clin Biochem 46: 38–43.
22. Wright LM, Huster D, Lutsenko S, Wrba F, Ferenci P, et al (2009) Hepatocyte GP73 expression in Wilson disease. J Hepatol 51: 557–564.
23. Maitra A, Thuluvath PJ (2004) GP73 and liver disease: a (Golgi) complex enigma. Am J Gastroenterol 99(6): 1096–1098.
24. Zoulim F, Perrillo R (2008) Hepatitis B: reflections on the current approach to antiviral therapy. J Hepatol 48 Suppl 1: S2–19.
25. Sebagh M, Samuel D, Antonini TM, Coilly A, Degli Esposti D, et al. (2012) Twenty-year protocol liver biopsies: Invasive but useful for the management of liver recipients. J Hepatol 56: 840–847.
26. Poynard T, Ngo Y, Perazzo H, Munteanu M, Lebray P, et al. (2011) Prognostic value of liver fibrosis biomarkers: a meta-analysis. Gastroenterol Hepatol (N Y) 7: 445–454.
27. Guha IN, Myers RP, Patel K, Talwalkar JA (2011) Biomarkers of liver fibrosis: what lies beneath the receiver operating characteristic curve? Hepatolog 54: 1454–1462.
28. Stabinski L, Reynolds SJ, Ocama P, Laeyendecker O, Ndyanabo A, et al. (2011) High prevalence of liver fibrosis associated with HIV infection: a study in rural Rakai, Uganda. Antivir The 16: 405–411.
29. Fung J, Lai CL, But D, Wong D, Cheung TK, et al. (2008) Prevalence of fibrosis and cirrhosis in chronic hepatitis B: implications for treatment and management. Am J Gastroenterol 103: 1421–1426.
30. Wong GL, Wong VW, Chim AM, Yiu KK, Chu SH, et al. (2011) Factors associated with unreliable liver stiffness measurement and its failure with transient elastography in the Chinese population. J Gastroenterol Hepatol 26: 300–305.
31. Wright LM, Yong S, Picken MM, Rockey D, Fimmel CJ (2009) Decreased survival and hepato-renal pathology in mice with C-terminally truncated GP73 (GOLPH2). Int J Clin Exp Pathol 2: 34–47.

Treatment of Naïve Patients with Chronic Hepatitis C Genotypes 2 and 3 with Pegylated Interferon Alpha and Ribavirin in a Real World Setting: Relevance for the New Era of DAA

Benjamin Heidrich[1,2,9], Steffen B. Wiegand[1,2,9], Peter Buggisch[3], Holger Hinrichsen[4], Ralph Link[5], Bernd Möller[6], Klaus H. W. Böker[7], Gerlinde Teuber[8], Hartwig Klinker[9], Elmar Zehnter[10], Uwe Naumann[11], Heiner W. Busch[12], Benjamin Maasoumy[1,2], Undine Baum[1,2], Svenja Hardtke[1,2], Michael P. Manns[1,2], Heiner Wedemeyer[1,2], Jörg Petersen[3], Markus Cornberg[1,2]*, for the HepNet Study Group

1 Department of Gastroenterology, Hepatology and Endocrinology, Hannover Medical School, Hannover, Germany, 2 German Liver Foundation, HepNet Study-House, Hannover, Germany, and German Center for Infection Research (DZIF), Partner Site Hannover-Braunschweig, Braunschweig, Germany, 3 IFI Institute for Interdisciplinary Medicine, Asklepios Klinik St Georg, Hamburg, Germany, 4 Gastroenterology, Gastroenterologische Schwerpunkt Praxis, Kiel, Germany, 5 St. Josefs hospital, Offenburg, Germany, 6 Medical Practice, Berlin, Germany, 7 Leberpraxis, Hannover, Germany, 8 Gastroenterological Practice, Frankfurt, Germany, 9 Dept. of Internal Medicine II, University of Würzburg, Würzburg, Germany, 10 Gastroenterological Practice, Dortmund, Germany, 11 Center for Addiction-Medicine, Hepatology and HIV, Praxiszentrum Kaiserdamm, Berlin, Germany, 12 Medical Practice, Münster, Germany

Abstract

Evidence based clinical guidelines are implemented to treat patients efficiently that include efficacy, tolerability but also health economic considerations. This is of particular relevance to the new direct acting antiviral agents that have revolutionized treatment of chronic hepatitis C. For hepatitis C genotypes 2/3 interferon free treatment is already available with sofosbuvir plus ribavirin. However, treatment with sofosbuvir-based regimens is 10–20 times more expensive compared to pegylated interferon alfa and ribavirin (PegIFN/RBV). It has to be discussed if PegIFN/RBV is still an option for easy to treat patients. We assessed the treatment of patients with chronic hepatitis C genotypes 2/3 with PegIFN/RBV in a real world setting according to the latest German guidelines. Overall, 1006 patients were recruited into a prospective patient registry with 959 having started treatment. The intention-to-treat analysis showed poor SVR (GT2 61%, GT3 47%) while patients with adherence had excellent SVR in the per protocol analysis (GT2 96%, GT3 90%). According to guidelines, 283 patients were candidates for shorter treatment duration, namely a treatment of 16 weeks (baseline HCV-RNA <800.000 IU/mL, no cirrhosis and RVR). However, 65% of these easy to treat patients have been treated longer than recommended that resulted in higher costs but not higher SVR rates. In conclusion, treatment with PegIFN/RBV in a real world setting can be highly effective yet similar effective than PegIFN± sofosbuvir/RBV in well-selected naïve G2/3 patients. Full adherence to guidelines could be further improved, because it would be important in the new era with DAA, especially to safe resources.

Editor: David R. Booth, University of Sydney, Australia

Funding: This registry was financially supported by MSD Sharp & Dohme GmbH (manufacturer of pegylated interferon alpha-2b) (http://www.msd.de/). The protocol and the contracts did not intend to influence the decision to treat patients with pegylated interferon alpha-2b. The HepNet study house of the German Liver Foundation, which was supported by the German Center for Infectious Disease Research (DZIF), coordinated and formally sponsored the registry. The funders had no role in study design, data collection and analysis, decision to publish, or preparation of the manuscript.

Competing Interests: Markus Cornberg has read the journal's policy and the authors of this manuscript have the following competing interests: Benjamin Heidrich: nothing to disclose; Steffen B. Wiegand: nothing to disclose; Peter Buggisch: Honoraria for consulting or speaking: Gilead, Roche, MSD, Janssen, BMS und AbbVie; Holger Hinrichsen: nothing to disclose; Ralph Link: nothing to disclose; Bernd Möller: nothing to disclose; Klaus H. W. Böker: Honoraria for speaking: Bristol-Myers-Squibb, Gilead, Roche Pharma, Merck (MSD Sharp & Dohme GmbH), Novartis; Janssen-Cilag Gilead; Gerlinde Teuber: received financial support for advise and talk from: Roche, MSD, Bristol-Myers Squibb, Janssen-Cilag, Gilead, AbbVie; Hartwig Klinker: received grants, Board membership fees and lecture fees from: AbbVie, Boehringer, Bristol-Myers Squibb, Gilead, Glaxo-SmithKline, Hexal, Janssen-Cilag, MSD, Roche, and ViiV Healthcare; Elmar Zehnter: nothing to disclose; Uwe Naumann: received financial support for research, advise and talk from: Roche, MSD, Bristol-Myers Squibb, Janssen-Cilag, Gilead, ViiV, AbbVie, Boehringer Ingelheim; Heiner W. Busch: Honoraria for speaking: Gilead, Janssen-Cilag, MSD Sharp & Dohme, Roche, ViiV; Benjamin Maasoumy: Honoraria for consulting or speaking: Roche Pharma, Roche Diagnostics, Abbott Molecular, Merck, MSD Sharp & Dohme, Janssen/Janssen TE, Fujirebio; Undine Baum: nothing to disclose; Svenja Hardtke: nothing to disclose; Michael P. Manns: received financial compensation for consultancy and/or lecture activities from: Roche, Bristol Myers Squibb, Boehringer Ingelheim, Novartis, Merck, Janssen, Idenix and GlaxoSmithKline, and research grants from: Roche, Gilead, Novartis, Boehringer Ingelheim, Bristol Myers Squibb, Merck and Janssen; Heiner Wedemeyer: Honoraria for consulting or speaking: Abbott, Abvie, Biolex, BMS, Boehringer Ingelheim, Gilead, ITS, JJ/Janssen-Cilag, Medgenics, Merck/Schering-Plough, Novartis, Roche, Roche Diagnostics, Siemens, Transgene, ViiV and research grants: Abbott, BMS, Gilead, Merck, Novartis, Roche Diagnostics, Siemens; Jörg Petersen: Grant/Research Support: BMS, Novartis, Roche and Consultant/Advisor: Abbott, AbbVie, BMS, Boehringer, Gilead, Kedrion, Janssen, Merck, MSD, Novartis, Roche and Sponsored lectures: Abbott, BMS, Boehringer, Gilead, Kedrion, Janssen, Merck, MSD, Novartis, Roche; Markus Cornberg: Lecture fees: Bristol-Myers-Squibb, Boehringer Ingelheim, Gilead, Roche Pharma, Roche Diagnostics, Merck (MSD Sharp & Dohme GmbH), Novartis, Falk and research support: Gilead, Roche Pharma, Roche Diagnostics, Merck (MSD Sharp & Dohme GmbH) and consultant fees: Abbvie, Boehringer Ingelheim, Gilead, Roche Pharma, Roche Diagnostics, Merck (MSD Sharp & Dohme GmbH), Novartis. This registry was financially supported by MSD Sharp & Dohme GmbH (manufacturer of pegylated interferon alpha-2b). The protocol and the contracts did not intend to influence the decision to treat patients with pegylated interferon alpha-2b.

* Email: Cornberg.Markus@mh-hannover.de

⊙ These authors contributed equally to this work.

Introduction

More than 150 million people world-wide and 8–11 million people in Europe are chronically infected with the hepatitis C virus (HCV) [1,2]. Patients with chronic hepatitis C are at risk to develop liver cirrhosis and hepatocellular carcinoma [3]. During the last 15 years there has been an enormous achievement in the diagnosis, management, and therapy of hepatitis C. Analysis of HCV-genotypes (GT), quantification of HCV-RNA viral load, and calculation of viral kinetics allow better management of patients with chronic hepatitis C. The standard treatment until recently consisted of pegylated interferon alpha (PegIFN) and ribavirin (RBV) [4]. Since 2011, the first direct acting antiviral agents (DAA) have been approved. The first generation protease inhibitors boceprevir and telaprevir were only approved for genotype 1 and combination with PegIFN and RBV was still necessary because monotherapy resulted in rapid emergence of drug resistance [5]. However, the availability of further DAA has already revolutionized the treatment of chronic hepatitis C. The main targets for DAA are the NS3/4A protease, NS5B polymerase and the NS5A replication complex. Combinations of different DAA from different classes will allow very potent treatments even without PegIFN [6]. In particular, therapy of GT2/3 has changed in 2014 with the approval of sofosbuvir (SOF). SOF is a new NS5B polymerase inhibitor with pangenotypic efficacy and extensive data were acquired in the treatment of GT2- and GT3-infected patients, which were the basis for the approval for the first interferon-free treatment of hepatitis C [7–9]. However, treatment with PegIFN/RBV dual therapy may be still considered depending on the health care system, especially for easy-to-treat GT2/3 patients. Treatment with SOF/RBV therapy for 12 to 24 weeks or SOF in combination PegIFN and RBV in HCV genotype 2 or 3 can be 10–20 times more expensive compared to PegIFN and RBV treatment [10].

For Peg-IFN/RBV a fixed duration of treatment (24 weeks) has been suggested [11], although the optimal results are likely to be achieved when the duration of therapy is adjusted based on viral kinetics. Many studies have investigated the reduction of treatment duration for HCV GT2/3 to 16, 14, or even 12 weeks [12–14]. Overall, reducing the treatment duration to less than 24 weeks increases the number of relapses. However, some HCV GT2/3 patients may indeed be treatable for 12–16 weeks if certain prerequisites are fulfilled, especially the rapid virologic response (RVR) by week 4 of therapy [15]. In addition to the RVR, the specific HCV genotype and the baseline viral load are associated with response [12]. Patients with low baseline viral load < 800.000 IU/ml and RVR have high SVR rates>85% after 16 weeks, 14 weeks, or even 12 weeks of therapy. Reducing treatment duration is not recommended for patients with advanced liver fibrosis or cirrhosis, insulin resistance, diabetes mellitus or BMI> 30 kg/m^2 [15]. Thus, recent clinical guidelines recommended that naïve patients with GT2/3 plus low viral load who achieve RVR can be treated shortly, i.e. 16 weeks according to the German Guidelines [15].

A major aim of this study was to find out if patients with GT2/3 were treated according to guidelines and if this treatment is efficient. We also discussed the results in the context of the new SOF-based treatment for GT2/3.

Materials and Methods

Patient population

The Competence Network for Viral Hepatitis in Germany (HepNet) implemented a nationwide multicenter prospective registry for naïve patients chronically infected with hepatitis C virus (HCV) genotype 2 and 3. MSD Merck Sharp & Dohme sponsored the registry (financial sponsorship only). The inclusion criteria (File S1) allowed treatment with both pegylated interferons (PegIFN a2a, PegIFN a2b).

Between June 2008 and December 2012 a total of 1006 patients were recruited in 72 centers in Germany. All patients at the age of 18 or older with chronic hepatitis C genotype 2 or 3 infection, detectable plasma HCV RNA and positivity of anti-HCV antibodies as well as no history of antiviral therapy were eligible (Figure 1).

HCV RNA quantification

HCV RNA was assessed at baseline, week 4, −12, end of treatment and 24 weeks after cessation of therapy. Samples were tested locally with different assays and thresholds. The Cobas-TaqMan assay with a lower limit of quantification (LoQ) of 15 IU/mL was used in 57%, the Abbott RealTime assay in 8% with a LoQ of 12 IU/mL and the Roche Amplicor assay with LoQ of 50 IU/mL in 5%. Additionally, in 24% the used assay was not indicated and in 7% others or in-house assays with different cut-offs were used. Assays were used according to manufacturer's instructions.

Laboratory results

Several Biochemical and hematological parameters at baseline were assessed locally. Biochemical markers included alanine aminotransferase (ALT), aspartate aminotransferase (AST), gamma-glutamyltransferase (GGT) and alkaline phosphatase (ALP) as well as bilirubin, creatinine and albumin. Hematological parameters included platelet counts and prothrombin time.

Definitions of response to therapy

Rapid virological response (RVR) was defined as HCV RNA below 15 IU/mL at week 4 of treatment with pegylated interferon alpha (PegIFN) and ribavirin (RBV), early virological response (EVR) was defined as ≥2 log10 decrease from baseline in HCV RNA or HCV RNA negativity at week 12; end of treatment response (EOT) and sustained virological (SVR) were defined as HCV RNA below detection limit at the end of treatment and 24 weeks after the end of treatment, respectively [15]. In the intention-to-treat (ITT) analysis all patients with at least one dose of PegIFN and RBV were included. Missing results for RVR and SVR were considered as negative results. For the per-protocol (PP) analysis, patients treated for at least 12 weeks and with available results at week 4 and/or 24 weeks after end of therapy were considered for each evaluation.

Definition of liver cirrhosis

Diagnosis of cirrhosis was either based on liver histology or non-invasive methods such as ultrasound, FibroScan or biochemical results. Liver cirrhosis in biopsies was defined as F4 in Metavir or F5-6 in ISHAK. In addition, diagnosis of liver cirrhosis was based

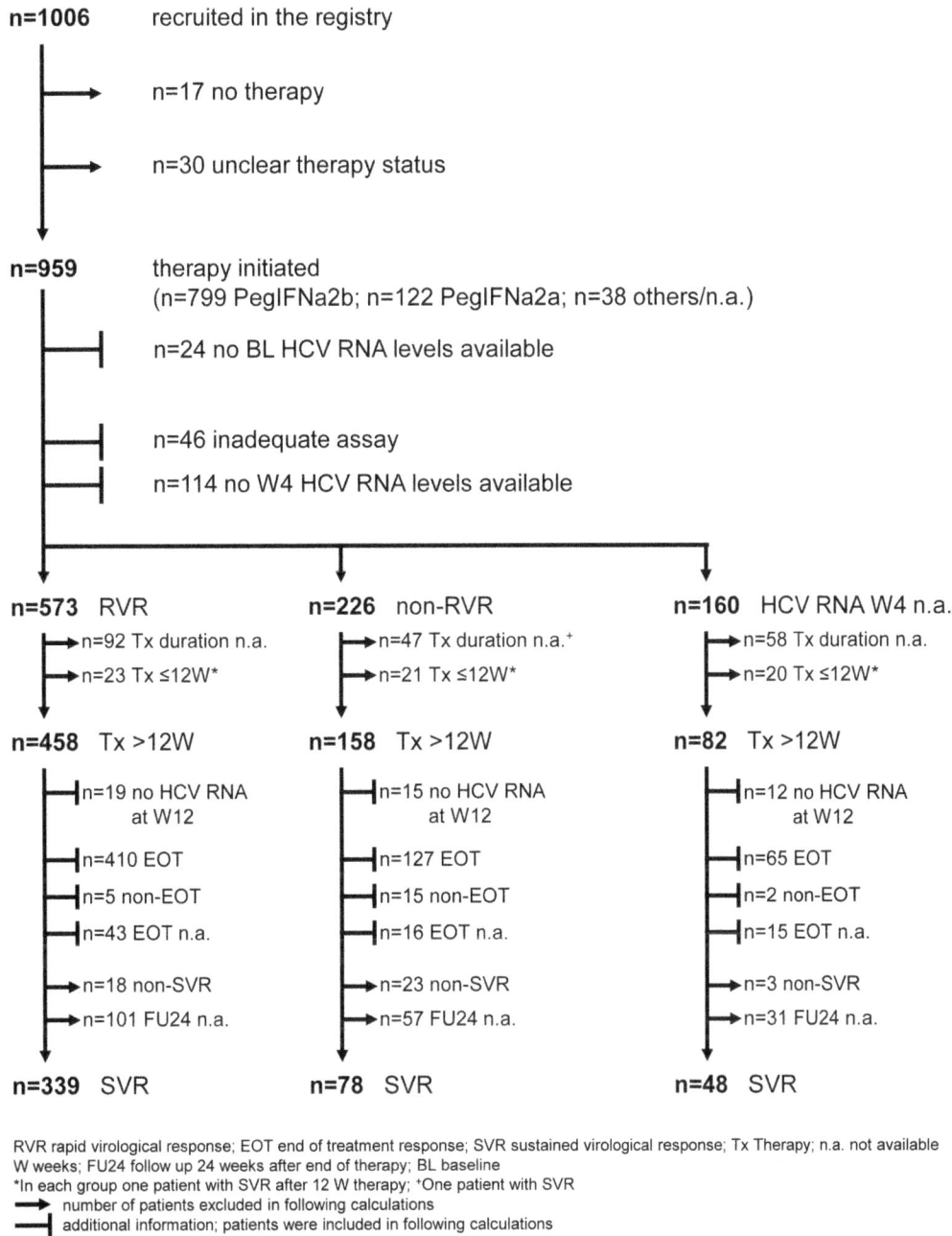

Figure 1. Flow chart of patients recruited in the HCV genotype 2/3 registry.

on ultrasound results assessed by the local physician. Liver stiffness ≥12.5 kPa was considered as cirrhosis [16]. Patients with at least two of the following criteria platelets <100/nL, AST/ALT ratio> 1, bilirubin>1.5 ULN and albumin <35 g/L fulfilled biochemical assessment of cirrhosis. Individuals were considered having cirrhosis if one of the definitions above was imbued.

Statistical analysis

For statistical analysis as well as for graphic design we used SPSS, version 15.0.1 (November 2006, SPSS, Munich, Germany) and GraphPad Prism 5 (GraphPad Software, Inc., La Jolla, CA, USA). Quantitative values are indicated in median and statistical differences were assessed by using Student t test. In case of analysis

of qualitative data we used Chi square test. Differences between clinical outcomes were determined using Cox regression analysis. Differences were considered significant at $p \leq 0.05$.

Ethical approval

Ethics committee at each participating institution approved the non-interventional patient registry of the German Competence Network for Viral Hepatitis (Hep-Net) and each patient signed a written informed consent form. The registry has been performed according to the World Medical Association Declaration of Helsinki (http://www.wma.net/e/policy/b3.htm). The procedures have been approved by the local ethics committee of the

Table 1. Baseline characteristics of all patients who started treatment with PegIFN/RBV.

Parameter*	Value	Range	n =
Male [%]	65.7		n = 617/939
Age [years]	43.8±10.6	20.1–81.8	n = 957
Weight [kg]	76.0±16.9	40.0–162.0	n = 931
BMI [kg/m²]	25.0±4.8	15.2–57.7	n = 919
CoO Germany [%]	60.0		n = 538
CoO EE/USSR [%]	30.8		n = 276
CoO Mediterranen [%]	6.1		n = 55
CoO Others [%]	3.0		n = 27
Genotype 3 [%]	82.7		n = 769
HCV RNA [log10 IU/mL]	5.8±1.0	1.2–8.7	n = 934
ALT [U/L]	89.0±107.7	11.0–1273.0	n = 909
Cirrhosis [%]	7.8		n = 75/959
Steatosis [%]	28.8		n = 225/782

Hannover Medical School (Vote No. 3860) and are in line with German law.

Results

Between June 2008 and December 2012 a total of 1006 patients were included. 959 patients received at least one dose of pegylated interferon alfa (PegIFN) and ribavirin (RBV). Two out of three patients were male with a median age of 43.8 years and BMI of 25.0 kg/m². The majority of patients originated from Germany and was infected with genotype (GT) 3. Hepatic steatosis was present in about one-third of patients and cirrhosis was diagnosed in 8.0% (Table 1, 2, and 3).

The Majority of patients received PegIFN-2b (n = 799; 83%) whereas 122 patients were treated with PegIFN-2a. For the remaining 38 patients the exact treatment regimen was not fully specified. In 24 patients (3%) baseline HCV RNA levels were not determined (Figure 1).

HCV RNA assays used for diagnosis and monitoring

Since our cohort consists of patients treated within a prospective registry in a real world setting in multiple centers several different HCV RNA assays were used. Overall, in the far majority of cases the used assays were indicated (n = 765; 76%). Importantly, in 46 cases out of 765 (6%) in-house PCRs were used instead of commercially available assays. Most of the patients (n = 691; 90%) were monitored with very sensitive assays with limits of quantification of 15 IU/mL. However, in 62 (8%) patients assays with moderate sensitivity (LoQ 50 IU/mL) and in 8 (1%) patients assays with low sensitivity (LoQ>50 IU/mL) were used.

Efficacy of treatment

The overall sustained virological response (SVR) was 49% in the intention-to-treat (ITT) analysis and 91% in the per-protocol (PP) analysis (Figure 2). Individuals with HCV GT2 had significantly higher SVR rates than GT3 patients in the ITT and PP analysis, respectively (ITT 61% vs. 48%; p = 0.0013; PP 96% vs. 90%; p = 0.0479) (Figure 2).

Table 2. Baseline characteristics of patients with HCV Genotype 2 who started treatment with PegIFN/RBV.

Parameter*	Value	Range	n =
Male [%]	63.4		n = 102/161
Age [years]	49.8±12.0	26.4–79.2	n = 160
Weight [kg]	78.0±16.4	47.0–149.0	n = 160
BMI [kg/m²]	26.1±4.9	16.7–45.0	n = 158
CoO Germany [%]	53.1		n = 85
CoO EE/USSR [%]	34.4		n = 55
CoO Mediterranen [%]	8.8		n = 14
CoO Others [%]	3.8		n = 6
HCV RNA [log10 IU/mL]	6.2±1.1	2.7–8.2	n = 154
ALT [U/L]	68.0±93.0	14.0–542.0	n = 152
Cirrhosis [%]	5.6		n = 9/161
Steatosis [%]	29.3		n = 41/140

Table 3. Baseline characteristics of patients with HCV Genotype 3 who started treatment with PegIFN/RBV.

Parameter*	Value	Range	n =	p#
Male [%]	66.0		n = 506/767	0.5250
Age [years]	42.2±9.9	20.1–81.8	n = 761	<0.0001
Weight [kg]	75.0±16.9	40.0–162.0	n = 760	0.0049
BMI [kg/m²]	24.6±4.7	15.2–57.7	n = 751	<0.0001
CoO Germany [%]	61.2		n = 447	0.0580
CoO EE/USSR [%]	30.5		n = 223	0.3440
CoO Mediterranen [%]	5.5		n = 40	0.1170
CoO Others [%]	2.7		n = 20	0.4920
HCV RNA [log10 IU/mL]	5.8±1.0	1.2–8.7	n = 753	0.0007
ALT [U/L]	93.0±109.4	11.0–1273.0	n = 745	0.0018
Cirrhosis [%]	8.6		n = 66/769	0.2050
Steatosis [%]	28.6		n = 182/636	0.8740

*Continuous values are indicated in median.
#Chi-Square or t-test results.
CoO = Country of Origin.

Rapid virological response (RVR) was achieved by 573 of all treated patients while 226 had HCV RNA levels above 15 IU/mL four weeks after therapy initiation. In the remaining 160 individuals HCV RNA quantification was not performed at week 4 or the sensitivity of the used assays was inadequate to define RVR (Figure 1). Thus, RVR was achieved in 573/799 (72%). In patients with GT3, 70% achieved RVR, while this happened more often in GT2 patients (70% vs. 78%; p = 0.052).

In the RVR group 340 patients achieved SVR, which is significantly higher compared to patients without RVR (ITT: 59% vs. 35% and PP: 95% vs. 77%; p<0.0001 for both) (Figure 3A). RVR was a predictor of SVR irrespective from the present GT 2 or 3 (Figure 3B). Individuals without or inadequate HCV RNA

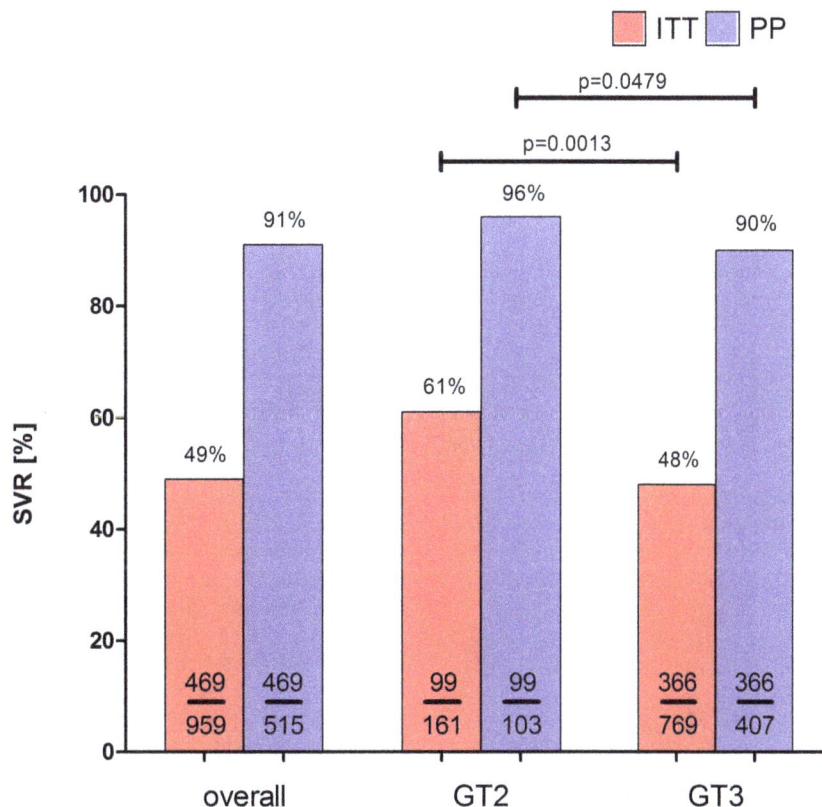

Figure 2. SVR rates in all patients with genotypes 2 and 3 (ITT and PP analysis).

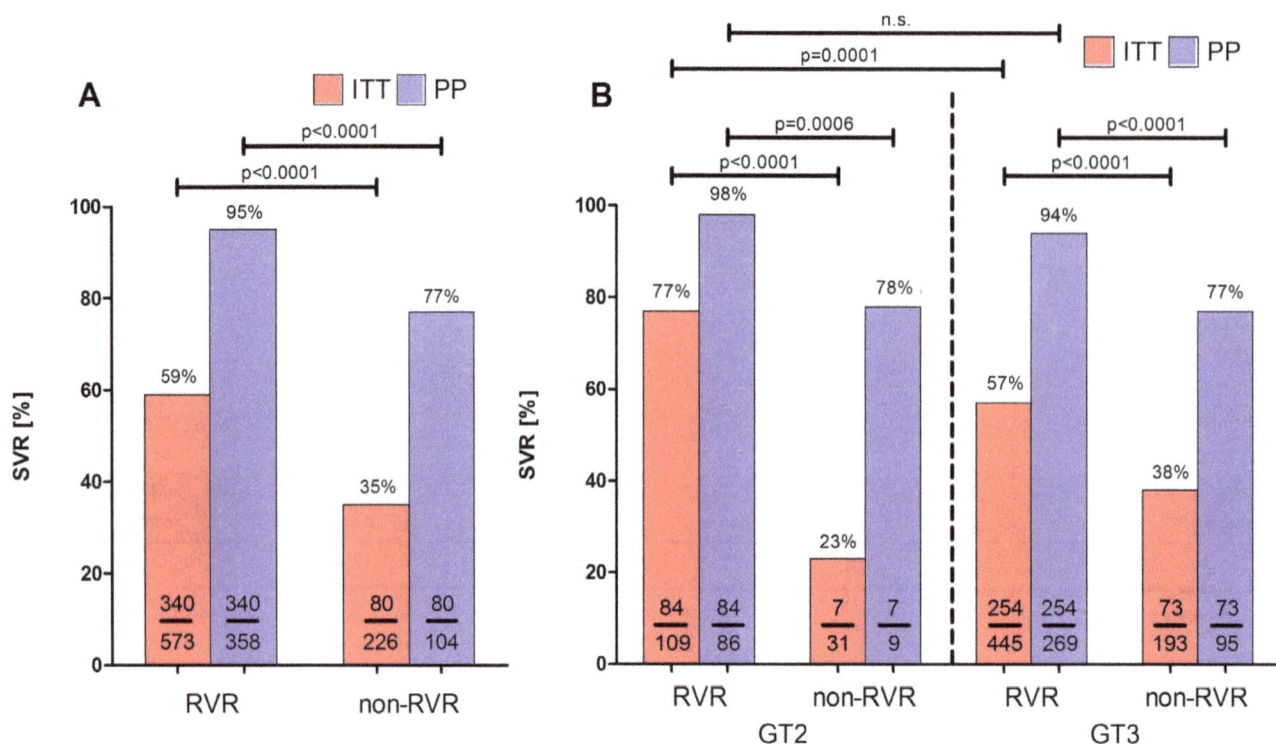

Figure 3. SVR rates according to HCV genotype and week 4 response. A: SVR rates in patients with or without RVR. B: SVR rates in patients with GT2 or 3 with or without RVR.

testing at week 4 achieved SVR rates of 31% and 92% in ITT and PP analysis, respectively. Patients with RVR were significantly younger (42.1 vs. 48.3 [years]; p<0.0001), had lower HCV RNA levels (5.8 vs. 6.1 [log 10 IU/mL]; p<0.0001) at baseline and had less often signs of cirrhosis (6% vs. 11%; p = 0.009) compared to patients without RVR (Table 4). Interestingly, no differences in the frequency of steatosis, dose of PegIFN and RBV, respectively, were observed (Table 4).

Compliance to the current German clinical guideline

According to the German clinical practice guideline patients chronically infected with hepatitis C virus genotype 2/3 should in principle be treated for 24 weeks. However, in naïve patients with low viral load (<800.000 IU/mL and no signs of cirrhosis) response-guided treatment (RGT) is strongly recommended. If these patients achieve RVR, a shortening of the treatment duration to 16 weeks is proposed with a grade A recommendation [15]. Patients with HCV RNA decline less than 2log10 after 12 weeks of therapy (no EVR) should be stopped immediately [15].

In our cohort, 459 patients fulfilled baseline criteria for RGT with PegIFN and RBV (Figure 4A). In 24 (3%) individuals HCV RNA testing was not performed at baseline. Out of 459 patients, 283 (62%) individuals achieved RVR, while 82 (18%) had HCV RNA levels above 15 IU/mL. Importantly, in 67 (15%) patients no HCV RNA quantification at week 4 was done. In 27 (6%) patients assays with low sensitivity were used, thus therapy shortening could not be decided. Overall, 283 patients treated in 48 centers fulfilled the criteria for RGT according to the German guideline. Interestingly, only 38 (13%) patients were treated for 16 weeks. In the majority of cases the physicians did not follow the recommended RGT criteria and patients were treated for 24 weeks (n = 157; 55%) (Figure 4B). Out of the 48 centers, there

were 9 centers with only one patient applicable for RGT. Therapy shortening was done in 2 out of 9 (22%) individuals. Out of 39 centers with at least 2 patients with option for shortening to 16 weeks only one center treated its patients for 16 weeks. Only 9 (23%) centers considered RGT in at least some of their patients. Thirty-three out of 39 (85%) centers treated their patients predominantly for 24 weeks or even longer up to 48 weeks. Importantly, the SVR rates in the 16-week as well as in the 24-week cohort were almost similar to more than 90% in the PP analysis (ITT: 71% vs. 79%; p = 0.294 and PP: 93% vs. 98%; p = 0.211) (Figure 5A). The same was true for GT3 (Figure 5B).

In addition, we analyzed non-cirrhotic patients with low baseline viral load who did not achieve RVR. Overall, 82 patients with low viral load and no signs of cirrhosis at baseline did not achieve RVR. According to the German guideline these patients may even be considered for longer treatment based on limited evidence [15]. In this registry 28 out of 82 (34%) were treated for 24 weeks (Figure 4A). About one third of patients (n = 26; 32%) received therapy longer than 24 weeks including 10 individuals treated for 48 weeks. For 15 patients treatment duration was not assessed. Importantly, the SVR rate was again above 90% in patients treated for 24 weeks and was comparable to all patients with RVR (data not shown). Therapy prolongation longer than 24 weeks did not lead to higher SVR rates in this registry with a relatively low number of patients (Tx 24 weeks 93% vs. Tx>24 weeks 82%; p = 0.3144). All patients, receiving therapy for more than 12 weeks, achieved EVR. Of note, 46 (7%) patients were not tested for HCV RNA at week 12.

Also patients with RVR and high viral load at baseline and/or liver cirrhosis had SVR rate of 94% and were comparable to patients with low viral load and no signs of cirrhosis (94% vs. 93%; p = 0.773).

Table 4. Baseline characteristics of patients with RVR and non-RVR.

Parameter*	RVR⁺ n = 573			non-RVR⁺ n = 226			p-value
	Value	Range	n =	Value	Range	n =	
Male [%]	65		n = 365/562	68		n = 151/223	0.4614
Age [years]	42.1±11.1	2.5–81.8	n = 560	48.3±9.7	20.1–66.4	n = 221	<0.0001
Weight [kg]	76.3±16.9	40.0–150.0	n = 557	76.0±16.3	47.0–140.0	n = 224	0.5197
BMI	25.2±4.8	15.2–51.2	n = 551	25.0±4.5	16.7–45.9	n = 221	0.5462
CoO Germany [%]⁺⁺	58		n = 311/540	63		n = 142/214	0.1374
Genotype 3 [%]	80		n = 445/554	86%		n = 193/224	0.0550
HCV RNA [log 10 IU/mL]	5.8±1.0	1.9–8.7	n = 563	6.1±0.8	2.7–7.5	n = 221	<0.0001
ALT [U/L]	2.3±2.5	0.3–27.8	n = 543	2.0±2.3	0.2–12.5	n = 219	0.5226
Cirrhosis [%]	6		n = 33/573	11		n = 25/226	0.0093
Steatosis [%]	29		n = 136/470	33		n = 60/184	0.3566
Dose of IFN** [μg/kg BW#]	1.5±0.7	0.5–13.8	n = 543	1.5±0.4	1.0–3.3	n = 221	0.4437
Dose of RBV⁻ [mg/kg BW#]	13.3±2.0	4.2–22.7	n = 539	13.5±2.2	1.8–28.6	n = 216	0.7976

*Continuous values are indicated in median.
⁺Not all parameters are available for each patient. Only available parameter were considered for calculations.
⁺⁺Country of Origin.
**Interferon.
⁻Ribavirin.
#body weight.

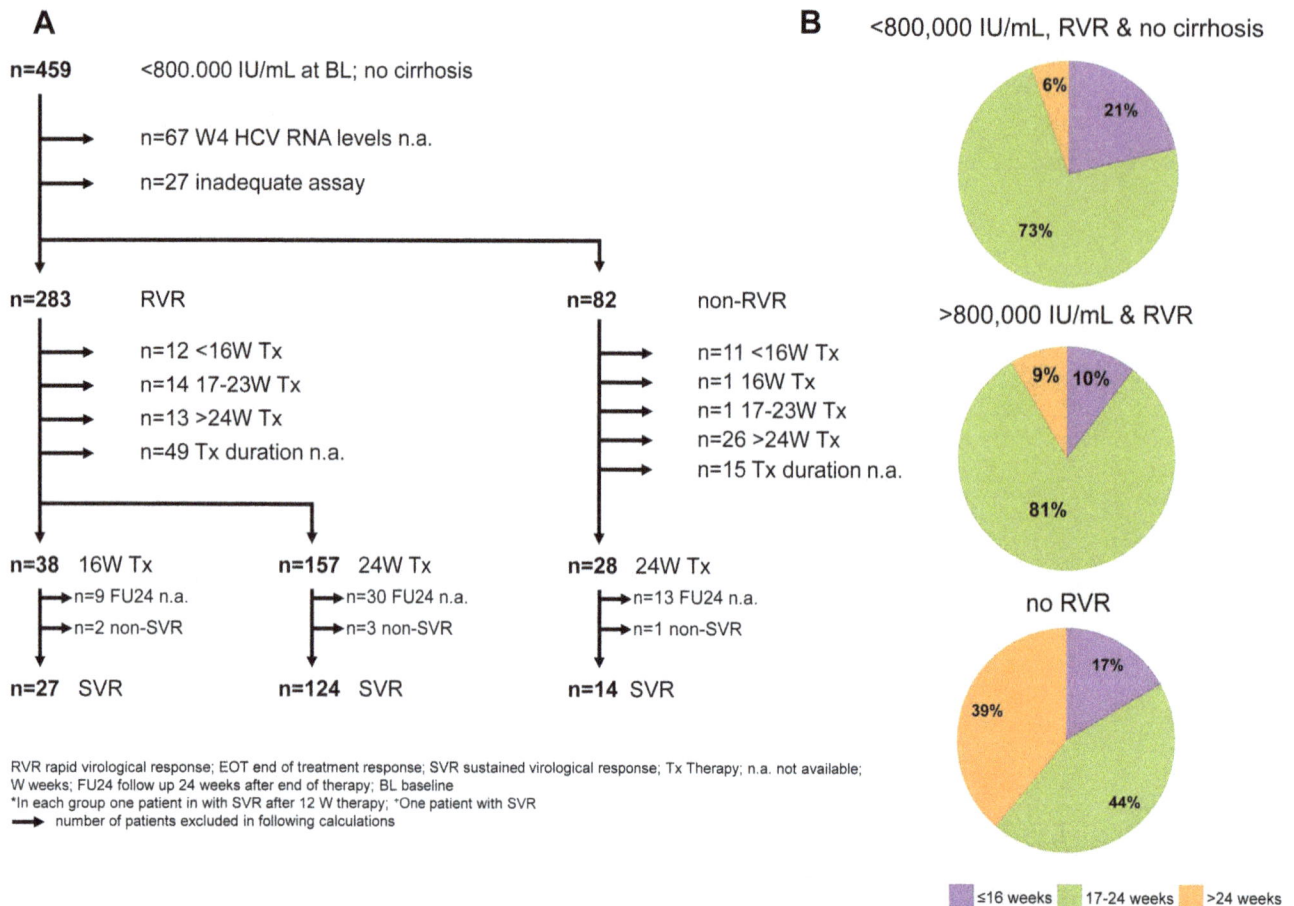

Figure 4. Therapy regimens and treatment durations in different groups of patients. A: Patients are divided in three different groups according to week 4 response and duration of therapy. B: The first group consists of the so called easy to treat patients with low viral load, no cirrhosis and RVR. In the second group are patients with RVR but high viral load irrespective of stage of liver fibrosis and the last group contains all patients with non-RVR.

Patients, who were treated with PEGIFN/RBV very efficacy, were patients with cirrhosis and non-RVR. In our registry only 20% (5/25) in the ITT and 50% (5/10) in the PP analysis achieved SVR. Median treatment duration was 24 weeks.

Additional costs due to over-treatment

Within our cohort many patients were treated longer than recommended in the German guideline due to different reasons, thus additional costs were generated. The majority of patients was treated with PegIFN-2b and had a mean weight of 77.4 kg. Based on these findings the approximate therapy costs for four weeks with 120 µg Peg-IFN-2b (PEGINTRON, MSD Whitehouse Station, NJ, USA) plus RBV (REBETOL, MSD Whitehouse Station, NJ, USA) are 2,346 €. In total 210 patients with low viral load and no signs of cirrhosis were treated longer than recommended (mean 22 weeks, median 24 weeks), which lead to additional costs of 897,589 € and 20 individuals with high viral load and/or signs of cirrhosis but with RVR were treated longer than 24 weeks (148,637 €) in contrast to the German guideline. Consequently over-treatment of patients with HCV GT2/3 resulted in further costs of 1,046,222 € in our cohort, 4,549 € per patient who was treated longer than recommended in agreement with the German guideline. Of note, 26 patients with neither high viral load nor signs of cirrhosis but no RVR were

treated longer than 24 weeks, which is based on limited evidence, resulting in extra costs of 238,344 €.

Discussion

Treatment of chronic hepatitis C is currently an area of dramatic changes. Since the approval of sofosbuvir (SOF), interferon free treatment is already available for genotypes 2 and 3 patients and suggested as standard of care by the new AASLD [17] and EASL guidelines [18]. However, this treatment revolution may be not available in all areas of the world at the same time and even if sofosbuvir is available everywhere, treatment may be not affordable for some health care systems. Thus it has to be discussed if the old standard of care, PegIFN and RBV may be considered for certain patients.

Our prospective patient registry revealed several very important findings: First, in a large, representative real-life cohort with more than 150 involved centers treatment with PegIFN and RBV was highly effective in naïve GT2/3 patients who were adherent to therapy. The overall per protocol analysis showed 91% SVR. However, in this real-world setting in Germany, the number of patients with low adherence or lost-to-follow up was high which resulted in poor intention-to treat SVR of just 49%. Our intention-to-treat SVR data are slightly lower compared to randomized trials where well-selected patients have been included by few

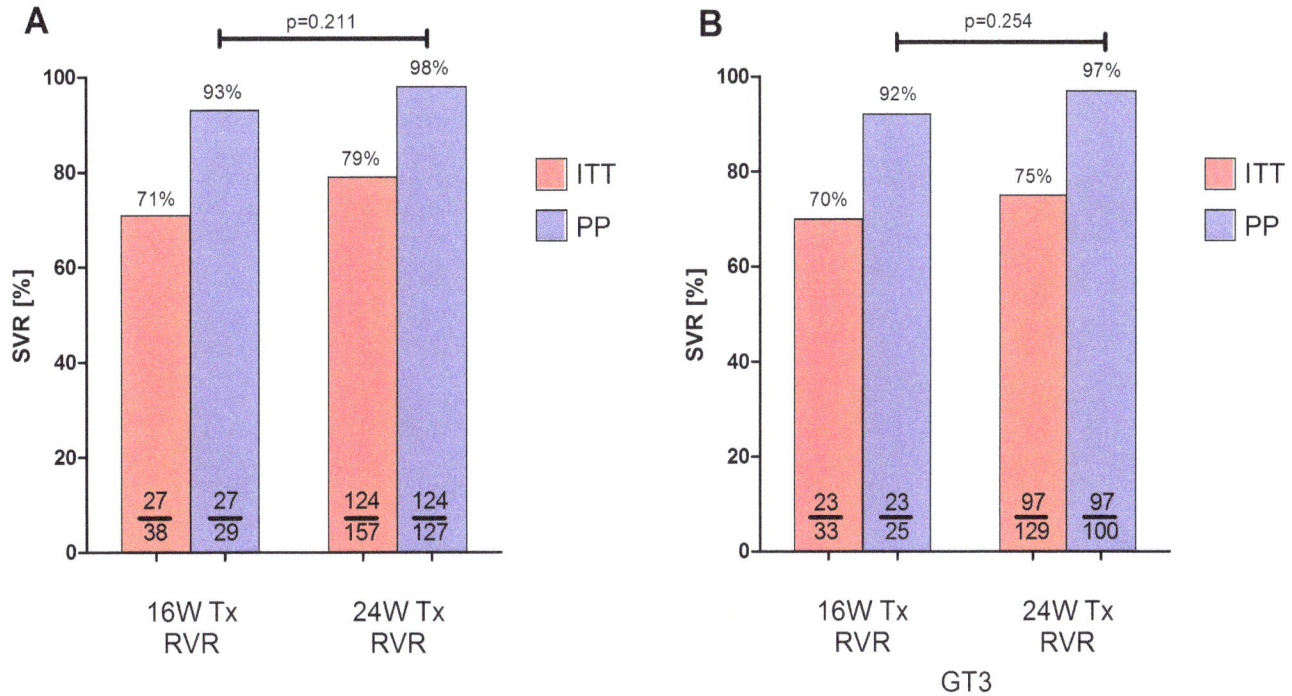

Figure 5. SVR rates in patients with RVR treated for 16 or 24 weeks in the overall cohort and in HCV genotype 3 patients. A: All patients had low viral, no signs of cirrhosis, RVR and were recommended for 16 weeks of treatment. B: All patients had low viral, no signs of cirrhosis, RVR and were recommended for 16 weeks of treatment.

well-selected study centers [11,13,19]. The recent HepNet REDD2/3 trial also showed a high discrepancy - 67% SVR versus 83% in the completer analysis. Also this trial was performed under real world-conditions involving 51 centers [20]. Reasons for the discrepancy between PP and ITT results are various. Treatment discontinuation due to side effects of PegIFN may be relevant, which call for IFN free therapies. However, in many cases patients were just non-compliant and did not return during or after treatment. Another major finding of our study was that treatment was unnecessarily prolonged or rather not shortened in a large portion of patients despite clear recommendations stated in national and international guidelines [15]. Only one center treated all easy to treat G2/3 patients with RVR for 16 weeks and just one fourth of centers considered RGT in the majority of patients. Importantly, over-treatment did not lead to an increase in SVR rates but may have increased the number of adverse events and certainly raised the costs of treatment dramatically. This suggests that the implementation of guidelines still needs to be improved. HCV therapy is a rapidly moving field and has seen tremendous changes in the recent years through the approval of different DAA. In some countries like Germany or the US sofosbuvir is already available and SOF/RBV ± PegIFN has become the new standard of care for most HCV GT2/3 patients and other DAA are already on the way. We think that our findings are indeed of great importance for this new era of DAA combination regimens. There cannot be a doubt that treatment of chronic hepatitis C with DAA will become highly expensive in most countries. Adherence to the exact treatment recommendations will be essential. One pill of sofosbuvir costs about 700 € in Germany or 1,000 US $ in the US (April 2014). Our data showed that only few centers followed guidelines very strictly. Current guidelines recommend 12 weeks SOF/RBV treatment for GT2 and either 24 weeks of SOF/RBV

or 12 weeks of PegIFN/RBV/SOF in GT3 patients [17,18]. If again treatment is prolonged in only some patients, costs will increase significantly, which will be an unacceptable burden for the national health care systems. Certainly, it has been considered that over-treatment with the IFN free SOF/RBV regimen may be very tempting due to very low frequency of side effects. Given the high costs of these modern therapies a dropout of more than 40% as documented in our study often due to poor compliance may not be acceptable. However, due to the better tolerability, treatment adherence may also improve. Nevertheless, the EASL recommends on-treatment HCV RNA testing at week 2 and 4 during SOF containing regimens to ensure patients adherence [18].

Finally, our data also confirmed that RGT treatment of naïve GT2/3 patients with low baseline viral load, no cirrhosis and RVR according to guidelines is possible and lead to high SVR in patients. Patients who are eligible to RGT and maintain on PegIFN/RBV therapy achieved SVR in 93%. SVR was not inferior to longer treatment of 24 weeks and saved 4,692 € per patient. This may be in particular relevant for GT3 patients who require 24 weeks of SOF/RBV. About 70% of IFN eligible and adherent GT3 patients achieved RVR with an SVR rate in>90% in our study. Similar data have been reported in randomized trials, i.e. 67% RVR with 85% SVR [19] or 71% RVR with 81%–90% SVR [13]. These SVR rates in GT3 are not inferior to SVR rates reported for 24 weeks SOF/RBV [9] or PegIFN/RBV/SOF [21] but therapy costs are about 50–100,000 € lower per patient (Table 5). As PegIFN based SOF therapy is recommended by recent guidelines, it also has to be discussed whether naïve PegIFN tolerant GT3 patients without cirrhosis and low baseline HCV RNA <800,000 IU/mL should be treated with dual PegIFN/ RBV. A pre-selection based on IFNL3 polymorphism may further increase the number of patients eligible for this approach [22].

Table 5. Costs per treatment schedule in naive GT2/3. *Valence trial [9] ** Lonestar-2 trial [21].

Patients	Treatment	Duration in weeks	ITT SVR (%)	PP SVR (%)	Costs in € per treated patient	Costs per ITT SVR	Costs per PP SVR
All G2	PegIFN/RBV	24	61	96	12,750	20,902	13,281
All G3	PegIFN/RBV	24	48	90	12,750	26,563	14,167
G3 LVL no cirrhosis	PegIFN/RBV RGT if RVR	16 (75%)	70	92	6,375	6,830	5,197
	PegIFN/RBV/SOF RGT if no RVR	4+12 (25%)	83	83	15,070	20,633	20,633
	combined				21,445	27,463	25,830
All G3	Peg-IFN/RBV/SOF**	12	83	83	66,500	80,120	80,120
All G3	SOF/RBV*	24	94	94	125,000	132,979	132,979

Patients without RVR can have low SVR [19] and may require an intensive treatment, which could be an add-on of SOF for 12 weeks. Recently, it has been shown that PegIFN/RBV plus SOF for 12 weeks resulted in 83% SVR in 24 difficult to treat GT3 patients from Texas [21]. An RGT approach would reduce treatment costs by more than 50,000 € per SVR in IFN eligible naïve patients compared with flat PegIFN/RBV/SOF for 12 weeks (Table 5). However, this approach has not been prospectively evaluated and four weeks longer exposure to PegIFN is required.

In summary, treatment of naïve patients with genotype 2 and 3 with PegIFN/RBV is highly effective in patients who tolerate PegIFN and maintain on treatment, especially in patients with low baseline HCV RNA <800,000 IU/mL, no cirrhosis and rapid virological response. Thus this selected group of patients should still be considered for PegIFN/RBV in particular in healthcare systems with limited resources even if sofosbuvir is available and still be co-administered with PegIFN. However, our data show that the majority of patients who are eligible for shorter treatment have been treated too long, which resulted in additional unnecessary costs and possible adverse events. On the other side, many patients are lost to-follow-up or discontinue treatment, which result in an overall low intention-to-treat SVR and especially increase the cost per SVR. If unchanged, overtreatment and non-compliance will raise the price of SVR to unacceptable values if SOF or other DAA with comparable costs are used. For all treatment concepts including IFN free regimens, adherence to guidelines needs further improvement, as this will not only optimize the efficacy but also the efficiency of treatment.

Acknowledgment

This registry was financially supported by MSD Sharp & Dohme GmbH (manufacturer of pegylated interferon alpha-2b). The protocol and the contracts did not intend to influence the decision to treat patients with pegylated interferon alpha-2b. We thank Renate Prinzing and Harald Blaak from MSD for their recommendations and support of this registry. The HepNet study house of the German Liver Foundation, which was supported by the German Center for Infectious Disease Research (DZIF), coordinated and formally sponsored the registry. We thank all patients recruited in this registry and the following contributors of the study: Sven Wollschläger – Dresden, Andreas Stallmach – Jena, Christine John – Berlin, Renate Heyne – Berlin, Thomas Berg – Berlin, Ansgar Lohse – Hamburg, Klaus Schmidt – Lübeck, Rainer Günther – Kiel, Joachim C. Arnold – Rotenburg/Wümme, Stefanie Holm – Hannover, Christoph Roggel – Minden, Peter Malfertheiner – Magdeburg, Christian Hoffmann – Hamburg, Dietrich Hüppe – Herne, Guido Gerken – Essen, Stefan Zeuzem – Frankfurt am Main, Frank Lammert – Homburg/Saar, Christoph Eisenbach – Heidelberg, Andreas Trein, Martin Rössle – Freiburg, Michael R. Kraus – Burghausen/Altötting, Nektarios Dikopoulos – Ulm, Reiner Wiest – Regensburg, Kurt Grüngreiff – Magdeburg, H.-J. Cordes – Frankfurt am Main, Bruno Tulaj – Aschaffenburg, A. Stoehr – Hamburg, Hartmut Bordel – Osnabrück, Armand von Lucadou – Nürnberg, Beate Quarterman – Neumarkt, Axel Baumgarten – Berlin, Karl-Heinz Kastner – Dillingen, Karl-Wilhelm Wiethold – Bremen, Rolf Zimmer – Ulm, Siegfried Köppe – Berlin, Heribert Renner – Nürnberg, Bernd Weber – Kassel, Reinhard Diedrich – Marburg, Lutwinus Weitner – Hamburg, Rajan Somasundaram – Berlin, Hans-Jörg Epple – Berlin, H. Lochs – Berlin, Wolfgang Klemm – Cottbus, Ann Michelsen – Rostock, Gunter Brauer – Cottbus, Christian Jellinek – Berlin, Torsten Hoheisel – Essen, Rüdiger Behrens – Halle/Saale, Wolfgang Steigleder – Filderstadt/Harthausen, M. Freitag – Karlsruhe, Karl-Heinz Hey – Paderborn, Annett Borkenhagen, Frank Doering – Bremen, Claus Niederau – Oberhausen,

Eugen Fürmann – Augsburg, Fajr Bannout – Augsburg, Katrin Heine – Wolfsburg, Kai U. Rehbehn – Solingen, Thomas Käser – Freudenstadt, Karl-Georg Simon – Leverkusen, Roland Reininghaus – Berlin, Johannes Benninger – Regensburg, Marcus Schuchmann – Mainz, Martin Hunstiger – Augsburg, Thomas Witthöft – Stade, Petra Sandow – Berlin, Geert Vogt – Leipzig

We thank Sandra Wiegand for proof-reading of the manuscript

References

1. Cornberg M, Razavi HA, Alberti A, Bernasconi E, Buti M, et al. (2011) A systematic review of hepatitis C virus epidemiology in Europe, Canada and Israel. Liver Int Off J Int Assoc Study Liver 31 Suppl 2: 30–60. doi:10.1111/j.1478-3231.2011.02539.x

2. Mohd Hanafiah K, Groeger J, Flaxman AD, Wiersma ST (2013) Global epidemiology of hepatitis C virus infection: new estimates of age-specific antibody to HCV seroprevalence. Hepatol Baltim Md 57: 1333–1342. doi:10.1002/hep.26141

3. Maasoumy B, Wedemeyer H (2012) Natural history of acute and chronic hepatitis C. Best Pract Res Clin Gastroenterol 26: 401–412. doi:10.1016/j.bpg.2012.09.009

4. Cornberg M, Deterding K, Manns MP (2006) Present and future therapy for hepatitis C virus. Expert Rev Anti Infect Ther 4: 781–793. doi:10.1586/14787210.4.5.781

5. Sarrazin C, Hézode C, Zeuzem S, Pawlotsky J-M (2012) Antiviral strategies in hepatitis C virus infection. J Hepatol 56 Suppl 1: S88 S100. doi:10.1016/S0168-8278(12)60010-5

6. Dusheiko G, Wedemeyer H (2012) New protease inhibitors and direct-acting antivirals for hepatitis C: interferon's long goodbye. Gut 61: 1647–1652. doi:10.1136/gutjnl-2012-302910

7. Lawitz E, Mangia A, Wyles D, Rodriguez-Torres M, Hassanein T, et al. (2013) Sofosbuvir for previously untreated chronic hepatitis C infection. N Engl J Med 368: 1878–1887. doi:10.1056/NEJMoa1214853.

8. Jacobson IM, Gordon SC, Kowdley KV, Yoshida EM, Rodriguez-Torres M, et al. (2013) Sofosbuvir for hepatitis C genotype 2 or 3 in patients without treatment options. N Engl J Med 368: 1867–1877. doi:10.1056/NEJMoa1214854

9. Zeuzem S, Dusheiko G, Salupere R, Mangia A, Flisiak R, et al. (2013) Sofosbuvir + Ribavirin for 12 or 24 Weeks for Patients with HCV Genotype 2 or 3: the VALENCE trial. Hepatol Baltim Md 58: 733A.

10. The price of good health (2014). Nat Med 20: 319. doi:10.1038/nm.3538

11. Hadziyannis SJ, Koskinas JS (2004) Differences in epidemiology, liver disease and treatment response among HCV genotypes. Hepatol Res Off J Jpn Soc Hepatol 29: 129–135. doi:10.1016/j.hepres.2004.02.011

12. Von Wagner M, Huber M, Berg T, Hinrichsen H, Rasenack J, et al. (2005) Peginterferon-alpha-2a (40KD) and ribavirin for 16 or 24 weeks in patients with genotype 2 or 3 chronic hepatitis C. Gastroenterology 129: 522–527. doi:10.1016/j.gastro.2005.05.008

13. Dalgard O, Bjøro K, Ring-Larsen H, Bjornsson E, Holberg-Petersen M, et al. (2008) Pegylated interferon alfa and ribavirin for 14 versus 24 weeks in patients with hepatitis C virus genotype 2 or 3 and rapid virological response. Hepatol Baltim Md 47: 35–42. doi:10.1002/hep.21975

14. Mangia A, Santoro R, Minerva N, Ricci GL, Carretta V, et al. (2005) Peginterferon alfa-2b and ribavirin for 12 vs. 24 weeks in HCV genotype 2 or 3. N Engl J Med 352: 2609–2617. doi:10.1056/NEJMoa042608

15. Sarrazin C, Berg T, Ross RS, Schirmacher P, Wedemeyer H, et al. (2010) [Prophylaxis, diagnosis and therapy of hepatitis C virus (HCV) infection: the German guidelines on the management of HCV infection]. Z Für Gastroenterol 48: 289–351. doi:10.1055/s-0028-1110008

16. Castéra L, Vergniol J, Foucher J, Le Bail B, Chanteloup E, et al. (2005) Prospective comparison of transient elastography, Fibrotest, APRI, and liver biopsy for the assessment of fibrosis in chronic hepatitis C. Gastroenterology 128: 343–350.

17. AASLD (2014) Recommendations for Testing, Managing, and Treating Hepatitis C. Available: http://www.hcvguidelines.org/fullreport

18. European Association for Study of Liver (2014) EASL Clinical Practice Guidelines: management of hepatitis C virus infection. J Hepatol 60: 392–420. doi:10.1016/j.jhep.2013.11.003

19. Shiffman ML, Suter F, Bacon BR, Nelson D, Harley H, et al. (2007) Peginterferon alfa-2a and ribavirin for 16 or 24 weeks in HCV genotype 2 or 3. N Engl J Med 357: 124–134. doi:10.1056/NEJMoa066403

20. Manns M, Zeuzem S, Sood A, Lurie Y, Cornberg M, et al. (2011) Reduced dose and duration of peginterferon alfa-2b and weight-based ribavirin in patients with genotype 2 and 3 chronic hepatitis C. J Hepatol 55: 554–563. doi:10.1016/j.jhep.2010.12.024

21. Lawitz E, Poordad F, Brainard D, Hyland RH, An D, et al. (n.d.) Sofosbuvir in Combination With PegIFN and Ribavirin for 12 Weeks Provides High SVR Rates in HCV-Infected Genotype 2 or 3 Treatment Experienced Patients with and without Compensated Cirrhosis: Results from the LONESTAR-2 Study. Hepatol Baltim Md 58: LB#4.

Author Contributions

Conceived and designed the experiments: MC HW MPM BH SBW. Performed the experiments: PB HH RL BM KHWB GT HK EZ UN HWB UB SH MPM HW JP MC BH SBW. Analyzed the data: BH SBW MC. Contributed reagents/materials/analysis tools: PB HH RL BM KHWB GT HK EZ UN HWB UB SH MPM HW JP MC BH SBW. Wrote the paper: BH SBW MC HW BM.

High Serum Levels of HDV RNA Are Predictors of Cirrhosis and Liver Cancer in Patients with Chronic Hepatitis Delta

Raffaella Romeo[1]*, **Barbara Foglieni**[2], **Giovanni Casazza**[3], **Marta Spreafico**[2], **Massimo Colombo**[1], **Daniele Prati**[2]

1 AM & A Migliavacca Center for Liver Disease, 1st Division of Gastroenterology, IRCCS Fondazione Cà Granda Ospedale Maggiore Policlinico, University of Milan, Milan, Italy, **2** Department of Transfusion Medicine and Hematology, Ospedale A. Manzoni, Lecco, Italy, **3** Dipartimento di Scienze Biomediche e Cliniche "L. Sacco", University of Milan, Milan, Italy

Abstract

Chronic infection with the hepatitis delta virus (HDV) is a risk factor for cirrhosis and hepatocellular carcinoma (HCC), but little is known whether the outcome of hepatitis is predicted by serum markers of HDV and hepatitis B virus (HBV) infection. The aim of the study was to investigate these correlations in 193 patients with chronic HDV infection who had been followed up for a median of 9.5 years (4.8–19.3). HDV-RNA was first measured by qualitative in-house nested RT-PCR and quantified by in-house real-time PCR. HDV RNA levels only appeared significantly associated to HCC (univariate analysis: OR 1.32, 95% CI 1.02–1.71; $p = 0.037$; multivariate analysis: OR 1.42, 95% CI 1.04–1.95; $p = 0.03$). In non-cirrhotics at first presentation ($n = 105$), HDV RNA levels were associated with progression to cirrhosis (univariate analysis: OR = 1.57, 95% CI 1.20–2.05, $p < 0.001$; multivariate analysis: OR = 1.60, 95% CI 1.20–2.12, $p = 0.007$) and development of HCC (univariate analysis: OR = 1.66, 95% CI 1.04–2.65, $p = 0.033$; multivariate analysis: OR = 1.88, 95% CI 1.11–3.19, $p = 0.019$). ROC analysis showed that approximately 600,000 HDV RNA copies/mL was the optimal cut-off value in our cohort of patients for discriminating the development of cirrhosis. High levels of HDV viremia in non-cirrhotic patients are associated with a considerable likelihood of progression to cirrhosis and the development of HCC. Once cirrhosis has developed, the role of HDV replication as a predictor of a negative outcome lessens.

Editor: Heiner Wedemeyer, Hannover Medical School, Germany

Funding: The authors have no support or funding to report.

Competing Interests: MC has the following interests: Grant and research support: Merck, Roche, BMS, Gilead Science Advisory committees: Merck, Roche, Novartis, Bayer, BMS, Gilead Science, Tibotec, Vertex, Janssen Cilag, Achillion, Lundbeck, Abbott, Boehringer Ingelheim, GSK, GenSpera, AbbVie Speaking and teaching: Tibotec, Roche, Novartis, Bayer, BMS, Gilead Science, Vertex. There are no patents, products in development or marketed products to declare.

* E-mail: raffaella.romeo@policlinico.mi.it

Introduction

Hepatitis delta virus (HDV) is a unique agent characterised by a single-stranded RNA genome encapsidated by the hepatitis B surface antigen (HBsAg) and a peculiar strategy of infection of the target organ [1]. In fact, HDV requires the helper functions provided by hepatitis B virus (HBV) in order to propagate to hepatocytes, it can only infect subjects with co-existing HBV infection due either to the simultaneous transmission of the two viruses or superinfection in an established HBV carrier [2,3]. Not surprisingly therefore, the incidence of HDV infection declined rapidly in Southern Europe and the Mediterranean basin after the early 1990s following the introduction of HBV vaccinations [4], but the many immigrants from highly endemic areas carrying chronic HDV infection has led to the emergence of a new scenario in Western Europe as a whole [5–7].

Chronic HDV infection has always been considered severe and rapidly progressive, leading to end-stage liver disease in just a few years, whereas a more slowly progressive form has been identified which evolved into cirrhosis in 30% of the patients followed up for periods of up to 28 years, with liver decompensation rather than

liver cancer (HCC) being the first cirrhosis-related complication to appear [8]. These observations suggest the existence of patient populations with heterogeneously evolving forms of chronic HDV infection, but the pathogenesis of HDV-related liver damage is still controversial. It seems unlikely that the virus has a direct cytopathic effect because studies have found liver grafts expressing HDAg alone without any tissue injury [9]. On the other hand, the so-called replication-associated cytopathogenicity of the virus might explain the tissue damage observed in patients with acute HDV infection, which is characterised by high levels of viral replication, whereas chronic infection is characterised by low levels of viral production and pathogenicity [2,10]. Furthermore, recent findings indicating the existence of a direct correlation between serum levels of HBsAg and HDV RNA in the absence of an inverse correlation with HBV DNA levels suggests an alternative interpretation of HDV pathogenicity that is more closely related to HBV biology [11].

The aim of this study was to investigate the correlations between viremia (serum HBsAg, HBV DNA and HDV RNA levels) and the clinical outcomes of chronic HDV infection, including the progression to cirrhosis, the development of HCC, decompensation, and liver-related death.

Patients and Methods

Patients

Patients were selected from the previously published cohort attending the Liver Centre of Ospedale Maggiore in Milan (Italy) [8]. The only selection criteria was the availability of multiple frozen serum samples (-70°C) collected at first visit at our division (baseline sample), as well as at least one frozen sample collected over follow-up. The study was approved by the Institutional Review Board of the Department of Internal Medicine at Maggiore Hospital. Patients gave their written informed consent to take blood for experiments and gave permission for use of their medical records.

Diagnosis of HDV Infection

HDV infection was defined as the presence of HDV antigen (HDAg) in liver tissue, or the detection of serum HDV RNA in anti-HDV/HBsAg seropositive patients as detailed elsewhere [12].

HDV RNA Extraction

HDV RNA was extracted from 200 μL of plasma using the High Pure Viral Nucleic Acid kit (Roche Applied Science, Basel, Switzerland). As many of the samples had very low concentrations of HDV RNA, it was essential to ensure efficient viral nucleic acid extraction. We therefore modified the extraction protocol including a preliminary step of one hour's incubation with the lysis/binding buffer supplied with the kit (chaotropic salt, poly(A), and proteinase K) at room temperature.

Quantitative HDV RNA Real-time PCR

An HDV RNA reference standard for the quantification of HDV RNA by Real Time PCR is not currently available. A 569 bp fragment of the HDV genome including the 5′ UTR HDV region has been cloned into a plasmid, which was used as positive control transcript for HDV Real Time PCR assay. Alignment of full-length HDV GenBank reference genomes representative of all HDV genotypes was used to locate conserved regions suitable for HDV RNA amplification, and the 5′ untranslated (UTR) region was identified as the most appropriate, as defined by others [13]. Thus, primers and probes were designed to amplify a 110 bp fragment of the 5′ UTR, taking into account the genetic variability of HDV genotypes. The assay was based on the use of fluorescence resonance energy transfer (FRET) probes, and included the forward primer HDV-s AGTGGCTCTCCCTTAGCCAT, the reverse primer HDV-as CGTCCTTCTTTCCTCTTCGGGT, the 3′-fluorescein-labelled probe HDV-FL TCCTCCTTCGG-ATGCCCAGGTCG, and the 5′-LC640-labelled probe HDV-LC CCGCGAGGAGGTGGAGATGCCAT. The reaction was performed using a LightCycler 2.0 instrument (Roche Diagnostics) and a 20 μL total volume containing 1× LightCycler RNA Master Hybridization Probe, 55 nM Mn(OAC)$_2$, 10 μM of each primer and probe, and 5 μL of RNA, and consisted of initial RNA retrotranscription (and Taq activation) for 25′ at 61°C followed by 30″ at 95°C, and then 45 amplification cycles (1″ at 95°C, 5″ at 62°C, and 4″ at 72°C) and a final melting curve analysis (30″ at 72°C, 20″ at 95°C, 30″ at 40°C, 1″ at 85°C, and 30″ at 40°C). All quantification were performed relatively to the plasmid standard described, which was used to define the 4-point quantification curve in each assay. Moreover, a real sample from the same patient was introduced in each Reverse Transcription-Real Time PCR analysis as positive internal control. The linearity of the PCR ranged from 10^3 to 10^8 copies/mL, and the sensitivity was 500 copies/mL. All samples were tested in duplicate and the mean of the two analysis was considered for statistical analysis. For the validation of the assay, a subset of 50 samples were also tested with a commercial CE IVD HVD Real Time PCR assay (LifeRiver Diagnostics, Shanghai, China), with concordant results (data not shown).

HBsAg Quantification

HBsAg was quantified by means of automated chemiluminescent microparticle immunoassays (Architect HBsAg, Abbott, Chicago, IL).

HBV DNA Quantification

For the purposes of this study, all of the patients were re-tested for HBV DNA by means of quantitative real-time PCR using a COBAS AmpliPrep/COBAS TaqMan automated system (HBV Test, Roche Diagnostics).

Liver Biopsy

Liver biopsies were obtained using a Tru-cut needle (16 gauge, Travenol, Hyland, CA; Uro-Cut 16G, TSK, Tokyo, Japan), and the sections were stained by means of conventional procedures. Liver cell necrosis, inflammation and fibrosis were graded on the basis of the METAVIR scoring system [14].

Disease Progression

Progression to cirrhosis in patients presenting with chronic hepatitis at entry was defined on the basis of fibrosis at liver histology (F 4) [14], a platelet count of <100,000 mm^3, the ultrasound (US) features of surface nodularity, splenomegaly, a portal vein diameter of >15 mm, endoscopically revealed oesophageal varices.

In the patients presenting with cirrhosis at entry, disease progression was defined as entry into a higher Child-Pugh class, and the development of clinical decompensation or HCC [15].

All of the patients with a clinical or histological diagnosis of cirrhosis underwent US surveillance and serum AFP determinations every 6 months as previously described [16]. HCC was diagnosed on the basis of the criteria used at the time of patient evaluation; since 2001, we used the guidelines published by the European Association for the Study of the Liver (EASL) [17]. In patients undergoing echo-guided liver biopsy, HCC was classified using internationally accepted criteria based on the pattern of invasive or replacing growth [18]. Complications of cirrhosis other than HCC, such as ascites, jaundice, hepatic encephalopathy and GI bleeding, were diagnosed and treated in accordance with established criteria [19,20].

Statistical Analysis

The categorical variables are given as numbers and percentages, and the continuous variables as mean values±standard deviation or median values and range, as appropriate. The serological variables were log-transformed (base 10 logarithm) before analysis. The chi-squared test and t test for independent samples were respectively used to compare proportions and mean values. The non parametric Mann–Whitney test was used in case of variables with non normal distributions. Univariate logistic regression models were used to assess the effect of the serological variables at the time of presentation and the risk of developing an event of interest (cirrhosis, HCC, liver decompensation, liver-related death, and "at least one of these") during the follow-up. In addition, multivariate logistic regression analyses were performed including in the above described univariate models some potential relevant confounders (age, sex, alcohol consumption, HBeAg and IFN). Finally, a subgroup analysis was performed to assess the effect of the variables of interest separately on the two subgroups of patients defined according to the clinical diagnosis at baseline (chronic hepatitis or cirrhosis). Odds ratios (ORs) with their 95% confidence intervals were calculated for the variables included in the models. In the logistic models, only patients with an available serological determination before the development of the event were included. A receiver operating characteristic (ROC) analysis was used to asses the ability of log-transformed HDV RNA to predict the development of cirrhosis in patients with chronic hepatitis. The area under the curve (AUC) was calculated as an overall assessment of the predictive ability of HDV RNA.

The sensitivity, specificity, positive predictive value (PPV) and negative predictive value (NPV) of the measurements were calculated, and the optimal HDV RNA cut-off value for predicting the development of cirrhosis was chosen on the basis of the maximum Youden index (the sum of sensitivity and specificity minus one). P values of <0.05 (two-tailed) were considered statistically significant. All of the statistical analyses were made using SAS statistical software (release 9.2) (SAS Institute Inc., Cary, NC, USA).

Results

We selected 193 patients for whom a baseline serum sample was available, as well as at least one sample collected over follow-up, with a median of three (2–6) samples/patient. We were able to select an homogeneous group of patients that reflected the original population of 299 patients. Indeed, among the 193 cases selected for the present study (65% of the original population), there were 35 patients who developed HCC (46 in the original cohort) and 35 who experienced liver decompensation (54 in the original cohort).

Table 1 shows the main epidemiological and virological characteristics of the 193 patients at the time of study entry, i.e. at the diagnosis of HDV infection, as compared to the general cohort of 299 patients [8], that also included patients who were diagnosed to have HDV infection in other institutions.,. The patients were prevalently Italians (94%), males (76%) with a mean age of 41 years. The modality of infection was sporadic in the vast majority of cases (146/193, 76%), and 15 patients (8%) were HBeAg positive. Thirty-eight cases (20%) had a previous history of an alcohol intake of >40 g/day. HBsAg could be quantified in 187 cases (97%), and HBV DNA was detectable in 169 cases (87%). All of the samples were HDV RNA positive upon qualitative testing, and viremia could be quantified in 157 samples (81%); the remaining 36 samples (19%) had concentrations that were below the detection limit of the quantitative assay. Liver cirrhosis was diagnosed at baseline in 88 cases (45%) by histological criteria in 75 (85%) and clinical criteria in the remaining 13 (15%). The proportion of cirrhosis was slightly higher in the current cohort because we are a referral centre for both HBV infection and advanced liver diseases. Therefore, we often received from other Italian institutions patients with HBV related cirrhosis before the diagnosis of HDV coinfection was made. The clinical criteria for diagnosing cirrhosis were platelets below 100.000 mm^3 in all the 13 patients, the ultrasound (US) features of surface nodularity in all patients, splenomegaly in eight, a portal vein diameter of >15 mm in five, presence of oesophageal varices in three. 82 (93%) patients were Child-Pugh class A, six (7%) were Child-Pugh class B.

We were not able to evaluate differences between the two cohorts in terms viral load, since baseline levels of HBsAg, HDV

RNA and HBV DNA could not be quantified in the general cohort. Finally, in the original cohort, mean age and median follow-up were calculated from the first evidence of chronic liver disease, while in the current cohort, mean age and follow-up were calculated at entry into the current study, corresponding to first access to our unit, when the first serum sample was stored.

Table 2 shows the main characteristics of the patients with and without liver cirrhosis. The patients with chronic hepatitis were significantly younger than those with cirrhosis (37.3 ± 11.0 vs 44.9 ± 10.3, p<0.001), had different modalities of infection (p = 0.024) and longer follow-up (p = 0.0003). There were no differences in terms of gender, alcohol intake, or baseline levels of HBsAg, HBV DNA or HDV RNA.

88 patients (45%) were previously treated with standard Interferon at doses between 6 and 9 MU, for a median of 18 months (6–94). 51/88 had chronic hepatitis at baseline but 20 of them progressed to cirrhosis over follow-up (histological diagnosis in all cases), after a median treatment of 24 months (6–56). 33/88 had a virological response (i.e. persistently negative serum HDV RNA or liver HDAg in at least 2-point analysis during 3 years of follow-up,18 with chronic hepatitis). However, in spite of the virological response, 5 chronic hepatitis progressed to cirrhosis documented at liver histology.

Considering the occurrence of HCC, liver decompensation and liver related death as clinical endpoints of the study, we performed the univariate and multivariate analysis of the principal epidemiological, clinical and virological variables. Among the 193 patients at baseline, 28 (14.5%) developed HCC, 26 (13.5%) developed liver decompensation and 25 (13%) died of liver related events. By univariate analysis, the virological variables only emerged as associated to the clinical outcome (Table 3). In particular, HDV RNA levels appeared significantly associated to HCC development (OR 1.32, 95% CI 1.02–1.71; p = 0.037) and occurrence of at least one unfavourable event (i.e. HCC, liver decompensation, liver related death) (OR 1.36, 95% CI 1.10–1.68; p = 0.004). Levels of HBsAg were significantly associated to the occurrence of liver decompensation (OR 2.31, 95% CI 1.09–4.91; p = 0.03). However, by multivariate analysis, serum HDV RNA levels only were confirmed as associated to HCC development (OR 1.42, 95% CI 1.04–1.95; p = 0.03) and occurrence of at least one unfavourable outcome (OR 1.41, 95% CI 0.99–3.21; p = 0.007).

We also performed univariate and multivariate analysis separately on patients with chronic hepatitis as well as in cirrhotic patients. Among the 105 patients with chronic hepatitis at baseline, 31 (29%) developed cirrhosis, 10 (9%) developed HCC, 7 (6%) developed liver decompensation and 7 (6%) died of liver related events. The results of the univariate analyses of patients with chronic hepatitis at baseline are summarised in Table 4. Univariate analysis showed that the baseline HDV RNA levels of the patients with chronic hepatitis were associated with progression to cirrhosis (OR = 1.57, 95% CI 1.20–2.05, p<0.001) and the development of HCC (OR = 1.66, 95% CI 1.04–2.65, p = 0.033). These findings were confirmed by the multivariate analysis (cirrhosis: OR = 1.56, 95% CI 1.14–2.12; p = 0.005; HCC: OR = 2.64, 95% CI 1.13–6.16; p = 0.025). Among the 88 patients with cirrhosis at baseline, 25 (28%) developed HCC, 28 (32%) developed liver decompensation and 28 (32%) died of liver related death. Univariate analysis showed no association between the serological parameters and the risk of any of the unfavourable events. Finally, with a view to identifying levels of HDV viremia correlated to a higher propensity of disease progression, we performed the ROC analysis in patients with chronic hepatitis. The ROC analysis identified 5.78 logHDV RNA (i.e. approximately 600,000 copies/mL) as the best cut-off value for predicting

Table 1. Comparison of the main epidemiological and virological characteristics of the 193 patients (current cohort) and 299 patients (general cohort [8]) at study entry.

	Current Cohort (n° = 193)	General Cohort (n° = 299)	p
Italian origin, n° (%)	181 (94)	290 (97)	ns
Males, n° (%)	147 (76)	230 (77)	ns
Mean age, years	40.8	30.5	na
Modality of infection, n° (%)			
Unknown	146 (76)	222 (74)	ns
Post-transfusion	14 (7)	27 (9)	ns
Intra venous drug use	24 (12)	38 (13)	ns
Sexual activity	9 (5)	12 (4)	ns
Alcohol >40 g/day, n° (%)	38 (20)	69 (23)	ns
HBsAg quantified, n° (%)	187 (97)	nd	
HBeAg +, n° (%)	15 (8)	27 (9)	ns
HDV-RNA positive, n° (%)	193 (100)	299 (100)	ns
HDV-RNA >500 cp/mL, n° (%)	157 (81)	nd	
HBV DNA >50 IU/mL, n° (%)	169 (87)	nd	
Liver cirrhosis, n° (%)	88 (45)	104 (35)	= 0.03*
Median follow-up, years	9.5 (4.8–19.3)	21 (1.2–43)	na

nd = not done. In the general cohort [8] HBsAg, HDV RNA and HBV DNA were not quantified.
na = not applicable. In the original cohort [8], mean age and median follow-up were calculated from the first evidence of chronic liver disease. In the current cohort, mean age and follow-up were calculated at entry into the current study, corresponding to first access to our unit as well as time of collection of the first serum sample available for testing.
*The proportion of cirrhosis was slightly higher in the current cohort because we are a referral centre for both HBV infection and advanced liver diseases. Therefore, we often received from other Italian institutions patients with HBV related cirrhosis before the diagnosis of HDV coinfection was made.

the development of cirrhosis (AUC = 0.73) in patients with chronic hepatitis (Fig. 1). This value was calculated in our patient cohort and with our HDV RNA quantification methods. This threshold had a sensitivity of 74%, a specificity of 64%, a PPV of 46.9%, and an NPV of 85.4%.

Table 2. Main baseline epidemiological and virological characteristics of the patients with and without cirrhosis.

	Chronic hepatitis (n = 105)	Cirrhosis (n = 88)	p
Males, No.	83 (79%)	64 (73%)	ns
Mean age ± SD, years	37.3 ± 11.0	44.9 ± 10.3	<0.001
Modality of infection, No.			p = 0.0236
Unknown	71 (68%)	75 (85%)	
Post-transfusion	9 (8%)	5 (6%)	
Intra venous drug use	17 (16%)	7 (8%)	
Sexual activity	8 (8%)	1 (1%)	
Median follow-up, years	12.5 (6.6–19.9)	6.8 (3.8–16.5)	p = 0.0003
Alcohol >40 g/day, No.	23 (22%)	15 (17%)	ns
Mean log HBsAg ± SD	3.4 ± 0.8	3.6 ± 0.6	ns
Mean log HBV-DNA ± SD	3.0 ± 1.6	3.0 ± 1.4	ns
Mean log HDV-RNA ± SD	5.0 ± 1.9	5.2 ± 1.6	ns
IFN treatment, No	51 (48%)	37 (42%)	ns
Virological Response, No	18 (17%)	15 (17%)	ns

Table 3. Results of univariate and multivariate analyses according to clinical outcomes in the 193 patients.

	HCC (28 patients)				Liver decompensation (26 patients)				Liver-related death (25 patients)				At least 1 event (48 patients)			
	Univariate		Multivariate		Univariate		Multivariate		Univariate		Multivariate		Univariate		Multivariate	
	OR	p	OR	p	OR	p	OR	p	OR	p	OR	p	OR	p	OR	p
HDV-RNA	1.32 (1.02–1.71)	0.037	1.42 (1.04–1.95)	0.026	1.26 (0.98–1.63)	0.076	1.12 (1.11–3.19)	0.140	1.16 (0.95–2.86)	0.251			1.36 (1.10–1.68)	0.004	1.41 (0.99–3.21)	0.007
HBV-DNA	1.0 (0.78–1.30)	0.961	0.98 (0.71–1.35)	0.903	1.23 (0.97–1.56)	0.081	1.16 (0.64–1.65)	0.233	1.21 (0.58–1.56)	0.131			1.14 (0.93–1.39)	0.199	1.14 (0.72–2.09)	0.293
HBsAg*	1.29 (0.68–2.46)	0.440	0.90 (0.38–2.13)	0.811	2.31 (1.09–4.91)	0.029	1.38 (0.19–1.38)	0.233	1.83 (0.36–1.73)	0.099			1.74 (0.99–3.06)	0.052	1.73 (0.13–1.05)	0.678

Multivariate models included HDV-RNA, HBV-DNA, HBsAg, age, sex, alcohol consumption, HBeAg and IFN.
*Seven patients with missing values.

Discussion

This study investigates a large cohort of patients followed up for a median period of 9.5 years, selected from a wider cohort already published [8]. The only criteria for selection was the availability of multiple frozen serum samples collected at baseline as well as during follow-up, in the respect of the overall characteristics of the original population. The study provides novel insights into the role and reciprocal interactions of HBV and HDV affecting the clinical outcome of HDV-related chronic liver disease. As cirrhosis is the major risk factor for late clinical complications, the non-cirrhotic patients with histological signs of chronic hepatitis alone, and those with histologically or clinically proven cirrhosis were analysed, whereas the levels of HDV RNA, HBV DNA and HBsAg were analysed in all of the samples collected at the time of clinical presentation, as well as in the samples collected from patients at the time of any subsequent development of cirrhosis or occurrence of any major event like HCC, clinical decompensation and liver related death.

The main finding of the study was that the clinical significance of HDV viremia is different in patients with chronic hepatitis alone and in those with established cirrhosis. Indeed, the univariate and multivariate analyses showed that the level of HDV viremia was the only virological parameter related to progression to cirrhosis and the end-stage complications of HDV, including HCC and clinical decompensation, in the patients who were not cirrhotic at the time of clinical presentation. This is the first study showing that the level of HDV viremia is the major driver of disease progression in patients with chronic hepatitis D, although our results are in line with previous findings that persistent HDV replication is the only predictor of an adverse outcome in patients with hepatitis delta [8]. Given the well-known inhibitory effect of HDV on HBV replication [21,22], it is not surprising that most of the circulating infectious viral particles contain HDV RNA instead of HBV DNA. In a study of patients with HBV infection alone whose design was similar to that of ours, Iloeje et al. found a close correlation between progression to cirrhosis and the level of circulating virus measured at the time of the first clinical observation, after censoring for important comorbidity factors such as age, gender, smoking and alcohol abuse [23].

Interestingly, we found similar baseline HDV RNA levels in our cirrhotic and non-cirrhotic patients, which suggests that, in addition to only predicting progression in the long term, quantifying HDV viremia has no value in cross-sectional evaluations. This hypothesis is supported by a recent cross-sectional analysis of 80 patients from different countries that showed no correlation between HDV RNA levels and histological necro-inflammation and fibrosis scores [11].

Another interesting finding of our study is that, once cirrhosis has developed, HDV RNA levels lose any significant relationship with disease progression, i.e. the occurrence of HCC, decompensation and liver related death. This finding may appear controversial from our previous results. As a matter of fact, in the previous publication we indicated that persistent HDV RNA over time was a risk factor associated to the occurrence of clinical decompensation, regardless from quantitative levels of HDV RNA. We found differences in terms of median follow-up, having chronic hepatitis patients significant longer observation time. One possible explanation is that for each patient we considered the first available sample as the baseline observation, regardless from the first evidence of liver disease. A previous study [24] has found that HDV viral replication tends to decline at the most advanced stages of liver disease, whereas serum HBV DNA levels may increase and, together with our data, this suggests that some factors not

Table 4. Results of univariate and multivariate analyses of serological parameters by clinical outcomes in 105 patients with chronic hepatitis.

| | Progression to cirrhosis (31 patients) | | | | HCC (10 patients) | | | | Liver decompensation (7 patients) | | | | Liver-related death (7 patients) | | | |
| | Univariate | | Multivariate | | Univariate | | Multivariate | | Univariate | | Multivariate | | Univariate | | Multivariate | |
	OR	p	OR	p	OR	p	OR	p	OR	p	OR	p	OR	p	OR	p
HDV-RNA	1.57 (1.20–2.05)	<0.001	1.56 (1.14–2.12)	0.005	1.66 (1.04–2.65)	0.033	2.64 (1.13–6.16)	0.025	1.65 (0.95–2.86)	0.074	2.01 (0.91–4.43)	0.083	1.44 (0.88–2.33)	0.144	1.82 (0.90–3.68)	0.095
HBV-DNA	1.00 (0.77–1.29)	0.983	1.09 (0.80–1.50)	0.580	0.95 (0.62–1.44)	0.801	1.29 (0.70–2.37)	0.410	0.95 (0.58–1.56)	0.831	1.06 (0.60–1.86)	0.843	1.03 (0.65–1.62)	0.913	1.19 (0.67–2.09)	0.5555
HBsAg*	1.26 (0.75–2.10)	0.385	0.97 (0.50–1.89)	0.939	0.91 (0.45–1.87)	0.802	0.33 (0.09–1.21)	0.094	0.79 (0.36–1.73)	0.552	0.49 (0.14–1.73)	0.269	0.70 (0.33–1.49)	0.360	0.37 (0.12–1.2)	0.099

Multivariate models included HDV-RNA, HBV-DNA, HBsAg, age, sex, alcohol consumption, HBeAg and IFN.
*Four patients with missing values.

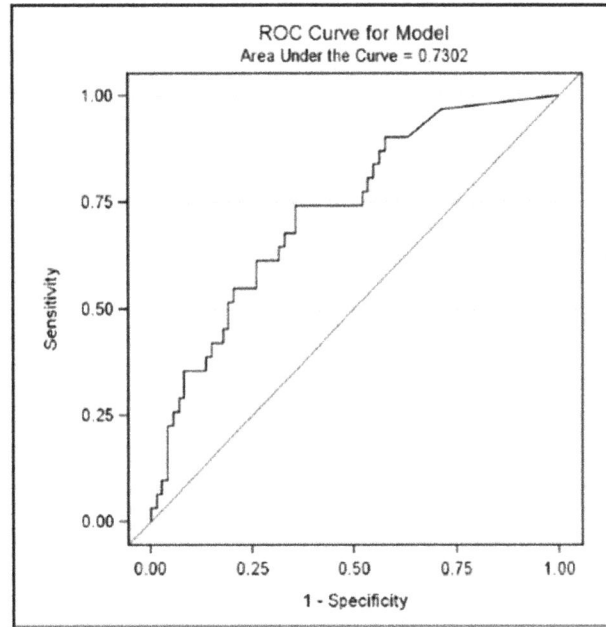

Figure 1. ROC analysis of HDV RNA levels. With a view to identifying levels of HDV viremia correlated to a higher propensity of disease progression, the ROC analysis identified 5.78 logHDV RNA (i.e. approximately 600,000 copies/mL) as the best cut-off value for predicting the development of cirrhosis (AUC = 0.73) in patients with chronic hepatitis.

included in the present analysis, including comorbidities, lifestyles and genetic predisposition, may influence the onset of complications in cirrhotic patients. This interpretation is supported by our finding that serum HDV RNA is independently associated with progression to cirrhosis and the development of HCC in patients with chronic hepatitis alone.

When we analysed the serological variables against the risk of developing at least one unfavourable event like progression to cirrhosis, HCC, clinical decompensation or liver-related death in these patients, there was a clear-cut trend towards a quantitative relationship between viremia and the risk of liver complication. A HDV RNA levels of >600,000 copies/mL predict in our cohort a risk of cirrhosis in about 50% of patients with chronic hepatitis (PPV = 46.9%) whereas lower values are a useful means of excluding the development of cirrhosis in a large number of cases (NPV = 85.4%). One possible explanation for higher levels of HDV RNA being associated with a greater risk of disease progression in patients with chronic hepatitis delta, is the influence of virus replication on cell immune responses against HDV-infected liver cells, as recently suggested by studies of host T cell immune responses in hepatitis delta genotypes 1 and 2 [25,26]. The possibility that genetic diversity of HDV plays a role in hepatitis progression is less likely since in our cohort of mainly Italian patients (95%), HDV genotype 1 was the most prevalent infecting strain [27].

While our findings clearly need to be validated in prospective studies of larger patient populations, still they underline the importance of treatment before cirrhosis occurs because, once it has developed, our results indicate that there is no association between any of the serological parameters and the occurrence of at least one unfavourable event, like the development of HCC, liver decompensation or liver-related death.

We did not find any direct or indirect correlation between HDV RNA and HBV DNA levels. As HDV proteins p24 and p27 repress the HBV enhancer by inhibiting HBV replication, and HDV p27 transactivates the interferon alpha-inducible MxA gene, which also inhibits HBV replication [28], it was no surprise to find that most of our patients had no detectable HBV. The same was found in long-term clinical study of potentially highly viremic HBeAg positive patients with chronic hepatitis delta [29], which demonstrated that most of the patients had HBV DNA levels of < 200,000 IU/mL at least once during follow-up, and 60% had levels of <2,000 IU/mL. It has recently been found that HDV patients carrying mutations at nucleotide positions 1762, 1764 and 1896 in the basal core promoter/precore region also have low HBV levels [30].

Consistent with the epidemiology of HDV in the Mediterranean basin, only 8% of the patients in our cohort were HBeAg positive at baseline, and there was no significant correlation with clinical outcome, as previously reported [29]. However, our findings and those from Spain [31] conflict with a recent finding from Turkey

of the existence of a correlation between serum HBsAg levels and HDV viremia, regardless of histological staging and the grading of liver disease in patients with chronic hepatitis delta [11].

In conclusion, chronic hepatitis D is highly likely to progress to cirrhosis and HCC in Italy, and this propensity is greater the higher the level of HDV viremia at the time of presentation. However, once cirrhosis has developed, the role of high HDV levels as a predictor of a negative outcome becomes attenuated.

Acknowledgments

The results of this study were presented in part at the 2012 Annual Meeting of the American Association for the Study of Liver Diseases (AASLD) and were awarded as Presidential Poster of Distinction.

Author Contributions

Conceived and designed the experiments: RR DP. Performed the experiments: BF MS. Analyzed the data: GC. Contributed reagents/materials/analysis tools: BF. Wrote the paper: RR MC DP.

References

1. Rizzetto M (1983) The delta agent. Hepatology 3: 729–737.
2. Farci P (2003) Delta hepatitis: an update. J Hepatol 39 (Suppl 1): S212–219.
3. Hadziyannis SJ (1997) Review: hepatitis delta. J Gastroenterol Hepatol 12: 289–298.
4. Gaeta GB, Stroffolini T, Chiaramonte M, Ascione T, Stornaiuolo G, et al (2000) Chronic hepatitis D: a vanishing disease? An Italian multicenter study. Hepatology 32: 824–827.
5. Wedemeyer H, Heidrich B, Manns MP (2007) Hepatitis D virus infection – not a vanishing disease in Europe. Hepatology 45: 1331–1332.
6. Erhardt A, Knut R, Sagir A, Kirschberg O, Heintges T, et al. (2003) Socioepidemiological data on hepatitis delta in a German university clinic – increase in patients from Eastern Europe and the former Soviet Union. Z Gastroenterol 41: 523–526.
7. Cross TJ, Rizzi P, Horner M, Jolly A, Hussain MJ, et al. (2008) The increasing prevalence of hepatitis Delta virus (HDV) infection in South London. J Med Virol 80: 277–282.
8. Romeo R, Del Ninno E, Rumi MG, Russo A, Sangiovanni A, et al. (2009) A 28-year study of the course of hepatitis D infection: a risk factor for cirrhosis and hepatocellular carcinoma. Gastroenterology 136: 1629–1638.
9. Ottobrelli A, Marzano A, Smedile A, Recchia S, Salizzoni M, et al. (1991) Patterns of hepatitis delta virus reinfection and disease in liver transplantation. Gastroenterology 101: 1649–1655.
10. Taylor JM (2006) Hepatitis delta virus. Virology 344: 71–76.
11. Zachou K, Yurdaydin C, Drebber U, Dalekos GN, Erhardt A, et al. (2010) Quantitative HBsAg and HDV-RNA levels in chronic delta hepatitis. Liver International 30: 430–437.
12. Colombo M, Cambieri R, Rumi MG, Ronchi G, Del Ninno E, et al. (1983) Long-term Delta superinfection in hepatitis B surface antigen carriers and its relationship to the course of chronic hepatitis. Gastroenterology 85: 235–239.
13. Kodani M, Martin A, Mixson-Hayden T, Drobeniuc J, Gish RR, et al. (2013) One-step real-time PCR assay for the detection and quantitation of hepatitis D virus RNA. J Virol Methods 193: 531–535.
14. The French METAVIR cooperative study group (1994) Intraobserver and interobserver variations in liver biopsy interpretation in patients with chronic hepatitis C. Hepatology 20: 15–20.
15. Pugh RN, Murray-Lyon IM, Dawson JL, Pietroni MC, Williams R (1973) Transection of the oesophagus for bleeding oesophageal varices. Br J Surgery 60: 643–649.
16. Colombo M, de Franchis R, Del Ninno E, Sangiovanni A, De Fazio C, et al. (1991) Hepatocellular carcinoma in Italian patients with cirrhosis. N Engl J Med 325: 675–680.
17. Bruix J, Sherman M, Llovet JM, Beaugrand M, Lencioni R, et al. (2001) Clinical management of hepatocellular carcinoma. Conclusions of the Barcelona EASL Conference. J Hepatol 35: 421–430.
18. Peters RL (1976) Pathology of hepatocellular carcinoma. In: Okuda K, Peters RL, eds. Hepatocellular Carcinoma. New York: John Wiley. 107p.
19. Portal hypertension III (2001) Proceedings of the Third Baveno International Consensus Workshop on Definition, Methodology and Therapeutic Strategies. De Franchis R, ed. London: Blackwell Science. 1p.
20. Salerno F, Angeli P, Bernardi M, Laffi G, Riggio O, et al. (1999) Clinical practice guidelines for the management of cirrhotic patients with ascites. Committee on Ascites of the Italian Association for the Study of the Liver. Ital J Gastroenterol Hepatol 7: 626–634.
21. Sakugawa H, Nakasone H, Nakayoshi T, Kawakami Y, Yamashiro T, et al. (2001) Hepatitis B virus concentrations in serum determined by sensitive quantitative assays in patients with established chronic hepatitis delta virus infection. J Med Virol 65: 478–484.
22. Hadziyannis SJ, Sherman M, Lieberman HM, Shafritz DA (1985) Liver disease activity and hepatitis B virus replication in chronic delta antigen-positive hepatitis B virus carriers. Hepatology 5: 544–547.
23. Iloeje UH, Yang HI, Su J, Jen CL, You SL, et al. (2006) Predicting cirrhosis risk based on the level of circulating hepatitis B viral load. Gastroenterology 130: 678–686.
24. Wu JC, Chen TZ, Huang YS, Yen FS, Ting LT, et al. (1995) Natural history of hepatitis D viral superinfection: significance of viremia detected by polymerase chain reaction. Gastroenterology 108: 796–802.
25. Aslan N, Yurdaydin C, Bozkaya H, Baglan P, Bozdayi AM, et al. (2003) Analysis and function of delta-hepatitis virus-specific cellular immune responses. J Hepatol (S2); 38: 15–16.
26. Huang YH, Tao MH, Hu CP, Syu WJ, Wu JC (2004) Identification of novel HLA-A*0201-restricted CD8+ T-cell epitopes on hepatitis delta virus. J Gen Virol 85: 3089–3098.
27. Niro GA, Smedile A, Andriulli A, Rizzetto M, Gerin JL, et al. (1997) The predominance of hepatitis Delta virus genotype I among chronically infected Italian patients. Hepatology 25: 728–734.
28. Williams V, Brichler S, Radjef N, Lebon P, Goffard A, et al. (2009) Hepatitis delta virus proteins repress hepatitis B virus enhancers and activate the alpha/beta interferon-inducible MxA gene. J Gen Virol 90: 2759–2767.
29. Heidrich B, Serrano BC, Idilman R, Kabaçam G, Bremer B, et al. (2012) HBeAg-positive hepatitis delta: virological patterns and clinical long-term outcome. Liver International epub 1–11.
30. Pollicino T, Raffa G, Santantonio T, Gaeta GB, Iannello G, et al. (2011) Replicative and transcriptional activities of hepatitis B virus in patients coinfected with hepatitis B and hepatitis delta virus. J Virol 85: 432–439.
31. Schaper M, Rodriguez-Frias F, Jardi R, Tabernero D, Homs M, et al. (2010) Quantitative longitudinal evaluations of hepatitis delta virus RNA and hepatitis B virus DNA shows a dynamic, complex replicative profile in chronic hepatitis B and D. J Hepatol 52: 658–664.

The Association of HMGB1 Expression with Clinicopathological Significance and Prognosis in Hepatocellular Carcinoma: A Meta-Analysis and Literature Review

Lu Zhang[1,9], Jianjun Han[2,9], Huiyong Wu[3], Xiaohong Liang[4], Jianxin Zhang[5], Jian Li[6], Li Xie[7], Yinfa Xie[8], Xiugui Sheng[9]*, Jinming Yu[10]*

1 Department of Gynecologic Oncology, Shandong Cancer Hospital and Institute, School of Medicine and life Science, University of Jinan-Shandong Academy of Medical Science, Jinan, Shandong, P.R. China, 2 Department of Cancer Interventional Radiology, Shandong Cancer Hospital and Institute, Jinan, Shandong, P.R. China, 3 Department of Cancer Interventional Radiology, Shandong Cancer Hospital and Institute, Jinan, Shandong, P.R. China, 4 Department of Immunology, Shandong University School of Medicine, Jinan, Shandong, China, 5 Department of Cancer Interventional Radiology, Shandong Cancer Hospital and Institute, Jinan, Shandong, P.R. China, 6 Department of Cancer Interventional Radiology, Shandong Cancer Hospital and Institute, Jinan, Shandong, P.R. China, 7 Provincial Key Laboratory of Radiation Oncology, Shandong Cancer Hospital and Institute, Jinan, Shandong, P.R. China, 8 Department of Cancer Interventional Radiology, Shandong Cancer Hospital and Institute, Jinan, Shandong, P.R. China, 9 Department of Gynecologic Oncology, Shandong Cancer Hospital and Institute, Jinan, Shandong, P.R. China, 10 Department of Radiation Oncology, Shandong Cancer Hospital and Institute, Jinan, Shandong, P.R. China

Abstract

Background: Hepatocellular carcinoma (HCC) is the fifth most common cancer, and it is the second most common cancer-related mortality globally. The prognostic value of high mobility group box 1 (HMGB1) remains controversial. The purpose of this study is to conduct a meta-analysis and literature review to evaluate the association of HMGB1 expression with the prognosis of patients with HCC.

Methods: A detailed literature search was made in Medline, Google Scholar and others for related research publications. The data were extracted and assessed by two reviewers independently. Analysis of pooled data were performed, Hazard Ratio (HR) and mean difference with corresponding confidence intervals (CIs) were calculated and summarized respectively.

Results: 10 relevant articles were included for this meta-analysis study. HMGB1 mRNA levels in HCC were significantly higher than those in normal (p<0.00001) and para-tumor tissues (p = 0.002) respectively. The protein levels of HMGB1 in HCC were significantly higher than those in para-tumor tissues (p = 0.005). Two studies reported the serum HMGB1 levels in patients with HCC of TNM stages, and indicating significantly different between stage I and II, stage II and III, as well as stage III and IV (two studies showed p<0.01 and p<0.001 respectively). The overall survival (OS) was significantly shorter in HCC patients with high HMGB1 expression compared those with low HMGB1 expression and the pooled HR was 1.31 with 95% CI 1.20–1.44, Z = 5.82, p<0.0001. Two additional studies showed that there were higher serum HMGB1 levels in patients with chronic hepatitis than those in healthy people (p<0.05).

Conclusions: The results of this meta-analysis suggest that HMGB1 mRNA and protein tissue levels in the patients with HCC are significantly higher than those in para-tumor and normal liver tissues respectively. Tissue HMGB1 overexpression is a potential biomarker for HCC diagnosis, and it is significantly associated with the prognosis of patients with HCC.

Editor: Erica Villa, University of Modena & Reggio Emilia, Italy

Funding: Funding from Jinan Municipal Science and Technology Development Plan (201401246) and Natural Science Foundation of Shandong Province (ZR2013H047). The funders had no role in study design, data collection and analysis, decision to publish, or preparation of the manuscript.

Competing Interests: The authors have declared that no competing interests exist.

* Email: xiuguisheng@yahoo.com (XS); jinmingyu70@yahoo.com (JY)

❾ These authors contributed equally to this work.

Introduction

Hepatocellular carcinoma (HCC) is the fifth most common cancer in men, worldwide, and seventh among women, and it is the second leading cause of cancer-related mortality globally [1].

HCC commonly occurs in Asia and Africa, and its incidence rate is starting to increase in Western countries [2,3]. Due to lack of effective biomarkers for diagnosis and prognosis, HCC is frequently found in late stages, when curative therapy approaches

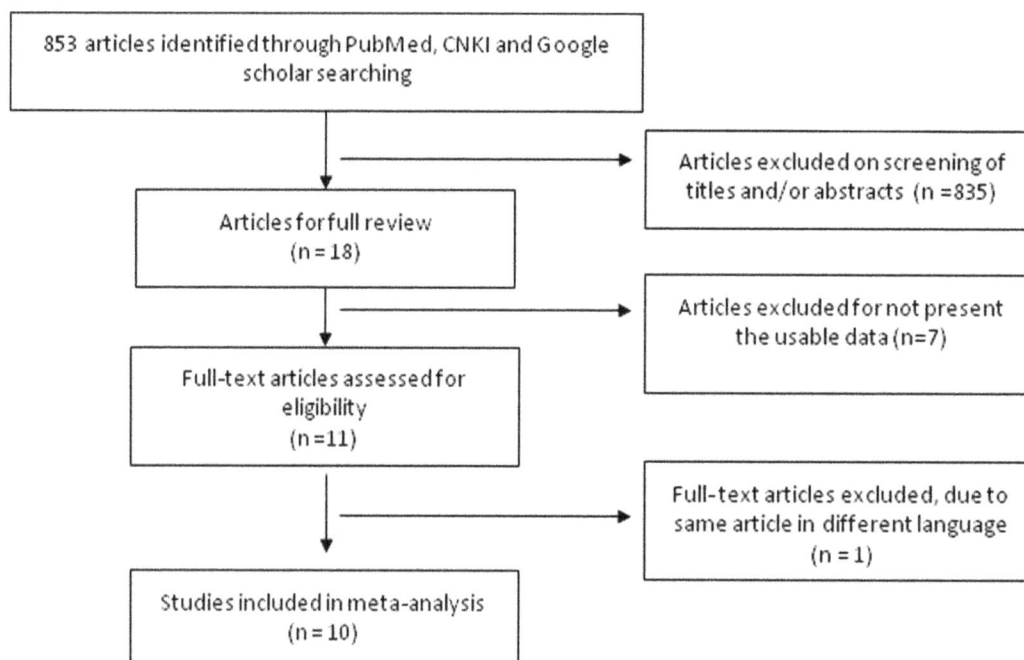

Figure 1. Schematic flow diagram for selection of included studies.

like resection, liver transplantation, radio frequency ablation (RFA), and transarterial chemoembolization (TACE) don't produce satisfactory clinical outcomes. HCC patients present with high recurrence and metastasis [4,5], the 5-year survival rate after surgery for HCC has been only 25%–39% [6]. Therefore, it is critical to identify the biomolecular markers for the diagnosis and prognosis to monitor recurrence of HCC.

The serum a-fetoprotein (AFP) has been widely used as a risk assessment factor in patients with cirrhosis and a screening method for early detection of HCC patients, and a prognostic factor for prediction of tumor recurrence. AFP is the only HCC biomarker that has been studied through to phase 5 of biomarker development [7]. However, its sensitivity and specificity vary significantly ranging from 40%–65% and 76%–96%, respectively [8,9,10]. Recent studies have identified other potential biomarkers for early detection of HCC, including the circulating AFP isoform AFP-L3 [11,12], des-gamma-carboxy prothrombin (DCP) [12],

Golgi protein-73 (GP73) [13] and circulating miRNA [14]. However, most of them are only in phase 1 or 2 stages, further studies are needed to determine whether these biomarkers can be translated from bench works to clinical settings. The effects of other biomarkers to predict the prognosis for HCC such as vascular endothelial growth factor (VEGF), Cyclin-dependent Kinases(CDK), β-catenin/Wnt pathway and microRNAs [15] have been controversial and again none of them has been applied to the clinical settings.

HMGB1 was discovered in calf thymus in 1973 and named for its electrophoretic mobility in polyacrylamide gels [16,17]. HMGB1 is encoded on human chromosome 13q12-13 and consists of 215 amino acids. It is a highly conserved protein containing two DNA binding domains A and B as well as a negatively charged C-terminal tail domain [18,19]. HMGB1 has different functions depending on its subcellular locations. HMGB1 is normally located in the nucleus where it acts as a DNA

Table 1. Main Characteristics of included studies.

Author	Year	HCC Sample size	Comments
Liu et al. [31]	2012	161	High expression of HMGB1 predicts poor prognosis for HCC
Jiang et al. [30]	2012	34	HMGB1 is associated with clinicopathologic features in patients with HCC
Cheng et al. [70]	2008	161	Serum HMGB1 is associated with clinicopathologic features in patients with HCC
Xiao et al. [56]	2014	208	The association of HMGB1 Gene with the prognosis of HCC
Ueno et al. [32]	2011	36	Significance of HMGB1 expression in HCC
Han et al. [71]	2014	13	Changes of HMGB1 expression in HCC
Gou et al. [72]	2013	82	Detection and clinical significance of HMGB1 in HCC
Wang et al. [73]	2013	39	Increased HMGB1 expression in HCC and its mechanism
Feng et al. [74]	2011	40	The expression and clinical significance of HMGB1 in HCC
Wang et al. [57]	2013	155	Expression, subcellular location and prognostic relevance of HMGB1 in HCC

Table 2. Serum HMGB1 levels (ng/ml) in TNM stages of patients with HCC.

Author	Sample size	I	II	III	IV	P	Detect method
Gou [72]	82	29.1±5.0	57.7±14.2	101.6±14.8	176.0±32.5	<0.01	Elisa
Cheng [70]	161	30.2±5.9	58.9±20.0	100.9±23.4	175.8±47.6	<0.0001	Western-blot

chaperon by regulating transcription, replication, recombination, repair, and genome stability [20]. In 2011, Hanahan and Weinberg proposed a new model to define the ten hallmarks for the tumor requirements [21]. Recent findings indicate that HMGB1 dysfunction is associated with every hallmark of cancer and contributes to cancer initiation and development [22]. HMGB1 overexpression and cytoplasmic localization have been observed in some cancer cells such as in colon cancer [23], gastrointestinal stromal tumors [24], cervical carcinomas [25] and melanoma [26]. Moreover, recent studies demonstrate that HMGB1 expression is a useful prognostic maker for colorectal cancer and diffuse malignant peritoneal mesothelioma [27,28,29]. Higher HMGB1 expression has been observed in HCC compared to normal liver tissues [30,31,32]. HMGB1 could be a potential biomarker that may be used to detect HCC at early stage and predict its prognosis. However, the prognostic value of HMGB1 for survival remains controversial due to limited statistic power. There is no meta-analysis study to reveal the association between HMGB1 expression and clinicopathological parameters of HCC. Therefore, we performed a meta-analysis to evaluate the association of HMGB1 expression with the clinicopathological parameters and prognosis in HCC.

Methods

Search strategy and selection criteria

The following electronic databases were searched for relevant articles without any language restrictions: Web of Science (1945 ~ 2014), the Cochrane Library Database (Issue 12, 2014), PubMed (1966 ~ 2014), EMBASE (1980 ~ 2014), CINAHL (1982 ~ 2014), CNKI, Google scholar, and the Chinese Biomedical Database (CBM) (1982 ~ 2014). We searched articles using the following terms: HMGB1 or high motility group box 1 and hepatocellular carcinoma, liver cancer or HCC. There were 27 articles identified from PubMed, 31 articles from Web Science, 33 articles from EMBASE, 262 articles from CNKI. 5950 articles from Google scholar were identified, however, only 500 of them were screened by titles and abstracts since the rest of them were not relevant. Finally total 853 articles were screened by titles and abstracts.

The inclusion criteria included: 1) The articles which the association between HMGB1 expression and the clinicopathological significance of HCC was evaluated; 2) The articles which the association of HMGB1 expression and prognosis in patients with HCC was evaluated; 3) The studies which utilized RT-PCR for detection of HMGB1 mRNA, ELISA for serum HMGB1 and Western Blot for tissue HMGB1 expression. The exclusion criteria included: 1) The studies which used the same population or overlapping database; 2) The studies of in vitro cell culture models (Figure 1). The search identified 18 articles of which 10 were eligible for quantitative analysis in this meta-analysis. The detailed information of 10 relevant citations was listed in Table 1.

Data extraction and study assessment

Two reviewers (Zhang and Han) independently extracted data and reviewed the contents of the manuscripts to determine whether they met the criteria for inclusion. Any discontent was discussed and resolved by a consensus including a third investigator (Wu). A data extract form was developed accordingly. One review author (Zhang) extracted the following data from the included studies: first author's name, year of publication, number of patients, stage of HCC, grade of HCC, and HMGB1 expression. The second author (Han) checked the extracted data,

Table 3. Serum HMGB1 levels (ng/ml) in patients with hepatitis and normal controls.

Author	Sample size (Heptitis/Normal)	Chronic Hepatitis	Normal control	P	Detect method
Wang [73]	39/48	13.5±6.3	3.9±1.4	<0.01	Elisa
Feng [74]	38/23	48.6±18.38	36.6±7.07	<0.05	Elisa

and disagreement was resolved by the discussion with the third author (Wu) for all issues.

Statistics analysis

All analysis was performed with Review Manager 5.2. Heterogeneity between studies was assessed using the Q-test and I^2 index. Mean differences with 95% confidence intervals were calculated by using a fixed or random effect model depending on heterogeneity (a fixed effect model for $I^2 < 50\%$, a random effect model for $I^2 > 50\%$). Meta-analysis was performed to compare HMGB1 mRNA expression between HCC and normal tissue, HMGB1 mRNA and protein expression levels between HCC and para-tumor tissue. Two studies investigated serum HMGB1 protein levels in TNM stages of HCC that were listed in Table 2. Another two studies detected serum HMGB1 levels in patients with hepatitis and normal controls, the data were listed in Table 3. The multivariate HRs were collected and the log HRs and its standard errors were calculated for individual study. Pooled hazard ratio (HR) with a 95% confidence interval was calculated for the association between HMGB1 expression and prognosis. All p values were two sided. Funnel plots were used for detection of publication bias. A sensitivity analysis, in which one study was removed at a time, was conducted to assess the result stability.

Results

Total 853 articles were screened by titles and abstracts. The search identified 18 articles of which 10 were eligible for quantitative analysis in this meta-analysis. 7 articles were excluded due to different detect methods used. One article was excluded due to duplication. 10 relevant articles were included for full review in detail and 6 of them were conducted with meta-analysis (Figure 1). The following items were collected from each study: first author's name, year of publication, number of patients, stages of HCC, detect methods, HMGB1 expression and prognosis (Table 1 and 2).

HMGB1 mRNA level in HCC was significantly higher than in normal and para-tumor tissues respectively. The pooled mean difference for HCC versus normal liver tissue was 0.38, (95% CI

0.22–0.54, Z = 4.59, p<0.00001, heterogeneity $I^2 = 91\%$, Figure 2) and for HCC versus para-tumor, mean difference was 0.31, (95% CI 0.12–0.51, Z = 3.12, p = 0.002, heterogeneity $I^2 = 93\%$, Figure 3). The protein level of HMGB1 in HCC was significantly higher than those in para-tumor tissues, the pooled mean difference was 0.51 with 95% CI 0.16–0.86, (Z = 2.83, p = 0.005, heterogeneity $I^2 = 98\%$, Figure 4). Figure 5 showed the result of a meta-analysis of hazard ratios (HR) of HMGB1 high expression and low expression in the survival of patients with HCC. The overall survival (OS) was significantly shorter in HCC patients with high HMGB1 expression compared those with low HMGB1 expression, and the pooled HR was 1.31 with 95% CI 1.20–1.44, (Z = 5.82, p<0.0001, heterogeneity $I^2 = 20\%$, Figure 5).

Four of included studies were fully reviewed without performing meta-analysis due to less number of patients in the selected articles. Two studies reported the serum HMGB1 levels in patients with HCC of TNM stage I, II, III, IV (Table 2). The differences were significant between stage I and II, stage II and III, as well as stage III and IV groups (two studies showed p<0.01 and p<0.0001 respectively). Another two studies investigated the serum HMGB1 levels, suggesting there were higher serum HMGB1 levels in patients with chronic hepatitis than in healthy people (p<0.01 and p<0.05 respectively) (Table 3).

A sensitivity analysis, in which one study was removed at a time, was conducted to assess the result stability. The pooled HR was not significantly changed, indicating the stability of our analyses. The funnel plots were largely symmetric (Figure 6) suggesting there were no publication biases in the meta-analysis of HMGB1 expression and clinicopathological features.

Discussion

For the first time, we conducted a meta-analysis and evaluated HMGB1 mRNA and protein expression levels in tissues from patients with HCC and normal liver or para-tumor tissues. The heterogeneity between studies was assessed using the Q-test and I^2 index. All I^2 indexes for comparisons of mRNA and protein expression between HCC and normal or para-tumor tissue were

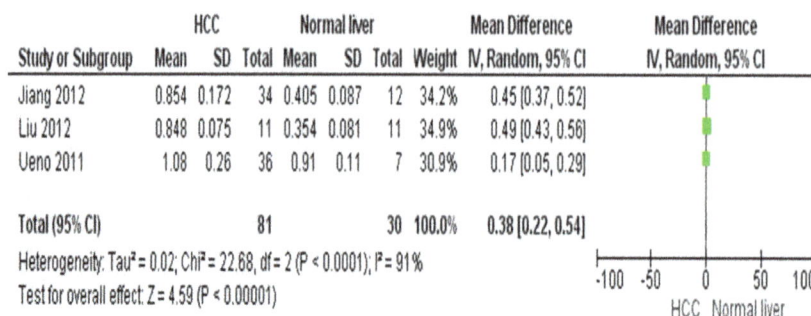

Figure 2. Forest plot for HMGB1mRNA/GADPH in HCC and normal liver tissue.

Study or Subgroup	HCC Mean	SD	Total	Para tumor Mean	SD	Total	Weight	Mean Difference IV, Random, 95% CI	Mean Difference IV, Random, 95% CI
Jiang 2012	0.854	0.172	34	0.527	0.155	34	34.4%	0.33 [0.25, 0.40]	
Liu 2012	0.848	0.075	11	0.354	0.081	11	34.9%	0.49 [0.43, 0.56]	
Ueno 2011	1.08	0.26	36	0.99	0.34	36	30.7%	0.09 [-0.05, 0.23]	
Total (95% CI)			81			81	100.0%	0.31 [0.12, 0.51]	

Heterogeneity: Tau² = 0.03; Chi² = 29.95, df = 2 (P < 0.00001); I² = 93%
Test for overall effect: Z = 3.12 (P = 0.002)

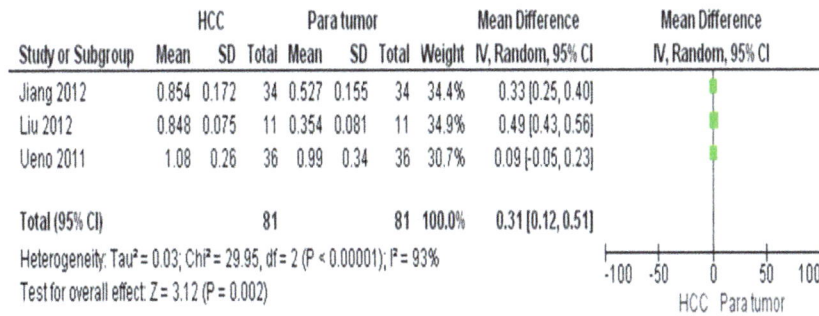

Figure 3. Forest plot for HMGB1mRNA/GADPH in HCC and para-tumor tissue.

great than 75%, indicating that there was significant heterogeneity between studies. All p values for test of overall effect were equal or less than 0.005, indicating mRNA and protein expression levels in HCC were significantly increased compared to those in the normal and para-tumor tissues respectively. This suggests that HMGB1 plays an important role in the pathogenesis of HCC. HMGB1 is a potential tissue biomarker for HCC diagnosis.

Cancer development is a multistep process. Accumulated evidences indicate that HMGB1 is associated with ten functional capabilities of cancers as Hanahan and Weinberg described in 2011 [21]. Its function depends on the subcellular locations. Within the nucleus, HMGB1 acts as a DNA chaperon to bind to the minor groove of DNA, stabilizing nucleosides and facilitating the assembly of site-specific DNA-binding proteins such as the nuclear hormone/nuclear hormone receptor complex and p53, p73, as well as retinoblastoma protein (Rb) transcription complexes [33,34]. When HMGB1 releases outside of the cell, it interacts with a wide range of proteins, such as the receptor of advanced glycation end products (RAGE), Toll-like receptors (TLRs: TLR2, TLR4 and TLR9), mitogen-activated protein kinase (MAPK), NF (nuclear factor)-κB, and coordinates immune system activation, cell migration, cell growth, angiogenesis, and tissue repair as well as regeneration [35,36,37,38,39,40].

Recent studies report that the expression of HMGB1 is upregulated in several types of malignancies including gastric cancer [41], breast cancer [33], nasopharyngeal carcinoma [42], and squamous cell carcinoma of the head and neck [43,44]. HMGB1 is not only constitutively expressed in the nucleus of cancer cells, but also is released by the tumor cells, macrophages, monocytes, dendritic cells (DCs), and T cells [45]. Released HMGB1 that acts as a proinflammatory cytokine from necrotic tumor cells creates a microenvironment and triggers signaling

pathway, such as the NF-κB and inflammasome, to induce proinflammatory cytokine release. This loop accelerates inflammatory response and tumor formation [22,46,47]. Therefore, serum HMGB1 levels could be prediction for progression of patients with HCC.

Two studies reported the serum HMGB1 levels in patients with HCC of TNM stage I, II, III, IV. The differences were significant between stage I and II, stage II and III, as well as stage III and IV groups (two studies showed p<0.01 and p<0.0001 respectively). Higher HMGB1 expression was detected in advanced stages of HCC patients. This suggests that HMGB1 plays an important role in the invasion, metastasis and progression of HCC. In support of this, recent evidences indicated HMGB1 was co-localized with RAGE, suggesting their potential contribution to cellular migration and tumor invasion. The expression of RAGE was closely associated with the invasive and metastatic behavior in different types of cancer such as gastric [48] and colorectal cancer [49]. The interaction of HMGB1 with RAGE leads to activation of the NF-κB, MAPK, and type IV collagenase (MMP-2/MMP-9) signaling pathways, all of which degrade extracellular matrix protein and play a major role in tumor invasion and metastasis [50,51,52,53]. Furthermore, tumor growth and metastasis were suppressed by blocking RAGE-HMGB1 complex in human and murine cancer cells [52,54]. Knockdown of HMGB1 gene also inhibited liver cancer growth and metastasis [31,55]. Therefore, the overexpression of HMGB1 is not only a potential biomarker for initial diagnosis of HCC, but it also could be a predictor of prognosis in patients with HCC. More studies are needed for a meta-analysis in the future to confirm the progression value of HMGB1 in the patients with HCC.

A few of studies reported controversial results of the association between HMGB1 expression and the prognosis of patients with

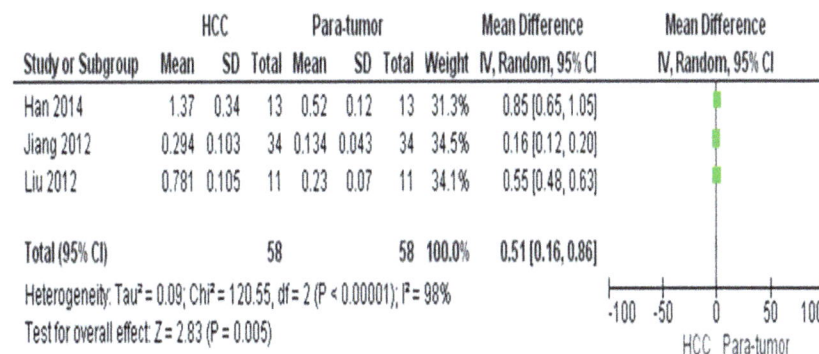

Study or Subgroup	HCC Mean	SD	Total	Para-tumor Mean	SD	Total	Weight	Mean Difference IV, Random, 95% CI	Mean Difference IV, Random, 95% CI
Han 2014	1.37	0.34	13	0.52	0.12	13	31.3%	0.85 [0.65, 1.05]	
Jiang 2012	0.294	0.103	34	0.134	0.043	34	34.5%	0.16 [0.12, 0.20]	
Liu 2012	0.781	0.105	11	0.23	0.07	11	34.1%	0.55 [0.48, 0.63]	
Total (95% CI)			58			58	100.0%	0.51 [0.16, 0.86]	

Heterogeneity: Tau² = 0.09; Chi² = 120.55, df = 2 (P < 0.00001); I² = 98%
Test for overall effect: Z = 2.83 (P = 0.005)

Figure 4. Forest plot for HMGB1 protein/GADPH in HCC and para-tumor tissue.

Study or Subgroup	log[Hazard Ratio]	SE	Weight	Hazard Ratio IV, Fixed, 95% CI	Hazard Ratio IV, Fixed, 95% CI
Liu 2012	0.263399	0.05559	70.2%	1.30 [1.17, 1.45]	
Wang 2013	0.322633	0.088	28.0%	1.38 [1.16, 1.64]	
Xiao 2014	-0.25026	0.35535	1.7%	0.78 [0.39, 1.56]	
Total (95% CI)			100.0%	1.31 [1.20, 1.44]	

Heterogeneity: Chi² = 2.51, df = 2 (P = 0.28); I² = 20%
Test for overall effect: Z = 5.82 (P < 0.00001)

0.01   0.1   1   10   100
High HMGB1   Low HMGB1

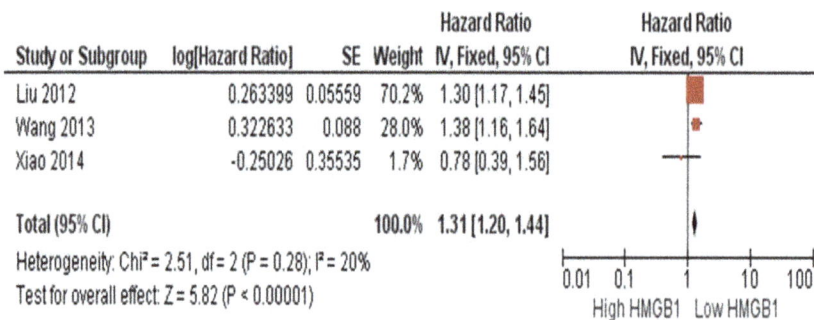

Figure 5. Forest plot for the association of HMGB1expression level and the risk of HCC

HCC [31,56,57]. Those studies on prognostic significance of HMGB1 expression were limited by low statistical power. We performed a meta-analysis for the first time and pooled three studies together (n = 524). The low heterogeneity ($I^2 = 20\%$) could be due to different methods to measure HMGB1 intensity in immunohistochemistry. Our pooled HR was 1.31 with 95% CI 1.20–1.44, test for overall effect p<0.0001, suggesting that high HMGB1 expression was significantly associated with the mortality of patients with HCC. Compared with low HMGB1 expression, HMGB1 high expression was associated with more than 1.3 times

the risk of mortality. HMGB1 affects the prognosis of HCC through complicated pathways. HMGB1 has the following abilities to induce tumorigenesis: 1). tumor cells and tumor-infiltrating leukocytes secret HMGB1 in tumor microenvironment which activates NK-κB and inflammatory pathways, promoting tumor growth, invasion and metastasis [46,47,58]; 2). HMGB1 also has the ability to increase the production of ATP and provide more energy for tumor growth [59]; 3). In addition, HMGB1 promotes angiogenesis [60,61,62,63] for tumor growth and metastasis; 4). Lastly, HMGB1 inhibits antitumor immunity for tumor survival

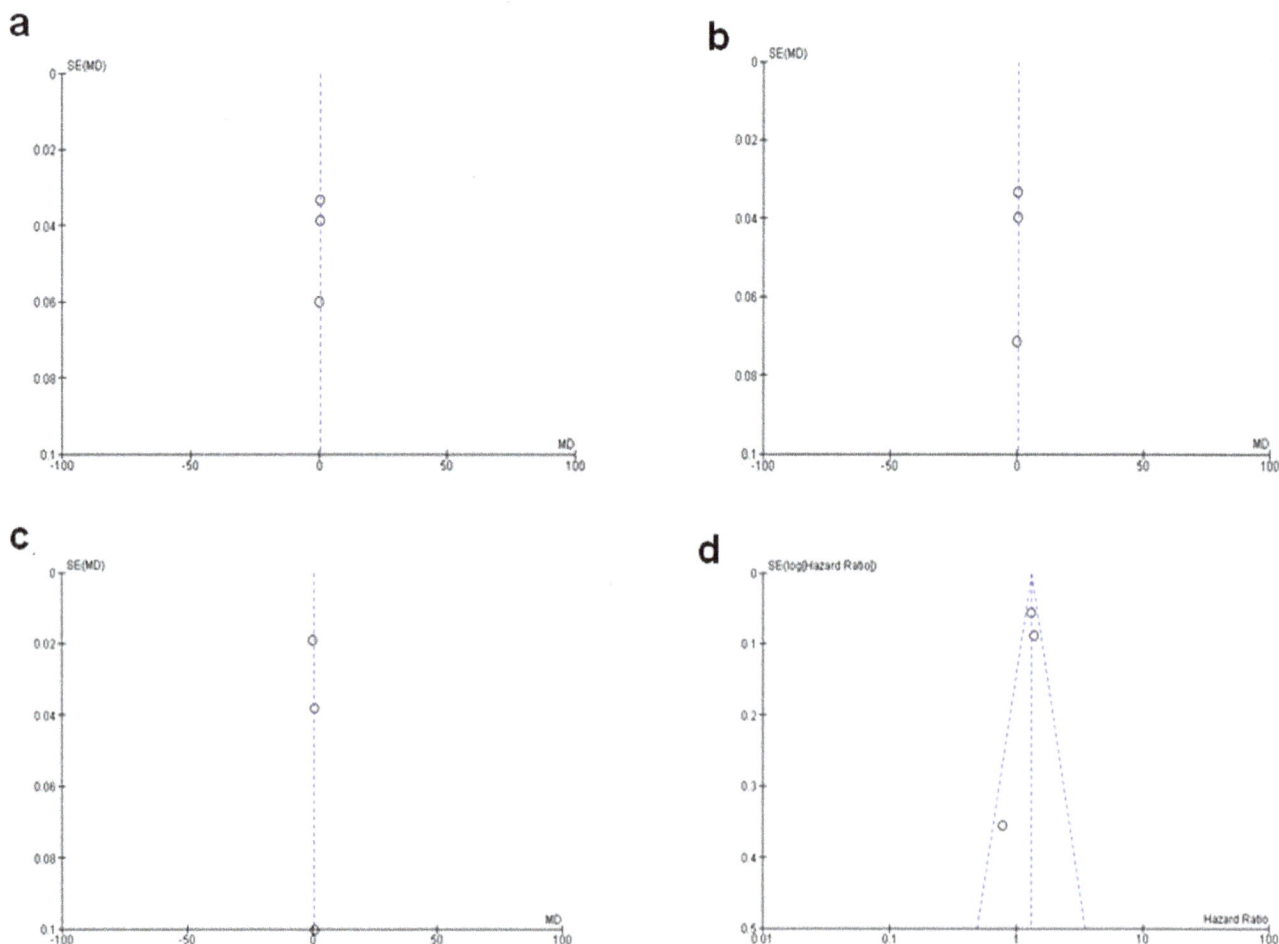

Figure 6. Funnel plot for publication bias. a: HMGB1 mRNA/GADPH in HCC and normal liver tissue; b: HMGB1 mRNA/GADPH in HCC and para-tumor tissue; c: HMGB1 protein/GADPH in HCC and para-tumor tissue; d: the association of HMGB1expression and the risk of HCC.

[64,65,66]. All these activities contribute to poor prognosis of HCC patients with high expression of HMGB1. Therefore, HMGB1 overexpression predicts a poor prognosis in patients with HCC.

Interestingly, two studies investigated serum HMGB1 in patients with chronic hepatitis (the precursor of HCC) and healthy people. Significantly higher serum HMGB1 was detected in the patients with chronic hepatitis compared to those detected in healthy people. The difference of serum HMGB1 levels between the two studies could be due to that different methods were used to detect the serum concentration of HMGB1. HMGB1 lacks a classic signal sequence. During infection, HMGB1 is translocated from the nucleus to the cytoplasm and is subsequently released into the extracellular milieu by HCV or HBV infection [67,68,69]. HMGB1 is likely to be crucial in initiating and mediating hepatitis. Further studies are needed to verify its role in the pathogenesis of chronic hepatitis and subsequently in HCC.

We evaluated the HMGB1 expression in patients with HCC (both tumor and para-tumor tissues) and normal liver tissues. Further studies should be focused on finding cut-offs for the diagnosis of HCC and determination of its stages. In the future,

more studies are needed to verify if HMGB1 blockage can be used in the development of new therapeutic agents for HCC. Finally, our study only selected the published articles, but it did not include some relevant unpublished papers which may result in certain publication bias. Thus the result should be interpreted carefully.

In conclusion, HMGB1 mRNA and protein tissue levels in the patients with HCC are significantly higher than in those of para-tumor and normal liver tissues respectively. HMGB1 overexpression is a potential biomarker for HCC diagnosis, and it significantly associated with the prognosis of patients with HCC.

Author Contributions

Conceived and designed the experiments: JY LZ JH. Performed the experiments: LZ JH HW XL. Analyzed the data: JZ JL LX YX. Wrote the paper: XS JY.

References

1. Jemal A, Bray F, Center MM, Ferlay J, Ward E, et al. (2011) Global cancer statistics. CA Cancer J Clin 61: 69–90.
2. Parkin DM, Bray F, Ferlay J, Pisani P (2005) Global cancer statistics, 2002. CA Cancer J Clin 55: 74–108.
3. Bosch FX, Ribes J, Diaz M, Cleries R (2004) Primary liver cancer: worldwide incidence and trends. Gastroenterology 127: S5–S16.
4. El-Serag HB, Marrero JA, Rudolph L, Reddy KR (2008) Diagnosis and treatment of hepatocellular carcinoma. Gastroenterology 134: 1752–1763.
5. Forner A, Bruix J (2008) Locoregional treatment for hepatocellular carcinoma: From clinical exploration to robust clinical data, changing standards of care. Hepatology 47: 5–7.
6. Thomas MB, Zhu AX (2005) Hepatocellular carcinoma: the need for progress. J Clin Oncol 23: 2892–2899.
7. Zhang BH, Yang BH, Tang ZY (2004) Randomized controlled trial of screening for hepatocellular carcinoma. J Cancer Res Clin Oncol 130: 417–422.
8. Trevisani F, D'Intino PE, Morselli-Labate AM, Mazzella G, Accogli E, et al. (2001) Serum alpha-fetoprotein for diagnosis of hepatocellular carcinoma in patients with chronic liver disease: influence of HBsAg and anti-HCV status. J Hepatol 34: 570–575.
9. Yoshida S, Kurokohchi K, Arima K, Masaki T, Hosomi N, et al. (2002) Clinical significance of lens culinaris agglutinin-reactive fraction of serum alpha-fetoprotein in patients with hepatocellular carcinoma. Int J Oncol 20: 305–309.
10. Khien VV, Mao HV, Chinh TT, Ha PT, Bang MH, et al. (2001) Clinical evaluation of lentil lectin-reactive alpha-fetoprotein-L3 in histology-proven hepatocellular carcinoma. Int J Biol Markers 16: 105–111.
11. Yamamoto K, Imamura H, Matsuyama Y, Kume Y, Ikeda H, et al. (2010) AFP, AFP-L3, DCP, and GP73 as markers for monitoring treatment response and recurrence and as surrogate markers of clinicopathological variables of HCC. J Gastroenterol 45: 1272–1282.
12. Nakamura S, Nouso K, Sakaguchi K, Ito YM, Ohashi Y, et al. (2006) Sensitivity and specificity of des-gamma-carboxy prothrombin for diagnosis of patients with hepatocellular carcinomas varies according to tumor size. Am J Gastroenterol 101: 2038–2043.
13. Tian L, Wang Y, Xu D, Gui J, Jia X, et al. (2011) Serological AFP/Golgi protein 73 could be a new diagnostic parameter of hepatic diseases. Int J Cancer 129: 1923–1931.
14. Qi J, Wang J, Katayama H, Sen S, Liu SM (2013) Circulating microRNAs (cmiRNAs) as novel potential biomarkers for hepatocellular carcinoma. Neoplasma 60: 135–142.
15. Pinato DJ, Pirisi M, Maslen L, Sharma R (2014) Tissue biomarkers of prognostic significance in hepatocellular carcinoma. Adv Anat Pathol 21: 270–284.
16. Goodwin GH, Johns EW (1973) Isolation and characterisation of two calf-thymus chromatin non-histone proteins with high contents of acidic and basic amino acids. Eur J Biochem 40: 215–219.
17. Goodwin GH SC, Johns EW (1973) A new group of chromatin-associated proteins with a high content of acidic and basic amino acids. Eur J Biochem 38: 14–19.
18. Weir HM, Kraulis PJ, Hill CS, Raine AR, Laue ED, et al. (1993) Structure of the HMG box motif in the B-domain of HMG1. EMBO J 12: 1311–1319.
19. Read CM, Cary PD, Crane-Robinson C, Driscoll PC, Norman DG (1993) Solution structure of a DNA-binding domain from HMG1. Nucleic Acids Res 21: 3427–3436.
20. Liu Y, Prasad R, Wilson SH (2010) HMGB1: roles in base excision repair and related function. Biochim Biophys Acta 1799: 119–130.
21. Hanahan D, Weinberg RA (2011) Hallmarks of cancer: the next generation. Cell 144: 646–674.
22. Tang D, Kang R, Zeh HJ, 3rd, Lotze MT (2010) High-mobility group box 1 and cancer. Biochim Biophys Acta 1799: 131–140.
23. Volp K, Brezniceanu ML, Bosser S, Brableltz T, Kirchner T, et al. (2006) Increased expression of high mobility group box 1 (HMGB1) is associated with an elevated level of the antiapoptotic c-IAP2 protein in human colon carcinomas. Gut 55: 234–242.
24. Choi YR, Kim H, Kang HJ, Kim NG, Kim JJ, et al. (2003) Overexpression of high mobility group box 1 in gastrointestinal stromal tumors with KIT mutation. Cancer Res 63: 2188–2193.
25. Hao Q, Du XQ, Fu X, Tian J (2008) [Expression and clinical significance of HMGB1 and RAGE in cervical squamous cell carcinoma]. Zhonghua Zhong Liu Za Zhi 30: 292–295.
26. Poser I, Golob M, Buettner R, Bosserhoff AK (2003) Upregulation of HMG1 leads to melanoma inhibitory activity expression in malignant melanoma cells and contributes to their malignancy phenotype. Mol Cell Biol 23: 2991–2998.
27. Tabata C, Shibata E, Tabata R, Kanemura S, Mikami K, et al. (2013) Serum HMGB1 as a prognostic marker for malignant pleural mesothelioma. BMC Cancer 13: 205.
28. Fahmueller YN, Nagel D, Hoffmann RT, Tatsch K, Jakobs T, et al. (2013) Immunogenic cell death biomarkers HMGB1, RAGE, and DNAse indicate response to radioembolization therapy and prognosis in colorectal cancer patients. Int J Cancer 132: 2349–2358.
29. Chiharu Tabata ES, Rie Tabata, Shingo Kanemura, Koji Mikami, Yoshitaka Nogi, et al. (2013) Serum HMGB1 as a prognostic marker for malignant pleural mesothelioma. BMC Cancer 13: 1–6.
30. Jiang W, Wang Z, Li X, Fan X, Duan Y (2012) High-mobility group box 1 is associated with clinicopathologic features in patients with hepatocellular carcinoma. Pathol Oncol Res 18: 293–298.
31. Liu F, Zhang Y, Peng Z, Gao H, Xu L, et al. (2012) High expression of high mobility group box 1 (hmgb1) predicts poor prognosis for hepatocellular carcinoma after curative hepatectomy. J Transl Med 10: 135.
32. Ueno S HK, Sakoda M, Iino S, Kurahara H MK, Ando K, et al. (2011) Significance of High Mobility Group Box-1 (HMGB1) Expression in Hepatocellular Carcinoma. Med J Kago Shima Univ 62: 27–35.
33. Brezniceanu ML, Volp K, Bosser S, Solbach C, Lichter P, et al. (2003) HMGB1 inhibits cell death in yeast and mammalian cells and is abundantly expressed in human breast carcinoma. FASEB J 17: 1295–1297.
34. Thomas JO, Travers AA (2001) HMG1 and 2, and related 'architectural' DNA-binding proteins. Trends Biochem Sci 26: 167–174.
35. Ghavami S, Rashedi I, Dattilo BM, Eshraghi M, Chazin WJ, et al. (2008) S100A8/A9 at low concentration promotes tumor cell growth via RAGE ligation and MAP kinase-dependent pathway. J Leukoc Biol 83: 1484–1492.
36. Palumbo R, Galvez BG, Pusterla T, De Marchis F, Cossu G, et al. (2007) Cells migrating to sites of tissue damage in response to the danger signal HMGB1 require NF-kappaB activation. J Cell Biol 179: 33–40.
37. Dong Xda E, Ito N, Lotze MT, Demarco RA, Popovic P, et al. (2007) High mobility group box I (HMGB1) release from tumor cells after treatment: implications for development of targeted chemoimmunotherapy. J Immunother 30: 596–606.

38. Scaffidi P, Misteli T, Bianchi ME (2002) Release of chromatin protein HMGB1 by necrotic cells triggers inflammation. Nature 418: 191–195.

39. Tian J, Avalos AM, Mao SY, Chen B, Senthil K, et al. (2007) Toll-like receptor 9-dependent activation by DNA-containing immune complexes is mediated by HMGB1 and RAGE. Nat Immunol 8: 487–496.

40. Wang H, Bloom O, Zhang M, Vishnubhakat JM, Ombrellino M, et al. (1999) HMG-1 as a late mediator of endotoxin lethality in mice. Science 285: 248–251.

41. Akaike H, Kono K, Sugai H, Takahashi A, Mimura K, et al. (2007) Expression of high mobility group box chromosomal protein-1 (HMGB-1) in gastric cancer. Anticancer Res 27: 449–457.

42. Wu D, Ding Y, Wang S, Zhang Q, Liu L (2008) Increased expression of high mobility group box 1 (HMGB1) is associated with progression and poor prognosis in human nasopharyngeal carcinoma. J Pathol 216: 167–175.

43. Liu Y, Xie C, Zhang X, Huang D, Zhou X, et al. (2010) Elevated expression of HMGB1 in squamous-cell carcinoma of the head and neck and its clinical significance. Eur J Cancer 46: 3007–3015.

44. Lotze MT, Tracey KJ (2005) High-mobility group box 1 protein (HMGB1): nuclear weapon in the immune arsenal. Nat Rev Immunol 5: 331–342.

45. Naglova H, Bucova M (2012) HMGB1 and its physiological and pathological roles. Bratisl Lek Listy 113: 163–171.

46. Gebhardt C, Riehl A, Durchdewald M, Nemeth J, Furstenberger G, et al. (2008) RAGE signaling sustains inflammation and promotes tumor development. J Exp Med 205: 275–285.

47. Mittal D, Saccheri F, Venereau E, Pusterla T, Bianchi ME, et al. (2010) TLR4-mediated skin carcinogenesis is dependent on immune and radioresistant cells. EMBO J 29: 2242–2252.

48. Kuniyasu H, Oue N, Wakikawa A, Shigeishi H, Matsutani N, et al. (2002) Expression of receptors for advanced glycation end-products (RAGE) is closely associated with the invasive and metastatic activity of gastric cancer. J Pathol 196: 163–170.

49. Sasahira T, Akama Y, Fujii K, Kuniyasu H (2005) Expression of receptor for advanced glycation end products and HMGB1/amphoterin in colorectal adenomas. Virchows Arch 446: 411–415.

50. Dumitriu IE, Baruah P, Manfredi AA, Bianchi ME, Rovere-Querini P (2005) HMGB1: guiding immunity from within. Trends Immunol 26: 381–387.

51. Evans A, Lennard TW, Davies BR (2004) High-mobility group protein 1(Y): metastasis-associated or metastasis-inducing? J Surg Oncol 88: 86–99.

52. Taguchi A, Blood DC, del Toro G, Canet A, Lee DC, et al. (2000) Blockade of RAGE-amphoterin signalling suppresses tumour growth and metastases. Nature 405: 354–360.

53. Takada M, Hirata K, Ajiki T, Suzuki Y, Kuroda Y (2004) Expression of receptor for advanced glycation end products (RAGE) and MMP-9 in human pancreatic cancer cells. Hepatogastroenterology 51: 928–930.

54. Huttunen HJ, Fages C, Kuja-Panula J, Ridley AJ, Rauvala H (2002) Receptor for advanced glycation end products-binding COOH-terminal motif of amphoterin inhibits invasive migration and metastasis. Cancer Res 62: 4805–4811.

55. Dong YD, Cui L, Peng CH, Cheng DF, Han BS, et al. (2013) Expression and clinical significance of HMGB1 in human liver cancer: Knockdown inhibits tumor growth and metastasis in vitro and in vivo. Oncol Rep 29: 87–94.

56. Xiao J, Ding Y, Huang J, Li Q, Liu Y, et al. (2014) The association of HMGB1 gene with the prognosis of HCC. PLoS One 9: e89097.

57. Wang Y (2013) Expression,Subcellular Location and Prognostic Relevance of High Mobility Group Box 1(HMGB1) in Hepatocellular Carcinoma. University of Science and Technology Graduation Thesis 2013: 11-14. Available: http://cdmd.cnki.com.cn/Article/CDMD-10487-1013273569.htm

58. Jube S, Rivera ZS, Bianchi ME, Powers A, Wang E, et al. (2012) Cancer cell secretion of the DAMP protein HMGB1 supports progression in malignant mesothelioma. Cancer Res 72: 3290–3301.

59. Kang R, Tang D, Schapiro NE, Loux T, Livesey KM, et al. (2014) The HMGB1/RAGE inflammatory pathway promotes pancreatic tumor growth by regulating mitochondrial bioenergetics. Oncogene 33: 567–577.

60. Yan W, Chang Y, Liang X, Cardinal JS, Huang H, et al. (2012) High-mobility group box 1 activates caspase-1 and promotes hepatocellular carcinoma invasiveness and metastases. Hepatology 55: 1863–1875.

61. Tafani M, Schito L, Pellegrini L, Villanova L, Marfe G, et al. (2011) Hypoxia-increased RAGE and P2X7R expression regulates tumor cell invasion through phosphorylation of Erk1/2 and Akt and nuclear translocation of NF-{kappa}B. Carcinogenesis 32: 1167–1175.

62. van Beijnum JR, Nowak-Sliwinska P, van den Boezem E, Hautvast P, Buurman WA, et al. (2013) Tumor angiogenesis is enforced by autocrine regulation of high-mobility group box 1. Oncogene 32: 363–374.

63. Sasahira T, Kirita T, Bhawal UK, Ikeda M, Nagasawa A, et al. (2007) The expression of receptor for advanced glycation end products is associated with angiogenesis in human oral squamous cell carcinoma. Virchows Arch 450: 287–295.

64. Kusume A, Sasahira T, Luo Y, Isobe M, Nakagawa N, et al. (2009) Suppression of dendritic cells by HMGB1 is associated with lymph node metastasis of human colon cancer. Pathobiology 76: 155–162.

65. Liu Z, Falo LD, Jr., You Z (2011) Knockdown of HMGB1 in tumor cells attenuates their ability to induce regulatory T cells and uncovers naturally acquired CD8 T cell-dependent antitumor immunity. J Immunol 187: 118–125.

66. He Y, Zha J, Wang Y, Liu W, Yang X, et al. (2013) Tissue damage-associated "danger signals" influence T-cell responses that promote the progression of preneoplasia to cancer. Cancer Res 73: 629–639.

67. Liu HB, Fan XG, Huang JJ, Li N, Peng JP, et al. (2007) [Serum level of HMGB1 in patients with hepatitis B and its clinical significance]. Zhonghua Gan Zang Bing Za Zhi 15: 812–815.

68. Jung JH, Park JH, Jee MH, Keum SJ, Cho MS, et al. (2011) Hepatitis C virus infection is blocked by HMGB1 released from virus-infected cells. J Virol 85: 9359–9368.

69. Zhou RR, Zhao SS, Zou MX, Zhang P, Zhang BX, et al. (2011) HMGB1 cytoplasmic translocation in patients with acute liver failure. BMC Gastroenterol 11: 21.

70. Cheng BQ, Jia CQ, Liu CT, Lu XF, Zhong N, et al. (2008) Serum high mobility group box chromosomal protein 1 is associated with clinicopathologic features in patients with hepatocellular carcinoma. Dig Liver Dis 40: 446–452.

71. Han F WT, Chen X (2014) Changes of high mobility group box 1 expression in hepatocellular carcinoma tissues. Journal of Medical Postgraduates 4.

72. Gou H SL, Han L (2013) Detection and clinical significance of high mobility group box protein 1 in liver cancer. Journal of Preventive Medicine 40.

73. Wang T HF, Liang J, Wang F, Chen G (2013) Increased HMGB1 expression in primary hepatic carcinoma and its mechanism Chinese Journal of Laboratory Diagnosis 17: 1783–1785.

74. Feng H (2011) The Expression and Clinical Significance of High Mobility Group Protein B 1 in Hepatocellular Carcinoma Chongqing Medical University Graduation Thesis: 11–17. Available: http://cdmd.cnki.com.cn/Article/CDMD-10631-1011173410.htm

Cys34-Cysteinylated Human Serum Albumin Is a Sensitive Plasma Marker in Oxidative Stress-Related Chronic Diseases

Kohei Nagumo[1], Motohiko Tanaka[2], Victor Tuan Giam Chuang[3], Hiroko Setoyama[2], Hiroshi Watanabe[1,4], Naoyuki Yamada[5], Kazuyuki Kubota[5], Motoko Tanaka[6], Kazutaka Matsushita[6], Akira Yoshida[7], Hideaki Jinnouchi[7], Makoto Anraku[8], Daisuke Kadowaki[1,4], Yu Ishima[1,4], Yutaka Sasaki[2], Masaki Otagiri[8,9], Toru Maruyama[1,4]*

1 Department of Biopharmaceutics, Graduate School of Pharmaceutical Sciences, Kumamoto University, Chuo-ku, Kumamoto, Japan, **2** Department of Gastroenterology and Hepatology, Graduate School of Medical Sciences, Kumamoto University, Chuo-ku, Kumamoto, Japan, **3** School of Pharmacy, Curtin Health Innovation Research Institute, Faculty of Health Sciences, Curtin University, Perth, Western Australia, Australia, **4** Center for Clinical Pharmaceutical Science, Kumamoto University, Chuo-ku, Kumamoto, Japan, **5** Institute of Innovation, Ajinomoto Co., Inc., Kawasaki-ku, Kawasaki, Japan, **6** Department of Nephrology, Akebono Clinic, Minami-Ku, Kumamoto, Japan, **7** Jinnouchi Clinic, Diabetes Care Center, Chuo-ku, Kumamoto, Japan, **8** Faculty of Pharmaceutical Sciences, Sojo University, Nishi-ku, Kumamoto, Japan, **9** DDS Research Institute, Sojo University, Nishi-ku, Kumamoto, Japan

Abstract

The degree of oxidized cysteine (Cys) 34 in human serum albumin (HSA), as determined by high performance liquid chromatography (HPLC), is correlated with oxidative stress related pathological conditions. In order to further characterize the oxidation of Cys34-HSA at the molecular level and to develop a suitable analytical method for a rapid and sensitive clinical laboratory analysis, the use of electrospray ionization time-of-flight mass spectrometer (ESI-TOFMS) was evaluated. A marked increase in the cysteinylation of Cys34 occurs in chronic liver and kidney diseases and diabetes mellitus. A significant positive correlation was observed between the Cys-Cys34-HSA fraction of plasma samples obtained from 229 patients, as determined by ESI-TOFMS, and the degree of oxidized Cys34-HSA determined by HPLC. The Cys-Cys34-HSA fraction was significantly increased with the progression of liver cirrhosis, and was reduced by branched chain amino acids (BCAA) treatment. The changes in the Cys-Cys34-HSA fraction were significantly correlated with the alternations of the plasma levels of advanced oxidized protein products, an oxidative stress marker for proteins. The binding ability of endogenous substances (bilirubin and tryptophan) and drugs (warfarin and diazepam) to HSA purified from chronic liver disease patients were significantly suppressed but significantly improved by BCAA supplementation. Interestingly, the changes in this physiological function of HSA in chronic liver disease were correlated with the Cys-Cys34-HSA fraction. In conclusion, ESI-TOFMS is a suitable high throughput method for the rapid and sensitive quantification of Cys-Cys34-HSA in a large number of samples for evaluating oxidative stress related chronic disease progression or in response to a treatment.

Editor: Rizwan H. Khan, Aligarh Muslim University, India

Funding: The authors have no support or funding to report.

Competing Interests: The authors have declared that no competing interests exist.

* E-mail: tomaru@gpo.kumamoto-u.ac.jp

Introduction

Post-translationally modified proteins can be used as biomarkers for the diagnosis of diseases or for the assessment of treatment responses. A prime example of this is the quantification of glycated hemoglobin and glycoalbumin for the diagnosis and treatment of diabetes mellitus [1,2]. Recent studies have demonstrated an association between oxidative stress and the development of chronic diseases. There is growing interest in developing diagnostic tools to monitor the extent of oxidative damage in tissues or organs, and the use of novel anti-oxidants for the treatment or prevention of such oxidative stress-related diseases [3–5]. However, at present, a rapid and sensitive clinical laboratory testing method for the rapid assessment of oxidative stress in humans is lacking.

Era's group and our laboratory have both developed a high performance liquid chromatography (HPLC) method to monitor the redox status of cysteine (Cys) 34 in human serum albumin (HSA) (Figure 1) [6,7]. Since the redox status of thiol (SH) groups sensitively reflects the oxidation-reduction status of its surrounding environment, this HPLC analytical method has been shown to be useful for assessing the level of oxidative stress in diseased states and for evaluating the anti-oxidative activity of a therapeutic agent [8–11].

Previous studies of Cys34 have shown that Cys34 can be modified by treatment with cysteine, glutathione, homocysteine or drugs that contain a SH group. Cys34 can also be oxidized to a sulfonic acid and a sulfinic acid, but information on the degree of each modified form of Cys34 under diseased conditions is not available [12–16]. Unfortunately, the HPLC analytical method

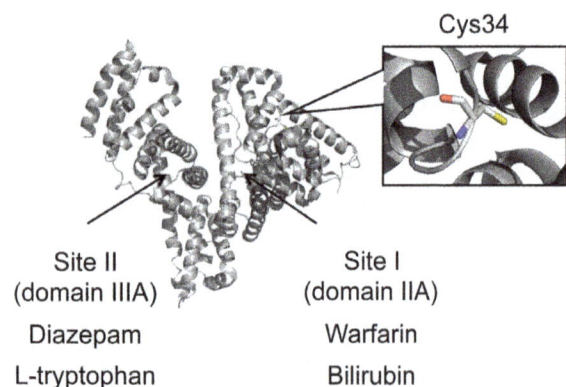

Figure 1. The structure of HSA. Superposition of the Cys34 and the location of two major ligand binding sites, Site I and II are shown.

does not provide any molecular structural information regarding the oxidized form of Cys34. Therefore, we attempted to establish an analytical method that allows the quantitative and qualitative evaluation of the redox state of Cys34 with a high degree of sensitivity using electrospray ionization time-of-flight mass spectrometer (ESI-TOFMS) to analyze HSA that is cysteinylated at Cys34 (Cys-Cys34-HSA) in vitro using plasma samples obtained from healthy subjects [17,18]. Moreover, recent analyses using ESI-TOFMS indicate that a significant amount of Cys-Cys34-HSA is present in the amniotic fluid of patients with gestational diabetes mellitus and in the plasma of dialysis patients [19,20]. If Cys-Cys34-HSA accounts for the majority of the oxidized forms of Cys34, the fraction of Cys-Cys34-HSA, as estimated by ESI-TOFMS should correspond to the degree of oxidized Cys34-HSA determined by HPLC reported in previous studies, and this may permit the fraction of Cys-Cys34-HSA to be used as a novel marker for oxidative stress in the blood circulation.

Nevertheless, correlations between the fraction of Cys-Cys34-HSA determined by ESI-TOFMS and the degree of oxidized Cys34-HSA determined by HPLC have not been reported. Furthermore, the impact of the cysteinylation of Cys34 on HSA functions in a diseased state, and the progression of the disease or response to treatment remain unknown.

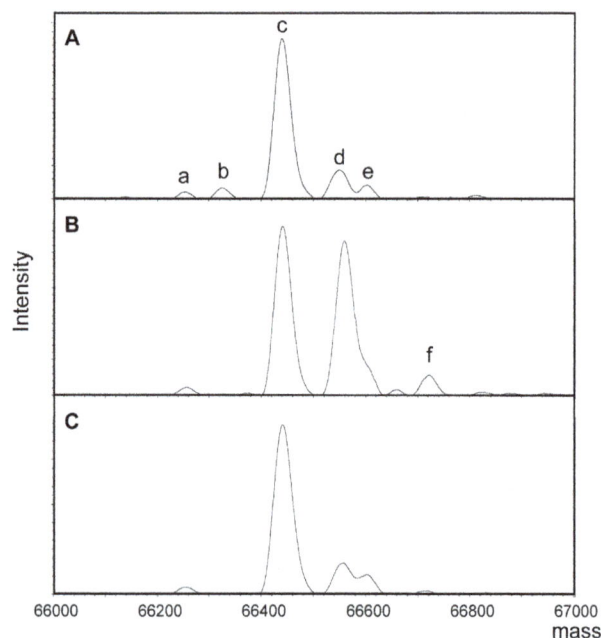

Figure 2. Deconvoluted ESI-TOFMS spectra of HSA. (A) Spectrum of HSA from healthy subject. (B) Spectrum of HSA from patient with chronic liver disease. (C) Spectrum of HSA from the same patient that (B) after DTT treatment. The peaks correspond to the following: (a) Asp-Ala truncation from N-terminal of HSA, (b) Leu truncation from C-terminal of HSA, (c) reduced HSA, (d) Cys-Cys34-HSA, (e) glycated HSA and (f) glycated Cys-Cys34-HSA.

Materials and Methods

Chemicals

Blue Sepharose 6 Fast Flow was from GE Healthcare (Tokyo, Japan). Potassium warfarin (Eisai Co., Tokyo, Japan), L-tryptophan (Wako Pure Chemical Industries, Ltd., Osaka, Japan) and diazepam (Nippon Roche K.K., Tokyo, Japan) were obtained. All other chemicals were of the highest grade commercially available, and all solutions were prepared using deionized and distilled water.

Table 1. General characteristics of the study participants.

	Healthy Subjects	Patients		
		Chronic Liver Disease	Chronic Kidney Disease (HD)	Diabetes Mellitus
Category	N = 9	N = 139	N = 38	N = 52
Gender (M/F)	6/3	60/79	20/18	21/31
Age (years)	61.4±4.4	57.4±15.0	58.6±16.1	59.0±16.1
Albumin (g/dl)	N/A	3.3±0.5	N/A	N/A
Bilirubin (mg/dL)	N/A	1.5±1.3	N/A	N/A
BUN (mg/dL)	N/A	N/A	63.6±11.8	N/A
SCr (mg/dL)	N/A	N/A	11.2±1.9	N/A
HbA1c (%)	N/A	N/A	N/A	7.9±1.6

Mean ± SD value are shown. BUN; blood urea nitrogen, SCr; serum creatinine, HD; hemodialysis.

Ethics statement

The study was approved by the institutional review board of Kumamoto University, and each of the institutional review boards of the hospitals where samples were collected ("Ethics Committee of the Hospital Akebono Clinic, "Ethics Committee of the Hospital Jinnouchi Clinic"). All samples were obtained with written informed consent reviewed by the ethical board of the corresponding hospital.

Clinical study of the correlation of Cys-Cys34-HSA and oxidized Cys34-HSA

9 mL blood samples were collected from individual study subjects and the samples were subjected to only one freeze thaw cycle, based on our previous work [18]. The collected blood was immediately diluted with 0.5 M sodium citrate buffer (pH 4.3) to stabilize for reduced albumin. Each plasma fraction was separated by centrifugation (4°C for 15 min, 2000 g). After collection, plasma samples were stored at −80°C until batch analysis.

Chronic liver disease. 139 patients with liver cirrhosis who had been admitted to the Kumamoto University Medical School Hospital of Japan, between March 2011 and May 2013 were enrolled in this study. The stratified Child-Pugh class was used to estimate the severity of liver disease The liver cirrhosis patients were divided into 3 groups according to their Child-Pugh classification: Child-Pugh grade A (n = 79; 68.20 ± 12.88 yrs), Child-Pugh grade B (n = 44; 62.71 ± 11.93 yrs), and Child-Pugh grade C (n = 16; 54.73 ± 7.27 yrs) (Table 1).

Chronic kidney disease. 38 patients with chronic renal failure who had been admitted to the Department of Nephrology of the Akebono Clinic of Japan, between March 2011 and May 2012 were enrolled in this study (58.55 ± 16.06 yrs). End-stage renal failure in hemodialysis (HD) patients were caused by glomerulonephritis (n = 8), nephrosclerosis (n = 5) or diabetic nephropathy (n = 14) (Table 1). At the time of their enrollment, all of the HD patients were receiving regular bicarbonate HD

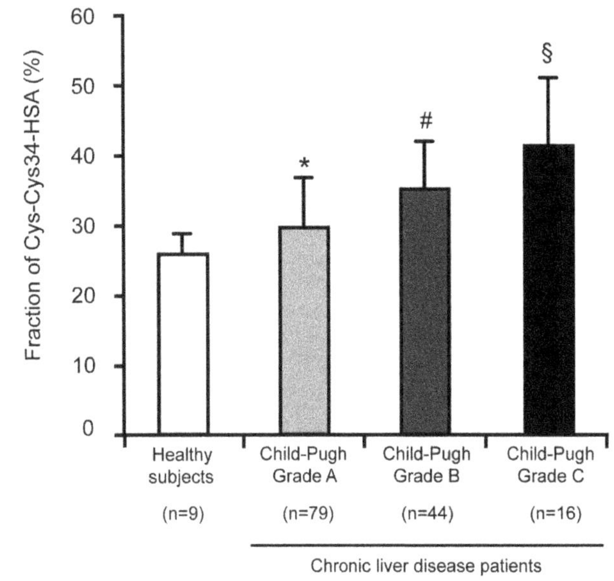

Figure 4. Effect of disease progression on the Cys-Cys34-HSA fraction in chronic liver disease patients. The Cys-Cys34-HSA fraction was measured by ESI-TOFMS. Values are expressed as mean ± SD (n = 9–79). *P<0.05 as compared with healthy subjects, #P<0.05 as compared with Child-Pugh Grade A, and §P<0.05 as compared with Child-Pugh Grade B.

therapy (4 to 5 hours per session, 3 times per week) using high-flux polysulfone hollow-fiber dialyzers.

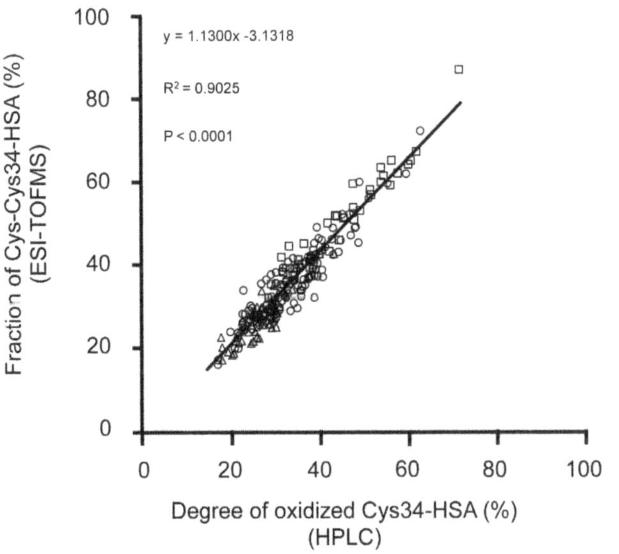

Diabetes mellitus. 52 patients with type 2 diabetes who had been admitted to the Jinnouchi Clinic, Diabetes Care Center of Japan, between March 2011 and May 2013 were enrolled in this study (58.98 ± 16.06 yrs) (Table 1). Eligible patients were 21–86 years old, HbA1C>7% and suffering from type 2 diabetes for at least 1 year but no longer than 5 years.

Effect of branched-chain amino acid (BCAA) treatment on Cys-Cys34-HSA in chronic liver disease patients. 60 patients with liver cirrhosis who had been admitted to the Kumamoto University Hospital of Japan, between March 2011 and May 2012 were enrolled in this study. The study population used for assessing the effect of BCAA treatment status is a sub-set of the patient population used for chronic liver diseases. These patients were given oral BCAA granules containing 952 mg of L-isoleucine, 1904 mg of L-leucine and 1144 mg of L-valine (LIVACT® Granules, AJINOMOTO PHARMACEUTICALS CO., LTD., Tokyo, Japan) at 4.15 g/sachet three times a day after meals. Plasma sample were collected at before, 3 and 5 months after treatment. The average albumin concentrations at before, 3 and 5 months after BCAA treatment were 2.85 ± 0.48 g/dl, 3.21 ± 0.43 g/dl and 3.36 ± 0.40 g/dl respectively. Plasma samples from age and sex-matched nine healthy subjects as controls were obtained from Kumamoto University Hospital (Table 1).

Determination of the degree of oxidized Cys34-HSA by HPLC

The SH redox status of HSA was determined with the HPLC system reported previously [8]. Briefly, 5 μL of aliquots of plasma were analyzed using a Shodex Asahipak ES-502N 7C column (Showa Denko, Tokyo, Japan). From the HPLC profile, the content of the oxidized form (HNA) and the un-oxidized form (HMA) of HSA was estimated as the area of each fraction divided

Figure 3. Relationship between the Cys-Cys34-HSA fraction (ESI-TOFMS) and the degree of oxidized Cys34-HSA (HPLC). The measured samples were 229 patients with chronic disease (including 139 patients with liver disease (circle), 38 patients with kidney disease (square) and 52 patients with diabetes mellitus (triangle)) (R^2 = 0.9025, P<0.001).

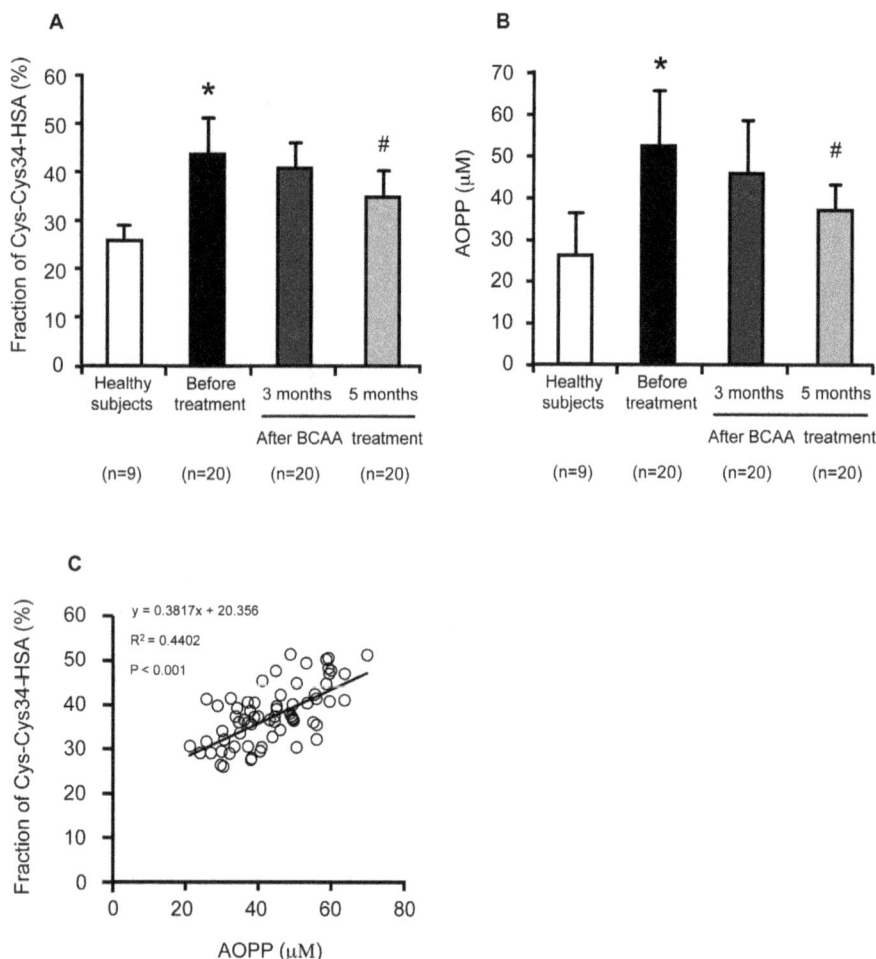

Figure 5. Change in the Cys-Cys34-HSA fraction and oxidative stress marker, AOPP, by BCAA treatment. (A) Change in the Cys-Cys34-HSA fraction. The Cys-Cys34-HSA fraction was measured by ESI-TOFMS. (B) Change in plasma AOPP level. (C) Correlation between the Cys-Cys34-HSA fraction and plasma AOPP level in chronic liver disease (n = 69). Values are expressed as mean ± SD (n = 20). *P<0.01 as compared with healthy subjects, #P<0.05 as compared with before treatment.

by the total area of the plasma HSA peak. Using the levels of HNA and HMA, the degree of oxidized Cys34-HSA, (HNA/(HNA + HMA)) ×100, which is considered to be a reliable marker for the extent of systematic oxidative damage in uremic patients was estimated [10,21].

Solid phase extraction and ESI-TOFMS measurement of plasma samples

5 μL of plasma was added to 495 μL of 50 mM sodium phosphate buffer (pH 6.0). A solid phase extraction (SPE) column (Bond Elute-C18 EWP 200 mg/3cc, Varian, Inc., CA) was initialized with 10/90 water/acetonitrile containing 0.1% formic acid, then equilibration was performed with water (1 mL). The above-mentioned diluted plasma sample was applied to the equilibrated SPE column. The column was washed with 10% acetonitrile (2 mL) containing 0.1% formic acid, and albumin was eluted with 90% acetonitrile containing 0.1% formic acid.

2 μL of eluent was flow injected into the ESI-TOFMS (microTOF®; Bruker Daltonics Inc. USA) at a flow rate of 15 μL/min with 10/90 water/acetonitrile containing 0.1% formic acid using the auto sampler of Ultimate 3000 (Dionex, Idstein, Germany).

The data were acquired by the MicroTOF® software (Bruker-Daltonics) and processed for Maxent deconvolution using DataAnalysis® software (Bruker-Daltonics). The deconvolution mass range was set to be from 66000 to 68000 Da. And the mass peak of HSA and its modified molecules such as Cys-Cys34-HSA or glycated HSA, was automatically assigned and converted to an output text file using script with a resolving power of 10000 m/dm and absolute intensity threshold of 1000. The fraction of Cys-Cys34-HSA (%) was calculated by (Cys-Cys34-HSA/(Cys-Cys34-HSA + reduced HSA)) ×100.

Purification of HSA from the plasma of chronic liver disease patients

HSA was purified from plasma samples using a previously reported method [21]. Briefly, HSA samples were isolated by Blue Sepharose 6 Fast Flow column (GE HealthcareTokyo, Japan). The samples were then dialyzed against deionized water for 48 h at 4°C, followed by lyophilization. The purity of the HSA samples was at least 95%, as evidenced by sodium dodecyl sulfate polyacrylamide gel electrophoresis (SDS-PAGE) and native-PAGE, respectively [21].

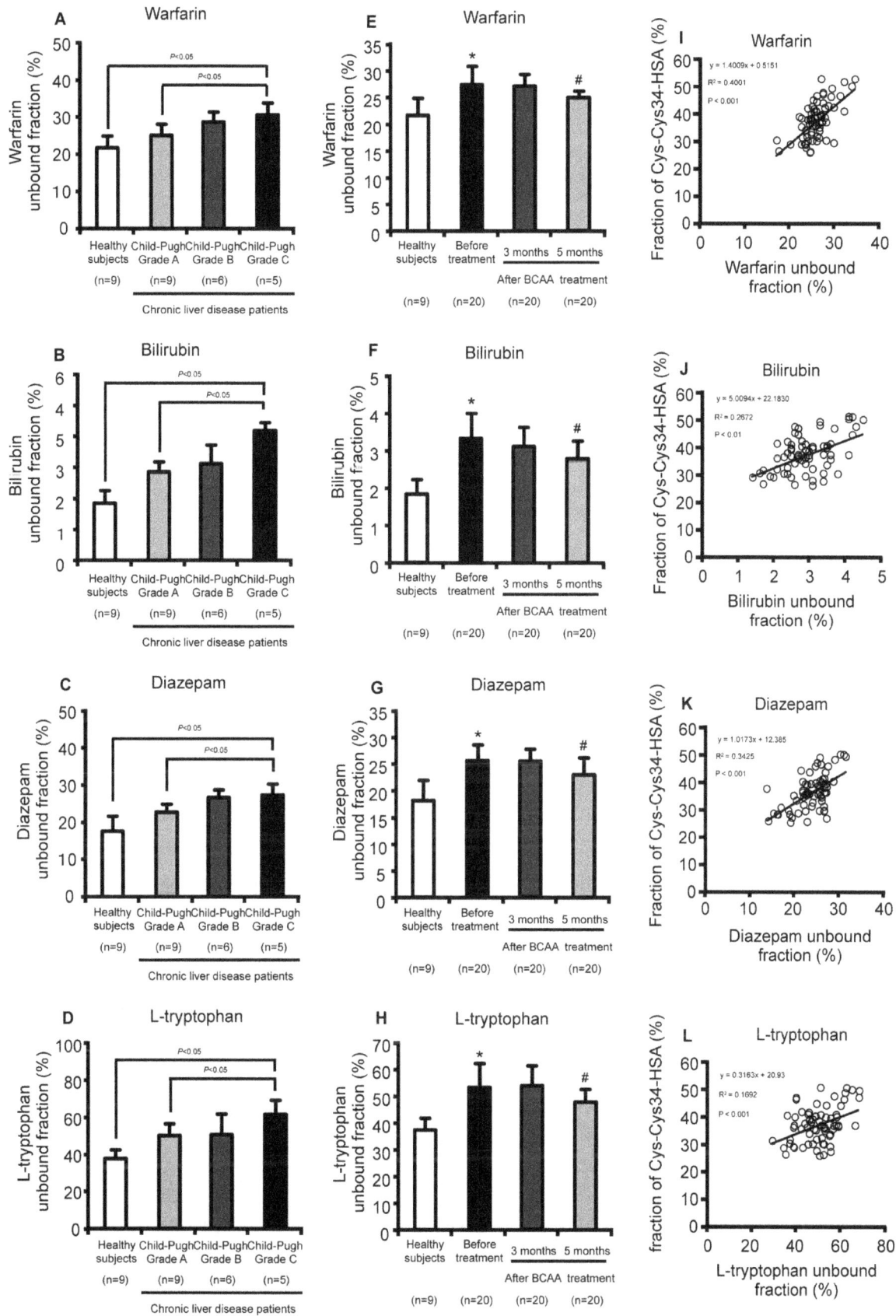

Figure 6. Relationship between the Cys-Cys34-HSA fraction and the ligand unbound fraction in chronic liver disease patients. Effect of disease progression on the unbound fraction Is of warfarin (A), bilirubin (B), diazepam (C) and L-tryptophan (D) to purified HSA. Effect of BCAA treatment on the unbound fraction of warfarin (E), bilirubin (F), diazepam (G) and L-tryptophan (H) to purified HSA. Correlation between the Cys-

Cys34-HSA fraction and the unbound fraction of warfarin (I), bilirubin (J), diazepam (K) and L-tryptophan (L) to purified HSA in chronic liver disease. Values are expressed as mean ± SD. *P<0.01 as compared with healthy subjects, #P<0.05 as compared with before treatment.

Determination of the unbound fraction of L-tryptophan, warfarin or diazepam to purified HSA

The binding of L-tryptophan, warfarin or diazepam (12.5 μM) to HSA (25 μM) purified from the plasma of chronic liver disease patients and healthy subjects in 67 mM sodium phosphate buffer (pH 7.4) was examined by ultrafiltration at 37°C. The ultrafiltration was carried out using a YM-30 ultrafiltration device (Amicon/ Millipore Inc., Bedford, MA, USA). HSA and the ligands were dissolved in 67 mM sodium phosphate buffer (pH 7.4). Samples of 250 μL were centrifuged at 10,000 g at 37°C for 3 min. Free (unbound) ligand concentrations in the filtrates were quantified by HPLC [22–24].

Determination of the unbound fraction of bilirubin to purified HSA

The unbound bilirubin concentrations were determined using a modified horseradish peroxidase (HRP) assay [25]. 15 μM bilirubin was added to 30 μL HSA purified from the plasma of chronic liver disease patients and healthy subjects dissolved in 67 mM phosphate buffer (pH 7.4). 200 μL aliquots of the bilirubin/HSA complexes were placed in a 96 well-plate and the samples allowed to equilibrate for 20 min at 37°C. 10 μL of freshly diluted 1.75 mM hydrogen peroxide was then added to each well, followed by incubation for 3 min. The reaction was initiated by adding 10 μL of 1 ng/mL HRP. The rate of oxidative destruction of the unbound bilirubin was monitored by the reduction in the absorbance of the mixture at 450 nm for 10 min. The concentrations of unbound bilirubin were determined by extrapolating the rate of oxidation of bilirubin to a standard curve prepared by plotting the oxidation rate versus the concentration of bilirubin. It was assumed that only the unbound bilirubin was available as a substrate for HRP so that there was a linear relationship between the rate of destruction of bilirubin and the concentration of the unbound species.

Determination of advanced oxidation protein products

Advanced oxidation protein products (AOPP) levels were determined spectrophotometrically by measuring the absorbance of the samples at 340 nm and expressed as chloramine-T equivalents after five-fold dilution of 200 μL of plasma with 20 mmol/L of pH 7.4 phosphate-buffered saline (PBS) and the subsequent addition of 80 μL of acetic acid, and reading against a blank PBS solution [26].

Statistical analysis

All data were expressed as the mean ± SD. Differences between groups were examined for statistical significance using the Wilcoxon signed-rank test with Bonferroni correction, and the magnitude of each correlation were evaluated using Spearman rank-correlation coefficient. A P-value <0.05 denoted the presence of a statistically significant difference. The StatView 5.0 software was used for data analysis.

Results

Detection of Cys-Cys34-HSA in patients with chronic liver disease by ESI-TOFMS

Two major peaks, corresponding to Cys-Cys34-HSA and reduced Cys34-HSA, so-called HMA, were identified when plasma samples obtained from healthy subjects were analyzed by ESI-TOFMS (Figure 2A). We previously evaluated the reproducibility of the redox state of Cys34 measurement in human plasma. As a result, Cys-Cys34-HSA had high reproducibility values with a CV% of below 0.5% (intra-day, n = 4) and 1.55% (inter-day, n = 4) [18]. In agreement with previous findings, an increased Cys-Cys34-HSA peak accompanied by a decreased HMA peak was observed in patients with diabetes mellitus or chronic renal failure (data not shown) [19,27]. Similar changes in the HSA mass spectra (MS) profile were also found for patients with chronic liver disease (Figure 2B). The HSA MS profile of chronic liver disease after dithiothreitol (DTT) treatment (Figure 2C) was similar to that for HSA profiles of healthy subjects (Figure 2A), indicating that the DTT treatment resulted in a reversal of the peaks for Cys-Cys34-HSA and HMA. These results confirm that the oxidative modification of Cys34 that occur in chronic liver disease patients are largely a reversible reaction, and that the most common oxidized form of Cys34 is cysteinylation.

Correlation between Cys-Cys34-HSA and oxidized Cys34-HSA

The degree of oxidized Cys34-HSA and the Cys-Cys34-HSA fraction of plasma samples obtained from 229 patients with chronic disease (including 139 patients with liver disease, 38 patients with kidney disease and 52 patients with diabetes mellitus) was determined by HPLC and ESI-TOFMS respectively and the correlation between these two parameters was examined. As shown in Figure 3, a significant correlation was observed between the fraction of Cys-Cys34-HSA and the degree of oxidized Cys34-HSA. A significant correlation was also observed for each of the disease groups such as chronic liver disease, chronic kidney disease and diabetes mellitus (data not shown).

Effect of disease severity or BCAA treatment on the Cys-Cys34-HSA fraction in patients with chronic liver disease

The relationship between the Cys-Cys34-HSA fraction and Child-Pugh classification in patients with chronic liver disease was examined. As shown in Figure 4, an increase in the severity of the disease was associated with an increase in the fraction of Cys-Cys34-HSA, suggesting an association between the progression of chronic liver disease and oxidative stress.

The effect of BCAA treatment on the Cys-Cys34-HSA fraction in patients with chronic liver disease was examined. As shown in Figure 5A, the Cys-Cys34-HSA fraction was decreased as the result of the BCAA treatment, with a significant improvement compared to the pre-treatment level observed 5 months after the treatment. Figure 5B shows the effect of BCAA treatment on plasma AOPP levels, a marker of oxidative stress for proteins in patients with chronic liver disease. The plasma AOPP levels were also decreased as the result of the BCAA treatment at 5 months after the treatment (Figure 5B). The Cys-Cys34-HSA fraction was significantly correlated with plasma AOPP levels (Figure 5C), further supporting the conclusion that the Cys-Cys34-HSA fraction is, in fact, an appropriate marker for oxidative stress in the general circulation.

Effect of the cysteinylation of Cys34 on ligand binding ability of HSA purified from the plasma of chronic liver disease patients

HSA has two major ligand bindings sites, so-called Site I and Site II where localized in subdomain IIA and IIIA on HSA, respectively (Figure 1). To investigate the effect of cysteinylation on ligand binding property, binding experiments by ultrafiltration technique were carried out using endogenous and exogenous substances. Bilirubin and L-tryptophan, which preferentially bind to Site I and Site II, respectively, were selected as models for endogenous ligands related to liver disease. On the other hand, warfarin and diazepam, representative drugs that bind to Site I and Site II respectively, were used as exogenous ligands.

As reported previously, the HSA purified from the patients showed an increased unbound fraction for all four ligands compared to HSA purified from healthy subjects. As shown in Figure 6A–D, the increases in the unbound fraction of all of the four ligands were associated with the progression of liver disease. In contrast, as shown in Figure 6E–H, the decreases in the unbound fraction of all of the four ligands observed in patients with chronic liver disease were significantly improved by the BCAA treatment. Interestingly, a moderate correlation was observed for the unbound fraction of warfarin and diazepam and a causal relationship was shown in the case of the unbound fraction of bilirubin and L-tryptophan with the Cys-Cys34-HSA fraction (Figure 6I–L), suggesting that, the cysteinylation of Cys34 affected the microenvironment of the ligand binding sites.

Discussion

Oxidative stress may cause the reversible and/or irreversible modification of sensitive proteins [17,21,28,29]. Since the redox status of a free thiol group in proteins can be a very important indicator of oxidative stress, determining the redox status of Cys34 in HSA may allow the degree of organ damage by oxidative stress and the development of new anti oxidative therapeutic approaches. The utility of monitoring the redox status of Cys34 in HSA as a marker for oxidative stress in the circulation was demonstrated in a previous study by determining the degree of oxidized Cys34-HSA by HPLC [30].

However, in order to be able to examine alterations in the function of albumin by conventional procedures, the protein must be purified from at least several mL of plasma which may not be feasible in routine laboratory tests. Therefore, an analytical method that requires only a small amount of plasma under a clinical setting for the rapid measurement of the marker would be desirable. Compared to HPLC, ESI-TOFMS is a high throughput method that can be used to analyze large numbers of samples rapidly and sensitively, and thus may be suitable for use in clinical laboratory testing. Furthermore, the ESI-TOFMS method offers an additional advantage of having the capability of characterizing the different forms of Cys34 oxidized forms of Cys34 that are produced by oxidation by a variety of endogenous substances.

Using ESI-TOFMS, the present study provides evidence that the most common oxidized form is cysteinylated Cys34 (Figure 2B). As shown in Figure 3, a significant positive correlation with a slope of nearly 1 was observed between the degree of oxidized Cys34-HSA estimated by HPLC and the fraction of Cys-Cys34-HSA determined by ESI-TOFMS. These results suggest that the fraction of Cys-Cys34-HSA is a more sensitive marker for oxidative stress in plasma, than the degree of oxidized Cys34-HSA determined by HPLC. The present study is the first to show a marked oxidation, predominantly cysteinylation, of Cys34 in oxidative stress-related diseases such as chronic liver and kidney

diseases and diabetes mellitus. The present study also found that the Cys-Cys34-HSA fraction increased in proportion to the Child-Pugh classification of cirrhotic patients. This is in agreement with the findings that oxidative stress plays an important role in the progression of chronic liver disease.

Recent studies have shown that the functional loss of HSA due to post-translational modification could influence homeostasis, which may contribute to the progression of chronic disease. Jalan et al. proposed that the loss of ligand binding capacity of albumin may be associated with an increased mortality of patients with decompensated cirrhosis [31]. Very recently, Oettl et al. reported that, in advanced liver disease, oxidative damage impairs the binding properties of HSA [32]. This reduced binding capacity of HSA is mainly related to impaired liver function. The decreased binding of toxic endogenous compounds to HSA may result in increased tissue distribution of these toxins, possibly enhancing the risk of tissue damage related to complications. In this study, a decreased binding affinity of bilirubin and tryptophan that might be related to liver disease was observed with increasing severity of liver disease. The present findings can be extrapolated to predict the binding of bile acids, another endogenous substance associated with disease progression, in chronic liver disease because bile acids bind Site I or Site II [33].

Interestingly, the changes in ligand binding were correlated with the alterations in the Cys-Cys34-HSA fraction. It is possible that the cysteinylation of Cys34 caused the changes in the microenvironment of the ligand binding sites, especially Site II, which could result in decreased ligand binding. On the other hand, the cysteinylation of Cys34 may further induce oxidative modifications to other amino acid residues that play an important role in ligand binding [17,21]. Our previous in vitro examination showed that the cysteinylation of Cys34 could induce structural changes in the regions surrounding ligand binding sites [17]. Meanwhile, an increased cysteinylation of Cys34 was found to be accompanied by an increase in the carbonyl content of HSA [9], suggesting that other residues in addition to Cys34, especially arginine, lysine, histidine, tyrosine and tryptophan that significantly contribute to ligand binding to Site I and Site II are oxidized. In fact, we previously demonstrated that oxidative stress modified residues Lys195, Lys190, Arg218, Trp211 and Arg222 that are involved in the ligand binding to Site I, and Arg410 and Tyr411 residues, which play a crucial role in the binding of ligands to Site II [12]. Thus, both direct and indirect mechanisms appear to be responsible for the impaired ligand bindings accompanied with cysteinylation of Cys34.

BCAA treatment improves hypoalbuminemia in chronic liver disease patients by increasing the biosynthesis of HSA [34]. Recent studies have revealed that this effect is mediated by the activation of the mTOR pathway [35,36]. The findings of this study indicate that the fraction of Cys-Cys34-HSA was significantly improved by BCAA treatment, most likely due to the increased biosynthesis of HMA. In addition to this indirect mechanism, recent studies have also demonstrated that BCAA per se has antioxidant activity [37]. It is thus possible that a reduction of oxidative stress caused by BCAA treatment led to a corresponding reduction in the cysteinylation of Cys34. On the other hand, the decreased binding affinity to bilirubin and tryptophan was recovered by a BCAA treatment, which is likely to be the result of an increased concentration of reduced Cys34 resulting from increased biosynthesis. Since the loss of ligand binding properties of HSA against these endogenous substances might contribute to an acceleration or inhibition of disease progression, the correlation between the Cys-Cys34-HSA fraction and the fraction of ligand binding to HSA suggests that the Cys-Cys34-HSA fraction might also serve as a marker for estimating changes in the physiological functions of albumin.

Recent studies revealed that albumin is an antioxidant in plasma and plays an important role in the homeostasis of the intravascular environment. Terawaki et al. reported that a low concentration of albumin with reduced Cys34 is associated with an increased incidence of severe cardiovascular disorders in dialysis patients due to a decreased antioxidative capacity [38]. This is because antioxidants are not as abundant in the plasma as they are in the cell, and albumin, which is abundant in plasma, serves as a dominant antioxidant in plasma. This is supported by the fact that about 80% of the total SH groups, a powerful ROS scavenger, present in plasma originate from Cys34 [15]. In a previous study, we reported that Cys34 accounted for approximately 40% of the total radical scavenging activity of HSA [39,40]. Thus, the observed changes in the Cys-Cys34-HSA fraction with increasing severity of liver disease or BCAA treatment are likely to reflect an alternation in available SH groups resulting from the cyteinylation or de-cysteinylation of Cys34. Such changes in the cysteinylation

of Cys34 could influence to the antioxidative capacity in general circulation, which may contribute to the progression of chronic disease.

Conclusion

Cys-Cys34-HSA is a useful marker for estimating binding properties of HSA and monitoring oxidative stress in the plasma of chronic oxidative stress-related disease patients and ESI-TOFMS can be used in clinical laboratory testing.

Author Contributions

Conceived and designed the experiments: KN HW TM. Performed the experiments: KN HW TM. Analyzed the data: KN HW NY TM. Contributed reagents/materials/analysis tools: KN Motohiko Tanaka HS HW NY KK Motoko Tanaka KM AY HJ MA DK YI YS MO TM. Wrote the paper: KN Motohiko Tanaka VT GC HS HW NY MA YI YS MO TM.

References

1. Association AD (2013) Diagnosis and classification of diabetes mellitus. Diabetes Care 36 Suppl 1: S67–74.
2. Furusyo N, Hayashi J (2013) Glycated albumin and diabetes mellitus. Biochim Biophys Acta.
3. Poli G (2000) Pathogenesis of liver fibrosis: role of oxidative stress. Mol Aspects Med 21: 49–98.
4. Descamps-Latscha B, Witko-Sarsat V (2001) Importance of oxidatively modified proteins in chronic renal failure. Kidney Int Suppl 78: S108–113.
5. Pergola PE, Raskin P, Toto RD, Meyer CJ, Huff JW, et al. (2011) Bardoxolone methyl and kidney function in CKD with type 2 diabetes. N Engl J Med 365: 327–336.
6. Sogami M, Era S, Nagaoka S, Kuwata K, Kida K, et al. (1985) High-performance liquid chromatographic studies on non-mercapt in equilibrium with mercapt conversion of human serum albumin. II. J Chromatogr 332: 19–27.
7. Terawaki H, Yoshimura K, Hasegawa T, Matsuyama Y, Negawa T, et al. (2004) Oxidative stress is enhanced in correlation with renal dysfunction: examination in the redox state of albumin. Kidney Int 66: 1988–1993.
8. Anraku M, Kitamura K, Shinohara A, Adachi M, Suenga A, et al. (2004) Intravenous iron administration induces oxidation of serum albumin in hemodialysis patients. Kidney Int 66: 841–848.
9. Anraku M, Kitamura K, Shintomo R, Takeuchi K, Ikeda H, et al. (2008) Effect of intravenous iron administration frequency on AOPP and inflammatory biomarkers in chronic hemodialysis patients: a pilot study. Clin Biochem 41: 1168–1174.
10. Shimoishi K, Anraku M, Kitamura K, Tasaki Y, Taguchi K, et al. (2007) An oral adsorbent, AST-120 protects against the progression of oxidative stress by reducing the accumulation of indoxyl sulfate in the systemic circulation in renal failure. Pharm Res 24: 1283–1289.
11. Kadowaki D, Anraku M, Tasaki Y, Kitamura K, Wakamatsu S, et al. (2007) Effect of olmesartan on oxidative stress in hemodialysis patients. Hypertens Res 30: 395–402.
12. Yamasaki K, Chuang VT, Maruyama T, Otagiri M (2013) Albumin-drug interaction and its clinical implication. Biochim Biophys Acta.
13. Sengupta S, Chen H, Togawa T, DiBello PM, Majors AK, et al. (2001) Albumin thiolate anion is an intermediate in the formation of albumin-S-S-homocysteine. J Biol Chem 276: 30111–30117.
14. Alvarez B, Carballal S, Turell L, Radi R (2010) Formation and reactions of sulfenic acid in human serum albumin. Methods Enzymol 473: 117–136.
15. Oettl K, Stauber RE (2007) Physiological and pathological changes in the redox state of human serum albumin critically influence its binding properties. Br J Pharmacol 151: 580–590.
16. Narazaki R, Otagiri M (1997) Covalent binding of a bucillamine derivative with albumin in sera from healthy subjects and patients with various diseases. Pharm Res 14: 351–353.
17. Kawakami A, Kubota K, Yamada N, Tagami U, Takehana K, et al. (2006) Identification and characterization of oxidized human serum albumin. A slight structural change impairs its ligand-binding and antioxidant functions. FEBS J 273: 3346–3357.
18. Kubota K, Nakayama A, Takehana K, Kawakami A, Yamada N, et al. (2009) A simple stabilization method of reduced albumin in blood and plasma for the reduced/oxidized albumin ratio measurement. Int J Biomed Sci 5: 293–301.
19. Regazzoni L, Del Vecchio L, Altomare A, Yeum KJ, Cusi D, et al. (2013) Human serum albumin cysteinylation is increased in end stage renal disease patients and reduced by hemodialysis: mass spectrometry studies. Free Radic Res 47: 172–180.
20. Boisvert MR, Koski KG, Skinner CD (2010) Increased oxidative modifications of amniotic fluid albumin in pregnancies associated with gestational diabetes mellitus. Anal Chem 82: 1133–1137.
21. Mera K, Anraku M, Kitamura K, Nakajou K, Maruyama T, et al. (2005) The structure and function of oxidized albumin in hemodialysis patients: Its role in elevated oxidative stress via neutrophil burst. Biochem Biophys Res Commun 334: 1322–1328.
22. Jagannathan V, March C, Venitz J (1995) Determination of unbound L-tryptophan in human plasma using high-performance liquid chromatography with fluorescence detection. Biomed Chromatogr 9: 305–308.
23. Mera K, Takeo K, Izumi M, Maruyama T, Nagai R, et al. (2010) Effect of reactive-aldehydes on the modification and dysfunction of human serum albumin. J Pharm Sci 99: 1614–1625.
24. Watanabe H, Tanase S, Nakajou K, Maruyama T, Kragh-Hansen U, et al. (2000) Role of arg-410 and tyr-411 in human serum albumin for ligand binding and esterase-like activity. Biochem J 349 Pt 3: 813–819.
25. Minomo A, Ishima Y, Kragh-Hansen U, Chuang VT, Uchida M, et al. (2011) Biological characteristics of two lysines on human serum albumin in the high-affinity binding of 4Z,15Z-bilirubin-IXα revealed by phage display. FEBS J 278: 4100–4111.
26. Witko-Sarsat V, Friedlander M, Capeillère-Blandin C, Nguyen-Khoa T, Nguyen AT, et al. (1996) Advanced oxidation protein products as a novel marker of oxidative stress in uremia. Kidney Int 49: 1304–1313.
27. Borges CR, Oran PE, Buddi S, Jarvis JW, Schaab MR, et al. (2011) Building multidimensional biomarker views of type 2 diabetes on the basis of protein microheterogeneity. Clin Chem 57: 719–728.
28. Musante L, Candiano G, Petretto A, Bruschi M, Dimasi N, et al. (2007) Active focal segmental glomerulosclerosis is associated with massive oxidation of plasma albumin. J Am Soc Nephrol 18: 799–810.
29. Carballal S, Radi R, Kirk MC, Barnes S, Freeman BA, et al. (2003) Sulfenic acid formation in human serum albumin by hydrogen peroxide and peroxynitrite. Biochemistry 42: 9906–9914.
30. Anraku M, Chuang VT, Maruyama T, Otagiri M (2013) Redox properties of serum albumin. Biochim Biophys Acta.
31. Jalan R, Schnurr K, Mookerjee RP, Sen S, Cheshire L, et al. (2009) Alterations in the functional capacity of albumin in patients with decompensated cirrhosis is associated with increased mortality. Hepatology 50: 555–564.
32. Oettl K, Birner-Gruenberger R, Spindelboeck W, Stueger HP, Dorn L, et al. (2013) Oxidative Albumin Damage in Chronic Liver Failure: Relation to Albumin Binding Capacity, Liver Dysfunction and Survival. J Hepatol.
33. Takikawa H, Sugiyama Y, Hanano M, Kurita M, Yoshida H, et al. (1987) A novel binding site for bile acids on human serum albumin. Biochim Biophys Acta 926: 145–153.
34. Kawaguchi T, Izumi N, Charlton MR, Sata M (2011) Branched-chain amino acids as pharmacological nutrients in chronic liver disease. Hepatology 54: 1063–1070.
35. Nishitani S, Ijichi C, Takehana K, Fujitani S, Sonaka I (2004) Pharmacological activities of branched-chain amino acids: specificity of tissue and signal transduction. Biochem Biophys Res Commun 313: 387–389.
36. Kuwahata M, Yoshimura T, Sawai Y, Amano S, Tomoe Y, et al. (2008) Localization of polypyrimidine-tract-binding protein is involved in the regulation of albumin synthesis by branched-chain amino acids in HepG2 cells. J Nutr Biochem 19: 438–447.
37. Ichikawa K, Okabayashi T, Shima Y, Iiyama T, Takezaki Y, et al. (2012) Branched-chain amino acid-enriched nutrients stimulate antioxidant DNA

repair in a rat model of liver injury induced by carbon tetrachloride. Mol Biol Rep 39: 10803–10810.

38. Terawaki H, Matsuyama Y, Matsuo N, Ogura M, Mitome J, et al. (2012) A lower level of reduced albumin induces serious cardiovascular incidence among peritoneal dialysis patients. Clin Exp Nephrol 16: 629–635.

39. Iwao Y, Ishima Y, Yamada J, Noguchi T, Kragh-Hansen U, et al. (2012) Quantitative evaluation of the role of cysteine and methionine residues in the antioxidant activity of human serum albumin using recombinant mutants. IUBMB Life 64: 450–454.

40. Anraku M, Takeuchi K, Watanabe H, Kadowaki D, Kitamura K, et al. (2011) Quantitative analysis of cysteine-34 on the anitioxidative properties of human serum albumin in hemodialysis patients. J Pharm Sci 100: 3968–3976.

Histological Changes in Kidney and Liver of Rats Due to Gold (III) Compound [Au(en)Cl₂]Cl

Ayesha Ahmed[1]*, Dalal M. Al Tamimi[1], Anvarhusein A. Isab[2]*, Abdulaziz M. Mansour Alkhawajah[3], Mohamed A. Shawarby[1]

1 Department of Pathology, College of Medicine, University of Dammam & King Fahd Hospital of the University, Al-Khobar, Saudi Arabia, 2 Department of Chemistry, King Fahd University of Petroleum and Minerals, Dhahran, Saudi Arabia, 3 Department of Pharmacology, College of Medicine, University of Dammam, Dammam, Saudi Arabia

Abstract

Introduction: Development of novel metallodrugs with enhanced anti-proliferative potential and reduced toxicity has become the prime focus of the evolving medicinal chemistry. In this regards, gold (III) complexes with various ligands are being extensively investigated. In the current study renal and hepatic toxicity of a newly developed gold (III) compound [Au(en)Cl₂]Cl was assessed by histopathological evaluation of liver and kidney specimens of rats exposed to the compound.

Methods: Male rats (n = 42) weighing 200–250 gram were injected single, varying doses of gold (III) compound [(dichlorido(ethylenediamine)aurate((III)]chloride [Au(en)Cl₂]Cl in the acute toxicity component of the study. In the sub-acute toxicity part, a dose of 32.2 mg/kg (equivalent to 1/10 of LD50) was administered intraperitoneally for 14 consecutive days before sacrificing the animals. After autopsy, the renal and hepatic tissues were preserved in buffered formalin. Processing of the samples was followed by histopathological evaluation. The results were compared with the normal controls (n = 11).

Results: A dose of 32.2 mg/kg (1/10 of LD_{50}) revealed no renal tubular necrosis. The predominant histopathological finding was mild pyelitis, a prominence of eosinophils and mild congestion. The hepatic lesions comprised varying extents of ballooning degeneration with accompanying congestion and focal portal inflammation.

Conclusion: Gold (III) compound [Au(en)Cl₂]Cl causes minimal histological changes in kidney and liver of rats, reflecting its relative safety as compared to other clinically established antineoplastic drugs.

Editor: Dermot Cox, Royal College of Surgeons, Ireland

Funding: The funding agency is King Abdulaziz City for Science and Technology through the Science & Technology Unit at King Fahd University of Petroleum & Minerals through project No. 08-BIO94-4 as part of the National Science, Technology and Innovation Plan (Kingdom of Saudi Arabia). The funders had no role in study design, data collection and analysis, decision to publish, or preparation of the manuscript.

Competing Interests: The authors have declared that no competing interests exist.

* E-mail: ayesash@hotmail.com (AA); aisab@kfupm.edu.sa (AI)

Introduction

Gold is a noble metal and a commonly used material due to its oxidation resistance and unique electrical, magnetic, optical and physical characteristics. It exists in multiple oxidation states ranging from −1 to +5; the predominant form being Au (I) and Au (III) [1]. Metallic gold is known to be an inert and nontoxic metal. It is only the gold salts and radioisotopes that have pharmacological significance [1].

The use of gold compounds as medicinal agents is referred to as chrysotherapy [2]. Medical and therapeutic use of gold dates back to thousands of years [3]. In ancient cultures, around 2500 BC, gold was considered an integral component in the treatment of diseases such as measles, skin ulcers, and smallpox [4,5]. In the 16th century, gold was recommended for the treatment of epilepsy. Its rational medicinal use began in the early 1920's when it was introduced as a treatment of tuberculosis [6]. Gold as an anti rheumatic agent was first reported in 1929 [7]. Gold and gold compounds are now mostly used for the treatment of various diseases including psoriasis, palindromic rheumatism, juvenile arthritis and discoid lupus erythematosus [8,9]. However, following the body's extensive exposure to gold compounds, it can diffuse to various organs like liver, kidney and spleen. Skin irritation, mouth ulcers, nephrotoxicity, liver toxicity and blood disorders have been associated with prolonged exposure to gold compounds [10].

Currently gold complexes have gained considerable attention due to their strong antiproliferative[11–14] and antiangiogenic potential [10]. The spectrum of gold complexes with documented cell growth inhibiting properties include a large variety of different ligands attached to gold in the oxidation states +1 or +3, that is gold (I) and gold (III) compounds [15,16]. Gold (I) complexes proved to be unsuitable for clinical practice due to accompanying cardiotoxicity [17,18], while studies on gold (III) complexes are comparatively scarce [8]. Gold (III) bears homology to cisplatin as it is isoelectronic with platinum (II) and tetracoordinate gold (III) complexes have the same square-planar geometries as cisplatin [3]. Cisplatin [*cis*-diamminedichloroplatinum(II)] is one of the most widely employed drugs in cancer chemotherapy, discovered more

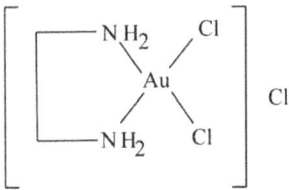

Figure 1. Dichlorido(ethylenediamine)-aurate(III) ion.

than 40 years ago [13], and it became the first FDA-approved platinum anticancer compound in 1978 [19]. Its effectiveness in solid tumoral lesions is markedly hampered by severe toxic side effects comprising predominantly nephrotoxicity [20,21], development of tumor resistance[22–25] and occurrence of secondary malignancies [3,12,14] that contributes a high treatment failure ratio in clinical management.

Current studies aim towards designing newer compounds showing enhanced anti-proliferative potential and less associated toxicity than cisplatin. In this regards, gold (III) complexes with various ligands like Au–N, Au–S or Au–C bonds are being extensively investigated for their bioactivities as antiproliferative agents [26] and simultaneously new combinations of complexes are being developed. Milovanovic et al have studied the cytotoxicity studies of $[Au(en)Cl_2]^+$ and $[Au(SMC)Cl_2]^+$ where SMC = S-methyl-L-cysteine and $[Au(DMSO)_2Cl_2]^+$ (DMSO = dimethyl sulphoxide). They concluded that gold (III) complexes are much faster to react with nucleophiles compare to Pt(II) complexes. They also demonstrated that gold (III) complexes exhibit relevant cytotoxic properties when tested on chronic lymphocytic leukemia cells (CLL). This conclusion indicates that gold(III) complexes have good potential for the treatment of cancer. In addition $[Au(en)Cl_2]^+$ complex shows cytotoxicity profiles comparable to cisplatin [27].

This study has led us to investigate further the conclusion achieved by the in vitro studies of Milovanovic et al [27]. The title compound is a newly developed gold (III) compound $[Au(en)Cl_2]Cl$, gold complexed with N-substituted ethylenediamine. **(Fig.1).**

It has been prepared and fully characterized by spectroscopic techniques such as UV–Vis, Far-IR, IR spectroscopy, solution, X-ray and solid NMR. The solution NMR was measured in D2O, implicating that it is water soluble [28,29]. In the current study we evaluated the histopathological toxicity of this compound in renal and hepatic tissues of rats.

Materials and Methods

This study was carried out in Pathology Department, College of Medicine, University of Dammam in 2010–2011. It was compartmentalized into two segments comprising acute toxicity and subacute toxicity studies. For both segments, Albino Wistar male rats (n = 42), weighing 200–250 gram were obtained from the College of Veterinary Medicine, King Faisal University, Al-Hassa, Saudi Arabia. They were placed in an animal house under standardized conditions, fed standard chow and exposed to an optimized environment one week before the start of the experiment.

Acute Toxicity Study

In acute toxicity, 5 groups of rats (A/I-E/I), with each group comprising 5 animals, were administered gold compound intraperitoneally in doses of 1500 mg/kg, 750 mg/kg, 375 mg/kg, 187.5 mg/kg and 93.75 mg/kg, respectively. A control group of 5 animals (F/I) was simultaneously administered 0.2 ml water intraperitoneally.

After 24 hours, the number of deceased rats was counted in each group and LD_{50} (dose that kills 50% of animals) was calculated (322 mg/kg) by the method of Miller and Tainter [30].

Autopsy was carried out in all animals and renal as well as hepatic tissues were preserved in 10% buffered formalin for subsequent evaluation of histopathological alterations.

Sub-acute Toxicity Study

The rats in this component of the study were divided into two treatment groups, A/II and B/II, with six rats in each. Group "A/II" served as the experimental group while group "B/II" served as the control. Rats in the experimental group (A/II) were injected with 32.2 mg/kg (1/10 of LD_{50}) body weight of the gold compound while rats in the control group (B/II) were injected with normal saline daily for 14 days.

Autopsy was carried out in all the rats. Renal and hepatic tissues were preserved in 10% buffered formalin until subjected to histopathological evaluation.

Histopathological Work Up

a) Fixation and tissue processing. The formalin preserved hepatic and renal tissue samples of $[Au(en)Cl_2]Cl$ dosed rats and controls were processed in an automated tissue processor (Tissue–tek VIP-5, from SAKURA). The processing consisted of an initial 2 step fixation comprising tissue immersion in 10% buffered formalin for two hours each, followed by removal of fixative in distilled water for 30 minutes. Dehydration was then carried out by running the tissues through a graded series of alcohol (70%, 90%, and 100%). The tissue was initially exposed to 70% alcohol

Table 1. Histological categorization of drug-induced hepatic lesions.

Acute hepatitis and cholestatic hepatitis	
Acute liver failure	Necrosis with marked inflammation, Necrosis with little or no inflammation
Cholestasis	Bland cholestasis, Cholestatic hepatitis
Chronic Hepatitis	
Granulomatous hepatitis	
Steatosis/Steatohepatitis	Macrovesicular, Microvesicular, Steatohepatitis
Vascular Abnormalities	Sinusoidal obstruction syndrome

Table 2. Acute toxicity, salient hepatic microscopic findings.

Groups	Ballooning degeneration			Hepatocellular necrosis/degeneration		Sinusoidal Obstruction syndrome	Inflammation portal/lobular			Congestion	
	Mild	Mod	marked	Individual cell degeneration	Necrosis with inflammation		Mild	Mod	Marked	Mild	Mod/marked
A/I (n = 5)	–	–	–	20% (1)	–	80% (4)	60%(3)	–	–	–	–
B/I (n = 5)	–	–	–	40% (2)	–	20% (1)	20%(1)	–	–	–	80%(4)
C/I (n = 5)	–	–	–	–	–	–	–	–	–	40%(2)	60%(3)
D/I* (n = 5)	–	–	–	–	–	–	40%(2)	–	–	–	100% (5)
E/I ** (n = 5)	–	20%(1)	–	–	20%(1)	–	20%(1)	–	–	20%(1)	60%(3)
F/I (n = 5)	–	60%(3)	40% (2)	–	–	–	40%(2)	–	–	20%(1)	40%(2)

*Capsular inflammation with peritonitis was discerned in 40% of cases.(fibrinopurulent exudates on the surface).
**An occasional microgranuloma was present in 20% of cases.

for 30 minutes followed by 90% alcohol for 1 hour and then two cycles of absolute alcohol, each for one hour.

Dehydration was then followed by clearing the samples in several changes of xylene. It consisted of tissue immersion for an hour in a mixture comprising 50% alcohol and 50% xylene, followed by pure xylene for one and a half hour. Samples were then impregnated with molten paraffin wax, then embedded and blocked out. Paraffin sections (4–5 um) were stained with hematoxylin and eosin, the conventional staining technic [31].

Stained sections were examined for necrosis, apoptosis, inflammation and vascular changes in renal tissue.

The hepatic tissue was evaluated for any alterations in the architecture, portal or lobular inflammation, sinusoidal dilatation and congestion along with presence of granulomas, degeneration, necrosis and fatty change.

b) Histopathological grading for renal lesions. Renal lesions in [Au(en)Cl$_2$]Cl dosed rats were assessed by light microscopy and graded into five categories by utilizing a scale of 0 to 5 as mentioned and adopted by Zhang et al [32]:

0 = normal histology,

1 = tubular epithelial cell degeneration, without significant necrosis/apoptosis;

2–5 = <25%, <50%, <75% and >75% of the tubules showing tubular epithelial cell necrosis/apoptosis, respectively, accompanied by other concomitant alterations.

c) Histopathological categorization of hepatic lesions. The hepatic lesions were categorized according to the criteria mentioned below by Ramchandran et al [33] (**table 1**).

Results

The results of the study are depicted in tables 2, 3, 4 and Figures 2, 3, 4, 5, 6, 7, -8.

Acute Toxicity

Renal Microscopic Findings. The renal lesion in all groups of this batch demonstrated variable extent of renal tubular necrosis/apoptosis (Fig. 2) with one grade showing slight predominance over the other. No single group specific necrosis grade was evident in the entire series.

All the 5 rats in group A/I (Dose: 1500 mg/kg) died before sacrificing. The renal microscopy revealed normal histology in three animals and tubular necrosis of grade 2 severity i.e. comprising less than 25% of the total tubular tissue, in the remaining two cases (Fig. 3a and 3b). Scattered occasional tubules with vacuolated cytoplasm were also seen along with one of the case showing cells with strongly eosinophilic cytoplasm.

In group B/I (Dose: 750 mg/kg), four out of five animals died before sacrificing. Again, a large range of necrosis was discerned, with three animals revealing grade 1 (Fig. 3c and 3d), one grade 4 and the last grade 5 tubular necrosis.

In group C/I (Dose: 375 mg/kg), three out of five animals died before sacrificing. All animals showed renal tubular necrosis comprising 75% or more of the total renal tissue examined (grade 5, Fig. 3e and 3f).

Group D/I (Dose: 187.5 mg/kg) had two dead animals out of five, before sacrificing. A wide range of renal tubular necrosis comprising around 25% to more than 75% of total tissue (predominantly grade 2) was discerned.

Group E/I (Dose: 93.75 mg/kg) with all 5 animals alive at necropsy, revealed renal tubular necrosis varying in range from individual cell necrosis/apoptosis to necrosis constituting less than 50% of the total renal tissue examined (predominantly grade 2–3).

Table 3. Sub-acute toxicity, salient renal microscopic findings.

Groups (n = 6 in each group)	Dosage mg/kg	Death %	Pyelitis/interstitial inflammation		Congestion	
			Mild	Mod/marked	Mild	Mod/Marked
A/II (n = 6)	32.2	0	100% (6)	–	100% (6)	–
B/II (n = 6)	0	0	83.33% (5)	16.66% (1)	100% (6)	–

Table 4. Sub-acute toxicity, salient hepatic microscopic findings.

Group	Dosage mg/kg	Death %	Ballooning degeneration			Inflammation portal/lobular			Congestion	
			Mild	Moderate	Marked	Mild	Moderate	Marked	Mild	Mod/marked
A/II**/*** (n = 6)	32.2	0	16.66% (1)	16.66% (1)	66.66% (4)	83.33% (5)	–	–	83.33% (5)	16.66% (1)
B/II (n = 6)	0	0	16.66% (1)	16.66% (1)	16.66% (1)	66.66% (4)	–	–	33.33% (2)	66.66% (4)

**100% (6) cases revealed capsular inflammation.
***16.66% (1) case revealed an occasional microgranuloma.

The control group (F/I) with all animals alive revealed normal renal tubular histology (Fig. 4a).

Varying extent of congestion dominated the entire histopathological spectrum.

Hepatic microscopic findings. The hepatic specimens of almost all 5 animals of each group, A/I, B/I, C/I, D/I and E/I revealed variable extent of micro and macro-vesicular steatosis (Fig. 5 and Fig. 6a). Varying extent of congestion (Fig. 6b and 6c) along with few cases showing sinusoidal obstruction syndrome were also present. In A/I and B/I, one and two cases respectively, revealed scattered individual hepatocytic cell degeneration without inflammation. One case showing focal necrosis with inflammation

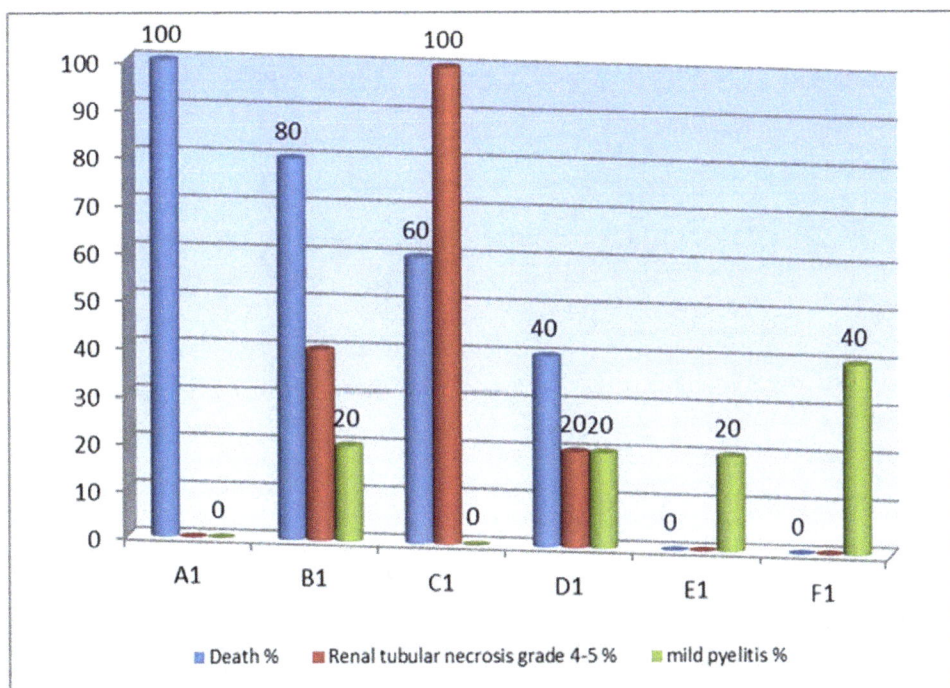

Concentration of the drug administered in different groups A1-F1

(A1:1500 mg/kg B1:750 mg/kg C1:375 mg/kg D1:187.5 mg/kg E1:93.75 mg/kg F1:control)

Figure 2. Spectrum of renal tubular necrosis seen in acute toxicity study of a gold (III) compound [Au(en)Cl₂]Cl.

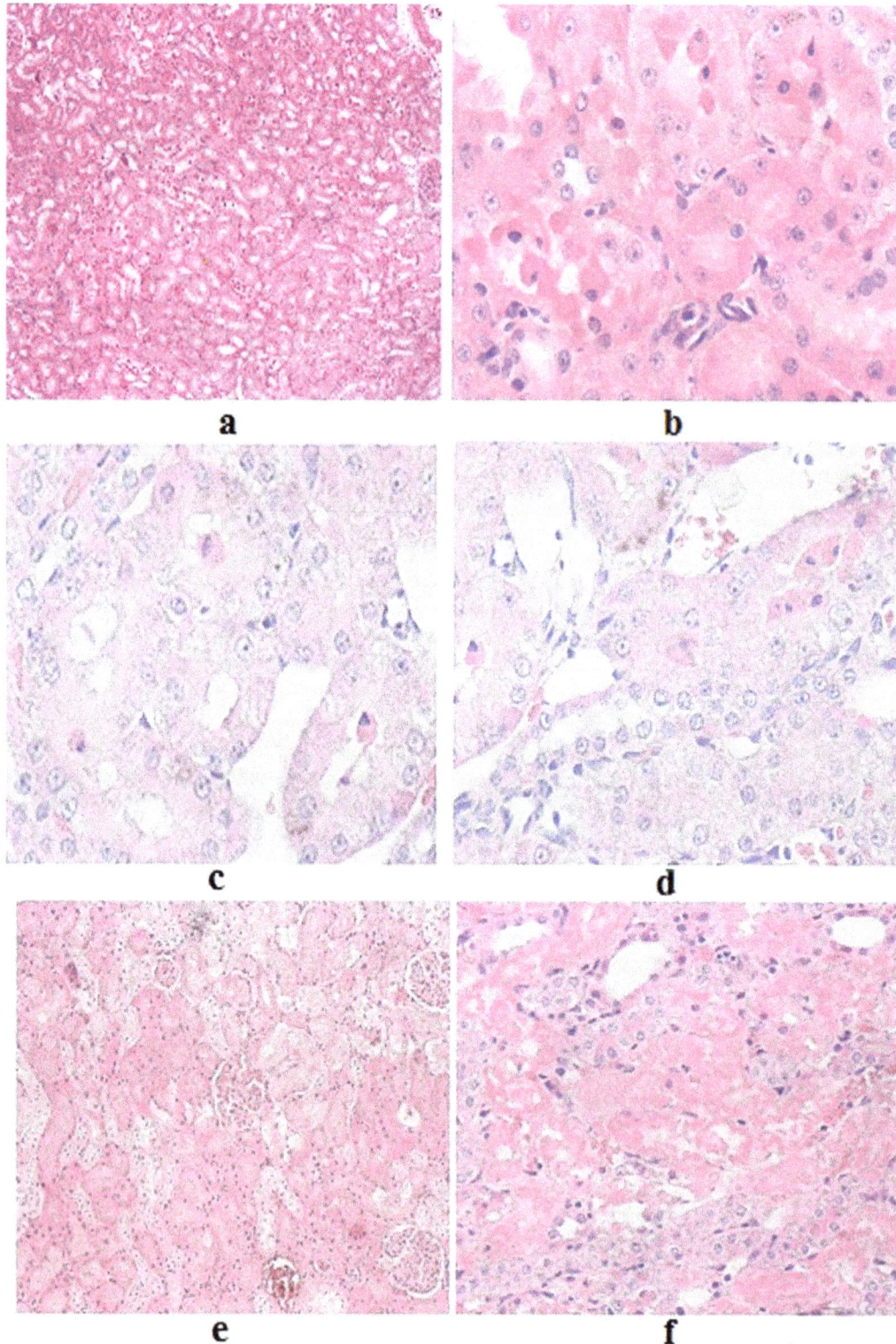

Figure 3. Microscopic findings of renal tubules showing different grades of renal tubular necrosis as seen in the acute toxicity study of a gold (III) compound [Au(en)Cl₂]Cl. a & b: Grade 2 as seen in H&E ×20 and ×40. Necrotic tubules are seen amongst viable renal tubules. The necrosis is less than 25% of the total material examined. In ×40 magnification, more abundant, necrotic cells are seen along with normal renal tubules. **c & d:** Grade 1 as seen in H&E ×40 magnification. Scattered individual apoptotic/necrotic cells with strongly eosinophilic cytoplasm and pyknotic nuclei are seen. **e & f:** Grade 5 as seen in H&E ×20 and ×40 The entire field shows mostly necrotic renal tubules.

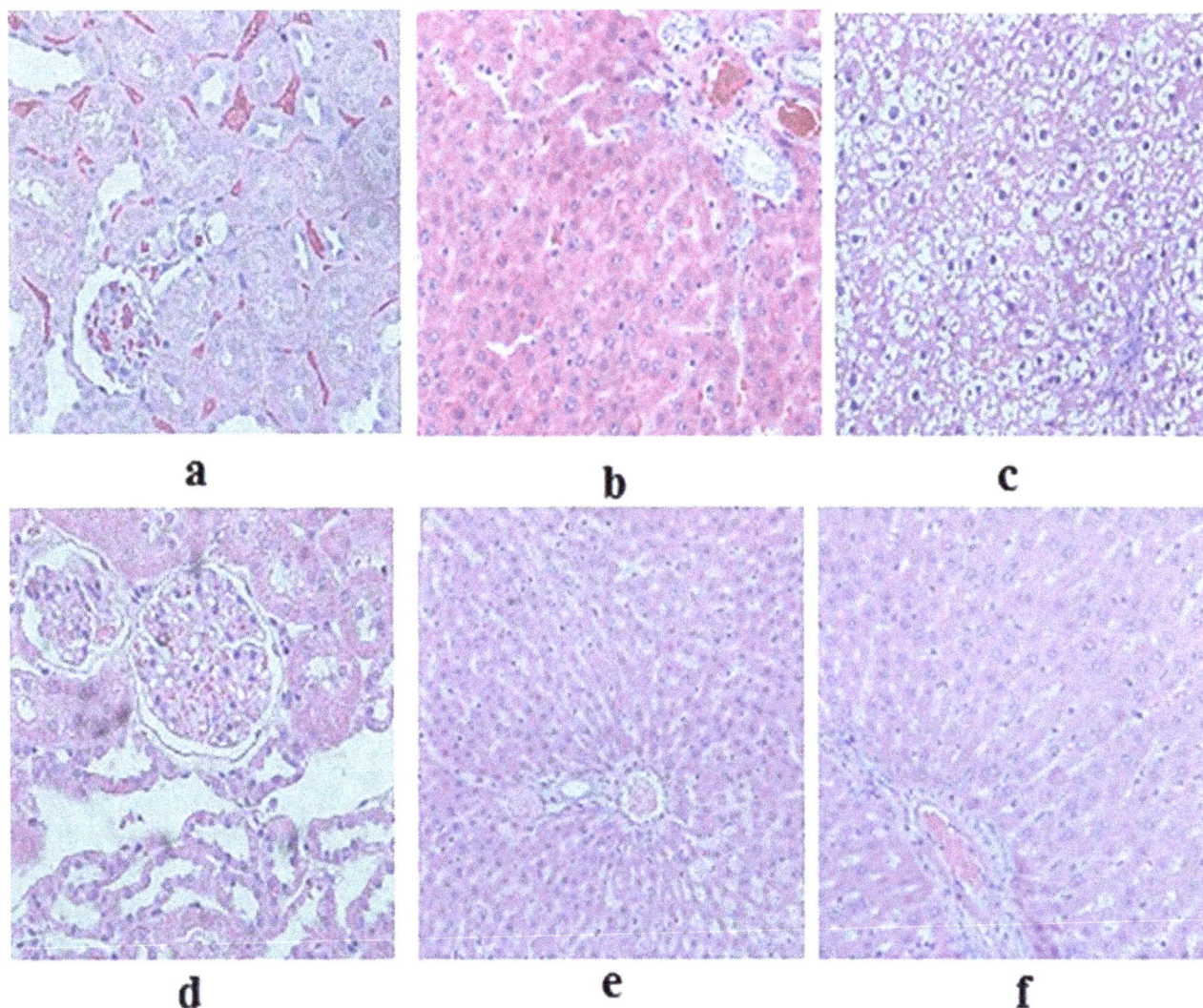

Figure 4. Renal and hepatic tissues in the controls used in acute (a,b,c) and sub-acute (d,e,f) toxicity parts of study. a: Renal tissue showing mild congestion with no other pathological change as seen in acute toxicity controls (H&E x40). **b:** Hepatic tissue as seen in acute toxicity controls (H&E x40) showing mild congestion. No other pathological change is seen in this focus. **c:** Marked ballooning degeneration as seen in acute toxicity controls (H&E x40). **d:** Unremarkable renal tubules as seen in sub-acute toxicity controls (H&E x40). **e:** Unremarkable hepatic tissue as seen in sub-acute toxicity controls (H&E x20). **f:** Unremarkable hepatic tissue as seen in sub-acute toxicity controls (H&E x40).

and another one revealing moderate ballooning degeneration with an occasional microgranuloma was seen in group E/I (Fig. 6d). The hepatic picture in F/I (control, drug free group, Fig. 4b and 4c) comprised moderate to marked ballooning degeneration (percentages of hepatic lesions are shown in table 2).

Sub-Acute Toxicity

This batch had two groups, each comprising 6 animals. The first group (A/II) was dosed with 32.2 mg/kg (1/10 of LD_{50}) for two weeks and the second (group B/II) was the drug free control group.

Group A/II had no animal dead before necropsy. As a whole, the renal tissue was unaffected as far as tubular necrosis (Fig. 7) was concerned. Varying extents of pyelitis with prominence of eosinophils and mild congestion spanned the entire histological picture (percentages are shown in table 3). The hepatic lesion comprised mild to marked ballooning degeneration (Fig. 8) and congestion, with one case revealing an occasional microgranu-

loma. Capsular inflammation, focal portal inflammation and an occasional focus of lobular inflammation completed the entire histological spectrum (percentages are shown in table 4).

In Group B/II the renal histology was within normal limits (Fig. 4d) with pyelitis, congestion and focal pigment deposition constituting the consistent microscopic findings (table 3). The hepatic picture ranged from normal, unaffected liver (Fig. 4e and 4f) in three cases to mild, moderate and marked ballooning degeneration, respectively, in the remaining three cases in this group (table 4). No steatosis was present in animals of this group.

Discussion

This study demonstrated minimal renal and hepatic toxicity by a newly developed gold (III) compound, [Au(en)Cl$_2$]Cl. In the sub-acute toxicity part of the study, this compound showed dose dependent renal toxicity but with a much extended nephrogenic safety range and also exhibited a notably higher safe upper limit compared to toxicity levels of clinically established antineoplastic

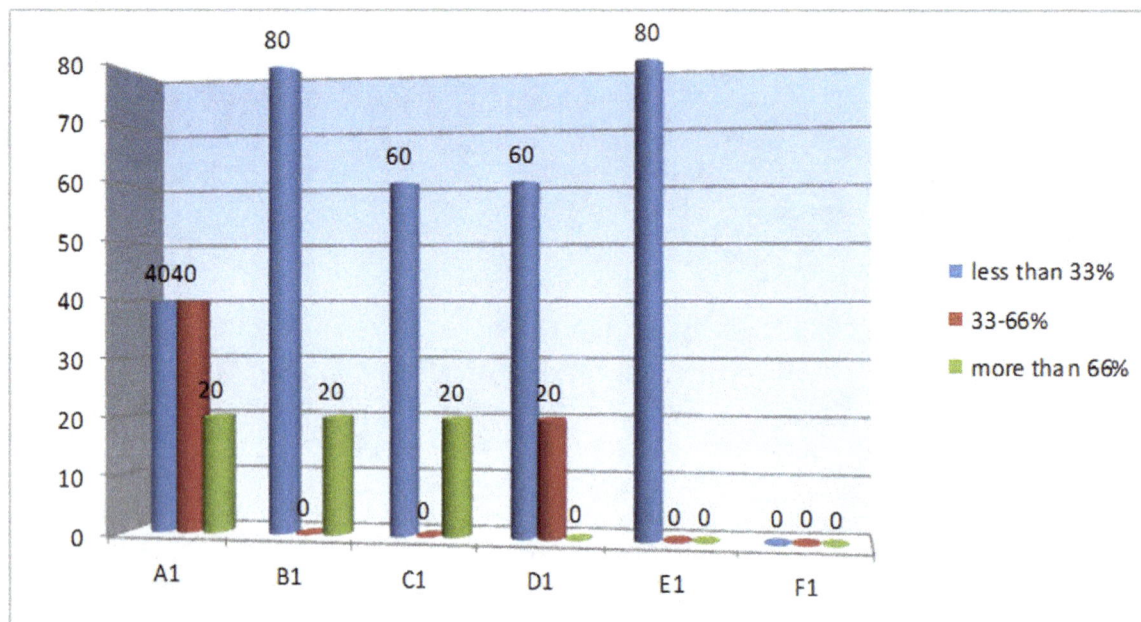

Concentration of the drug administered in different groups A1-F1

(A1:1500 mg/kg B1:750 mg/kg C1:375 mg/kg D1:187.5 mg/kg E1:93.75 mg/kg F1:control)

Figure 5. Extent of hepatic steatosis seen in acute toxicity study of a gold (III) compound [Au(en)Cl$_2$]Cl.

drugs like cisplatin, doxyrubicin and 5-Florouracil(5-FU) as reported in other studies. Comparative analysis with other gold compounds was limited by paucity of toxicity studies. Many studies report gold(III) complexes as emerging, potential anticancer agents [34,35,36,37] with elaboration of their mechanisms of action and antiproliferative activity [27,35] against many different cancer stem lines, but their toxicity data as regards detailed renal and hepatic histopathological manifestations have not been adequately described.

In our study a dose of 32.2 mg/kg (1/10 of LD$_{50}$) revealed normal renal tubular histology with no evidence of tubular necrosis. Mild pyelitis with a prominence of eosinophils and mild congestion was a consistent finding. Varying extent and grade of renal tubular necrosis was only seen with the administration of the gold(III) compound at very high dosages (range of 187.5–1500 mg/kg), administered in the acute toxicity component of the study.

Other antineoplastic drugs are seen to exhibit a significantly low renal tolerance. In a study comprising multi drug analysis by Hanigan et al, rats dosed intraperitoneally with 15 mg/kg of body weight cisplatin revealed grade 4 tubular necrosis [38]. Atasyara et al described remarkable epithelial vacuolation, necrosis, and desquamation of cells with protein casts in renal tubules after a single intraperitoneal dose of 7.5 mg/kg of cisplatin [39].In a study by Ravindra et al, rats injected intraperitoneally with 0.4 mg/kg of cisplatin for a period of 8 weeks showed different alterations comprising marked proximal tubular dilation and desquamation along with acute tubular necrosis [40]. Other drugs like methrotrexate and cyclosporine have been reported to have a nephrotoxic effect culminating to cell death by direct tubular toxicity and intratubular precipitation [41,42] along with proximal tubular apoptosis and necrosis [43] respectively, but studies evaluating their dose dependent renal histopathological manifestations are not available.

Nephrotoxicity is an integral and inherent accompaniment of multiple anti-neoplastic drugs [23,24,44–46] which usually have a narrow therapeutic index and the minimum dosage required to significantly decrease tumor burden is usually associated with substantial nephrotoxicity. The significantly diminished renal toxicity of N-substituted ethylenediamine complexes of gold could be attributed to their different anti-proliferative mechanism of action and selective sparing of the proximal tubular epithelial cells. Their mechanism although not precisely delineated, comprises a cumulative impact on induction of cell cycle blockage, interruption of the cell mitotic cycle, programmed cell death (apoptosis) or premature cell death (necrosis) [47].

Hepatotoxicity is an entity not as extensively explored as nephrotoxicity as it does not manifest itself as a dose limiting factor [48]. With our ethylenediamine derivative of gold, in the acute toxicity component of the study, varying extent of steatosis was the main finding. In the sub acute toxicity component, varying extent of ballooning degeneration with accompanying congestion and focal portal inflammation comprised the predominant histopathological lesion. One of the samples revealed an occasional focus of lobular inflammation. Capsular inflammation was also a consistent finding. Other drugs like cisplatin produce hepatoxicity in high doses [49,50]. El-Sayyad et al investigated the effects of cisplatin, doxorubicin and 5-FU belonging to different chemical classes on rats liver and showed that groups receiving cisplatin and doxorubicin exhibited increased hepatoxicity in comparison to 5-FU treatment. The most pronounced histopathlogical abnormalities observed were hepatic cord dissolution [51]. Avci et al demonstrated that a dose of 10 mg/kg cisplatin could induce sinusoidal congestion, hydropic and vacuolar degeneration, extensive disorganization in hepatocytes, and significant fibrosis around central venules and expanded periportal areas [48]. In another multidrug, multimodal study by Kart et al, moderate to severe hydropic degeneration in centrilobular zones extending

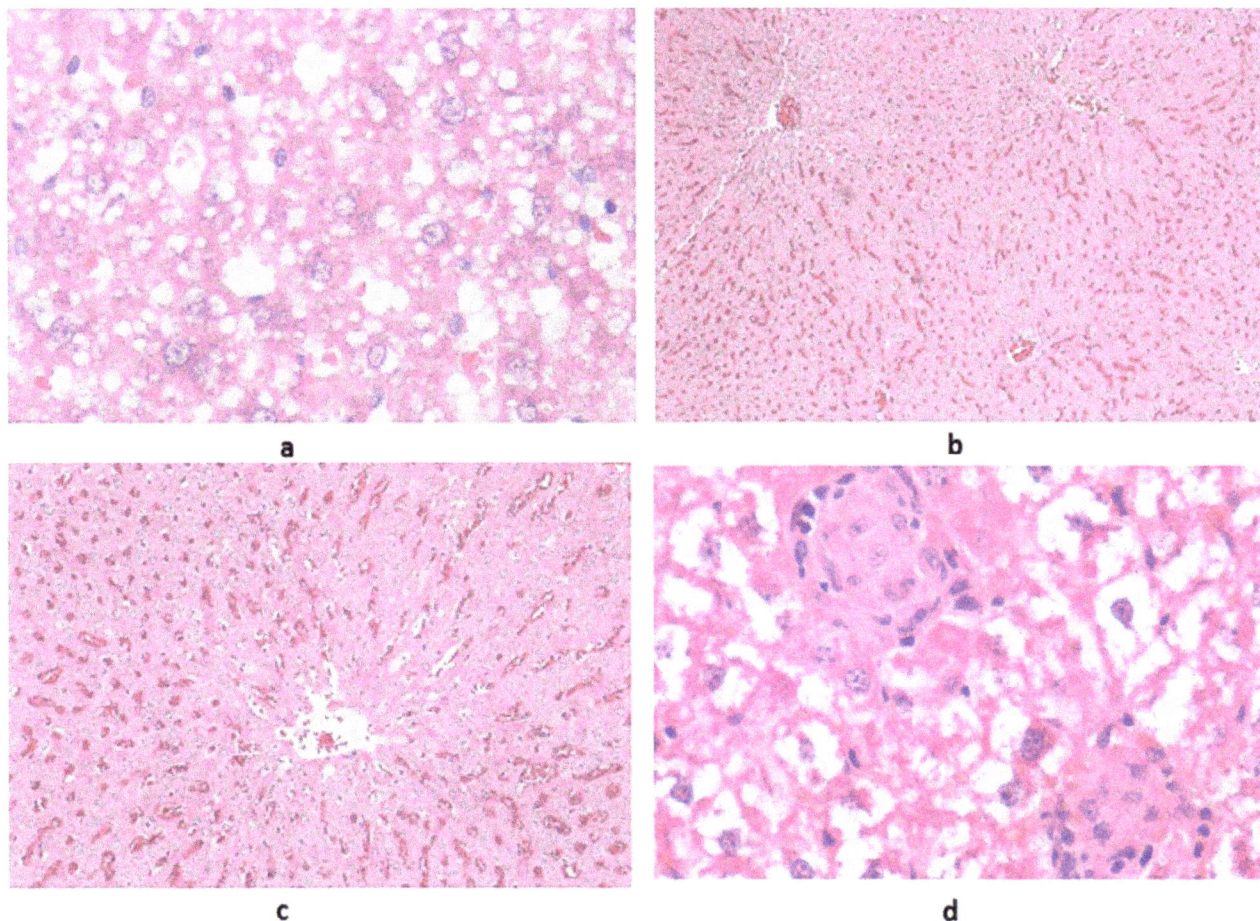

Figure 6. Spectrum of hepatic microscopic findings as seen in the acute toxicity study of a gold (III) compound [Au(en)Cl$_2$]Cl. a: Marked mixed micro and macrovesicular steatosis, H&E ×40. b & c: Marked sinusoidal congestion and dilatation, H & E ×20 and ×40 respectively. d: Marked ballooning degeneration along with two microgranulomas, H & E ×40.

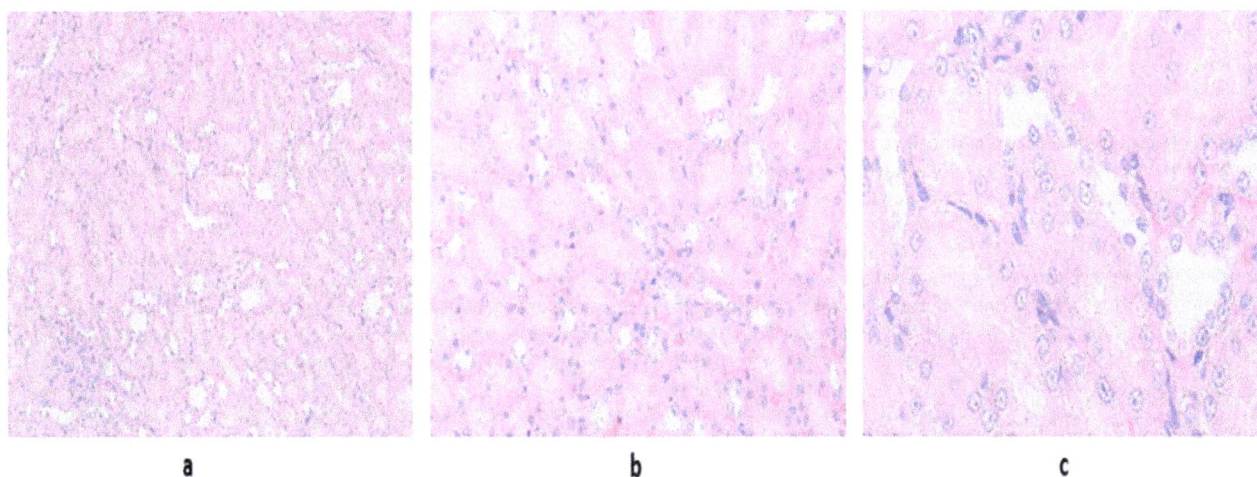

Figure 7. Microscopic pictures of renal tubules, with no evidence of necrosis as seen in sub-acute toxicity study of a gold (III) compound [Au(en)Cl$_2$]Cl, H&E at magnifications of : a. ×10. b. ×20. c. ×40.

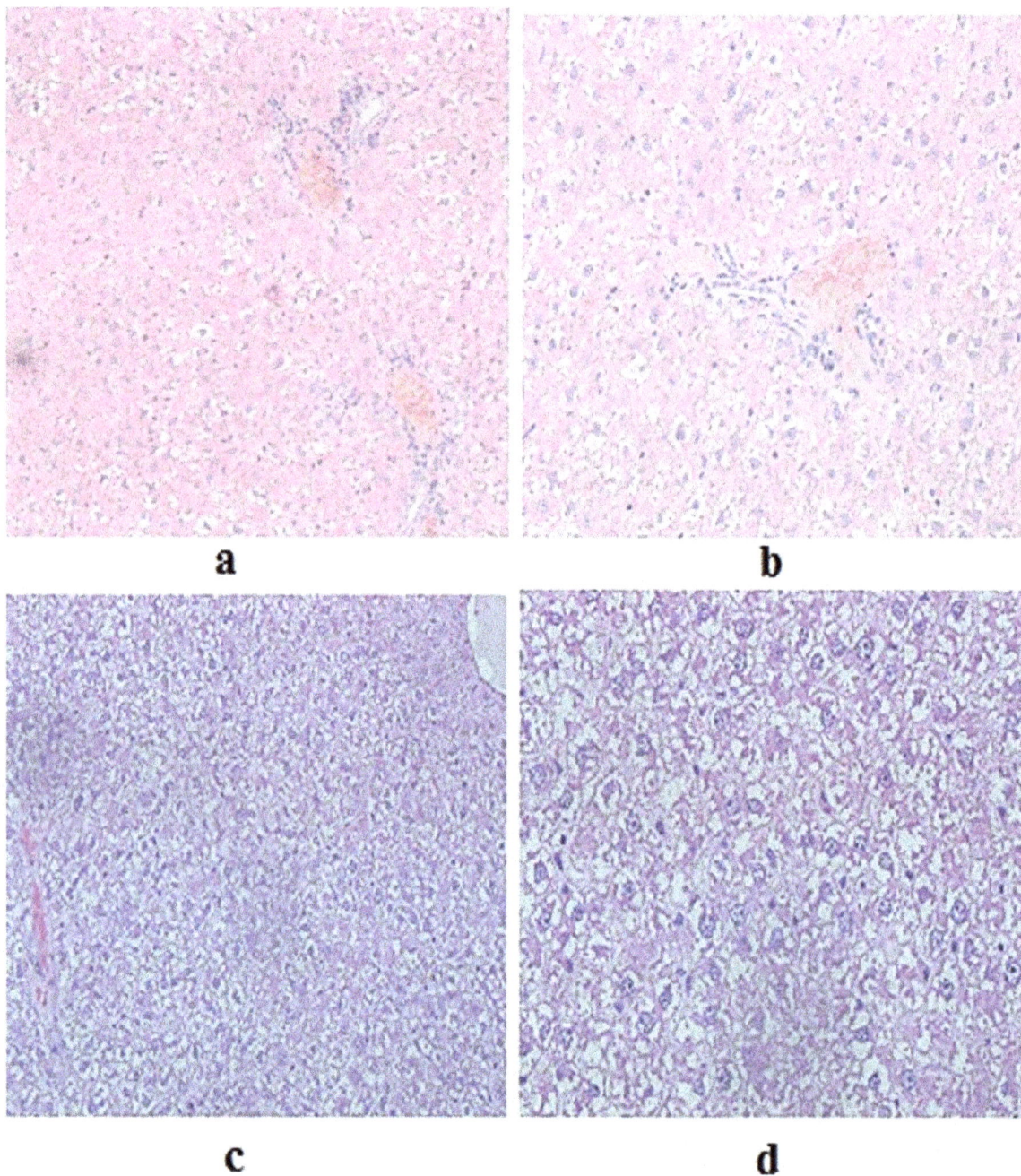

Figure 8. Hepatic microscopic findings in sub-acute toxicity study of a gold (III) compound [Au(en)Cl₂]Cl. a: Mild ballooning degeneration, H&E ×20. **b:** Mild ballooning degeneration, H&E × 40. **c:** Marked ballooning degeneration, H&E ×20. **d:** Marked ballooning degeneration, H&E ×40Toxicity.

towards the portal region was obtained with a single intraperitoneal 6.5 mg/kg dose of cisplatin. Necrotic hepatocytes, especially concentrated around the central veins, were observed in the severely affected cases [52].

Ballooning degeneration was a finding that was also evident in the control group of animals as well. As regards ballooning degeneration, the non significant difference between controls and drug dosed rats in hepatic toxicity in the sub-acute group reflects that drug toxicity may not be the only reason for the hepatic lesion.

The hepatic lesion produced by N-substituted ethylenediamine complexes with gold was substantially milder than cisplatin with no evidence of apoptosis or necrosis in the entire series of animals receiving a drug dose of 32.2 mg/kg for 14 days.

Conclusions

Gold (III) compound [Au(en)Cl₂]Cl in sub-acute toxicity study, produced less renal and hepatic toxicity as compared to other clinically established antineoplastic drugs. In the entire series of animals, no renal tubular necrosis was seen. Mild pyelitis and congestion dominated the histopathological picture. In hepatic tissue, ballooning degeneration of varied extent and severity prevailed in the drug dosed animals with no evidence of hepatocytic degeneration and necrosis.

Acknowledgments

We acknowledge services of Mrs Khalda Al Johy, Mrs Zainab Al Najar, Mr Shakir Ahmad and Mrs Maria Rosario Lazaro in conducting the laboratory work.

Author Contributions

Conceived and designed the experiments: AA AI AMMA. Performed the experiments: AA DT MS. Analyzed the data: AA MS. Contributed reagents/materials/analysis tools: AA AI AMMA DT MS. Wrote the paper: AA AI MS. Designing and writing grant proposal: AI AA AMMA MS DT. Developing the drug: AI AMMA. Treating the animals: AMMA. Preparing the tissue, histological evaluation: AA MS DT. Analysis and preparing manuscript: AA AI AMMA MS DT.

References

1. Nagender RP, Eladia MP, Josef H (2009) Gold and nano-gold in medicine: overview, toxicology and perspectives. J Appl Biomed 7(2): 75–91.
2. Pacheco EA, Tiekink E, Whitehouse MW (2009) Biomedical Applications of Gold and Gold Compounds. In: Cort C, Holliday R (Editors) Gold Science and Applications. World Gold Council, London, CRC Press 217–230.
3. Milacic V, Fregona D, Dou QP (2008) Gold complexes as prospective metal-based anticancer drugs. Histol Histopathol 23(1): 101–8.
4. Kean WF, Forestier F, Kassam Y, Buchanan WW, Rooney PJ (1985) The history of gold therapy in rheumatoid disease. Semin Arthritis Rheum 14(3): 180–6.
5. Mahdihassan S (1985) Cinnabar-gold as the best alchemical drug of longevity, called Makaradhwaja in India. Am J Chin Med: 13(1–4): 93–108.
6. Daniel MC, Astruc D (2004) Gold Nanoparticles: assembly, supramolecular chemistry, quantum-size related properties, and applications toward biology, catalysis, and nanotechnology. Chem Rev 104(1): 293–346.
7. Kean WF, Gerecz E, Hogan MG (1987) Gold therapy II. Historical, chemical, pharmacological and biological profile of anti-arthritic gold compounds. Singapore Med J 28(2): 117–25.
8. Felson DT, Anderson JJ, Meenan RF (1990) The comparative efficacy and toxicity of second-line drugs in rheumatoid arthritis. Results of two meta analyses. Arthritis Rheum 33(10): 1449–61.
9. Shaw IC (1999) Gold-based therapeutic agents. Chem Rev 99(9): 2589–2600.
10. Bhattacharya R, Mukherjee P (2008) Biological properties of "naked" metal nanoparticles. Adv Drug Deliv Rev 60: 1289–1306.
11. Wu ML, Tsai WJ, Ger J, Deng JF, Tsay SH, et al. (2001) Cholestatic hepatitis caused by acute gold potassium cyanide poisoning. Clin Toxicol 39: 739–43.
12. Cattaruzza L, Fregona D, Mongiat M, Ronconi L, Fassina A, et al. (2011) Antitumor activity of gold(III)-dithiocarbamato derivatives on prostate cancer cells and xenografts. Int J Cancer 128(1): 206–15.
13. Rosenberg B, VanCamp I, Krigas T (1965) Inhibition of Cell Division in Escherichia coli by Electrolysis Products from a Platinum Electrode. Nature 205: 698–9.
14. Rosenberg B, VanCamp I, Trosko JE, Mansour VH (1969) Platinum compounds: a new class of potent antitumour agents. Nature 222(5191): 385–6.
15. Galanski M, Jakupec MA, Keppler BK (2005) Update of the Preclinical Situation of Anticancer Platinum Complexes: Novel Design Strategies and Innovative Analytical Approaches. Curr Med Chem 12(18): 2075–94.
16. Ott I (2009) Review On the medicinal chemistry of gold complexes as anticancer drugs. Coord Chem Rev 253(11–12): 1670–81.
17. Schmidbauer H (1999) Gold-progress in chemistry, biochemistry and technology. Chichester, John Wiley & Sons.
18. Hoke GD, Macia RA, Meunier PC, Bugelski PJ, Mirabelli CK, et al. (1989) In vivo and in vitro cardiotoxicity of a gold containing antineoplastic drug candidate in the rabbit. Toxicol Appl Pharmacol 100(2): 293–306.
19. Tiekink ER (2002) Gold derivatives for the treatment of cancer. Crit Rev Oncol Hematol 42: 225–48.
20. Kelland L (2007) The resurgence of platinum-based cancer chemotherapy. Nat Rev Cancer 7: 573–84.
21. Meijer S, Mulder NH, Sleijfer DT, de Jong PE, Sluiter WJ, et al. (1982) Nephrotoxicity of cis-diamminedichloride platinum [CDDP] during remissio-ninduction and maintenance chemotherapy of the testicular carcinoma. Cancer Chemother Pharmacol 8: 27–30.
22. Brock PR, Koliouska DE, Baratt TM, Yeomans E, Pritchard J (1991) Partial reversibility of cisplatin nephrotoxicity in children. J Pediatr 118: 531–4.
23. Chao S, Chiang J, Huang A, Chang W (2011) An integrative approach to identifying cancer chemoresistance-associated pathways. BMC Medical Genomics 4(1): 23–37.
24. Yamashita T, Miyamoto S, O'Malley B, Li D (2010) The Role of PARP 1 for Cisplatin-Based Chemoresistance. Otolaryngol Head Neck Surg 143(2): 54–60.
25. Oliver TG, Mercer KL, Sayles LC, Burke JR, Mendus D, et al. (2010) Chronic cisplatin treatment promotes enhanced damage repair and tumor progression in a mouse model of lung cancer. Genes & Dev 24: 837–852.
26. Ott I, Gust R (2007) Non Platinum Metal Complexes as Anti-cancer Drugs. Arch Pharm Chem Life Sci 340: 117–126.
27. Milovanović M, Djeković A, Volarević V, Petrović B, Arsenijević N, et al. (2010) Ligand substitution reactions and cytotoxic properties of [Au(L)Cl$_2$]$^+$ and [AuCl$_2$(DMSO)$_2$]$^+$ complexes (L = ethylenediamine and S-methyl-l-cysteine). J Inorg Biochem 104(9): 944–9.
28. Al-Maythalony BA, Wazeer MIM, Isab AA (2009) Synthesis and characterization of gold(III) complexes with alkyldiamine ligands. Inorg Chim Acta 362: 3109–13.
29. Zhu S, Gorski W, Powell DR, Walmsley JA (2006) Synthesis, Structure, and Electrochemistry of Gold(III) Ethylenediamine Complexes and Interactions with Guanosine 5'-Monophosphate. Inorg. Chem 45 (6): 2688–94.
30. Miller LC, Tainter MI (1937) Estimation of LD$_{50}$ or ED$_{50}$ values and their errors using Log-Probit graph paper. Proc Soc Expt. Biol. Med 57: 261–264.
31. Underwood JCE (1985) Histochemistry. Theoretical and applied. Vol. 2: Analytical technology Pearse AGE. Fourth edition. Churchill Livingstone, Edinburgh.
32. Zhang J, Brown RP, Shaw M, Vaidya VS, Zhou Y, et al. (2008) Immunolocalization of Kim-1, RPA-1, and RPA-2 in Kidney of Gentamicin-, Mercury-, or Chromium-treated Rats: Relationship to Renal Distributions of iNOS and Nitrotyrosine. Toxicol Pathol 36(3): 397–409.
33. Ramachandran R, Kakar S (2009) Histological patterns in drug-induced liver disease. J Clin Pathol 62: 481–92.
34. Bindoli A, Rigobello MP, Scutari G, Gabbiani C, Casini A, et al. (2009) Thioredoxin reductase: a target for gold compounds acting as potential anticancer drugs. Coord Chem Rev 253(11–12): 1692–07.
35. Magherini F, Modesti A, Bini L, Puglia M, Landini I, et al. (2010) Exploring the biochemical mechanisms of cytotoxic gold compounds: a proteomic study. J Biol Inorg Chem 15(4): 573–82.
36. Chow KH, Sun RW, Lam JB, Li CK, Xu A, et al. (2010) A gold(III) porphyrin complex with antitumor properties targets the Wnt/beta-catenin pathway. Cancer Res 70(1): 329–37.
37. Yan JJ, Chow AL, Leung CH, Sun RW, Ma DL, et al. (2010) Cyclometalated gold(III) complexes with N-heterocyclic carbene ligands as topoisomerase I poisons. Chem Commun (Camb) 46(22): 3893–5.
38. Hanigan MH, Lykissa ED, Townsend DM, Ou C, Barrios R, et al. (2010) γ-Glutamyl Transpeptidase-Deficient Mice Are Resistant to the Nephrotoxic Effects of Cisplatin. Am J Pathol 159(5): 1889–94.
39. Atasayara S, Gürer-Orhanb H, Orhanb H, Gürelc B, Girgina G, et al. (2009) Preventive effect of aminoguanidine compared to vitamin E and C on cisplatin - induced nephrotoxicity in rats. Exp Toxicol Pathol 61(1): 23–32.
40. Ravindra P, Bhiwagade DA, Kulkarni S, Rataboli PV, Dhume CY (2010) Cisplatin induced histological changes in renal tissue of rat. J Cell Animal Bio 4(7): 108–11.
41. Grönroos M, Chen M, Jahnukainen T, Capitanio A, Aizman RI, et al. (2006) Methotrexate induces cell swelling and necrosis in renal tubular cells. Pediatr Blood Cancer 1;46(5): 624–9.
42. Rollino C, Beltrame G, Ferro M, Quattrocchio G, Tonda L, et al. (2010) Cancer treatment-induced nephrotoxicity: BCR-Abl and VEGF inhibitors. G ItalNefrol 50: S70–4.
43. Healy E, Dempsey M, Lally C, Ryan MP (1998) Apoptosis and necrosis: mechanisms of cell death induced by cyclosporine A in a renal proximal tubular cell line. Kidney Int 54(6): 1955–66.
44. Yao X, Panichpisal K, Kurtzman N, Nugent K (2007) Cisplatin Nephrotoxicity: A Review: oxygen species. Am J Med Sci 334(2): 115–24.
45. Arany I, Safirstein RL (2010) Cisplatin nephrotoxicity. Semin Nephrol 2003;23: 460–4.
46. Basu A, Krishnamurthy S (2010) Cellular responses to Cisplatin-induced DNA damage. J Nucleic Acids. doi:10.4061/2010/201367.
47. Isab AA, Sheikh MN, Monim-ul-Mehboob M, Al-Maythalony BA, Wazeer MIM (2011) Synthesis, characterization and anti proliferative effect of [Au(en)$_2$]Cl$_3$ and [Au(N-propyl-en)$_2$]Cl$_3$ on human cancer cell lines: Spectrochimica acta Part A Molecular and biomolecular spectroscopy 79(5): 1196–1201.

48. Avci A, Cetin R, Erguder IB, Devrim E, Kilicoglu B, et al. (2008) Cisplatin Causes Oxidation in Rat Liver Tissues:Possible Protective Effects of Antioxidant Food Supplementation. Turk J Med Sci 38 (2): 117–120.

49. Liu J, Liu Y, Habeebu SS, Klaassen CD (1998) Metallothionein (MT)-null mice are sensitive to cisplatin-induced hepatotoxicity. Toxicol Appl Pharmacol 149: 24–31.

50. Martins NM, Santos NA, Curti C, Bianchi ML, Santos AC (2008) Cisplatin induces mitochondrial oxidative stress with resultant energetic metabolism impairment, membrane rigidification and apoptosis in rat liver. J Appl Toxicol 28(3): 337–44.

51. El-Sayyad HI, Ismail MF, Shalaby FM, Abou-El-Magd RF, Gaur RL, et al. (2009) Histopathological effects of cisplatin, doxorubicin and5-flurouracil (5-FU) on the liver of male albino rats. Int J Biol Sci 28;5(5): 466–73.

52. Kart A, Cigremis Y, Karaman M, Ozen H (2010) Caffeic acid phenethyl ester (CAPE) ameliorates cisplatin-induced hepatotoxicity in rabbit. Exp Toxicol Pathol 62(1): 45–52.

A Serum MicroRNA Signature Is Associated with the Immune Control of Chronic Hepatitis B Virus Infection

Maurizia Rossana Brunetto[1]*, Daniela Cavallone[1], Filippo Oliveri[1], Francesco Moriconi[1], Piero Colombatto[1], Barbara Coco[1], Pietro Ciccorossi[1], Carlotta Rastelli[1], Veronica Romagnoli[1], Beatrice Cherubini[1], Maria Wrang Teilum[2], Thorarinn Blondal[2], Ferruccio Bonino[3]

1 Laboratory of Molecular Genetics and Pathology of Hepatitis Viruses, Hepatology Unit, Reference Center of the Tuscany Region for Chronic Liver Disease and Cancer, University Hospital of Pisa, Pisa, Italy, 2 Division of Dx and Services, Exiqon A/S, Copenhagen, Denmark, 3 Digestive and Liver Disease, General Medicine II Unit, University Hospital of Pisa, Pisa, Italy

Abstract

Background and Aims: The virus/host interplay mediates liver pathology in chronic HBV infection. MiRNAs play a pivotal role in virus/host interactions and are detected in both serum and HBsAg-particles, but studies of their dynamics during chronic infection and antiviral therapy are missing. We studied serum miRNAs during different phases of chronic HBV infection and antiviral treatment.

Methods: MiRNAs were profiled by miRCURY-LNA-Universal-RT-miRNA-PCR (Exiqon-A/S) and qPCR-panels-I/II-739-miRNA-assays and single-RT-q-PCRs. Two cohorts of well-characterized HBsAg-carriers were studied (median follow-up 34–52 months): a) training-panel (141 sera) and HBsAg-particles (32 samples) from 61 HBsAg-carriers and b) validation-panel (136 sera) from 84 carriers.

Results: Thirty-one miRNAs were differentially expressed in inactive-carriers (IC) and chronic-hepatitis-B (CHB) with the largest difference for miR-122-5p, miR-99a-5p and miR-192-5p (liver-specific-miRNAs), over-expressed in both sera and HBsAg-particles of CHB (ANOVA/U-test p-values: $<0.000001/0.000001$; $<0.000001/0.000003$; $<0.000001/0.000005$, respectively) and significantly down-regulated during- and after-treatment in sustained-virological-responders (SVR). MiRNA-profiles of IC and SVR clustered in the heatmap. Liver-miRNAs were combined with miR-335, miR-126 and miR-320a (internal controls) to build a MiR-B-Index with 100% sensitivity, 83.3% and 92.5% specificity (-1.7 cut-off) in both training and validation cohorts to identify IC. MiR-B-Index (-5.72, $-20.43/14.38$) correlated with ALT (49, 10/2056 U/l, $\rho = -0.497$, p<0.001), HBV-DNA (4.58, undetectable/>8.3 Log_{10} IU/mL, $\rho = -0.732$, p<0.001) and HBsAg (3.40, 0.11/5.49 Log_{10} IU/mL, $\rho = -0.883$, p<0.001). At multivariate analysis HBV-DNA (p = 0.002), HBsAg (p<0.001) and infection-phase (p<0.001), but not ALT (p = 0.360) correlated with MiR-B-Index. In SVR to Peg-IFN/NUCs MiR-B-Index improved during-therapy and post-treatment reaching IC-like values (5.32, $-1.65/10.91$ vs 6.68, 0.54/9.53, p = 0.324) beckoning sustained HBV-immune-control earlier than HBsAg-decline.

Conclusions: Serum miRNA profile change dynamically during the different phases of chronic HBV infection. We identified a miRNA signature associated with both natural-occurring and therapy-induced immune control of HBV infection. The MiR-B-Index might be a useful biomarker for the early identification of the sustained switch from CHB to inactive HBV-infection in patients treated with antivirals.

Editor: Isabelle A. Chemin, CRCL-INSERM, France

Funding: The study was supported in part by the 2010 CUCCs-grant of Tuscany Region Italy (FB). All the additional source of support were internal to our organization (i.e. funding dedicated to research internal to our Liver Unit). The funders had no direct role in the study design, data collection and analysis, decision to publish, or preparation of the manuscript.

Competing Interests: The authors' have read the journal's policy and the authors of this manuscript have the following competing interests: Maurizia Rossana Brunetto: speakers' bureau Abbott, BMS, Gilead, Janssen, MSD, Novartis, Roche; Maria W Teilumm, Thorarinn Blondal: current employees of Exiqon AS, Denmark; Ferruccio Bonino: advisory boards and/or speakers' bureau for Abbvie, BMS, Fuijrebio, Gilead, Janssen, MSD and Roche.

* Email: brunettomaurizia@gmail.com

Introduction

Hepatitis B Virus (HBV) is not cytopathic and liver pathology is mediated by the interplay between virus and immune system; accordingly, 3 major phases are identified in chronic HBV infection: immune tolerance, activation and immune control [1–3]. High viral load and circulating hepatitis B "e" antigen (HBeAg) in absence of virus induced liver disease characterize the immune tolerance phase, that is lost when the antiviral immune reaction tries to taper HBV replication causing liver inflammation, namely

HBeAg positive chronic hepatitis B (CHB) [1–3]. An effective immune activation leads to the immune control of HBV replication (HBV-DNA<2000 IU/mL) and HBeAg/anti-HBe seroconversion, that identifies the inactive HBeAg-negative, HBsAg carrier (IC). When the control of viral replication is ineffective HBeAg-defective HBV-variants are selected with progression to HBeAg-negative, anti-HBe-positive CHB, the most prevalent form of HBV disease worldwide [4–6]. Antiviral therapy is aimed to halt disease progression suppressing viral replication with indefinite nucleos(t)ide analogs (NUCs) treatment or achieving a sustained off-therapy immune control after finite courses of Pegylated-interferon (Peg-IFN) [1–3]. In recent years monitoring of HBV-DNA and HBsAg serum levels significantly improved the management of antiviral treatment [7–9]. However, the decline of HBV-DNA serum levels during Peg-IFN therapy does not help to distinguish responders (SVR) from relapsers (REL) and early HBsAg kinetics are predictive of response in Peg-IFN, but non in NUC treated patients [8]. In addition the kinetics of constitutive HBV markers are the biological hallmark of viral expression, but not the expression of the host's response to antivirals. Thus, serum biomarkers of the effective control of HBV infection are currently unsatisfactory and remain an unmet need in the clinical management of chronic HBV carriers [1–3]. MicroRNAs (miRNAs), are small endogenous single-stranded RNAs that modulate the expression of cellular genes and play key roles in vital biological processes and immunity [10]. Host- and/or virus-encoded miRNAs appear to regulate the outcome of both infections and diseases [11–12], as shown for the liver-specific miRNA, miR-122, that is essential for the replication of hepatitis C virus (HCV) [13]. In chronic HBV infection several miRNAs are up-regulated in the serum of HBsAg carriers as compared to controls and circulating HBsAg particles carry specific hepatocellular miRNAs [14–15]. Preliminary reports suggest that serum miRNA profiling may contribute to characterize chronic HBV carriers with or without HCC [16–18]. However, studies focused on the relations between serum miRNAs and the different phases of chronic HBV infection and during antiviral therapy are missing: in the present study we analysed the dynamics of miRNA profiles in sera and circulating HBsAg particles of IC and CHB according to treatment response.

Patients and Methods

Study population

Training cohort. Serum samples (141) were obtained from 61 (40 males, median age 50 years, 21–79) well characterized HBsAg carriers, 57 infected with HBV genotype D and 4 genotype A (Table 1). In case of low HBV-DNA levels (<20000 IU/mL) and normal transaminases (ALT) at presentation, they were followed for at least 1 year with monthly blood tests for classification [1,6], thereafter every 3/6 months (m) as all the other HBV carriers. The HBV carriers were followed-up (median follow-up 34, 18–144 m) at the Hepatology Unit of the University Hospital of Pisa. The study was approved by the local Ethic Committee of the University Hospital of Pisa. All patients provided informed written consent.

HBsAg carriers were classified according to their biochemical and viral profiles [1,6]: a) 5 HBeAg positive carriers [1 immune tolerant, IT (HBV-DNA>8.3 $\log_{10}$ IU/mL, HBsAg>4.39 $\log_{10}$ IU/mL, normal ALT) and 4 with chronic hepatitis B]; b) 16 IC (HBV-DNA persistently <2000 IU/mL and normal ALT); c) 36 HBeAg negative CHB patients [HBV-DNA>2000 IU/mL with evidence of HBV induced liver disease (at histology and/or liver elastometry and ultrasound)]; d) 4 HBeAg negative, anti-HDV

(Hepatitis D Virus) positive carriers with chronic hepatitis (IgM anti-HDV and HDV-RNA positive).

Thirty-two HBeAg negative CHB patients underwent to antiviral treatment: 21 received Peg-IFN 180 µg/week ± NUCs for 12–36 m and 11 NUCs for a median period of 60 m (36–114 m); in 2 patients who cleared HBsAg, NUCs were discontinued after 36 and 112 m, respectively. Response to Peg-IFN was defined as: a) end of treatment (EOT) response if HBV-DNA was <2000 IU/mL at EOT (18 cases); b) non response (NR) if HBV-DNA was >2000 IU/mL at EOT (3 cases); c) relapse (REL) when florid viral replication recurred after an EOT response (5 cases); d) sustained virologic response (SVR) if viral load persisted <2000 IU/mL at every 3 month controls for at least 12 months after EOT (13 cases). Sera were obtained at baseline (BL) and week 24 post-treatment (post-T-FU) in all Peg-IFN treated patients; additional sampling (week 12 and 24 during treatment, EOT) were obtained in 14 patients. In NUCs treated patients (all achieved undetectable on treatment serum HBV-DNA) serum samples were obtained at BL and at their last available on treatment follow-up (EOF) or 24 weeks after NUCs discontinuation (post-T-FU). In 5 HBeAg positive carriers, 16 IC carriers and 4 HBV/HDV patients sera were obtained at a single time point; in 4 HBeAg negative CHB patients with fluctuating disease profiles the sampling was performed during spontaneous remission (ALT range 19–28 U/L; HBV-DNA 3.71–4.57 $\log_{10}$ IU/mL) and at the time of HBV reactivation (ALT range 210–550 U/L; HBV-DNA 4.35–7.18 $\log_{10}$ IU/mL). MiRNA profiling was obtained from whole serum in all samples; in addition, to target specifically hepatocellular miRNAs, the profiling was performed in HBsAg immune precipitated (IP) particle from 32 sera [6 from IC and 26 from 13 HBeAg negative CHB patients, with SVR (5), REL (5) or NR (3) to Peg-IFN].

Validation cohort

A second well characterized cohort of 84 HBV carriers (59 males, median age 54 years, 17–79) followed-up for 52 m (18–159 m) and classified according to the above defined criteria was used to generate the validation serum panel (overall 136 sera) of the MiR-B-Index (Table 1). Serum samples were obtained at a single point in 23 IC, 5 IT and 4 untreated HBeAg negative CHB patients. In 52 (16 HBeAg positive) treated patients, samples were collected at BL and 24 week Post-T-FU in the 15 Peg-IFN ± NUC treated patients [9 HBeAg positive: 5 with SVR (HBeAg/anti-HBe seroconversion and HBV-DNA<2000 IU/mL at EOT and in post-T-FU); 6 HBeAg negative: 1 SVR, 4 REL, 1 NR] and at BL and EOF in the 37 patients (7 HBeAg positive) treated with NUCs (all achieved undetectable on treatment HBV-DNA, none cleared HBsAg). In addition, 15 serum samples of the study cohort were retested together with the validation cohort.

Serological tests

HBsAg qualitative and quantitative, anti-HBs, anti-HBc, IgM anti-HBc HBeAg and anti-HBe, anti-HCV, anti-HDV and anti-HIV were detected by commercially available immunoassays (Abbott laboratories, N. Chicago, IL, USA). Serum HBV DNA levels were quantified by COBAS TaqMan assay, sensitivity 6 IU/mL, dynamic range 6–1.70×10^8 IU/mL (Roche Diagnostic Systems Inc, Mannheim, Germany). HBV genotyping was performed by direct sequencing of the small HBs region. Serum ALT levels were tested by routine biochemistry (normal range: < 45 U/L and <33 U/L for male and female respectively). Circulating HBsAg particles were obtained by immunoprecipitation as previously reported [14].

Table 1. Baseline and treatment features of study (A) and validation (B) cohorts.

Cohort	Group	Patients n.	Sera samples n.	Age years	Gender M/F	ALT U/L	HBsAg Log₁₀ UI/mL	HBV-DNA Log₁₀ UI/mL	Treatment	Response
A	Overall	61	141	50 (21–79)	40/21	52 (11–558)	3.46 (0.18–5.49)	4.45 (n.d. −>8.23)	29 Untreated, 21 IFN±NUCs, 11 NUCs	IFN: 13 SVR, 5 Rel, 3 NR. NUCs: 2 SVR, 9 OTR.
	IC	16	16	54 (32–79)	12/4	20 (11–34)	1.58 (0.18–3.22)	1.91 (n.d. −3.10)	No	
	HDV	4	4	38 (25–59)	3/1	179 (86–207)	4.25 (4.17–4.39)	1.76 (n.d. −1.98)	No	
	HBeAg pos carriers	5	5	36 (21–71)	3/2	64 (26–84)	4.84 (3.71–5.49)	7.88 (7.05–>8.23)	No	
	HBeAg neg CHB	36	116	49 (33–62)	22/14	57 (17–558)	3.57 (1.13–4.09)	4.94 (n.d −8.12)	4 Untreated, 21 IFN±NUCs, 11 NUCs	IFN: 13 SVR, 5 Rel, 3 NR. NUCs: 2 SVR, 9 OTR.
B	Overall	84	136	54 (17–79)	59/25	48 (10–2056)	3.38 (0.11–5.49)	4.87 (n.d. −>8.23)	32 Untreated, 15 IFN±NUCs, 37 NUCs	IFN: 6 SVR, 4 Rel, 5 NR. NUCs: 30 OTR.
	IC	23	23	55 (26–74)	16/7	22 (10–42)	1.43 (0.11–3.14)	1.67 (n.d. −3.13)	No	
	HBeAg pos IT	5	5	27 (19–46)	4/1	27 (19–41)	4.60 (4.41–5.49)	>8.23	No	
	HBeAg pos CHB	16	32	45 (22–67)	14/2	81 (21–374)	4.58 (2.92–5.22)	8.04 (4.53 −>8.23)	9 IFN±NUCs, 7 NUCs,	IFN: 5 SVR, 4 NR. NUCs: 4 SC, 3 OTR.
	HBeAg neg CHB	40	76	55 (17–79)	25/15	101 (13–2056)	3.47 (2.57–4.56)	5.23 (n.d. −>8.23)	4 Untreated, 6 IFN±NUCs, 30 NUCs	IFN: 1 SVR, 4 Rel, 1 NR NUCs: 30 OTR

n.d. = not detectable, SVR = Sustained virologic response, SC = HBeAg to anti-HBe seroconversion, Rel = relapse, NR = no response, OTR = on treatment response.

RNA-isolation, cDNA-synthesis and RT-q-PCR

Total RNA was extracted from 200 µL serum or HBsAg-IP (resuspended in PBS) using miRNeasy-Mini-kit (Qiagen-Inc.) as described [19]. RNA (16 µL) was reverse-transcribed and profiled on q-PCR panels in 80 µL reactions using the miRCURY-LNA Universal-RT-cDNA-Synthesis and RT-miRNA-PCR (Exiqon-A/S). The cDNA was diluted 1:50 and assayed in 10 µL PCR reactions; each miRNA was assayed once by qPCR on the Ready-to-use microRNA-PCR panels I/II containing 739-miRNA-assays. The amplification was performed in a LightCycler 480-System (Roche-Applied-Science) in 384-well-plates.

Single RT-q-PCR for each of the 6 miRNAs (miR-122-5p, miR-99a-5p, miR-192-5p, miR-126-3p, miR-335-5p and miR-320a) were used for the MiR-B-Index evaluation. Briefly, total RNA was extracted from 200 µL serum using miRCURY RNA Isolation kit (Exiqon). RNA (2 µL) was reverse-transcribed using the miR-CURY-LNA Universal-RT-cDNA-Synthesis. The cDNA was diluted 1:50 and amplified in 10 µL PCR reactions using RT-miRNA-PCR (Exiqon-A/S). The amplification was performed on LightCycler 2.0 System (Roche-Applied-Science) using specific primers to quantify each miRNA.

Data analysis and statistics

The amplification curves of miRNAs were analyzed using the Roche LC software for the quantification of cycles (Cq), by the second derivative max method, according to the recommendations of the Minimum Information for Publication of Quantitative Real-time PCR Experiments (MIQE) [20] and for the melting curve analysis. The amplification efficiency was calculated using the LinReg algorithm with criteria between 0.8–1.1 [21–22]. All assays were inspected for distinct melting curves and the Tm was checked to be within known specifications for each particular assay. Furthermore any sample assay data point to be included in the data analysis had to be detected with 5 Cq less than the corresponding negative control assay data point and with a Cq < 37 for serum samples, but 3 Cq less than the corresponding negative control assay data point and with a Cq < 37 for IP HBsAg samples due to lower signal. Data that did not pass these criteria were omitted from any further analysis. Normfinder was used to find the best normalizer candidates which in this study was the Global Mean of all assays expressed in all samples tested [23–24]. By this approach we normalised all miRNAs Cq, obtaining for each miRNA the ΔCq. In all statistical comparison we used a number of assays based on the criteria that the smallest groups of analysed cases needed data present in all samples. We subtracted the microRNAs value from the sample average (global mean), thus the larger the value, the higher is the miRNA expression in reported results. For example when we obtain a positive ΔΔCq value after subtraction, a control group mean value from an affected group mean value $2^{(\Delta Cq(affected) - \Delta Cq(Ctrl))}$ then a value of one means $2^{(1)}$, namely double as much expression for the given miRNA, on average, in the affected group. Statistics and data presentation were performed in Microsoft Excel, GraphPad Prism 6.03 and TIGR's Multiple Experiment Viewer (MEV) version 4.8 [25–26]. Correlations of miRNA profiling, MiR-B-Index and their variation over time in the different groups of HBsAg carriers were analysed by Spearman test, Mann-Whitney U-Test, Kruskal-Wallis test, Student t test, analysis of variance (ANOVA) and ANOVA for repeated measures, when appropriate. When values per group were few for ANOVA or other statistics we used the fold-change-method to evaluate up- or down-regulations using a 2-fold-change as threshold [27]. Linear regression analysis was performed to evaluate the independent variables associated with MiR-B-Index and its Δ-variation. The diagnostic performance of

Mir-B-Index for the identification of IC versus CHB patients was evaluated by ROC curve analysis; the selection of cut-off value was aimed to maximize the sensitivity (100% of IC). The statistical analyses were performed using SPSS version 19.0 (IBM Corp., Armonk, NY). The statistical significance was defined as p < 0.05, after Bonferroni correction when required.

Results

HBsAg particles miRNA profiling

A 44 miRNAs average yield was obtained from each HBsAg-pellet with an overall mean Cq of 34 after quality control (QC) and background filtering. No miRNA was expressed in all samples, therefore, normalization was performed adding the UniSp4 spike-in (RNA-spike-in-kit, Exiqon-AS) in the RNA purification process to monitor small RNA yields. When comparing the different groups (IC, untreated and treated HBeAg-negative CHB patients), we analyzed 32 miRNAs with 15 or more values across the 32 samples (37 Cq background filter value was given for missing or filtered values). Differences in the miRNAs expression (ΔCq) were observed comparing IC samples with that of BL-CHB (SVR, REL, NR) and REL/NR-post-T-FU, but not between IC and SVR-post-T-FU ones, that showed major difference with the other groups (Table 2, Figure 1). The most differentially expressed miRNAs (ΔΔCq) comparing SVR-BL-CHB to both SVR-post-T-FU and IC were miR-122-5p (ΔΔCq 2.77 and 3.34), miR-192-5p (ΔΔCq 2.35 and 2.04), miR-125b-5p (ΔΔCq 1.71 and 1.56), miR-30c-5p (ΔΔCq 1.66 and 0.92) and miR-99a-5p (ΔΔCq 1.57 and 1.30). The same miRNAs were up-regulated in all BL-CHB and REL/NR-post-T-FU. Let-7g-5p (ΔΔCq −0.33 and −0.96), miR-223-3p (ΔΔCq −0.36 and −2.22), miR-16-5p (ΔΔCq −0.43 and −1.21), miR-15a-5p (ΔΔCq −0.98 and −1.37) and miR-451a (ΔΔCq −2.07 and −1.91) were down-regulated. Differences were more evident (Table 2; Figure 1) after compiling the miRNA data of BL-CHB with REL/NR-post-T-FU and comparing them with IC and/or SVR-post-T-FU. Overall 18 miRNAs were over-expressed (ΔΔCq > 1) in all BL-CHB and in REL/NR-post-T-FU samples when compared to SVR-Post-T-FU, and 12 miRNAs when compared to IC. Only 1 and 2 miRNAs were down-regulated (ΔΔCq < −1) after comparison with SVR-post-T-FU and IC respectively. MiR-122-5p, miR-192-5p, miR-125b-5p and miR-99a-5p showed the highest up-regulation; miR-451a was down regulated in 1 of the 2 comparisons (Table 2). An unsupervised two-way hierarchical clustering of miRNAs and samples showed the clustering of IC with SVR-post-T-FU (Figure 1). Finally, we compared the most differentially expressed miRNAs (32) in ours and in the study of Novellino et al. [14] (31 miRNAs): in spite of the different platforms which were used, 9 miRNAs were consistently detected in both series, miR-19b, miR-24, miR-26a, miR-27a, miR-30b, miR-30c, miR-106b, miR-122, miR-223.

Serum miRNA profiling

In total we profiled 141 whole sera from 61 chronic carriers in different phases of HBV infection and at different time points during antiviral therapy. The overall miRNA yields were good, 152 of the 739 tested miRNAs passed background filtering and QC and 26 miRNAs were expressed in all samples after excluding only two samples because of low yields (<50 miRNAs passing filtering and QC). Of those 26 microRNAs 7, 14 and 5 assays show standard deviation <0.5, 0.5–1.0 and >1.0 respectively, after normalization. Sixty-six of the 152 miRNAs that passed the QC criteria were expressed in all samples of the smallest groups (HDV, n = 4 and HBeAg Positive, n = 5), were used in the analysis.

Table 2. Mean ΔCq values (± standard deviation) of miRNAs from HBsAg particles per groups in Peg-IFN treated patients and inactive carriers [NR-BL (A); NR-Post-T-FU (B); REL BL (C); REL-Post-T-FU (D); SVR BL (E); SVR-Post-T-FU (F); IC (G); NR, REL, SVR BL and REL/NR Post-T-FU (H)].

Assay	ΔCq (mean ± SD) per group								Group comparisons (ΔΔ Cq)			
	A	B	C	D	E	F	G	H	F-E	G-E	F-H	G-H
	NR	NR	REL	REL	SVR	SVR	IC	A+B+C+D+E				
	Baseline	Follow up	Baseline	Follow up	Baseline	Follow up						
hsa-miR-122-5p	29.91±0.58	29.78±0.36	30.55±0.98	30.14±0.90	30.89±1.14	33.67±2.05	34.23±1.66	30.33±0.91	2.77	3.34	3.34	3.90
hsa-miR-192-5p	33.38±0.62	33.10±0.72	33.46±0.97	33.30±0.86	34.10±1.41	36.44±0.56	36.14±1.41	33.51±0.97	2.35	2.04	2.93	2.63
hsa-miR-125b-5p	34.41±0.04	34.70±0.90	34.59±0.81	34.78±0.72	35.29±1.21	37.00±0.00	36.86±0.32	34.79±0.84	1.71	1.56	2.21	2.06
hsa-miR-122-3p	34.12±0.62	34.32±0.67	35.14±1.93	34.31±1.35	35.53±1.31	36.74±0.73	36.95±0.55	34.77±1.36	1.21	1.42	1.97	2.18
hsa-miR-99a-5p	34.23±0.80	33.90±0.05	35.03±1.24	34.58±1.13	35.19±1.20	36.76±0.23	36.49±0.72	34.69±1.07	1.57	1.30	2.07	1.80
hsa-miR-30c-5p	35.15±0.66	34.99±0.55	35.63±1.12	34.58±0.50	35.26±1.44	36.92±0.19	36.18±1.84	35.13±0.96	1.66	0.92	1.79	1.05
hsa-miR-27b-3p	35.35±0.68	35.49±1.32	35.54±1.14	34.87±0.83	35.56±0.83	37.12±0.27	36.21±1.76	35.35±0.91	1.56	0.66	1.77	0.86
hsa-miR-23b-3p	34.91±0.43	35.28±0.86	35.39±1.16	35.52±1.11	35.43±1.33	36.90±0.20	36.30±1.47	35.35±1.00	1.47	0.86	1.56	0.95
hsa-miR-215	34.86±1.21	34.56±0.73	35.60±0.93	35.52±1.16	36.23±0.82	37.09±0.35	37.00±0.00	35.53±1.01	0.86	0.77	1.56	1.47
hsa-miR-30b-5p	34.89±0.76	34.99±0.31	35.59±1.38	34.29±1.11	35.50±1.53	36.73±0.38	36.04±2.16	35.07±1.20	1.23	0.54	1.66	0.96
hsa-miR-26a-5p	34.78±0.62	34.84±0.34	35.50±0.95	35.32±1.32	35.41±0.96	36.90±0.34	35.84±2.59	35.24±0.92	1.49	0.43	1.66	0.60
hsa-miR-148a-3p	35.10±0.82	35.47±0.57	35.80±0.96	35.31±1.21	35.80±1.36	36.71±0.64	36.69±0.91	35.53±1.01	0.91	0.89	1.18	1.16
hsa-miR-194-5p	35.49±0.98	35.79±0.76	35.70±1.02	35.50±1.17	36.50±0.52	37.18±0.29	37.00±0.00	35.33±0.92	0.68	0.50	1.36	1.17
hsa-miR-21-5p	33.87±0.33	34.16±0.37	34.52±1.46	34.03±1.71	35.44±1.48	35.72±1.80	35.55±3.24	34.48±1.35	0.28	0.11	1.24	1.07
hsa-miR-19b-3p	34.57±0.34	34.04±0.35	35.80±1.13	34.41±1.22	35.32±1.19	35.98±1.48	35.24±2.95	34.93±1.14	0.66	-0.08	1.06	0.32
hsa-miR-92a-3p	34.47±1.30	34.71±0.99	35.26±1.01	33.81±0.42	35.17±1.18	35.29±1.33	35.56±3.05	34.70±1.06	0.12	0.40	0.58	0.86
hsa-miR-20a-5p	35.31±1.21	35.24±0.98	35.87±1.10	35.01±0.86	35.93±1.33	36.50±1.09	35.79±2.69	35.51±1.07	0.57	-0.13	0.99	0.28
hsa-miR-101-3p	34.64±0.70	34.45±0.72	34.66±1.20	34.29±0.89	35.18±1.45	35.42±1.39	35.26±2.25	34.66±1.04	0.24	0.08	0.76	0.60
hsa-miR-103a-3p	36.08±0.61	35.72±0.64	36.50±0.59	35.33±1.18	35.86±1.20	36.74±0.58	35.84±2.74	35.50±0.94	0.88	-0.02	0.84	-0.06
hsa-miR-125a-5p	35.63±1.76	34.95±1.80	35.63±1.31	35.61±2.15	35.34±1.54	34.83±1.38	36.60±0.54	35.46±1.56	-0.51	1.26	-0.63	1.14
hsa-miR-24-3p	35.22±0.55	35.15±0.40	36.15±1.04	35.64±0.92	36.19±0.88	36.89±0.15	35.61±2.66	35.77±0.88	0.70	-0.58	1.12	-0.16
hsa-miR-107	36.26±0.68	36.85±0.23	36.50±0.59	35.57±1.16	36.30±0.79	37.00±0.01	36.01±2.25	36.25±0.84	0.71	-0.29	0.76	-0.24
hsa-miR-450b-3p	36.51±0.62	36.19±0.60	36.71±0.65	36.64±0.36	36.41±0.99	36.44±0.55	36.79±0.47	36.52±0.64	0.02	0.38	-0.08	0.27
hsa-miR-106a-5p	35.82±0.42	36.11±1.12	35.94±1.16	35.92±1.13	36.37±0.61	36.88±0.38	35.58±2.38	36.04±0.88	0.51	-0.79	0.83	-0.47
hsa-let-7b-5p	35.04±0.60	36.33±1.25	35.49±1.28	35.76±0.78	36.77±0.41	36.51±0.67	36.16±1.88	35.91±1.02	-0.26	-0.61	0.60	0.25
hsa-miR-27a-3p	36.56±0.60	36.31±0.27	36.69±0.57	36.09±0.51	36.50±0.92	36.89±0.26	35.87±2.52	36.43±0.62	0.38	-0.63	0.46	-0.56
hsa-miR-320a	36.07±0.89	35.70±1.24	35.89±1.20	34.79±0.82	35.93±0.91	36.09±0.99	35.29±2.40	35.64±1.03	0.16	-0.63	0.45	-0.34
hsa-let-7g-5p	35.89±0.83	35.95±1.02	36.56±0.46	36.10±0.76	36.92±0.18	36.59±0.69	35.96±2.15	36.35±0.71	-0.33	-0.96	0.23	-0.39
hsa-miR-16-5p	36.63±0.72	36.63±0.42	36.20±0.90	36.39±0.74	36.87±0.28	36.44±1.04	35.66±3.00	36.53±0.65	-0.43	-1.21	-0.09	-0.87
hsa-miR-15a-5p	36.00±0.98	36.41±1.03	35.95±0.75	35.39±0.56	36.79±0.70	35.81±1.71	35.42±2.95	36.09±0.86	-0.98	-1.37	-0.28	-0.67
hsa-miR-223-3p	34.90±1.42	36.16±0.93	36.59±0.66	35.86±1.35	35.94±1.12	35.58±1.80	33.73±3.41	35.96±1.13	-0.36	-2.22	-0.38	-2.23

Table 2. Cont.

Assay	ΔCq (mean ± SD) per group								Group comparisons (ΔΔ Cq)			
	A	B	C	D	E	F	G	H	F-E	G-E	F-H	G-H
	NR	NR	REL	REL	SVR	SVR	IC	A+B+C+D+E				
	Baseline	Follow up	Baseline	Follow up	Baseline	Follow up						
hsa-miR-451a	33.40±1.04	36.05±1.43	35.66±1.31	35.31±1.92	35.7¹ ±1.40	33.63±2.79	33.79±3.50	35.32±1.58	−2.07	−1.91	−1.69	−1.53

On the right comparisons between groups F and E; G and E; F and H; G and H.

The dataset was normalized using the global mean (n = 26 assays) method [24].

Untreated HBV Carriers. One way ANOVA (after Bonferroni correction, cut-off p = 0.000758) revealed 31 miRNAs with significantly different expression: the largest differences were primarily observed between IC and both HBeAg positive and negative CHB, secondly between HBeAg-positive and HBeAg-negative CHB (Table 3). Among HBeAg positive carriers the miRNA profiling of one immune tolerant carrier was comparable to those of the other 4 patients with CHB. The statistical power of comparisons between HBeAg-positive CHB and HDV/CHB was weakened by the small sample size. Since several miRNAs from HBeAg-negative-CHB failed the Shapiro-Wilk normality test (data not shown), we used individual Wilcoxon, Mann-Whitney U tests yielding very similar results (Table 3). Significant differences were found between IC and CHB patients and the most significant ones affected the same miRNAs showing the largest difference in HBsAg particles of CHB patients and IC, namely miRNA-122-5p (ANOVA and U test p-values: <0.000001 and 0.000001 respectively); miRNA-192-5p (ANOVA and U test p-values: < 0.000001 and 0.000005); miRNA-99a-5p (ANOVA and U test p-values: <0.000001 and 0.000003). Other miRNAs with the largest differences were miR-148a-3p (ANOVA and U test p-values: < 0.000001 and 0.000009) and miR-126-3p (ANOVA and U test p-values: <0.000001 and 0.003751). Overall CHB patients showed significantly more liver specific miRNAs than IC. The IC miRNA profile correlated with that of subjects without liver disease of Wang et al. [28] who used the miRCURY qPCR platform [correlations between (n = 47 assays) mean un-normalized-ΔCq values (40-Cq) Pearson-r = .9470, r^2 = .8968, p<0.000000001; Spearman-ρ = 0.9373, p<0.000000001, data not shown].

Peg-IFN treated patients. The effect of Peg-IFN on the circulating miRNA profile of HBeAg-negative-CHB was studied comparing BL and week 12 sera in 14 cases [6 SVR, 5 REL and 3 NR]: 8 miRNAs were differentially expressed, but only miR-30e-3p was significantly up-regulated in all patients' sera after Bonferroni adjustment (ΔΔCq 1.7, p = 0.000354, Table 4). Otherwise, only minor differences were seen, indicating that the overall whole serum miRNA profiling did not change significantly after 12 weeks of IFN treatment. Next we looked at the dynamic variation of miRNA profiles during (BL, week 12, 24 and EOT) and after therapy (week 24 post-T-FU) according to treatment response (Table 5). NR did not show, by ANOVA analysis, any significant changes throughout the entire observation period. REL revealed one miRNA, let-7b-5p, with significant differential expression over the 5 time-points. SVR during treatment had significant changes in 5 miRNAs, namely miR-122-5p, miR-21-5p, miR-99a-5p, miR-23a-3p and miR-192-5p. MiR-99a-5p and miR-192-5p were always down-regulated on treatment; miR-21-5p was up-regulated at weeks 12 and 24 and EOT, returning to baseline values at Post-T-FU. MiR-23a-3p was up-regulated over the course of treatment and subsequent follow-up. Comparing NR and REL to SVR, at the different time-points, by one-way ANOVA a total of 21 miRNA resulted significantly differentially expressed, after Bonferroni correction (Table 6): miR-320a and miR-320b and miR-335-5p at week 24 during treatment, but not at other time points; miR-99a-5p at EOT and at 24 week post-T-FU. At EOT additional miRNAs, like miR-122-3p and -5p, miR-192-5p and miR-194, were differentially expressed between the groups as compared to post-T-FU, but the differences did not achieve statistical significance after Bonferroni correction.

NUCs treated patients. All HBeAg negative CHB patients treated with NUCs had undetectable HBV-DNA and ALT within the normal range at EOF/post-T-FU evaluation, that was done 59

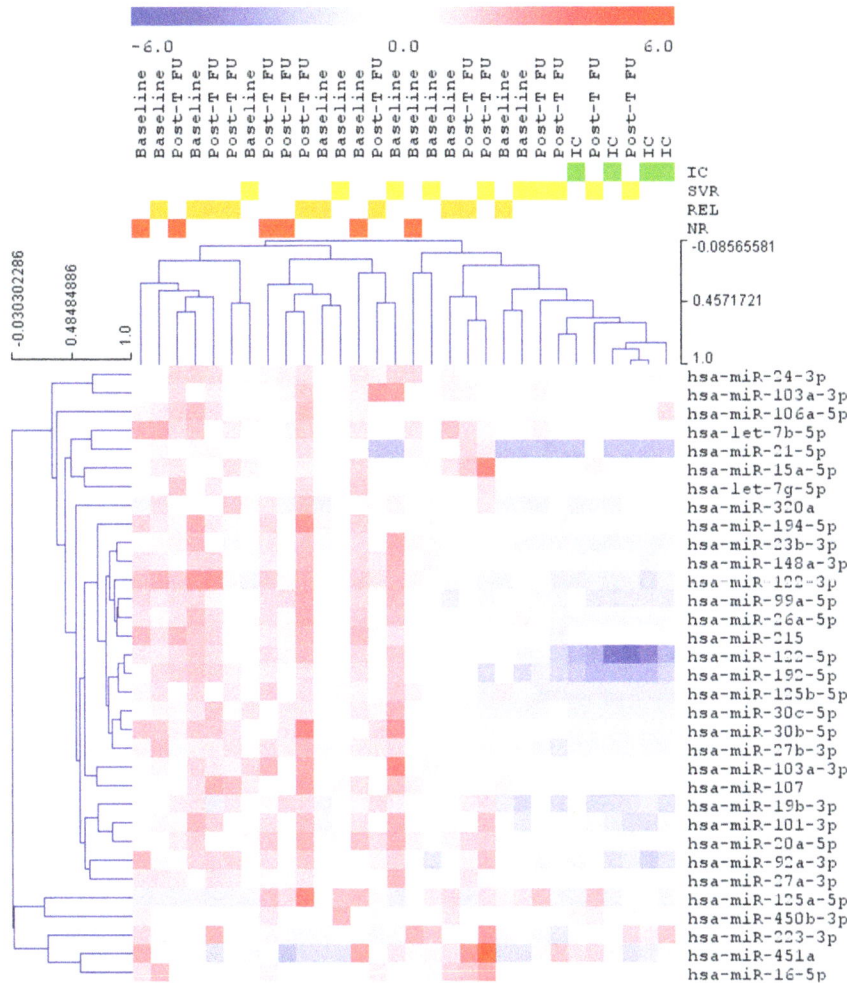

Figure 1. Hierarchical clustering of miRNAs from HBsAg particles and samples. The heatmap shows the result of the two-way hierarchical clustering of miRNAs from HBsAg particles and samples (zero centered). The colour scale shown at the top illustrates the relative expression level of a miRNA across all samples: red colour represents an expression level above mean, blue colour represents expression lower than the mean. The SVR post-T FU (Peg-IFN treated patients) group clusters with the IC group.

(33–144) months after treatment start. Comparing the miRNA profiling in baseline and end of follow-up sera we observed an overall reduction in liver specific miRNAs: miR-122, miR-192 and miR-99a ($\Delta\Delta$Cqs of 2.28, 1.77 and 1.35 and p = 0.02, 0.04 and 0.09 respectively). However, only miR-148a-3p showed a significant difference (p = 0.00072) after Bonferroni adjustment.

MiR-B-Index, miRNA calculator. We exploited the 3 hepatocellular miRNAs (miR-122-5p+miR-99a-5p+miR-192-5p) with the most significant differential expression in IC versus CHB to build a miRNA calculator. Three additional miRNAs: miR-335 (detected in all serum samples regardless of grouping, and not detected in IP-HBsAg samples), miRNA-126 (down-regulated in serum samples, CHB versus IC, and not detected in IP HBsAg samples) and miR-320a (stable across groups in both serum samples and IP HBsAg) were selected as endogenous controls to account for RNA input variation and other technical variations within the profiling platform. We define this miRNA panel calculator [(Cq miR-122-5p+Cq miR-99a-5p+Cq miR-192-5p) −(Cq miR-126-3p+Cq miR-335-5p+Cq miR-320a)] as MiR-B-Index.

Overall the median MiR-B-Index value in untreated HBV carriers was −4.52 (−16.12/10.91), with significant differences

among groups: −15.82 in IT carriers, −13.31 (−16.12/−11.27) in HBeAg positive CHB, −5.38 (−10.71/5.72) in HBeAg negative CHB, −7.36 (−8.85/4.86) in HBV/HDV CH and 5.28 (−1.65/10.91) in IC (p<0.001). Using MiR-B-Index as binary classifier we made a receiver operating characteristic (ROC) curve separating IC versus: a) patients with CHB either HBeAg positive, negative or HBV/HDV [Active Liver Disease group 1 (ALD1); Figure 2A] and b) HBeAg negative CHB [Active Liver Disease group 2 (ALD2); Figure 2B]. The AUROCs of MiR-B-Index to identify IC from ALD1 and ALD2 were 0.9520 (95% CI 0.903–1.000, p< 0.001, Figure 2A) and 0.954 (95% CI 0.902–1.000, p<0.001, Figure 2B), respectively. By using a cut-off value of −1.7 while classifying IC from ALD1 and ALD2, 100% sensitivity, 84.4 and 83.3% specificity, 69.6% and 72.7% PPVs, 100% NPVs, 88.5% diagnostic accuracy (DA) were achieved.

In the 21 Peg-IFN treated patients the median BL and post-T-FU MiR-B-Index values were significantly different [−5.81 (−10.71/5.72) and 3.76 (−12.99/9.53) respectively, p = 0.022]. At BL MiR-B-Index values were higher in SVR (−4.49, −10.71/5.72) as compared to REL (−7.23, −9.99/−5.81) and NR (−7.56, −7.93/−7.26), p = 0.047: the difference resulted from the MiR-B-Index values (median 3.70, −0.77/5.72) observed in 4

Table 3. One-way ANOVA and Wilcoxon Mann Whitney U test in 61 untreated HBV carriers: 31 miRNAs (out of 66 tested) showed significant differential expression after either ANOVA or the U test on the four group comparison (Bonferroni multiple testing cut-off = 0.000758).

| Assay | ANOVA | | | | | Wilcoxon Mann-Whitney U test | | | | | |
| | ΔCq (mean ± SD) per group | | | | p value | p value | | | | | |
	HBeAg Ne CHB	HDV	IC	HBeAg pos CHB		IC vs HBeAg Neg	HDV vs HBeAg Neg	HBeAg pos vs HBeAg Neg	HDV vs IC	HBeAg pos vs IC	HDV vs HBeAg pos
hsa-miR-122-5p	3.87±1.81	3.21±2.24	0.33±1.16	5.81±0.39	<0.000001	0.000001	0.429017	0.001182	0.035729	0.001063	0.014306
hsa-miR-148a-3p	-0.66±0.95	-0.92±0.99	-2.47±0.79	1.01±0.59	<0.000001	0.000009	0.557818	0.000708	0.031450	0.001357	0.014306
hsa-miR-192-5p	0.18±1.71	0.04±2.03	-3.33±1.60	2.39±0.46	<0.000001	0.000005	0.895133	0.000781	0.019472	0.001194	0.014306
hsa-miR-126-3p	1.03±0.60	0.88±0.15	1.66±0.61	-0.78±0.92	<0.000001	0.003751	0.455102	0.000588	0.016395	0.001063	0.014306
hsa-miR-99a-5p	-0.33±1.60	-0.95±2.11	-3.05±0.85	1.66±0.33	<0.000001	0.000003	0.470703	0.001250	0.071861	0.001063	0.014306
hsa-miR-142-3p	0.80±0.77	0.86±0.31	1.57±0.65	-1.11±0.80	<0.000001	0.001467	0.792069	0.001182	0.045500	0.001063	0.014306
hsa-miR-142-5p	-3.82±0.98	-3.86±0.50	-2.58±0.86	-5.92±0.92	<0.000001	0.000322	0.835705	0.001260	0.021448	0.001063	0.014306
hsa-miR-223-3p	2.01±0.95	2.63±0.82	3.06±0.38	0.05±1.15	<0.000001	0.000051	0.173178	0.004865	0.317311	0.001063	0.027486
hsa-miR-194-5p	-1.46±1.68	-1.59±1.90	-4.39±1.32	1.09±0.59	<0.000001	0.000074	0.758415	0.000509	0.036714	0.001837	0.014306
hsa-miR-424-5p	-1.61±0.78	-1.56±0.40	-0.84±0.33	-3.77±1.42	<0.000001	0.004321	0.958650	0.002351	0.016210	0.002200	0.014306
hsa-miR-215	-1.39±1.80	-1.58±2.15	-4.39±1.28	1.09±0.47	<0.000001	0.000067	0.929976	0.000898	0.026453	0.001837	0.014306
hsa-miR-378a-3p	-1.81±0.93	-2.20±1.22	-3.26±0.58	-0.63±0.42	0.000001	0.000026	0.475551	0.004282	0.141032	0.001357	0.027486
hsa-miR-30b-5p	-0.42±0.87	-0.44±0.63	-1.07±0.53	1.40±0.37	0.000001	0.004263	0.895133	0.000380	0.109599	0.001063	0.014306
hsa-miR-15b-5p	-1.31±0.82	-1.27±0.63	-0.40±0.41	-2.51±0.32	0.000002	0.000168	0.928155	0.003633	0.021448	0.001063	0.014306
hsa-miR-23a-3p	-0.41±0.57	0.17±0.33	0.37±0.41	-1.20±0.71	0.000004	0.000033	0.030464	0.065087	0.317311	0.007686	0.033895
hsa-miR-27b-3p	-0.50±0.77	-0.52±0.70	-1.25±0.39	0.80±0.40	0.000004	0.000220	0.964041	0.001087	0.071015	0.001194	0.014306
hsa-miR-23b-3p	-0.56±1.23	-1.01±1.02	-1.73±0.44	1.24±0.63	0.000008	0.000393	0.379537	0.001549	0.133614	0.001063	0.014306
hsa-miR-365a-3p	-3.15±1.48	-4.11±2.39	-5.47±0.61	-1.51±0.60	0.000011	0.000228	0.354539	0.007391	0.157299	0.002200	0.014306
hsa-miR-26b-5p	-1.49±0.57	-1.60±0.47	-1.89±0.62	-0.22±0.51	0.000012	0.026989	0.792069	0.000781	0.317311	0.001944	0.014306
hsa-miR-122-3p	-1.05±2.00	-1.52±2.02	-4.45±1.80	1.80±0.45	0.000012	0.000785	0.458902	0.000638	0.058782	0.004483	0.014306
hsa-miR-34a-5p	-3.22±1.53	-3.96±2.10	-5.62±0.71	-3.19±1.60	0.000190	0.000023	0.598020	0.861255	0.117185	0.001837	0.806496
hsa-miR-30c-5p	-0.42±1.01	-0.72±0.86	-1.19±0.51	1.22±0.37	0.000025	0.002531	0.356170	0.001031	0.161513	0.001063	0.014306
hsa-let-7i-5p	-3.07±1.02	-2.88±0.84	-2.26±0.54	-4.64±0.52	0.000038	0.001100	0.724571	0.003881	0.230139	0.001063	0.014306
hsa-miR-30d-5p	-4.42±0.47	-4.21±0.15	-4.72±0.46	-3.45±0.53	0.000043	0.093959	0.186630	0.003558	0.071015	0.004104	0.086411
hsa-miR-93-5p	-1.05±0.78	-0.58±0.93	-0.36±0.48	-1.54±0.13	0.002882	0.000051	0.235499	0.020837	0.548506	0.001063	0.141645
hsa-miR-16-5p	0.95±1.27	1.73±1.08	2.12±0.77	-0.81±1.25	0.000058	0.000771	0.202597	0.015205	0.271332	0.001063	0.014306
hsa-miR-30e-3p	-3.75±1.17	-4.15±0.69	-5.05±1.23	-2.21±0.25	0.000067	0.000654	0.211352	0.000859	0.111164	0.001194	0.014306
hsa-miR-21-5p	2.28±0.50	2.41±0.70	1.56±0.59	2.13±0.30	0.000345	0.000165	0.598020	0.521622	0.057433	0.026026	0.462433
hsa-miR-103a-3p	0.23±0.37	0.10±0.15	0.70±0.34	0.19±0.78	0.001603	0.000210	0.660390	0.268329	0.009322	0.073553	0.624206

Table 3. Cont.

Assay	ANOVA ΔCq (mean ± SD) per group					Wilcoxon Mann-Whitney U test p value					
	HBeAg Ne CHB	HDV	IC	HBeAg pos CHB	p value	IC vs HBeAg Neg	HDV vs HBeAg Neg	HBeAg pos vs HBeAg Neg	HDV vs IC	HBeAg pos vs IC	HBeAg pos vs HDV
hsa-miR-152	-3.68±0.64	-4.38±0.56	-4.44±0.64	-3.42±0.52	0.000682	0.000240	0.034097	0.380758	1.000000	0.007256	0.027486
hsa-miR-15a-5p	1.22±0.98	1.38±0.78	1.84±0.74	-0.29±0.40	0.000304	0.016691	0.792069	0.000898	0.230139	0.001063	0.014306

patients, whose HBV-DNA (4.45, 2.67–5.19 Log_{10} IU/mL) and HBsAg (2.48, 1.13–3.54 Log_{10} IU/mL) levels were lower than in the remaining 8 (HBV-DNA: 5.83, 0.78–7.42 Log_{10} IU/mL; HBsAg 3.5, 2.87–4.09 Log_{10} IU/mL, p = 0.123 and p = 0.045, respectively) with MiR-B-Index (−5.03, −10.71/−3.27) comparable to REL/NR (−7.41, −9.99/−5.81). At 24 week post-T-FU in SVR MiR-B-Index values were significantly higher (5.32, 0.54/9.53) as compared to REL (−7.41, −12.99/−1.87) and NR (−6.31, −7.37/−5.92), p = 0.001: all SVR had values above the −1.7 MiR-B-Index cut-off (Figure 2C–D). On treatment MiR-B-Index kinetics were studied in 14 patients: at EOT MiR-B-Index increase was observed in all SVR (2.02, −2.06/5.84), 4 with values >−1.7 (Figure 2C), but not in REL and NR (−9.49, −11.65/−3.58 and −8.82, −12.17/−3.99, respectively), p = 0.008.

Overall in the 11 NUCs treated patients MiR-B-Index showed a trend to improve [BL vs post-T-FU median values −5.86 (−13.39/6.57) vs 0.12 (−8.41/9.46), p = 0.071]. The MiR-B-Index increase did not correlate with treatment duration ($\rho = 0.127$, p = 0.709). In 5 patients whose MiR-B-Index increased above the −1.7 cut-off antiviral therapy was discontinued because of HBsAg/anti-HBs seroconversion in 2 while serum HBsAg levels dropped below 400 IU/mL (14.6, 300 and 380 IU/mL) in the remaining 3 who continued treatment. The MiR-B-Index of the 2 NUC-treated patients with HBsAg/anti-HBs seroconversion (9.46 and 7.08) were comparable with IFN-SVRs at post-T-FU (5.32, 0.54/9.53).

Validation of MiR-B-Index. The MiR-B-Index was retested in 15 samples of the training cohort using single microRNA specific RT-q-PCR and showed values highly comparable with those obtained by Ready to use micro-RNA-PCR panel I/II (data not shown). In untreated HBV carriers the median MiR-B-Index values were −6.07 (−20.43/14.38), with significant variation between groups: −11.17 (−20.43/−7.73) in IT, −14.20 (−18.06/−4.63) in HBeAg positive CHB, −6.82 (−18.42/−0.18) in HBeAg negative CHB and 7.29 (−1.41/14.38) in IC (p<0.001). We ran a ROC curve analysis to discriminate IC from HBeAg negative CHB and the AUROC value was 0.995 (95% CI 0.984–1.000; p<0.000001). The MiR-B-Index values ≥−1.7 identified IC with 100% sensitivity, 92.5% specificity, 88.5% PPV, 100% NPV and 95.2% diagnostic accuracy. In the 15 Peg-IFN treated patients (9 HBeAg positive) the MiR-B-Index at 24 week post-T-FU was significantly different from BL [−4.24 (−16.80/5.94) vs −14.20 (−18.06/−7.25), p<0.001] and showed significantly higher values in SVR patients as compared to REL/NR [2.9 (0.07/5.94) vs −7.04 (−16.80/−4.09), p = 0.001]. Overall, MiR-B-Index increased in the 37 NUCs treated patients [BL vs post-T-FU median values −6.73 (−18.42/−0.33) vs 0.07 (−9.54/4.17), p<0.000001].

MiR-B-Index and ALT, HBV-DNA and HBsAg serum levels. Because the MiR-B-Index performance was highly comparable in both training and validation cohorts, the correlation between its values and ALT, HBV-DNA and HBsAg serum levels were performed combining the 2 cohorts.

Overall at BL MiR-B-Index (−5.72, −20.43/14.38) showed a significant correlation with ALT (49, 10/2056 U/l, $\rho = -0.497$, p<0.001), HBV-DNA (4.58, undetectable/>8.3 Log_{10} IU/mL, $\rho = -0.732$, p<0.001) and HBsAg serum levels (3.40, 0.11–5.49 Log_{10} IU/mL, $\rho = -0.883$, p<0.001). When we considered ALT values by class (≤40, 41–80, 81–120, >120 U/L) we found that MiR-B-Index values in patients with ALT ≤40 U/L were significantly higher than the others (p<0.000001) whereas they were similar in the 3 groups with ALT>40 U/L [−7.23 (−20.43/6.57) vs −8.64 (−18.42/−2.21) vs −6.59 (−16.99/4.86), p = 0.102]. Immune Tolerant carriers in spite of normal ALT as

Inactive Carriers (26, 19–41 U/L vs 20, 10–42 U/L), had MiR-B-Index values significantly different from IC [−11.61 (−20.43/−7.73) vs 6.68 (−1.65/14.38), p<0.001], but comparable to those of HBeAg positive CHB patients [−14.47 (−18.06/−4.63), p = 1.00]. At multivariate analysis factors independently associated with MiR-B-Index were HBV-DNA (p = 0.002) and HBsAg (p<0.001) serum levels, phase of HBV infection (IC, IT, HBV/HDV, HBeAg positive and HBeAg negative CHB; p<0.001), but not ALT values (p = 0.360).

HBsAg serum levels were significantly correlated with MiR-B-Index in untreated carriers [IC, IT, HBeAg-positive and negative CHB at BL: HBsAg 3.38, 0.11–5.49 Log_{10} IU/mL and MiR-B-Index −5.61 (−20.43/14.38); $\rho = -0.904$, p<0.001), but not in the post-T-FU sera of IFN-SVR patients (HBsAg 1.29, undetectable/2.70 Log_{10} IU/mL; MiR-B-Index 4.96, 0.07/9.53; $\rho = -0.423$, p = 0.08). In NUC-treated patients MiR-B-Index increased significantly from BL to EOF independently of the extent of HBsAg decline [BL and EOF MiR-B-Index values in patients with >1 log HBsAg decline −6.56 (−18.42/0.37) vs 1.99 (−3.46/14.17), p<0.001; BL and EOF MiR-B-Index values in patients with <1 log HBsAg decline −6.62 (−15.18/6.57) vs −1.25 (−9.54/9.22), p<0.001]. The MiR-B-Index Δ-variation from BL to EOF was significantly higher in patients with HBsAg decline >1 log [12.56 (4.88/19.39) vs 5.03 (−5.97/15.95), p<0.001) and associated with BL MiR-B-Index values ($\rho = -0.450$, p = 0.001), NUC treatment duration ($\rho = 0.310$, p = 0.032), BL HBsAg serum levels ($\rho = -0.320$, p = 0.039) and HBsAg Δ-variation from BL to EOF ($\rho = -0.663$, p<0.0001), but not with BL ALT and HBV-DNA levels. At multivariate analysis only BL MiR-B-Index values (p = 0.007) and HBsAg Δ-variation between BL and EOF (p = 0.002) resulted independently associated with the Δ-decline of MiR-B-Index.

Discussion

The study of serum miRNA of well characterized HBsAg carriers shows important variations of their profiles across the different phases of chronic HBV infection: the major difference is observed between inactive carriers and chronic hepatitis patients, who show a highly significant over-expression of miR-122-5p, miR-99a-5p and miR-192-5p (Table 3). The same miRNAs reveal a consonant profile in circulating HBsAg-particles, where major differences in the expression of the 32 most commonly detected miRNAs, were observed when comparing IC to untreated CHB

patients. In patients with SVR to Peg-IFN the post-T-FU sera presented miRNA profiles highly similar to IC (Table 2) and the heatmap demonstrated the clustering of these 2 groups (IC and SVR-post-T-FU samples; Figure 1). On the contrary, in Relapsers and Non Responders the post-T-FU miRNAs patterns matched those of BL. These findings support the hypothesis that consistent changes in circulating miRNA profiles parallel the immune control of HBV infection. Accordingly, CHB patients with SVR to Peg-IFN, at variance with REL and NR, experienced the largest difference in their serum miRNA signature overtime, with major variations of the miRNA average signal (ΔCq) when comparing post-T-FU with BL samples (Table 2; Figure 1). In 14 patients whose miRNA profiles could be studied across their whole treatment course we observed that serum miRNA patterns did not change significantly during the first 12 weeks of Peg-IFN, with the exception of miR-30e-3p, that was up-regulated in all patients (Table 4; p = 0.000354). Our finding is in agreement with a previous report suggesting an early induction of the miRs-30 cluster by IFN independently of therapy response [26]. During the course of treatment, NR patients did not show any significant variation of additional miRNAs, whereas REL had significant differential expression over the 5 time-points of miRNA let-7b-5p (Table 5). The implications of such miRNA modulation deserve further investigation since the up-regulation of let-7 family during IFN therapy was reported to inhibit hepatitis C virus replication [29]. The comparison of NR/REL and SVR at every time point (Table 6) showed that 21 miRNAs were differentially expressed and 5 of them, miR-122-5p, miR-21-5p, miR-23a-3p, miR-99a-5p and miR-192-5p had the most significant changes during treatment in SVR. MiRNA-99a-5p and miRNA-192-5p were down-regulated throughout treatment and post-T-FU, whereas miRNA-21-5p was up-regulated at week 12, 24 and EOT and returned to BL-values at post-T-FU. Interestingly miR-122-5p, miR-99a-5p and miR-192-5p showed parallel differential patterns in whole serum and HBsAg-particles of IC and CHB patients once they achieved SVR as compared to untreated CHB and REL/NR. These 3 miRNAs are the 1st, 2nd and 6th most represented miRNAs of human liver [16,28]: serum miR-122 and miR-99 levels had been shown to be higher in HBsAg carriers than healthy controls [16] and miR-122 and miR-192 associated with liver necro-inflammation [30–34].

The findings prompted us to evaluate a combination of the most significant miRNAs to produce a MiR-B-Index to identify the sustained switch from active to inactive HBV infection in treated

Table 4. Differentially expressed miRNAs comparing Baseline (BL) and Week 12 (Wk 12) sera in 14 Peg-IFN HBeAg negative CHB patients.

Assay	ΔCq (mean ± SD)		ΔΔCq	Student's t test
	BL	Wk 12	Wk 12 - BL	p value
hsa-miR-30e-3p	−3.26±0.51	−1.52±1.35	1.74	0.000354
hsa-let-7b-5p	−0.51±0.27	−0.10±0.31	0.41	0.001731
hsa-miR-27a-3p	−0.56±0.46	−1.06±0.48	−0.50	0.014224
hsa-miR-142-5p	−4.41±0.55	−4.97±0.48	−0.56	0.019861
hsa-miR-29c-3p	−2.34±0.33	−2.02±0.35	0.32	0.027692
hsa-miR-590-5p	−4.01±0.69	−4.72±0.76	−0.71	0.030467
hsa-miR-32-5p	−3.73±0.78	−3.15±0.50	0.57	0.040616
hsa-miR-378a-3p	−1.17±0.65	−1.71±0.57	−0.54	0.042229

Of the 8 miRNAs presenting p<0.05 only miR-30e-3p passes the Bonferroni correction (cut-off <0.000758) for multiple testing (ΔΔCq 1.7 up-regulation, p = 0.000354).

Table 5. Dynamic variation of miRNA profiles at Baseline (BL), during (week 12, 24 and End of Treatment, EOT) and after therapy (week 24 post-treatment follow-up, PT-FU) according to treatment response (NR, REL, SVR) in 14 Peg-IFN treated patients.

Treatment response	Assay	ΔCq (mean ± SD)					ANOVA p-value
		BL	Wk 12	Wk 24	EOT	PT-FU	
NR	hsa-miR-24-3p	-0.18±0.25	0.42±0.18	0.47±0.17	0.07±0.33	-0.02±0.12	0.020606
	hsa-miR-335-5p	-3.49±0.29	-2.85±0.36	-3.58±0.27	-3.16±0.23	-2.63±0.52	0.032632
	hsa-miR-103a-3p	-0.07±0.11	-0.24±0.07	0.23±0.26	0.01±0.09	-0.20±0.21	0.035818
REL	hsa-let-7b-5p	-0.33±0.23	0.13±0.26	0.16±0.17	-0.19±0.28	-0.49±0.17	0.000054
	hsa-miR-451a	3.15±0.95	4.98±1.50	5.10±1.78	4.38±0.75	2.41±0.91	0.009256
	hsa-miR-92a-3p	2.36±0.55	2.33±0.62	2.39±0.60	1.99±0.21	1.43±0.27	0.022724
	hsa-miR-27a-3p	-0.72±0.33	-1.26±0.37	-1.01±0.52	-0.81±0.53	-0.32±0.32	0.028419
	hsa-miR-24-3p	0.52±0.34	0.08±0.26	0.23±0.17	0.26±0.12	0.13±0.05	0.038510
SVR	hsa-miR-122-5p	3.67±1.50	4.75±1.04	3.67±1.33	3.02±0.84	0.96±1.08	0.000001
	hsa-miR-21-5p	2.24±0.41	3.18±0.69	3.22±0.44	3.53±0.45	2.31±0.72	0.000026
	hsa-miR-99a-5p	-0.58±1.39	0.13±0.95	-1.03±1.09	-1.76±0.80	-2.49±0.51	0.000063
	hsa-miR-23a-3p	-0.26±0.50	-0.40±0.59	-0.04±0.54	0.32±0.23	0.55±0.28	0.000083
	hsa-miR-192-5p	-0.30±1.98	0.80±1.05	-0.40±1.57	-0.94±1.34	-2.96±1.46	0.000592
	hsa-miR-27a-3p	-0.31±0.43	-0.76±0.59	-0.61±0.57	-0.31±0.19	0.10±0.37	0.001911
	hsa-miR-23b-3p	-0.59±1.02	-0.74±0.92	-1.58±0.80	-2.04±0.60	-1.65±0.62	0.002195
	hsa-miR-215	-1.79±1.94	-0.63±1.29	-2.15±1.70	-2.93±1.55	-4.27±1.42	0.002369
	hsa-miR-142-3p	1.16±0.69	0.71±0.47	1.15±0.47	1.33±0.38	1.80±0.40	0.002439
	hsa-miR-223-3p	2.05±0.85	1.71±0.87	2.50±0.88	2.64±0.42	3.00±0.45	0.003421

Statistical analysis by one way ANOVA.

Table 6. Comparison of miRNA profile of SVR vs NR and REL at different time points by Student's t test analysis: a total of 21 miRNA (out of 66 tested) showed significant differential expression after Bonferroni correction (cut-off<0.000758).

| Assay | ΔCq values (mean±SD) at different time points in treated patients by response | | | | | | | | | | | | | | |
| | Baseline | | | Wk 12 | | | Wk 24 | | | EOT | | | PT-FU | | |
	NR/REL	SVR	p value	NR/REL	SVR	p value	NR/REL	SVR	p value	NR/REL	SVR	p value	NR/REL	SVR	p value
hsa-miR-99a-5p	0.75±0.61	−0.58±1.39	0.021340	0.61±0.49	0.13±0.95	0.243917	0.48±1.14	−1.03±1.09	0.027866	0.58±0.89	−1.76±0.80	0.000271	0.48±0.64	−2.49±0.51	<0.000001
hsa-miR-122-5p	4.83±0.44	3.67±1.50	0.048059	5.20±0.45	4.75±1.04	0.292392	4.84±1.24	3.67±1.33	0.116944	4.98±0.83	3.02±0.84	0.000949	4.62±0.80	0.96±1.08	<0.000001
hsa-miR-194-5p	−0.22±0.43	−1.78±1.88	0.032860	0.17±0.49	−0.90±1.07	0.028206	−0.09±1.23	−2.17±1.88	0.027077	−0.11±1.09	−2.80±1.23	0.001648	−0.40±0.85	−4.22±0.99	0.000001
hsa-miR-192-5p	1.34±0.45	−0.30±1.98	0.033972	1.79±0.59	0.80±1.05	0.044638	1.60±1.15	−0.40±1.57	0.016877	1.66±0.96	−0.94±1.34	0.001802	1.30±0.71	−2.96±1.46	0.000001
hsa-miR-122-3p	0.45±1.05	−1.60±2.33	0.032246	0.45±0.93	−0.60±1.91	0.196555	0.68±1.34	−2.63±2.34	0.005641	0.00±1.04	−3.26±1.95	0.002170	−0.02±0.94	−3.93±1.03	0.000002
hsa-miR-30b-5p	0.10±0.40	−0.45±0.75	0.077031	0.32±0.62	−0.43±0.96	0.100295	0.33±0.80	−0.94±0.96	0.018803	0.22±0.77	−1.35±0.85	0.003482	0.29±0.57	−1.28±0.50	0.000002
hsa-miR-23b-3p	0.25±0.84	−0.59±1.02	0.065659	−0.22±0.55	−0.74±0.92	0.213548	−0.16±0.87	−1.58±0.80	0.008788	−0.43±0.79	−2.04±0.60	0.001333	0.00±0.49	−1.65±0.62	0.000004
hsa-miR-215	0.00±0.68	−1.79±1.94	0.021694	0.26±0.59	−0.63±1.29	0.105766	−0.03±1.27	−2.15±1.70	0.020575	0.13±0.96	−2.93±1.55	0.000983	−0.41±0.87	−4.27±1.42	0.000008
hsa-miR-27b-3p	−0.02±0.52	−0.50±0.76	0.134757	−0.07±0.30	−0.04±0.51	0.903444	−0.06±0.87	−0.76±0.49	0.102072	−0.25±0.61	−0.92±0.43	0.039902	−0.14±0.55	−1.09±0.25	0.000053
hsa-miR-16-5p	0.24±0.94	0.93±0.81	0.087366	0.72±0.78	0.49±0.96	0.632638	0.53±1.04	1.30±0.79	0.155772	0.68±0.88	1.56±0.72	0.069830	0.41±0.71	1.68±0.43	0.000053
hsa-miR-30c-5p	0.39±0.67	−0.47±0.69	0.011765	0.16±0.52	−0.35±1.05	0.247105	0.23±0.91	−0.94±0.93	0.036705	0.02±0.69	−1.34±0.65	0.002911	0.20±0.56	−1.24±0.67	0.000068
hsa-miR-451a	4.21±1.66	5.14±1.55	0.219248	4.77±1.33	4.77±0.91	0.994832	4.27±2.25	5.65±1.16	0.196676	4.40±1.28	5.64±1.05	0.076776	2.98±1.14	5.54±1.12	0.000072
hsa-miR-335-5p	−3.08±0.57	−3.02±0.56	0.824538	−3.29±0.61	−2.85±0.71	0.236619	−3.45±0.43	−2.34±0.28	0.000129	−3.14±0.33	−2.27±0.60	0.004191	−2.66±0.46	−2.72±0.95	0.874613
hsa-miR-23a-3p	−0.63±0.36	−0.26±0.50	0.090519	−1.03±0.70	−0.40±0.59	0.099407	−0.84±0.74	−0.04±0.54	0.045330	−0.70±0.68	0.32±0.23	0.004114	−0.36±0.63	0.55±0.28	0.000189
hsa-miR-320a	1.39±0.52	1.47±0.63	0.768428	1.07±0.45	2.17±0.63	0.002283	0.94±0.44	2.09±0.35	0.000213	1.34±0.55	2.17±0.54	0.015648	0.91±0.45	1.38±0.58	0.070640
hsa-miR-148b-3p	−3.23±0.84	−2.55±0.49	0.028449	−2.81±0.69	−3.08±1.59	0.674942	−3.24±1.02	−2.49±0.72	0.152339	−3.01±0.62	−1.83±0.81	0.009116	−3.17±0.46	−2.02±0.66	0.000410
hsa-miR-148a-3p	0.05±0.52	−1.00±1.23	0.036910	−0.24±0.31	−0.08±0.78	0.590737	−0.23±0.86	−0.47±0.47	0.558978	−0.12±0.79	−0.86±0.62	0.081059	−0.14±0.81	−1.94±0.95	0.000465
hsa-miR-142-5p	−4.57±0.36	−3.58±1.30	0.091416	−5.18±0.44	−4.34±0.50	0.008481	−5.00±0.78	−4.19±0.50	0.051284	−4.93±0.73	−4.31±0.30	0.078933	−4.55±0.68	−2.94±0.84	0.000469
hsa-miR-223-3p	1.49±0.66	2.05±0.85	0.133044	1.06±0.50	1.71±0.87	0.102789	1.29±0.99	2.50±0.88	0.036023	1.32±1.14	2.64±0.42	0.019661	1.76±0.91	3.00±0.45	0.000484
hsa-miR-320b	1.00±0.35	1.15±0.71	0.583403	0.93±0.56	1.75±0.66	0.027984	0.86±0.45	1.87±0.31	0.000487	1.14±0.62	1.97±0.39	0.013767	0.75±0.57	1.20±0.53	0.081259
hsa-miR-484	−1.92±0.48	−1.80±0.57	0.638648	−2.06±0.64	−1.44±0.43	0.066611	−1.90±0.85	−1.15±0.30	0.063498	−1.91±0.59	−1.00±0.35	0.006027	−2.19±0.60	−1.34±0.36	0.000623

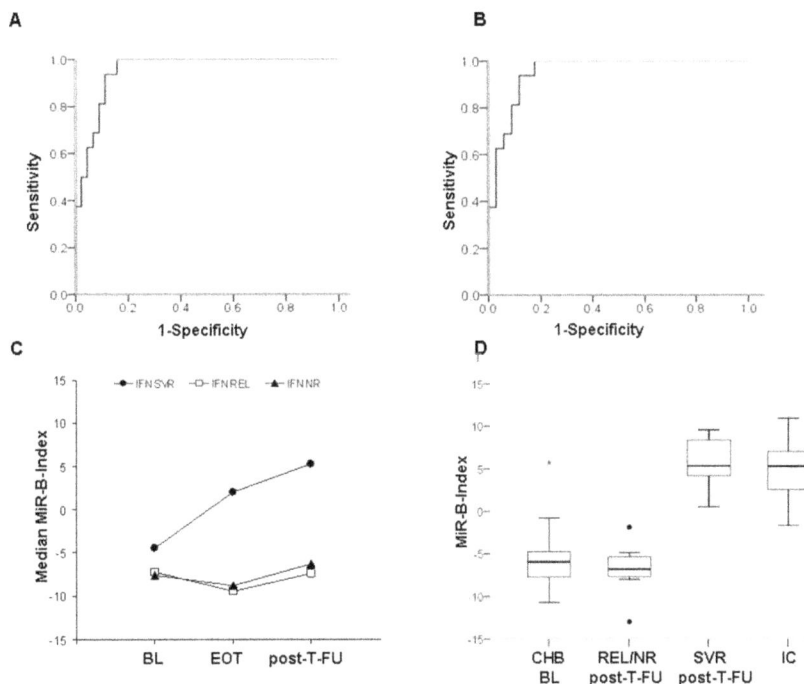

Figure 2. MiR-B-Index in HBV carriers: diagnostic performance to identify inactive carriers (AUROCs), index kinetics in Peg-IFN treated patients by outcome and distribution of the index values by treatment outcome and phase of HBV infection. A) Receiver operating characteristic curve for MiR-B-Index in IC vs patients with chronic hepatitis (HBeAg positive or negative CHB, HBV/HDV chronic hepatitis, ALD1): 0.9520 (95% CI 0.903 to 1.000, p<0.001); **B)** ROC for MiR-B-Index in IC vs HBeAg negative CHB (ALD2): 0.954 (95% CI 0.902 to 1.000, p<0.001; **C)** Kinetics of MiR-B-Index in 14 patients treated with Peg-IFN: MiR-B-Index values progressively increased in SVR, whereas they showed minor fluctuations in REL/NR (p<0.001); **D)** Whisker plot of the MiR-B-Index (y-axis) values in BL CHB patients treated with Peg-IFN (NR, REL and SVR), 24 week post-T-FU of REL/NR and SVR and IC, separately (CHB-BL vs IC p<0.001; SVR-BL vs SVR PT-FU p<0.001; REL/NR BL vs REL/NR PT-FU p = 0.462; SVR PT-FU vs IC p = 0.792).

patients with CHB and eventually to improve the inactive-carrier diagnostic accuracy. We combined the 3 liver-miRNAs with miR-335, miR-126 and miR-320a for internal normalization and, by using a cut-off of −1.7, the MiR-B-Index showed a high diagnostic performance both in the training (100% sensitivity, 83.3% specificity, 72.7% PPV, 100% NPV, 88.5% DA) and in the validation (100% sensitivity, 92.5% specificity, 88.5% PPV, 100% NPV and 95.2% DA) cohorts in identifying IC from CHB. In addition, all patients who achieved off-therapy SVR either after Peg-IFN or NUCs showed significant MiR-B-Index improvements during therapy with values at their post treatment follow-up highly comparable to those of IC (5.32 vs 6.68, p = 0.324). All these evidences propose the MiR-B-Index as a candidate biomarker to identify either spontaneous or therapy induced transition from active to inactive phase of chronic HBV infection. Accordingly, MiR-B-Index showed a significant correlation with those parameters (ALT, HBV-DNA and HBsAg; p<0.001 for all), that are currently used to manage HBV carriers, however it appears to provide additional information, contributing to a more stringent characterization at the single patient level. First of all, MiR-B-Index values in spite of being associated with ALT levels, resulted to be primarily influenced by the phase of HBV infection (p< 0.001): in fact, HBeAg positive immune-tolerant carriers, in spite of their normal ALT, had MiR-B-Index values comparable to those of HBeAg positive CHB patients. Furthermore, during NUCs treatment even though all the patients normalized ALT, only a proportion of them experienced a significant improvement of MiR-B Index. These findings do not support the hypothesis that the MiR-B-Index results from the amount of liver damage, but suggest that it could indeed mirror the extent of HBV infection

control. Indeed in untreated HBV carriers its values showed a very high correlation (ρ = −0.904, p<0.001) with HBsAg serum levels, that are inversely correlated with the extent of the immune control [6,8]. All NUC treated patients with HBsAg/anti-HBs seroconversion or decline of HBsAg serum levels <400 IU/mL showed a consistent MiR-B-Index improvement with values above the −1.7 cut-off. Overall, MiR-B-Index variations during NUC therapy appear closely linked with those of HBsAg, however our findings suggest that its variations beckon the effective achievement of sustained immune control of HBV with faster kinetics than HBsAg [5–6]. Accordingly, in SVR to Peg-IFN the correlation between MiR-B-Index and HBsAg serum levels at post-T-FU was not significant (ρ = −0.423, p = 0.08) and among the 6 patients with SVR in whom we tested EOT samples the MiR-B-Index was already improved with IC like values in 4 (66%). Thus, it appears that, during antiviral therapy, MiR-B-Index provides complementary information to HBsAg monitoring.

Furthermore, a few HBeAg negative CHB patients with SVR to Peg-IFN showed MiR-B-Index values comparable to IC already at baseline with further improvement during treatment, whereas this never occurred in NR and REL; during NUC therapy, the improvement of MiR-B-Index was influenced by baseline MiR-B-Index values. Both evidences suggest that MiR-B-Index could help to identify patients susceptible to respond to Peg-IFN and to achieve a sustained control of HBV infection during a time limited NUC treatment. Altogether these findings propose the MiR-B-Index as candidate biomarker to predict and to identify either spontaneous or therapy induced transition from active to inactive phase of chronic HBV infection. MiR-B-Index might be helpful to tailor antiviral treatment at the individual level, identifying NUCs treated patients who could stop therapy safely without risk of hepatitis B relapse once they achieve a sustained immune control of HBV infection or IFN treated patients who could benefit from prolonged treatment.

In conclusion our study shows for the 1st time that the dynamic change of a miRNA signature may identify both natural occurring and therapy induced immune control of HBV infection. The same signature qualifies as new diagnostic biomarker to satisfy the unmet need of the early identification of the sustained switch from chronic active hepatitis B to the inactive HBV infection in patients treated with antivirals. MiR-B-Index is worth being tested in larger cohorts of patients infected with different HBV genotypes, treated with different antivirals and with different therapy outcomes.

Author Contributions

Conceived and designed the experiments: MRB FB. Performed the experiments: TB MWT DC. Analyzed the data: TB MWT FB DC MRB FO. Contributed reagents/materials/analysis tools: MRB FB TB. Contributed to the writing of the manuscript: MRB FB TB. Data acquisition: MRB DC FM. Clinical management and follow-up of the patients: MRB FO P. Colombatto B. Coco P. Ciccorossi CR VR B. Cherubini. Critical review: MRB FB TB. Statistical analysis: TB MWT DC FO.

References

1. (2012) EASL-Clinical-Practice-Guidelines: Management of chronic HBV infection, J Hepatol 57: 167–185.
2. Lok ASK, BJ McMahon (2009) Chronic hepatitis B: update 2009. Hepatology 50(3): 661–2.
3. Liaw Y-F, Kao J-H, Piravitvisuth T, Chan HLY, Chien R-N, et al. (2012) Asian-Pacific consensus statement on the management of chronic hepatitis B: a 2012 update. Hepatol Int 6: 531–561.
4. Bonino F, Rosina F, Rizzetto M, Rizzi R, Chiaberge E, et al. (1986) Chronic hepatitis in HBsAg carriers with serum HBV-DNA and Anti-HBe. Gastroenterology 90: 1268–73.
5. Brunetto MR, Oliveri F, Coco B, Leandro G, Colombatto P, et al. (2002) Outcome of anti-HBe positive chronic hepatitis B in alpha-interferon treated and untreated patients: a long term cohort study. J Hepatol 36: 263–70.
6. Brunetto MR, Oliveri F, Colombatto P, Moriconi F, Ciccorossi P, et al. (2010) Hepatitis B surface antigen serum levels help to distinguish active from inactive hepatitis B virus genotype D carriers. Gastroenterology 139: 483–490.
7. Brunetto MR, Moriconi F, Bonino F, Lau GK, Farci P, et al. (2009) Hepatitis B virus surface antigen levels: a guide to sustained response to peginterferon alfa-2a in HBeAg-negative chronic hepatitis B. Hepatology 49: 1141–1150.
8. Janssen HL, Sonneveld MJ, Brunetto MR (2012) Quantification of serum HBsAg: is it useful for the management of chronic hepatitis B? Gut 61: 641–45.
9. Brunetto MR, Marcellin P, Cherubini B, Yurdaydin C, Farci P, et al. (2013) Response to peginterferon alfa-2a (40 KD) in HBeAg-negative CHB: on-treatment kinetics of HBsAg serum levels vary by HBV genotype. J Hepatol 59(6): 1153–9.
10. Ambros V (2004) The functions of animal microRNAs. Nature 431: 350–55.
11. Xiao C, Rajewsky K (2009) MicroRNA Control in the Immune System: Basic Principles. Cell 136: 26–36.
12. Cullen BR (2011) Viruses and microRNAs: RISCy interactions with serious consequences. Genes & Development 25: 1881–94.
13. Jopling CL, Yi M, Lancaster AM, Lemon SM, Sarnow P (2005) Modulation of hepatitis C virus RNA abundance by a liver-specific MicroRNA. Science 309: 1577–1581.
14. Novellino L, Rossi RL, Bonino F, Cavallone D, Abrignani S, et al. (2012) Circulating hepatitis B surface antigen particles carry hepatocellular micro-RNAs. PLoS One 7(3): e31952.
15. Hayes CN, Akamatsu S, Tsuge M, Miki D, Akiyama R, et al. (2012) Hepatitis B virus-specific miRNAs and Argonaute2 play a role in the viral life cycle. PLoS One 7: e47490.
16. Li LM, Hu ZB, Zhou ZX, Chen X, Liu FY, et al. (2010) Serum microRNA profiles serve as novel biomarkers for HBV infection and diagnosis of HBV-positive hepatocarcinoma. Cancer Res 70(23): 9798–807.
17. Ji F, Yang B, Peng X, Ding H, You H, et al. (2011) Circulating microRNAs in hepatitis B virus-infected patients. J Viral Hepat 18(7): e242–51.
18. Wang XW, Heegaard NHH, Orum H (2012) MicroRNAs in Liver Disease. Gastroenterology 142: 1431–43.
19. Blondal T, Nielsen JS, Baker A, Andreansen D, Mouritzen P, et al. (2013) Assessing sample and miRNA profile quality in serum and plasma or other biofluids. Methods 59: S1–6.
20. Bustin SA, Benes V, Garson AJ, Hellemans J, Huggett J, et al. (2009) The MIQE Guidelines: Minimum Information for Publication of Quantitative Real-Time PCR Experiments. Clinical Chemistry 55: 611–622.
21. Ramakers C, Ruijter JM, Deprez RHL, Moorman AF (2003) Assumption-free analysis of quantitative real-time polymerase chain reaction (PCR) data. Neurosci Lett 339(1): 62–66.
22. Ruijter JM, Ramakers C, Hoogaars WM, Karlen Y, Bakker O, et al. (2009) Amplification efficiency: linking baseline and bias in the analysis of quantitative PCR data. Nucleic Acids Res 37: e45.
23. Andersen CL, Ledet-Jensen J, Ørntoft T (2004) Normalization of real-time-quantitative-RT-PCR data: a model based variance estimation approach to identify genes suited for normalization applied to bladder- and colon-cancer data-sets. Cancer Research 64: 5245–50.
24. Mestdagh P, Van Vlierberghe P, De Weer A, Muth D, Westermann F, et al. (2009) A novel and universal method for microRNA RT-qPCR data normalization. Genome Biol 10: R64.
25. Saeed AI, Sharov V, White J, Li J, Liang W, et al. (2003) TM4: a free, open-source system for microarray data management and analysis. Biotechniques 34(2): 374–8.
26. Saeed Al, Bhagabati NK, Braisted JC, Liang W, Sharov V, et al. (2006) TM4 microarray software suite. Methods in Enzymology 411: 134–93.
27. Livak KJ, Schmittgen TD (2001) Analysis of relative gene expression data using Real-Time-Quantitative-PCR and the 22DDCT-Method. Methods 25: 402–48.
28. Wang K, Yuan Y, Cho J, McClarty S, Baxter D, et al. (2012) Comparing the microRNA spectrum between serum and plasma. PLoS-One 7: e41561.
29. Hu J, Xu Y, Hao J, Wang S, Li C, et al. (2012) MiR-122 in hepatic function and liver diseases. Protein Cell 3: 364–371.
30. Zhang X, Daucher M, Armistead D, Russel R, Kottilil S (2013) MicroRNA expression profiling in HCV-infected human hepatoma cells identifies potential anti-viral targets induced by interferon-α. PLoS-One. 8: e55733.
31. Cheng M, Si Y, Niu Y, Liu X, Li X, et al. (2013) High-throughput profiling of IFNα and IL-28B regulated microRNAs and identification of let-7s with anti-HCV activity by targeting IGF2BP1. J Virol 87: 9707–18.
32. Li D, Liu X, Lin L, Hou J, Li N, et al. (2011) MicroRNA-99a inhibits hepatocellular carcinoma growth and correlates with prognosis of patients with hepatocellular carcinoma. J Biol Chem 286: 36677–36685.
33. van der Meer AJ, Farid WR, Sonneveld MJ, de Ruiter PE, Boonstra A, et al. (2013) Sensitive detection of hepatocellular injury in chronic hepatitis C patients with circulating hepatocyte-derived microRNA-122. J Viral Hepat 20: 158–166.
34. Hu J, Wang Z, Tan CJ, Liao BY, Zhang X, et al. (2013) Plasma microRNA, a potential biomarker for acute rejection after liver transplantation. Transplantation 95: 991–99.

Genetic Association of Human Leukocyte Antigens with Chronicity or Resolution of Hepatitis B Infection in Thai Population

Nawarat Posuwan[1,3,4], Sunchai Payungporn[2,3], Pisit Tangkijvanich[2,3], Shintaro Ogawa[1], Shuko Murakami[1], Sayuki Iijima[1], Kentaro Matsuura[1], Noboru Shinkai[1], Tsunamasa Watanabe[1], Yong Poovorawan[4], Yasuhito Tanaka[1]*

1 Department of Virology and Liver Unit, Nagoya City University Graduate School of Medical Sciences, Nagoya, Japan, 2 Research Unit of Hepatitis and Liver Cancer, Faculty of Medicine, Chulalongkorn University, Bangkok, Thailand, 3 Department of Biochemistry, Faculty of Medicine, Chulalongkorn University, Bangkok, Thailand, 4 Center of Excellence in Clinical Virology, Faculty of Medicine, Chulalongkorn University, Bangkok, Thailand

Abstract

Background: Previous studies showed that single nucleotide polymorphisms (SNPs) in the *HLA-DP*, *TCF19* and *EHMT2* genes may affect the chronic hepatitis B (CHB). To predict the degree of risk for chronicity of HBV, this study determined associations with these SNPs.

Methods: The participants for this study were defined into 4 groups; HCC (n = 230), CHB (n = 219), resolved HBV infection (n = 113) and HBV uninfected subjects (n = 123). The *HLA-DP* SNPs (rs3077, rs9277378 and rs3128917), *TCF19* SNP (rs1419881) and *EHMT2* SNP (rs652888) were genotyped.

Results: Due to similar distribution of genotype frequencies in HCC and CHB, we combined these two groups (HBV carriers). The genotype distribution in HBV carriers relative to those who resolved HBV showed that rs3077 and rs9277378 were significantly associated with protective effects against CHB in minor dominant model (OR = 0.45, $p < 0.001$ and OR = 0.47, $p < 0.001$). The other SNPs rs3128917, rs1419881 and rs652888 were not associated with HBV carriers.

Conclusions: Genetic variations of rs3077 and rs9277378, but not rs3128917, rs1419881 and rs652888, were significantly associated with HBV carriers relative to resolved HBV in Thai population.

Editor: Man-Fung Yuen, The University of Hong Kong, Hong Kong

Funding: This work was supported by grants from The JSPS RONPAKU (Dissertation PhD) Program; the Ratchadapiseksompotch Endowment Fund of Chulalongkorn University [RES560530155-AM and RES560530093-HR]; Higher Education Research Promotion and National Research University Project of Thailand Office of the Higher Education Commission [HR1155A-55 and HR1162A-55]; Thailand Research Fund [DPG5480002 and BRG5580005]; Chulalongkorn University, Integrated Innovation Academic Center, Chulalongkorn University Centenary Academic Development Project [CU56-HR01]; King Chulalongkorn Hospital and the Office of the National Research Council of Thailand (NRCT); grant-in-aid from the Ministry of Health, Labour, and Welfare of Japan and the Ministry of Education, Culture, Sports, Science and Technology, Japan. The funders had no role in study design, data collection and analysis, decision to publish, or preparation of the manuscript.

Competing Interests: The authors have declared that no competing interests exist.

* E-mail: ytanaka@med.nagoya-cu.ac.jp

Introduction

The hepatitis B virus (HBV) is one of the most common causes of chronic hepatitis B (CHB), liver cirrhosis and hepatocellular carcinoma (HCC). Globally more than 2 billion people have been infected with HBV and 378 million are suffering from chronic hepatitis. Over 600,000 people die each year because of HBV infection. In high prevalence areas such as the central Asian republics, Southeast Asia, Sub-Saharan Africa and the Amazon basin over 8% of the population may be HBV carriers [1]. The main route of HBV infection is vertical transmission from mother to infant and horizontal transmission between children, whereby 90% will develop chronic hepatitis as infants or in early childhood and never clear the virus [1–3]. In contrast, 15% of HBV infections in adulthood develop into chronic hepatitis with viral persistence.

The frequency of HBV infection which develops into chronic hepatitis depends on the age at which the person is infected [1,2]. However, the factors determining HBV persistence or clearance are not clearly understood [4–6]. Risk factors for viral persistence include the following: virological factors (viral load, genotype, viral gene mutations and co-infection with another virus), host factors (age at infection, gender, immune status and genetic variability) and extrinsic factors (e.g. alcohol consumption and chemotherapy) [7]. Whether viral infection results in acute or chronic infection also depends on cellular immune responses influenced by human leukocyte antigen (*HLA*) class I and II molecules which must present the viral antigens to CD8+ T cells and CD4+ T cells, respectively [8]. The genes encoding *HLA* are the most polymorphic in the human genome, presumably in order to be able to respond to all potential foreign antigens [9].

Recently, many genome-wide association studies (GWAS) have been performed to seek associations between human genetic variation and the outcome of HBV infection [10–15]. Studies in the Japanese population showed that 11 single nucleotide polymorphisms (SNPs) located within or around the *HLA-DPA1* and *HLA-DPB1* loci are significantly associated with the occurrence of CHB. Of these 11 SNPs, the most strongly associated with the outcome of HBV infection were rs9277535 and rs3128917 in *HLA-DPB1* and rs3077 in *HLA-DPA1* [10].

Thereafter, GWAS studies in the Korean population confirmed the presence of these host factors related to HBV outcome and reported two new SNPs significantly associated with CHB within the *HLA* region, namely rs1419881 and rs652888 in transcription factor 19 (*TCF19*) and euchromatic histone-lysine methyltransferase 2 (*EHMT2*), respectively [16]. *TCF19* (or transcription factor SC1) is a *trans*-activating factor that mainly influences the transcription of genes required for late growth regulation at the G1-S checkpoint and during S phase [17]. *EHMT2* is a histone methyltransferase responsible for mono- and di-methylation of H3K9 (lysine at 9th residue of histone subunit 3) in euchromatin [18], which modifies the conformation of chromatin from its tightly packed form, heterochromatin, and thus influences gene repression or transcriptional silencing [19].

In the present study, we determined associations between the SNPs of *HLA-DPA1* (rs3077), *HLA-DPB1* (rs9277378 and rs3128917), *TCF19* (rs1419881) and *EHMT2* (rs652888) in HBV infected patients compared to those with resolved infections and those who had never been infected.

Materials and Methods

Ethics Statement

This study was approved by the Institutional Review Board of the Faculty of Medicine, University (Bangkok, Thailand) code IRB.455/54. Written informed consent was obtained from each patient and all samples were anonymized.

Sample Collection

All blood samples were negative for hepatitis C virus and human immunodeficiency virus. Subjects were defined into 4 groups: 230 hepatitis B surface antigen (HBsAg)-positive HCC, and 219 CHB who had been HBsAg-positive for at least 6 months were recruited at the King Chulalongkorn Memorial Hospital, whereas patients with resolved HBV and uninfected subjects were from the Thai Red Cross Society and from the north-eastern part of Thailand (age>40 years) which had been screened by Immunoassay (Architect i2000SR, Abbott, USA.) for HBsAg, antibody to hepatitis B surface antigen (anti-HBs) and antibody to hepatitis B core protein (anti-HBc). Of these subjects, 113 were negative for HBsAg but positive for anti-HBc and/or positive for anti-HBs after resolution of infection, while 123 uninfected subjects were all negative for HBsAg, anti-HBc and anti-HBs. All samples in this study were collected from subjects who have lived at the same area in Thailand, suggesting that the genetic background would be balanced between a case and control.

Genotyping assays

DNA was extracted from peripheral blood mononuclear cell using phenol-chloroform DNA extraction. The concentration of DNA was determined by NanoDrop 2000c spectrophotometer (Thermo Scientific, Wilmington, DE). We determined SNPs of *HLA-DPA1* (rs3077), *HLA-DPB1* (rs9277378 and rs3128917), and

the genes *TCF19* (rs1419881) and *EHMT2* (rs652888) by commercial TaqMan PCR assays (Applied Biosystems, USA). In this study we investigated *HLA-DPB1* (rs9277378) because this SNP had a high level of linkage disequilibrium with rs9277535 (D' = 1.00, $R^2 = 0.954$) [20] and was clearly detectable by the TaqMan assay rather than rs9277535.

Statistical analyses

In this study, Hardy-Weinberg equilibrium was performed on each SNP. The Chi-square test of independence and Odds Ratio (OR) from two-by-two tables for comparisons between case and control groups was performed using Microsoft Excel. Statistical significance was defined by $P<0.05$. The calculated of possibility level was established using Chi-square contingency table analysis.

Results

Subjects were defined into 4 groups: group 1) HCC (age = 58.2 ± 12 years, 190/230 (82.6%) male); group 2) CHB (age = 46.6 ± 10 years, 144/219 (65.7%) male); group 3) those with resolved HBV (age = 48.2 ± 6 years, 83/113 (73.5%) male); and group 4) HBV uninfected subjects (age = 46.7 ± 6 years, 73/123 (59.3%) male). The details are given in Table 1. To find the genetic factor associated with chronicity of HBV infection, however, the two groups (group 1 and 2) were combined (designated "HBV carriers"). Indeed, according to the frequencies of minor alleles of the SNPs in the *HLA-DP*, *TCF19* and *EHMT2* genes listed in Table 2, the frequencies of minor alleles of these 5 SNPs in HCC and CHB were similar (data shown in Table S1). The composite HBV carriers group had a minor allele frequency for rs3077 and rs9277378 lower than in groups 3 and 4 (OR = 0.57, 95% CI = 0.42–0.78, $p<0.001$ and OR = 0.63, 95% CI = 0.47–0.85, $p = 0.008$ for rs3077, OR = 0.59, 95% CI = 0.44–0.81, $p = 0.001$ and OR = 0.56, 95% CI = 0.42–0.75, $p<0.001$ for rs9277378, respectively). In contrast, the minor allele frequency for rs1419881 in HBV carriers was similar to group 3 (OR = 0.80, 95% CI = 0.60–1.08, $p = 0.142$) but lower than in group 4 (OR = 0.64, 95% CI = 0.48–0.85, $p = 0.002$). Moreover, minor allele frequency for rs3128917 and rs652888 in HBV carriers was comparable to groups 3 and 4 (OR = 1.14, 95% CI = 0.85–1.53, $p = 0.371$ and OR = 1.06, 95% CI = 0.80–1.41, $p = 0.673$ for rs3128917; OR = 1.14, 95% CI = 0.84–1.55, $p = 0.400$ and OR = 1.12, 95% CI = 0.83–1.50, $p = 0.471$ for rs652888, respectively).

The results of Hardy-Weinberg equilibrium analysis of each SNPs were shown in Table 3. All data were over 0.01 ($p>0.01$), indicating that the frequencies did not deviate from Hardy-Weinberg equilibrium. The genotype distribution in HBV carriers compared to subjects with HBV resolution showed that both rs3077 and rs9277378 were significantly associated with protective effects against CHB in minor dominant model (OR = 0.45, 95% CI = 0.30–0.69, $p<0.001$ for rs3077 and OR = 0.47, 95% CI = 0.31–0.72, $p<0.001$ for rs9277378, are described in Table 3), suggesting that major homozygous genotypes were risk factors with the chronicity of HBV. The other SNPs rs3128917, rs1419881 and rs652888 were not associated against HBV carrier status (OR = 1.22, 95% CI = 0.76–1.97, $p = 0.413$ for rs3128917, OR = 0.67, 95% CI = 0.42–1.06, $p = 0.084$ for rs1419881 and OR = 1.31, 95% CI = 0.87–2.00, $p = 0.198$ for rs652888, respectively).

The genotype frequencies for 5 SNPs are shown in Table 3. Comparing HBV carriers with uninfected subjects showed that rs3077, rs9277378 and rs1419881 were all protectively associated with chronic HBV infection (OR = 0.63, 95% CI = 0.42–0.95,

Table 1. Characteristics of participants in HCC, CHB, resolved HBV and HBV uninfected subjects in Thailand.

	HCC (n = 230)	CHBª (n = 219)	Resolvedᵇ (n = 113)	Uninfectedᶜ (n = 123)
Age (years)	58.2±12	46.6±10	48.2±6	46.7±6
Male	190 (82.6%)	144 (65.7%)	83 (73.5%)	73 (59.3%)
HBsAg positive	230 (100%)	219 (100%)	0	0
ALT>40 (IU/L)	43 (18.7%)	61 (27.8%)	-	-
Alb (g/dl)	3.7 (2.5–5.6)	4.5 (3–5.2)	-	-
TB (mg/dl)	1.2 (0.17–14.8)	0.56 (0.2–2.67)	-	-

Abbreviation: HCC, hepatocellular carcinoma; CHB, chronic hepatitis B; HBsAg, hepatitis B surface antigen;
ALT, Alanine transaminase; Alb, Albumin; TB, Total bilirubin.
ªDefined as chronic hepatitis B includes chronic HBV infection but not cirrhosis and HCC.
ᵇDefined as HBsAg negative but anti-HBc or/and anti-HBs positive.
ᶜDefined as any HBV serological markers negative.

$p = 0.025$ for rs3077 and OR = 0.55, 95% CI = 0.36–0.82, $p = 0.003$ for rs9277378 and OR = 0.57, 95% CI = 0.36–0.90, $p = 0.015$ for rs1419881, respectively). Comparing HBV carriers and uninfected subjects rather than those with resolved infection regarding rs1419881 was significantly protective association against CHB, but rs3128917 and rs652888 were not associated against CHB (OR = 1.58, 95% CI = 1.02–2.46, $p = 0.042$ for rs3128917 and OR = 1.09, 95% CI = 0.65–1.82, $p = 0.080$ for rs652888). When we consider the Bonferroni corrections (5 SNPs), however, the P value for rs1419881 did not reach the level of significant difference (0.015>0.05/5) between HBV carriers and HBV uninfected subjects. These data suggested that other SNPs, rs1419881, rs3128917 and rs652888 were not associated with HBV carriers in this study.

Results of meta-analysis for 3 SNPs (rs3077, rs9277378 and rs3128917) in the *HLA* gene were shown in Table S2 and S3; HBV carriers were compared to HBV resolved or HBV uninfected subjects, respectively. While the other 2 SNPs were published only from Korean population, thus the meta-analysis appeared only between HBV carriers and HBV uninfected subjects. All SNPs analyzed by the meta-analysis were significantly associated with HBV carriers.

The associations between these 5 SNPs and HBV status are depicted graphically in Figure S1. Each histogram compares HBV carriers with subjects that have resolved HBV infection or were never infected. The results showed that the minor dominant model of rs3077 and rs9277378 was highly protective associated against chronic HBV, while no significant associations were observed with rs3128917 and rs652888. Furthermore, comparing the frequency of rs1419881 between HBV carriers and uninfected subjects also revealed its association against chronic HBV infection but the association with resolved HBV did not achieve statistical significance.

Discussion

Genetic variations of rs3077 and rs9277378, but not rs3128917, rs1419881 and rs652888, were significantly associated with HBV carriers relative to resolved HBV in Thai population. In the human genome, single nucleotide polymorphisms are found in every 300–570 nucleotides. Many SNPs have no effect on the function of the encoded proteins, but some variants do appear in regulatory or coding part of the gene and affect gene expression level or protein function which can give rise to disease [21] such as the 3 SNPs including rs3077, rs9277378 and rs3128917 in *HLA-*

Table 2. Minor allele frequencies in HBV carriers, resolved HBV and uninfected subjects in Thailand.

SNPs	Gene	Minor allelesª	HBV carriersᵇ (2n = 898)	Resolved (2n = 226)	Uninfected (2n = 246)	HBV carriers vs. Resolved OR (95% CI)	P values	HBV carriers vs. Uninfected OR (95% CI)	P values
rs3077	HLA-DPA1	T	227 (25.3%)	84 (37.2%)	86 (35.0%)	0.57 (0.42–0.78)	<0.001	0.63 (0.47–0.85)	0.008
rs9277378	HLA-DPB1	A	237 (26.4%)	85 (37.6%)	96 (39.0%)	0.59 (0.44–0.81)	0.001	0.56 (0.42–0.75)	<0.001
rs3128917	HLA-DPB1	G	459 (51.1%)	108 (47.8%)	122 (49.6%)	1.14 (0.85–1.53)	0.372	1.06 (0.80–1.41)	0.673
rs1419881	TCF19	C	361 (40.2%)	103 (45.6%)	126 (51.2%)	0.80 (0.60–1.08)	0.142	0.64 (0.48–0.85)	0.002
rs652888	EHMT2	C	329 (36.6%)	76 (33.6%)	84 (34.1%)	1.14 (0.84–1.55)	0.400	1.11 (0.83–1.50)	0.478

Abbreviation: CI, confidence interval; OR, odds ratio.
ªDefined by using data from public database (NCBI).
ᵇDefined as the combination between HCC and CHB.

Table 3. Genotype frequencies in HBV carriers, resolved HBV and uninfected subjects in Thailand.

SNP	Genotype	HBV carriers[a] (n = 449)	Resolved (n = 113)	Uninfected (n = 123)	HBV carriers vs. Resolved		HBV carriers vs. Uninfected	
					OR (95% CI)	P values	OR (95% CI)	P values
rs3077	CC	259 (57.7%)	43 (38.1%)	57 (46.3%)	1.00	-	1.00	-
HLA-DPA1	CT	153 (34.1%)	56 (49.6%)	46 (37.4%)	0.45 (0.29–0.71)	<0.001	0.73 (0.47–1.13)	0.161
	TT	37 (8.2%)	14 (12.4%)	20 (16.3%)	0.44 (0.22–0.88)	0.018	0.41 (0.22–0.75)	0.003
	Dominant[b]				**0.45 (0.30–0.69)**	**<0.001**	**0.63 (0.42–0.95)**	**0.025**
	HWEp	0.038	0.516	0.049				
rs9277378	GG	242 (53.9%)	40 (35.4%)	48 (39.0%)	1.00	-	1.00	-
HLA-DPB1	AG	177 (39.4%)	61 (54.0%)	54 (43.9%)	0.48 (0.31–0.75)	0.001	0.65 (0.42–1.00)	0.051
	AA	30 (6.7%)	12 (10.6%)	21 (17.1%)	0.41 (0.20–0.87)	0.018	0.28 (0.15–0.54)	<0.001
	Dominant				**0.47 (0.31–0.72)**	**<0.001**	**0.55 (0.36–0.82)**	**0.003**
	HWEp	0.757	0.110	0.390				
rs3128917	TT	99 (22.0%)	29 (25.7%)	38 (30.9%)	1.00	-	1.00	-
HLA-DPB1	TG	241 (53.7%)	60 (53.1%)	48 (39.0%)	1.18 (0.71–1.94)	0.525	1.93 (1.19–3.13)	0.008
	GG	109 (24.3%)	24 (21.2%)	37 (30.1%)	1.33 (0.73–2.44)	0.355	1.13 (0.67–1.92)	0.648
	Dominant				**1.22 (0.76–1.97)**	**0.413**	**1.58 (1.02–2.46)**	**0.042**
	HWEp	0.117	0.496	0.015				
rs1419881	TT	162 (36.1%)	31 (27.4%)	30 (24.4%)	1.00	-	1.00	-
TCF19	TC	213 (47.4%)	61 (54.0%)	60 (48.8%)	0.67 (0.41–1.08)	0.097	0.66 (0.41–1.07)	0.088
	CC	74 (16.5%)	21 (18.6%)	33 (26.8%)	0.67 (0.36–1.25)	0.210	0.42 (0.24–0.73)	0.002
	Dominant				**0.67 (0.42–1.06)**	**0.084**	**0.57 (0.36–0.90)**	**0.015**
	HWEp	0.778	0.349	0.792				
rs652888	TT	169 (37.6%)	50 (44.2%)	57 (46.3%)	1.00	-	1.00	-
EHMT2	TC	231 (51.4%)	50 (44.2%)	48 (39.0%)	1.37 (0.88–2.12)	0.162	1.62 (1.05–2.50)	0.027
	CC	49 (10.9%)	13 (11.5%)	18 (14.6%)	1.12 (0.56–2.22)	0.756	0.92 (0.49–1.70)	<0.001
	Dominant				**1.31 (0.87–2.00)**	**0.198**	**1.09 (0.65–1.82)**	**0.080**
	HWEp	0.022	0.926	0.142				

Abbreviation: CI, confidence interval; OR, odds ratio ; HWEp, Hardy-Weinberg equilibrium analysis.
[a]Defined as the combination between HCC and CHB.
[b]Defined as a minor dominant according to the comparison between heterozygous+minor homozygous genotype and major homozygous genotype (eg. rs3077; CT+TT vs. CC).

DP region of MHC class II. The function of HLA-DP is to present bound peptide antigens, e.g. from HBV, at the surface of antigen-presenting cells. CD4+ T cells recognize these antigens and initiate the adaptive immune response. They assist the MHC class I-restricted CD8+ T cells which are the primary cellular effectors mediating HBV clearance from the liver during acute viral infection [22]. HBV infection will either be cleared by these means, or establish itself as a chronic infection. The reason for the latter is unclear but may be related to variation of *HLA-DP* alleles. Thus, the position of *HLA-DP* SNPs might be associated with possibility of clearance or chronicity. The rs3077 and rs9277535 SNPs are located within the 3′ untranslated region (UTR) of *HLA-DPA1* and *HLA-DPB1*, respectively while rs3128917 is located downstream of *HLA-DPB1*.

Recent investigations have identified 11 risk alleles for CHB related to mRNA expression of *HLA-DPA1* and *HLA-DPB1* [23]. The results showed that only these two alleles, rs3077 and rs9277535 were strongly associated with the risk of CHB and decreased expression of *HLA-DPA1* and *HLA-DPB1*, respectively. In contrast, while rs3128917 was associated with CHB, it was not associated with the level of HLA-DPB1 expression [23]. Variation

at 5′ and 3′ UTRs can alter the binding sites of regulatory proteins which protect and stabilize newly synthesized RNA, either increasing or decreasing binding [24,25]. Nevertheless, the present study showed that rs3128917 was not associated with HBV carrier status in Thailand. Because rs3128917 is located downstream of the direction of transcription of the gene, this suggests that it does not affect regulation or coding of the gene and would have no effect on HLA protein expression.

The results from the present study not only establish the importance of variation at the *HLA-DP* gene but also explore two new SNPs, rs1419881 located in *TCF19* and rs652888 in the *EHMT2* gene [16]. *TCF19* (or transcription factor SC1) is a late growth regulatory gene like histone, thymidine kinase etc, maximally expressed at the onset of DNA synthesis at the G1-S boundary and S phase of cell cycle. This protein is also involved in regulations of growth and transcription factors controlling the number and development of peripheral-blood monocytes and erythrocytes [26]. The *EHMT2* gene is a histone methyltransferase [18] mainly responsible for mono- and di-methylation of H3K9 in euchromatin. This changes the conformation of chromatin from euchromatin to heterochromatin and then affects gene repression

[19]. Histone methylation has a critical role in gene transcription and epigenetic events [27–30].

According to recently published GWAS data [11], two SNPs associated with the risk for CHB in the Korea population were identified. These were the top signals in the genome-wide significance level analysis and were independently associated with *HLA-DP* and *HLA-DQ*, respectively. The authors then confirmed the results in a replication sample, showing that the frequency of their two SNPs strongly associated with CHB; OR = 0.76, 95% CI = 0.68–0.86, p = 4.51E-11 for rs1419881 and OR = 1.26, 95% CI = 1.07–1.47, p = 2.78E-06 for rs652888 [16]. Furthermore, another GWAS study focused on HLA, of hepatitis B vaccinated people in Indonesia, showed that rs652888 was also associated with risk of CHB ($p \leq 0.0001$) in that population [31].

In the present study, however, we found that rs1419881 tended to be associated with chronic HBV infection, based on the results of a comparison between HBV carriers and uninfected subjects. Nonetheless, it did not reach the significance by the Bonferroni corrections, as well as when HBV carriers were compared with patients who had their HBV infection resolved, no association with rs1419881 was observed. The second SNP, rs652888, was not associated with chronic HBV infection in the Thai population. Although our study had sampling error due to small samples, it might be another effect that the result between rs652888 in *EHMT2* gene and chronic hepatitis B in Thai population was not associated. The reason for these negative findings for the two SNPs might be due to the affected gene functions that were not involved with the immune system or processes of persistent infection. Data supporting this notion are to be found in the GWAS data for the Korean population, where pathway analysis of genes involved in the regulation of immune function showed that *TCF19* and *EHMT2* genes are not significantly involved in human immunity [16].

Mapping the position of the two new SNPs showed that rs1419881 located at the 3′ UTR of exon 4, with a tendency towards association with CHB and rs652888 which is not associated with CHB located on an intron. The position of each SNP might affect the phenotype of gene expression and susceptibility to disease, explaining why some are associated with chronic HBV infection, and others not. According to previous publications, the 3′ UTR of the *HLA-DP* region is strongly involved with regulating HLA-DP expression and influences the outcome of HBV infection [32]. In addition, another study showed that variation of the 3′ UTR of HLA-C was strongly associated with HLA-C expression levels and with control of human immunodeficiency virus [33]. This illustrated the general principle that the position of SNPs affects association with diseases.

The prevalence of HBV in Eastern countries, i.e. Asia, sub-Saharan Africa and the Pacific is much higher than in Western Europe and America. Most people in Eastern countries are infected with HBV during childhood and 8–10% of these develop CHB. In contract, the frequency of chronic carriers in Western Europe and North America is ≤1%. Furthermore, previous GWAS and meta-analysis reported that A alleles at rs3077 and rs9277353 have protective effects against CHB. Asian and African populations, especially Chinese, have lower frequencies of A alleles than European and American populations [10,34,35]. Moreover, the previous study showed no associations of rs3077 and rs9277535 with progressive CHB infection; however rs3077 was highly significant associated with HBV infection but not associated with rs9277353 in Caucasian populations [36].

While the frequency of alleles at rs3128917 and rs1419881 in Asian and African populations are quite similar, Northern and Western European populations have high frequencies of the protective T allele at rs3128917 but have low T allele frequencies

(a risk allele for CHB) at rs1419881. The allele frequencies of populations in the worldwide for conspicuous details came from dbSNP Short Genetic Variations available at http://www.ncbi.nlm.nih.gov/projects/SNP/snp_ref.cgi. Lastly, both ethnic Eastern and Western populations have similar allele frequencies at rs652888, carrying a risk for CHB, with T allele frequencies very much higher than C allele frequencies, which has a protective effect. In addition, evolution of genomic characteristics, the migratory history of different populations, as well as HBV genotypes [37], HBV carrier rate [38] and pathological procession of liver disease [39] in each country may affect the distribution of *HLA* alleles. This was illustrated by a recent report in two Han Chinese populations (southern and northern) having different distributions of *HLA-DP* genes [39]. Thus, the genetics of the host is one of the factors influencing and predicting disease outcome [40].

According to less number of samples, it might influence statistical power in this study. Thus, we made another statistic meta-analysis of data obtained from previous reports and this study in Table S3. We compared HBV carriers with HBV uninfected subjects, because most previous studies also compared CHB with HBV clearance and/or healthy (negative for any HBV serological markers). Interestingly, all SNPs analyzed by the meta-analysis were significantly associated with HBV carriers. These results could support our data in Thailand. Additionally, no heterogeneity was observed between HBV carriers and HBV-resolved subjects (P_{het} = 0.10 for rs3077, 0.79 for rs9277378, and 0.07 for rs3128917), as well as between HBV carriers and HBV uninfected subjects (P_{het} = 0.10 for rs3077, 0.02 for rs9277378, 0.91 for rs1419881, and 0.04 for rs652888) except for rs9277378 (P_{het} = 0.000), for the minor allele frequency (MAF) of only rs9277378 was different between HapMap-CHB (MAF = 46.3% of G allele) and HapMap-JPT (MAF = 44.8% of T allele).

In the present study, we determined associations of variations at the *HLA-DP* gene with outcome in HBV infected Thai patients and the major homozygous genotypes of rs3077 and rs9277378, but not rs3128917, were significantly associated with HBV carrier status. Although genetic variation of two new SNPs, rs1419881 in the *TCF19* gene and rs652888 in the *EHMT2* gene, were not associated with the outcome of HBV infection in the Thai population, a large-scale study should be required.

Supporting Information

Figure S1 Association of 5 SNPs with HBV carriers, resolved HBV and uninfected subjects in Thailand. The results were compared between percentages of combination of heterozygous genotypes and minor homozygous genotypes (White square) with percentages of major homozygous genotypes (Grey square). Five SNPs applied in this study were rs3077, rs9277378 and rs3128917 in *HLA-DP* gene, rs1419881 in *TCF19* gene and rs652888 in *EHMT2* gene. OR, odds ratio; (lower-upper), 95% confidence interval.

Table S1 Minor allele frequencies in HCC, CHB, resolved HBV and uninfected subjects in Thailand.

Table S2 The meta-analysis of minor allele frequencies in HBV carriers and resolved HBV.

Table S3 The meta-analysis of minor allele frequencies in HBV carriers and uninfected subject.

Author Contributions

Conceived and designed the experiments: SP TW YP YT. Performed the experiments: NP. Analyzed the data: NP SP SI KM NS. Contributed reagents/materials/analysis tools: PT SO SM. Wrote the paper: NP.

References

1. Kao JH, Chen DS (2002) Global control of hepatitis B virus infection. Lancet Infect Dis 2: 395–403.
2. Zanetti AR, Van Damme P, Shouval D (2008) The global impact of vaccination against hepatitis B: a historical overview. Vaccine 26: 6266–6273.
3. Dandri M, Locarnini S (2012) New insight in the pathobiology of hepatitis B virus infection. Gut 61 Suppl 1: i6–17.
4. Pan CQ, Zhang JX (2005) Natural History and Clinical Consequences of Hepatitis B Virus Infection. Int J Med Sci 2: 36–40.
5. Tran TT, Martin P (2004) Hepatitis B: epidemiology and natural history. Clin Liver Dis 8: 255–266.
6. Pumpens P, Grens E, Nassal M (2002) Molecular epidemiology and immunology of hepatitis B virus infection - an update. Intervirology 45: 218–232.
7. Elgouhari HM, Abu-Rajab Tamimi TI, Carey WD (2008) Hepatitis B virus infection: understanding its epidemiology, course, and diagnosis. Cleve Clin J Med 75: 881–889.
8. Singh R, Kaul R, Kaul A, Khan K (2007) A comparative review of HLA associations with hepatitis B and C viral infections across global populations. World J Gastroenterol 13: 1770–1787.
9. Thio CL, Thomas DL, Karacki P, Gao X, Marti D, et al. (2003) Comprehensive analysis of class I and class II HLA antigens and chronic hepatitis B virus infection. J Virol 77: 12083–12087.
10. Kamatani Y, Wattanapokayakit S, Ochi H, Kawaguchi T, Takahashi A, et al. (2009) A genome-wide association study identifies variants in the HLA-DP locus associated with chronic hepatitis B in Asians. Nat Genet 41: 591–595.
11. Mbarek H, Ochi H, Urabe Y, Kumar V, Kubo M, et al. (2011) A genome-wide association study of chronic hepatitis B identified novel risk locus in a Japanese population. Hum Mol Genet 20: 3884–3892.
12. Wang L, Wu XP, Zhang W, Zhu DH, Wang Y, et al. (2011) Evaluation of genetic susceptibility loci for chronic hepatitis B in Chinese: two independent case-control studies. PLoS One 6: e17608.
13. An P, Winkler C, Guan L, O'Brien SJ, Zeng Z, Consortium HBVS (2011) A common HLA-DPA1 variant is a major determinant of hepatitis B virus clearance in Han Chinese. J Infect Dis 203: 943–947.
14. Nishida N, Sawai H, Matsuura K, Sugiyama M, Ahn SH, et al. (2012) Genome-wide association study confirming association of HLA-DP with protection against chronic hepatitis B and viral clearance in Japanese and Korean. PLoS One 7: e39175.
15. Hu L, Zhai X, Liu J, Chu M, Pan S, et al. (2012) Genetic variants in human leukocyte antigen/DP-DQ influence both hepatitis B virus clearance and hepatocellular carcinoma development. Hepatology 55: 1426–1431.
16. Kim YJ, Young Kim H, Lee JH, Jong Yu S, Yoon JH, et al. (2013) A genome-wide association study identified new variants associated with the risk of chronic hepatitis B. Hum Mol Genet : In press.
17. Ku DH, Chang CD, Koniecki J, Cannizzaro LA, Boghosian-Sell L, et al. (1991) A new growth-regulated complementary DNA with the sequence of a putative trans-activating factor. Cell Growth Differ 2: 179–186.
18. Shinkai Y, Tachibana M (2011) H3K9 methyltransferase G9a and the related molecule GLP. Genes Dev 25: 781–788.
19. Tachibana M, Sugimoto K, Fukushima T, Shinkai Y (2001) Set domain-containing protein, G9a, is a novel lysine-preferring mammalian histone methyltransferase with hyperactivity and specific selectivity to lysines 9 and 27 of histone H3. J Biol Chem 276: 25309–25317.
20. Barrett JC, Fry B, Maller J, Daly MJ (2005) Haploview: analysis and visualization of LD and haplotype maps. Bioinformatics 21: 263–265.
21. Prokunina L, Alarcon-Riquelme ME (2004) Regulatory SNPs in complex diseases: their identification and functional validation. Expert Rev Mol Med 6: 1–15.
22. Yang PL, Althage A, Chung J, Maier H, Wieland S, et al. (2010) Immune effectors required for hepatitis B virus clearance. Proc Natl Acad Sci U S A 107: 798–802.
23. O'Brien TR, Kohaar I, Pfeiffer RM, Maeder D, Yeager M, et al. (2011) Risk alleles for chronic hepatitis B are associated with decreased mRNA expression of HLA-DPA1 and HLA-DPB1 in normal human liver. Genes Immun 12: 428–433.
24. Miller GM, Madras BK (2002) Polymorphisms in the 3'-untranslated region of human and monkey dopamine transporter genes affect reporter gene expression. Mol Psychiatry 7: 44–55.
25. Di Paola R, Frittitta L, Miscio G, Bozzali M, Baratta R, et al. (2002) A variation in 3' UTR of hPTP1B increases specific gene expression and associates with insulin resistance. Am J Hum Genet 70: 806–812.
26. Ferreira MA, Hottenga JJ, Warrington NM, Medland SE, Willemsen G, et al. (2009) Sequence variants in three loci influence monocyte counts and erythrocyte volume. Am J Hum Genet 85: 745–749.
27. Cho HS, Kelly JD, Hayami S, Toyokawa G, Takawa M, et al. (2011) Enhanced expression of EHMT2 is involved in the proliferation of cancer cells through negative regulation of SIAH1. Neoplasia 13: 676–684.
28. Albert M, Helin K (2010) Histone methyltransferases in cancer. Semin Cell Dev Biol 21: 209–220.
29. Krivtsov AV, Armstrong SA (2007) MLL translocations, histone modifications and leukaemia stem-cell development. Nat Rev Cancer 7: 823–833.
30. Lu Z, Tian Y, Salwen HR, Chlenski A, Godley LA, et al. (2013) Histone-lysine methyltransferase EHMT2 is involved in proliferation, apoptosis, cell invasion, and DNA methylation of human neuroblastoma cells. Anticancer Drugs 24: 484–493.
31. Png E, Thalamuthu A, Ong RT, Snippe H, Boland GJ, el at. (2011) A genome-wide association study of hepatitis B vaccine response in an Indonesian population reveals multiple independent risk variants in the HLA region. Hum Mol Genet 20: 3893–3898.
32. Thomas R, Thio CL, Apps R, Qi Y, Gao X, et al. (2012) A novel variant marking HLA-DP expression levels predicts recovery from hepatitis B virus infection. J Virol 86: 6979–6985.
33. Kulkarni S, Savan R, Qi Y, Gao X, Yuki Y, et al. (2011) Differential microRNA regulation of HLA-C expression and its association with HIV control. Nature 472: 495–498.
34. Guo X, Zhang Y, Li J, Ma J, Wei Z, et al. (2011) Strong influence of human leukocyte antigen (HLA)-DP gene variants on development of persistent chronic hepatitis B virus carriers in the Han Chinese population. Hepatology 53: 422–428.
35. Yan Z, Tan S, Dan Y, Sun X, Deng G, et al. (2012) Relationship between HLA-DP gene polymorphisms and clearance of chronic hepatitis B virus infections: case-control study and meta-analysis. Infect Genet Evol 12: 1222–1228.
36. Vermehren J, Lotsch J, Susser S, Wicker S, Berger A, et al. (2012) A common HLA-DPA1 variant is associated with hepatitis B virus infection but fails to distinguish active from inactive Caucasian carriers. PLoS One 7: e32605.
37. Zeng G, Wang Z, Wen S, Jiang J, Wang L, et al. (2005) Geographic distribution, virologic and clinical characteristics of hepatitis B virus genotypes in China. J Viral Hepat 12: 609–617.
38. Hyams KC (1995) Risks of chronicity following acute hepatitis B virus infection: a review. Clin Infect Dis 20: 992–1000.
39. Li J, Yang D, He Y, Wang M, Wen Z, et al. (2011) Associations of HLA-DP variants with hepatitis B virus infection in southern and northern Han Chinese populations: a multicenter case-control study. PLoS One 6: e24221.
40. Wong DK, Watanabe T, Tanaka Y, Seto WK, Lee CK, et al. (2013) Role of HLA-DP polymorphisms on chronicity and disease activity of hepatitis B infection in Southern Chinese. PLoS One 8: e66920.

Effects of Nucleoside Analogue on Patients with Chronic Hepatitis B-Associated Liver Failure: Meta-Analysis

Feng Xie[9], Long Yan[9], Jiongjiong Lu, Tao Zheng, Changying Shi, Jun Ying, Rongxi Shen, Jiamei Yang*

Department of Special Treatment and Liver Transplantation, Eastern Hepatobiliary Surgery Hospital, The Second Military Medical University, Shanghai, China

Abstract

Purpose: The effectiveness of nucleoside analogue on patients with chronic hepatitis B-associated liver failure is still controversial. To address this issue, we did a review of the literatures and analyzed the data with emphasis on the survival and reduction in serum HBV DNA level.

Methods: We searched 11 randomized controlled trials that included 654 patients with chronic hepatitis B-associated liver failure. 340 patients adopted nucleoside analogue, such as lamivudine (LAM), entecavir (ETV), telbivudine (LdT), or tenofovir disoproxil fumarate (TDF), and the remaining 314 patients adopted no nucleoside analogue or placebo. A meta-analysis was carried out to examine the survival, HBV e antigen serologic conversion, and reduction in serum HBV DNA level. The pooled odds ratio (OR) was used to reflect the treatment effects.

Results: The overall analysis revealed nucleoside analogue significantly improved 1-month(OR = 2.10; 95% CI, [1.29, 3.41]; $p = 0.003$), 3-month (OR = 2.15; 95% CI, [1.26, 3.65]; $p = 0.005$), 12-month survival (OR = 4.62; 95% CI, [1.96, 10.89]; $p = 0.0005$). Comparison of 3-month HBV DNA showed significant reduction for adoptive nucleoside analogue patients (OR = 54.47; 95% CI, [16.37, 201.74]; $p < 0.00001$). Comparison of 3-month HBV e antigen serologic conversion showed a highly significant improvement of HBV e antigen lost for patients received adoptive antiviral therapy (OR = 6.57; 95% CI, [1.64, 26.31]; $p = 0.008$).

Conclusions: The benefits of nucleoside analogue on patients with chronic hepatitis B-associated liver failure is significant for improving patient survival, HBV e antigen serologic conversion, and rapid reduction of HBV DNA levels.

Editor: Sang-Hoon Ahn, Yonsei University College of Medicine, Republic Of Korea

Funding: This work was supported in part by grants from the China Postdoctoral Science Fund (20100470107), China Postdoctoral Science Special Fund (201104750), CSCO Fund (Y-B2011-006) and the Fund of the Ministry of Science and Technology of China (2008ZX10002-018). The funders had no role in study design, data collection and analysis, decision to publish, or preparation of the manuscript.

Competing Interests: The authors have declared that no competing interests exist.

* E-mail: jiameiyang@gmail.com

9 These authors contributed equally to this work.

Introduction

Chronic hepatitis B(CHB),caused by the hepatitis B virus (HBV), is a serious health problem worldwide, especially in China and other parts of Asia[1]. Chronic HBV infection is the most common cause of liver failure, which can develop as acute liver failure (ALF) (in the absence of any pre-existing liver disease), acute-on-chronic liver failure (ACLF) (an acute deterioration of known or unknown chronic liver disease), or a chronic decompensation of an end-stage liver disease[2]. Liver failure is a clinical syndrome that the major liver functions, particularly detoxification, synthetic functions and metabolic regulation, are impaired and it can lead to hepatic encephalopathy, ascites, jaundice, cholestasis, bleeding and hepatorenal syndrome (HRS)[3]. If the patients could not received effective treatments, they get poor prognosis because of the severity of the disease and the presence of active viral replication, which is considered as a determinant of prognosis recently[4].

As oral antiviral agents, nucleoside analogue, including lamivudine (LAM), adefovir dipivoxil (ADV), entecavir (ETV),

telbivudine (LdT), and tenofovir disoproxil fumarate (TDF), have activities conferring biochemical, virological, and serological improvement in CHB patients[5,6], and then generate the function of preventing cirrhosis and, consequently, liver failure and hepatocellular carcinoma, even for the decompensated liver disease patients[7].

Recently nucleoside analogue have been proved efficacious in improving the status of patients with severe decompensated chronic liver disease and acute-on-chronic liver failure (ACLF) related with CHB[8–13]. However, some effects for these patients are less conclusive, like the effect generated by using nucleoside analogue for a short-term time. Some studies reported they did not produce significant biochemical changes and slow down the progression of liver failure on patients with severe CHB liver disease and acute exacerbation of CHB[14–16]. Hence, we selected some randomized controlled trials (RCTs), and then conducted a review and meta-analysis to evaluate the efficacy of nucleoside analogue treatment on chronic liver failure patients.

Methods

Selection criteria

In the meta-analysis, we included studies from randomized controlled trials that compared the antiviral therapy adopted nucleoside analogue (included LAM, ADV, ETV, LdT, TDF) with no antiviral treatment for patients who were undergoing chronic hepatitis B-associated liver failure.

Though the concept of acute-on-chronic liver failure (ACLF) is well identified and the diagnostic criteria are unified[2], there isn't a clear general definition of liver failure induced by chronic hepatitis B. According to the consensus recommendations of the Asian Pacific Association for the study of the liver (APASL) about the acute-on-chronic liver failure, the criteria of chronic hepatitis B-associated liver failure and severe chronic hepatitis B formulated by Chinese Medical Association[17,18], we made a criteria for the patients with chronic hepatitis B-associated liver failure in the selected studies. Studies were included when the patients met the following criteria:

(1) previously diagnosed CHB or HBV induced cirrhosis;

(2) progressively raising in serum bilirubin level (>85 μmol/L or >5 mg/dL);

(3) prothrombin activity<40% or international normalized ratio (INR)≥1.5;

(4) HBV DNA level >10³ copies/ml;

And the exclusion criteria were:

(1) superinfection with human immunodeficiency virus(HIV) and/or other hepatitis viruses (hepatitis E, A, D, or C);

(2) other causes of chronic liver failure, like drug hepatitis, autoimmune hepatitis, alcoholic liver disease, et al;

(3) patients were receiving antiviral therapy at the moment when they were recruited or had received antiviral therapy in 6 months before the studies;

(4) evidence of hepatocellular carcinoma (HCC);

(5) patients had received artificial liver treatment during the studies

Search strategy

The investigators wrote a protocol and carried out a comprehensive search of Medline, PubMed, Embase, the Cochrane Center Register of Controlled Trials, Biological Abstracts, China National Knowledge Infrastructure, and the Chinese BioMedical Literature Database without language, publication, or date restrictions. However, when the Chinese literatures have no English abstracts, they would be excluded. In addition, reference lists of the trials selected before and relevant reviews were examined for other eligible trials. We also searched http://www.ClinicalTrials.gov website for the information of prospective and ongoing trials. Through the searching task, we used the terms 'nucleoside analog',' nucleoside analogue',' nucleotide analog',' nucleotide analogue',' lamivudine',' adefovir dipivoxil',' entecavir',' telbivudine',' tenofovir disoproxil fumarate',' liver failure',' hepatic failure',' chronic hepatitis B', and 'severe chronic hepatitis B'.

Data extraction and quality assessment

Data were extracted independently by two authors, Feng Xie and Long Yan. We screened abstracts of all retrieved articles and then matched the full texts of all articles selected during screening against the inclusion criteria. Disagreements on which articles met the inclusion criteria were resolved by discussion until a consensus was reached. Feng Xie and Long Yan completed the data extraction using a standardized approach that gathered the publication details and study characteristics: year of publication, the first author, number of patients, sex, methods and design, serum HBV DNA level and HBV DNA negative patients, seropositivity and seronegativity for HBV e antigen (HBeAg), alanine transarninase, albumin, serum bilirubin, prothrombin activity or international normalized ratio (INR), number of patients assessable for 1-, 3- and 12-month overall survival.

We used the Jadad score (maximum number of points is 5)[19] to assess the quality of the selected studies based on the description of adequate sequence generation, double blinding, description of deviations and withdrawals. The score was 4 for one study, 3 for one study and 2 for nine studies

Statistical analysis

The analyses were carried out using STATA 11.0 and Review Manager 5. P values at<0.05 were regarded as statistically significant. Since the study carried out by Yao-Li Cui had a three-arm design: it separately compared two regimens (ETV and LAM) to placebo, each antiviral arm was paired to the control arm independently[32].

The data of 1-, 3- and 12-months survival, patients with negative HBV DNA level, HBV e antigen serologic conversion in each arm were extracted from each study and combined using analysis method named Mantel and Haenszel [20] to calculate the pooled odds ratio (OR). The odds ratios (ORs) reflected the treatment effects. A pooled OR>1 indicated higher survival, HBV DNA negative and HBV e antigen serologic conversion in the antiviral arm. In order to identify the differences of effect of each nucleoside analogue, the subgroup analyses were adopted when the analysis was carried out.

Cochran's Q test(Chi-square X^2 test) and I^2 test were used for across studies to assess the variation across study results that is due to heterogeneity rather than chance. I^2 can be readily calculated from a typical meta-analysis as $I^2 = 100\% \times (Q-df)/Q$, where Q is Cochran's heterogeneity statistic and df is the degrees of freedom. Negative values of I^2 are equal to zero. A value of 0% indicates no observed heterogeneity, and larger values show increasing heterogeneity[21]. In our meta-analysis, P>0.01 in Cochran's Q test and I^2<25% would be considered as there was no or low-level heterogeneity, and the fixed-effects model was adopted when the data across studies was pooled. Otherwise, the random-effects model was used. I^2>50% was considered as significant heterogeneity. In addition to the use of subgroup and the random-effects model, some explanation would be made. Publication bias was assessed visually using a funnel plot.

Results

Selection of studies

A total of eleven studies met the inclusion criteria for this review[22–32], including 654 patients. The strategy summarized in Figure 1. Ten of these studies were from mainland China[22–30,32], and the remaining one[31] was from India. The patients of control arm in ten studies were required to take no nucleoside analogue, and only one[31] adopted placebo as the treatment of control arm. The oral antiviral agents adopted for the patients of the test groups were: 6 studies used ETV[22–26,32], 3 used LAM[27,28,32], 2 used LdT[29,30], and 1 used TDF[31]. One study[32] was three-arm design, and it had two test groups: one used LAM, another used ETV. In addition, excepted liver transplantation and artificial liver treatment, all patients were given standard medical treatment: intensive and care monitoring; supplements of enteral or parenteral nutrition; intravenous drop infusion albumin and plasma; maintenance water, electrolyte and acid–base equilibrium; prevention and treatment complications; etc. The characteristics of each study are listed in Table 1.

Survival

Four studies[24–26,32] reported the information of 1-month survival contained 332 patients (179 patients took nucleoside analogue). 145 patients in four studies used ETV and 34 patients used LAM. There was no person died in one study during the first 1 month[26]. The only test arm using LAM presented the same survival rate compared to control arm. The estimated pooled OR for both four studies showed a highly significant survival rate for patients receiving adoptive antiviral therapy (OR = 2.10; 95% CI, [1.29, 3.41]; p = 0.003; Figure 2). To assess the heterogeneity, the Cochran's Q test showed P = 0.32 and I^2 test had a value of 14%, what indicated the degree of variability between studies was consistent with what could be estimated to occur by chance. In order to identify the difference of treatment effectiveness between LAM and ETV, the subgroup analysis was adopted. The study in LAM subgroup showed no different survival rate between the test and control arms. The ETV subgroup presented even more highly significant survival rate for patients receiving antiviral therapy (OR = 2.66; 95% CI, [1.51, 4.68]; p = 0.0007), and the P = 0.69 in Cochran's Q test and I^2 = 0% when evaluated the heterogeneity.

Five studies[23,27,28,31,32] reported the information of 3-month survival including 282 patients (156 patients took nucleoside analogue). Among these studies, LAM was used in three studies (69 patients), ETV was used in two studies (73 patients), and TDF was used in one study (14 patients). The study carried

out by Zhao Rui had no person died in the first 3 months. The estimated pooled OR for five studies showed a highly significant survival rate for patients receiving antiviral therapy (OR = 2.15; 95% CI, [1.26, 3.65]; p = 0.005; Figure 3). The assessment of heterogeneity acquired P = 0.32 in Cochran's Q test and I^2 = 15%, meaning there was no significant variability of these studies. The subgroup of ETV and TDF had individual OR value of 1.38 (95% CI, [0.54, 3.56]) and 7.33 (95% CI, [1.16, 46.23]). The OR value was 2.24 (95% CI, [1.11, 4.51]) in the LAM subgroup, and it had no evidence of significant heterogeneity (P = 0.34 in Cochran's Q test and I^2 = 7%).

There were only two studies[22,23] reported the information of 12-month survival contained 140 patients. All the two studies adopted ETV as the oral antiviral agents for 70 patients. The result also indicated higher survival rate compared nucleoside analogue arms with control arms (OR = 4.62; 95% CI, [1.96, 10.89]; p = 0.0005; Figure 4).It had no evidence of significant heterogeneity (P = 0.25 in Cochran's Q test and I^2 = 24%).

Reduction in serum HBV DNA level

Four studies[27–29,31] reported the information of 3-month HBV DNA reduction. The concept of negative HBV DNA was used to assess the effects of reduction in serum HBV DNA, which meant the patients with undetectable HBV DNA level follow the lowest detection limit of the test equipment. The lowest detection limit was not mentioned in one study[27]. There was one study[31] used the lowest detection limit of 50 IU/mL (about 280 copies/mL), and at 3 months, undetectable HBV DNA was achieved in three of eight (37%) patients in the TDF-treated group (eight persons were survival at the end of 3 months), whereas none in the placebo group. The remaining two studies used the lower detection limit of 10^3 copies/mL (about 178 IU/mL). The pooled

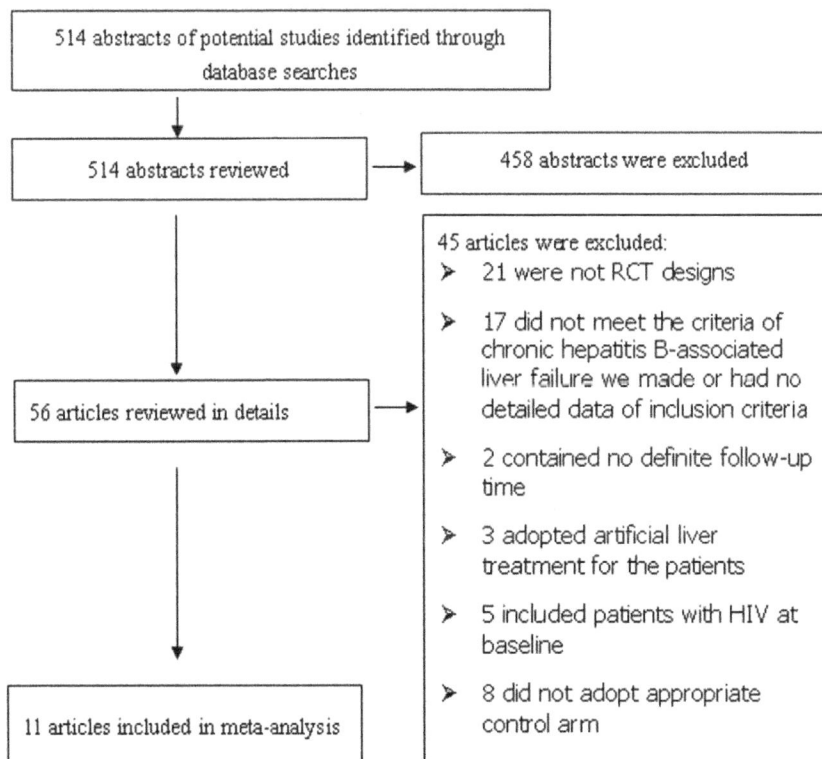

Figure 1. Identification process for eligible studies.

Table 1. Characteristics of included studies.

Study	Country	Study design	Blinding	Treatment	Number of patients	Age (mean±SD)	Sex (M:F)	HBeAg (positive)	PTA (mean±SD) (%)	INR
1 Zhong et al.(2009)	China	RCT	NA	entecavir (ETV)0.5 mg/d	30	NA	20:10	NA	31.41 ± 5.08	NA
				no nucleoside analogue	30	NA	20:10	NA	30.94 ± 5.87	NA
2 Zhao et al.(2009)	China	RCT	NA	entecavir (ETV)0.5 mg/	40	48.6	54:26	NA	<40	NA
				no nucleoside analogue	40	48.6	54:26	NA	<40	NA
3 Yang et al.(2008)	China	RCT	NA	entecavir (ETV)0.5 mg	55	28.5±8.9	72:38	NA	28.5 ± 13.8	NA
				no nucleoside analogue	55	28.5±8.9	72:38	NA	29.2 ± 12.8	NA
4 Guo et al.(2008)	China	RCT	NA	entecavir (ETV)0.5 mg/	37	34.8±8.5	27:10	18	31.3±6.1	NA
				no nucleoside analogue	45	36.4±9.1	29:16	20	30.1±7.4	NA
5 Han et al.(2009)	China	RCT	NA	entecavir (ETV)0.5 mg/	20	NA	30:6	NA	28.8±9.5	NA
				no nucleoside analogue	16	NA	30:6	NA	29.6±9.7	NA
6 Xu et al.(2004)	China	RCT	NA	lamivudine (LAM)100 mg/d	11	46.2±7.8	16:7	NA	38.31±5.69	NA
				no nucleoside analogue	12	46.2±7.8	16:7	NA	35.66±2.98	NA
7 Guo et al.(2003)	China	RCT	NA	lamivudine (LAM)100 mg/d	24	38±17.1	24:0	24	29.3±8.3	NA
				no nucleoside analogue	24	39±18.4	24:0	24	29.1±8.4	NA
8 Qiu et al.(2009)	China	RCT	NA	telbivudine (LdT)600 mg/d	30	41.45±10.9	48:12	21	34.29±22.29	NA
				no nucleoside analogue	30	41.45±10.9	48:12	20	35.58±24.23	NA
9 Qin et al.(2012)	China	RCT	NA	telbivudine (LdT)600 mg/d	12	48.65±7.3	15:9	NA	31.2±9.4	NA
				no nucleoside analogue	12	48.65±7.3	15:9	NA	29.4±7.6	NA
10 Hitendra Garg et al.(2011)	India	RCT	Double Blinding	tenofovir disoproxil fumarate (TDF)300 mg/d	14	47.5	10:4	8	NA	1.85
				placebo	13	45	10:3	7	NA	1.93
11 Yao et al.(2010)	China	RCT	NA	entecavir (ETV)0.5 mg/d	33	38.39±10.82	3:30	10	NA	2.27±0.55
				lamivudine (LAM)100 mg/d	34	39.35±10.61	3:31	13	NA	2.61±1.03
				no nucleoside analogue	37	41.03±11.48	6:31	11	NA	2.33±0.88

Study or Subgroup	nucleo s(t)ide analog(ue) Events	Total	no nucleo s(t)ide analog(ue) Events	Total	Weight	Odds Ratio M-H, Fixed, 95%CI	Odds Ratio M-H, Fixed, 95%CI
1.1.1 lamivudine							
Yao-Li Cui2 2010	23	34	25	37	33.7%	1.00 [0.37, 2.71]	
Subtotal (95% CI)		34		37	33.7%	1.00 [0.37, 2.71]	
Total events	23		25				
Heterogeneity: Not applicable							
Test for overall effect: Z = 0.01 (P = 0.99)							
1.1.2 entecavir							
Guo Yu-xiang 2008	33	37	32	45	13.6%	3.35 [0.99, 11.37]	
Han Zhi-qi 2009	20	20	16	16		Not estimable	
Yang Hai-min2008	40	55	26	55	30.9%	2.97 [1.34, 6.59]	
Yao-I Cui 2010	26	33	25	37	21.8%	1.78 [0.60, 5.26]	
Subtotal (95% CI)		145		153	66.3%	2.66 [1.51, 4.68]	
Total events	119		99				
Heterogeneity: Chi² = 0.74, df = 2 (P = 0.69); I² = 0%							
Test for overall effect: Z = 3.39 (P = 0.0007)							
Total (95% CI)		179		190	100.0%	2.10 [1.29, 3.41]	
Total events	142		124				
Heterogeneity: Chi² = 3.60, df = 3 (P = 0.32); I² = 14%							
Test for overall effect: Z = 3.00 (P = 0.003)							
Test for subgroup differences: Not applicable							

0.01   0.1   1   10   100
Favours experimental   Favours control

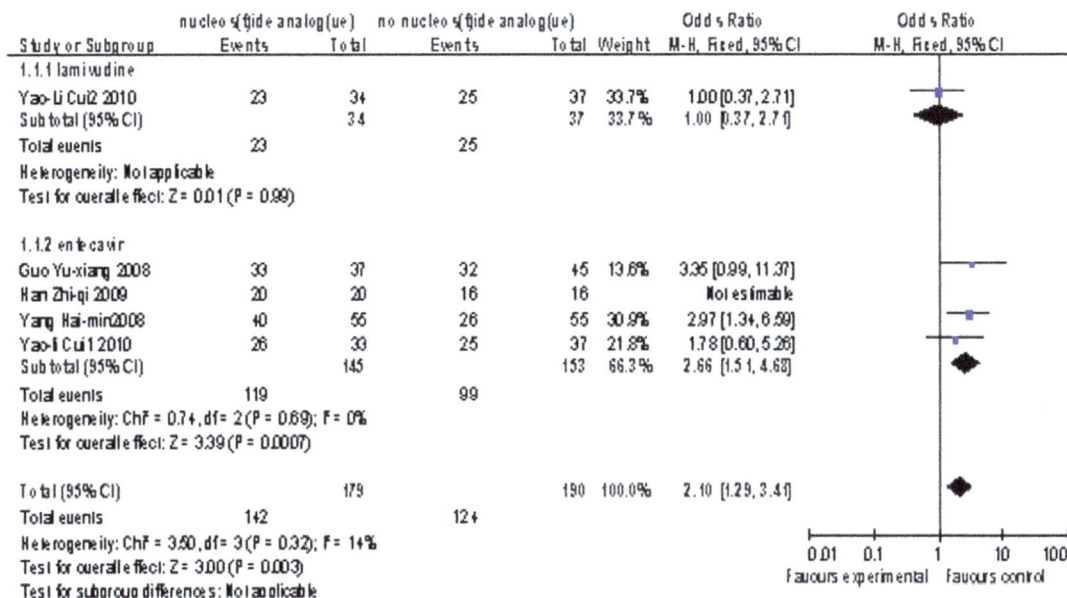

Figure 2. Comparison of 1-month survival of liver failure patients treated with nucleoside analogue or no nucleoside analogue.

OR for these two studies of negative HBV DNA patients showed significant reduction in HBV DNA for adoptive nucleoside analogue patients (OR = 54.47; 95% CI, [16.37, 201.74]; p<0.00001; Figure 5). There was no evidence of heterogeneity among the two individual studies (p = 0.63 in Cochran's Q test; I² = 0%).

HBV e antigen serologic conversion

Three studies [28,29,31] reported the information of 3-month HBV e antigen serologic conversion. There was one study used LAM as the oral antiviral agents (including 24 patients) and one study used LdT (including 30 patients). The remaining one having 14 patients used TDF. According to patients lost HBV e antigen in these three studies, the estimated pooled OR value showed a

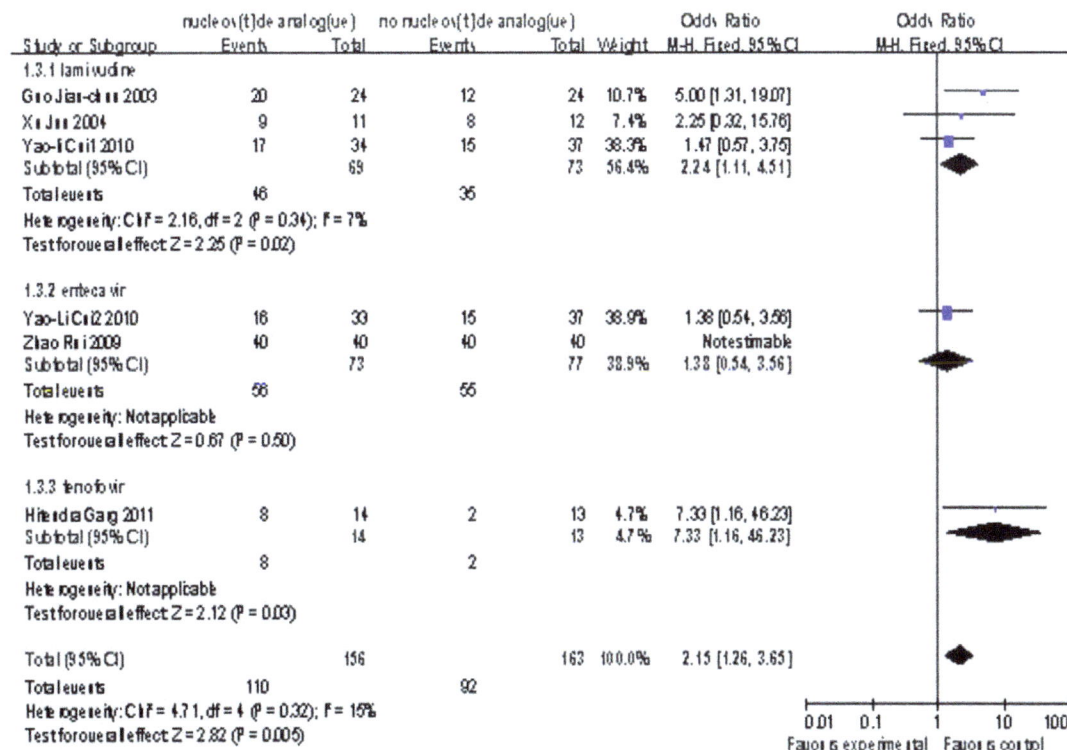

Study or Subgroup	nucleos(t)ide analog(ue) Events	Total	no nucleos(t)ide analog(ue) Events	Total	Weight	Odds Ratio M-H, Fixed, 95%CI	Odds Ratio M-H, Fixed, 95%CI
1.3.1 lamivudine							
Guo Jian-chu 2003	20	24	12	24	10.7%	5.00 [1.31, 19.07]	
Xi Jun 2004	9	11	8	12	7.4%	2.25 [0.32, 15.76]	
Yao-I Cui 2010	17	34	15	37	38.3%	1.47 [0.57, 3.75]	
Subtotal (95% CI)		69		73	56.4%	2.24 [1.11, 4.51]	
Total events	46		35				
Heterogeneity: Chi² = 2.16, df = 2 (P = 0.34); I² = 7%							
Test for overall effect Z = 2.25 (P = 0.02)							
1.3.2 entecavir							
Yao-Li Cui2 2010	18	33	15	37	38.9%	1.38 [0.54, 3.56]	
Zhao Rui 2009	40	40	40	40		Not estimable	
Subtotal (95% CI)		73		77	38.9%	1.38 [0.54, 3.56]	
Total events	58		55				
Heterogeneity: Not applicable							
Test for overall effect Z = 0.67 (P = 0.50)							
1.3.3 tenofovir							
Hierda Gang 2011	8	14	2	13	4.7%	7.33 [1.16, 46.23]	
Subtotal (95% CI)		14		13	4.7%	7.33 [1.16, 46.23]	
Total events	8		2				
Heterogeneity: Not applicable							
Test for overall effect Z = 2.12 (P = 0.03)							
Total (95% CI)		156		163	100.0%	2.15 [1.26, 3.65]	
Total events	110		92				
Heterogeneity: Chi² = 4.71, df = 4 (P = 0.32); I² = 15%							
Test for overall effect Z = 2.82 (P = 0.005)							

0.01   0.1   1   10   100
Favours experimental   Favours control

Figure 3. Comparison of 3-month survival of liver failure patients treated with nucleoside analogue or no nucleoside analogue.

Study or Subgroup	nucleo\(t)de analog(ue) Events	Total	no nucleo\(t)de analog(ue) Events	Total	Weight	Odds Ratio M-H, Fixed, 95% CI	Odds Ratio M-H, Fixed, 95% CI
Zhao Rui 2009	38	40	27	40	25.7%	9.15 [1.91, 43.90]	
Zhong Xiu-hua 2009	21	30	13	30	74.3%	3.05 [1.05, 8.84]	
Total (95% CI)		70		70	100.0%	4.62 [1.96, 10.89]	
Total events	59		40				

Heterogeneity: Chi² = 1.31, df = 1 (P = 0.25); I² = 24%
Test for overall effect: Z = 3.50 (P = 0.0005)

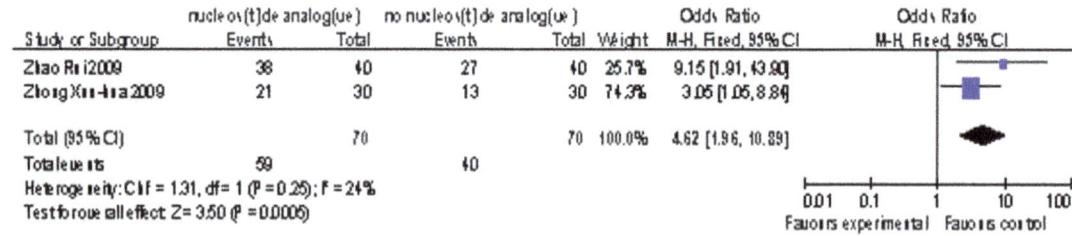

Figure 4. Comparison of 12-month survival of liver failure patients treated with nucleoside analogue or no nucleoside analogue.

highly significant improvement of HBV e antigen lost for patients received adoptive antiviral therapy (OR = 6.57; 95% CI, [1.64, 26.31]; p = 0.008; Figure 6). It had no evidence of significant heterogeneity in these three studies (P = 0.32 in Cochran's Q test and $I^2 = 12\%$).

Safety

None of these studies reported patients developed significant adverse reaction, or need for dose modification, early discontinuation. Only one study observed two patients had mild gastrointestinal reaction after they took ETV[25], and that was tolerated well and did not disturb the therapy.

Publication bias

A funnel plot of the studies used in the meta-analysis reporting on 1-month survival is shown in Figure 7. None of the studies lay outside the limits of the 95% CI, and there was no evidence of publication bias.

Discussion

The result clearly indicated nucleoside analogue significant improve survival, HBV e antigen serologic conversion, and rapid reduction of HBV DNA levels. The effects of nucleoside analogue for severe liver disease have been demonstrated by plenty of previous trails. But most of them were not RCTs, and the conclusions of many articles, even guidelines, originated from them. What we wanted to do was to get a stricter conclusion. Now that liver failure is considered as a complication of chronic hepatitis B infection, and of course it would provoke concern in recruiting a sufficient number of patients to conduct a controlled trial using no antiviral treatment (even in areas of high endemicity). What's more, for patients with chronic hepatitis B-associated liver failure, liver transplantation is currently regarded as a primary and complementary measure[33], and withholding antiviral treatment would have been considered as unethical,

which also made the RCTs have not enough participants. However, in China and India, liver transplantation is not readily available nor feasible due to the lack of organs and facilities for liver transplantation. This had made some RCT studies were conducted in these areas.

For patients with severe liver disease associated with CHB, the severity of liver disease at the time of initiating antiviral therapy, like elevated base-line serum bilirubin and creatinine levels and detectable baseline serum HBV DNA level, is a more relevant determinant of short-term mortality than the virological response[34] That may be the reason for not all patients got benefits from nucleoside analogue treatment.

In our selected RCTs, eight of the eleven searched studies published the survival data after using nucleoside analogue for a short-term time. All of the eight studies showed positive results. Nucleoside analogue can markedly suppress HBV replication by suppression of HBV-polymerase activity, leading to improvement of liver function and reduced incidence of fibrosis, cirrhosis in CHB patients[7,35]. Recent data suggest that the prognosis of patients with chronic hepatitis B-associated severe liver disease may be related to pretreatment HBV DNA load[36]. The rapidly suppression of HBV DNA load can stabilize or halt disease progression, and thereby improves prognosis, despite when the heightened immune response in the liver is ongoing[32]. From our analysis we found nucleoside analogue also had significant positive effects for the short-term HBV DNA reduction. Probably it caused the improvement of liver function and even the benefit of survival.

Data regarding the efficacy of long-term treatment with nucleoside analogue for those patients with liver failure was lack in previous literatures. The severity of liver disease, the poor prognosis of patients and the high mortality rate[37] has restrict the conducted of long-term trails. One previous study followed up patients who suffered from severe acute hepatitis B for at least one year to observe the effect of LAM, found that there was no significant difference in the clinical outcome, biochemical and HBV e antigen serologic conversion between the LAM treated and

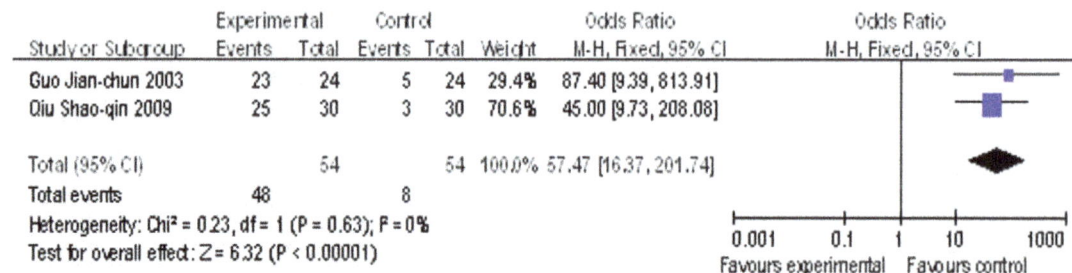

Study or Subgroup	Experimental Events	Total	Control Events	Total	Weight	Odds Ratio M-H, Fixed, 95% CI	Odds Ratio M-H, Fixed, 95% CI
Guo Jian-chun 2003	23	24	5	24	29.4%	87.40 [9.39, 813.91]	
Qiu Shao-qin 2009	25	30	3	30	70.6%	45.00 [9.73, 208.08]	
Total (95% CI)		54		54	100.0%	57.47 [16.37, 201.74]	
Total events	48		8				

Heterogeneity: Chi² = 0.23, df = 1 (P = 0.63); I² = 0%
Test for overall effect: Z = 6.32 (P < 0.00001)

Figure 5. Comparison of 3-month HBV DNA reduction of liver failure patients treated with nucleoside analogue or no nucleoside analogue.

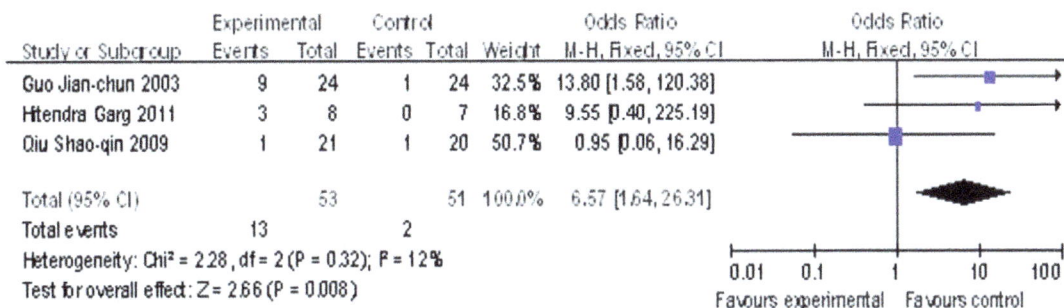

Figure 6. Comparison of 3-month HBV e antigen serologic conversion of liver failure patients treated with nucleoside analogue or no nucleoside analogue.

the placebo treated groups[13]. Two of our selected studies had the data of 12-month survival, and when compared with no antiviral treatment group, the nucleoside analogue treated group had a higher survival rate (OR = 4.62). However, these two studies were insufficient. Definite conclusion should be further studied and discussed. Especially the risks of drug resistance on these patients could only be acquired from long-term studies.

When we compared the effects of nucleoside analogues, the strategy of subgroup was adopted in our statistical analysis. But the selected studies can only provide the data of two or three nucleoside analogues during the same period of time, the comparision of effects brought by each drugs could not obtain a definite conclusion. Previously some nonRCT studies had provided information about the effects of nucleoside analogue drugs for patients with HBV-related decompensated liver disease[8,12,13,16,38]. Though all of these nucleoside analogue drugs have been confirmed having positive effects of improvement on survival rate, liver functions, reduction of HBV DNA, for the severe liver disease patients, When taking efficacy and drug resistance into consideration, ETV and TDF would be chosen for the first-line therapy[38]. Due to the weaker activity against LAM-resistant hepatitis B virus of ETV, and the fact that patients with LAM resistance would get a high rate of drug resistance if using ETV 1 mg/day for long-term, TDF could be considered as a better choice than ETV for LAM experienced patients.

When initiating antiviral therapy, the severity of liver disease, like elevated base-line serum bilirubin and creatinine levels and detectable baseline serum HBV DNA level could affect the results of patients[14,16,34]. It suggested us that antiviral therapy should be initiated as early as possible before the liver disease become too severe to be rescued.

In conclusion, though liver transplantation is currently regarded as a primary measure for patients with chronic hepatitis B-associated liver failure, the early initiation of adaptive nucleoside analogue drugs for antiviral therapy is also necessary.

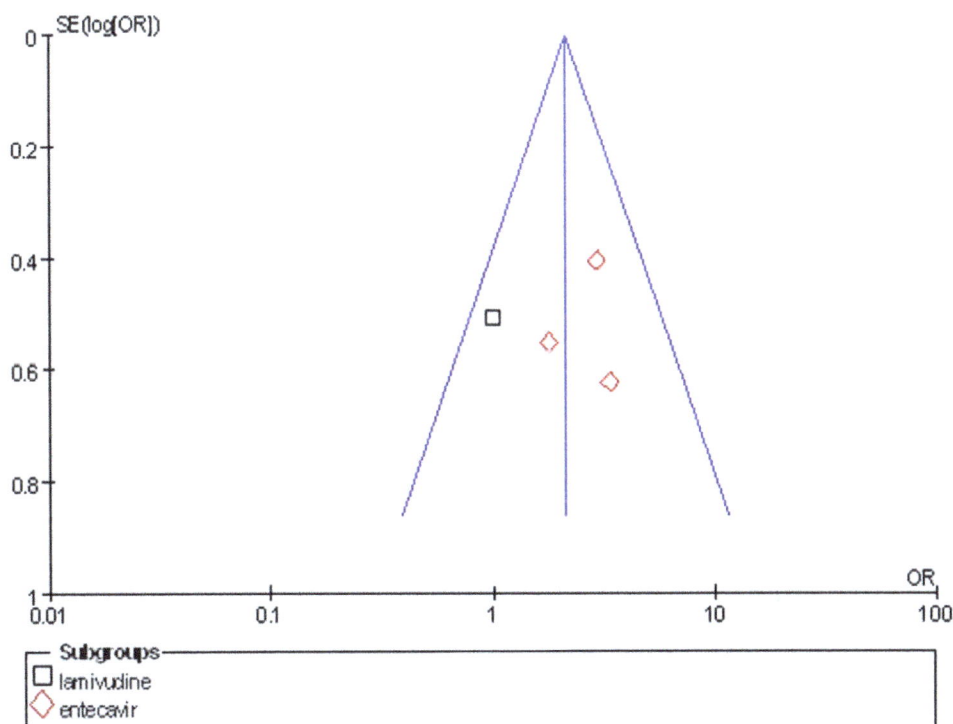

Figure 7. The funnel plot of OR value for 1-month survival of liver failure patients.

Finally, we had to mention the weaknesses of these selected studies. The low quality and the conducted areas must be the main shortages. When they were assessed using the Jadad score, the score was 4 for one study, 3 for one study and 2 for nine studies. And all the studies belonged to Asia (ten studies belonged to the mainland of China, and one belonged to India). Obviously these weaknesses could bring some limitations. Under ideal conditions, more double blinding, and large scale randomised control trials should be carried out.

References

1. Hepatitis B: fact sheet N°204. Geneva: World Health Organization, July 2012. (Accessed September 13, 2004, at http://www.who.int/mediacentre/factsheets/fs204/en/).
2. Sarin SK, Kumar A, Almeida JA, Chawla YK, Fan ST, et al. (2009) Acute-on-chronic liver failure: consensus recommendations of the Asian Pacific Association for the study of the liver (APASL). Hepatol Int 3:269–282.
3. Marrero J, Martinez FJ, Hyzy R (2003) Advances in critical care hepatology. Am J Respir Crit Care Med 168: 1421–1426.
4. Fontana RJ (2004) Management of decompensated HBV cirrhosis:lamivudine and beyond. Am J Gastroenterol 99: 64–67.
5. European Association for the Study of the Liver (2012) EASL Clinical Practice Guidelines: Management of chronic hepatitis B virus infection. J Hepatol 57:167–185.
6. Lok AS, McMahon BJ (2009) Chronic hepatitis B: update 2009. Hepatology 50:661–662.
7. Everhart JE, Hoofnagle JH (1992) Hepatitis B-related end-stage liver disease. Gastroenterology 103:1692–1694.
8. Liaw YF, Sung JJ, Chow WC, Farrell G, Lee CZ, et al. (2004) Lamivudine for patients with chronic hepatitis B and advanced liver disease. N Engl J Med 351:1521–1531.
9. Sun LJ, Yu JW, Zhao YH, Kang P, Li SC (2010) Influential factors of prognosis in lamivudine treatment for patients with acute-on-chronic hepatitis B liver failure. J Gastroenterol Hepatol 25:583–590.
10. Schiff ER, Lai CL, Hadziyannis S, Neuhaus P, Terrault N, et al. (2003) Adefovir dipivoxil therapy for lamivudine-resistant hepatitis B in pre- and post-liver transplantation patients. Hepatology 38:1419–1427.
11. Shim JH, Lee HC, Kim KM, Lim YS, Chung YH, et al. (2010) Efficacy of entecavir in treatment-naive patients with hepatitis B virus-related decompensated cirrhosis. J Hepatol 52:176–182.
12. Liaw YF, Sheen IS, Lee CM, Akarca US, Papatheodoridis GV, et al. (2011) Tenofovir disoproxil fumarate (TDF), emtricitabine/TDF, and entecavir in patients with decompensated chronic hepatitis B liver disease. Hepatology 53:62–72.
13. Chan HLY, Chen YC, Gane EJ, Sarin SK, Suh DJ, et al. (2012) Randomized clinical trial: efficacy and safety of telbivudine and lamivudine in treatment-naïve patients with HBV-related decompensated cirrhosis. J Viral Hepat 19:732–743.
14. Tsubota A, Arase Y, Suzuki Y, Suzuki F, Sezaki H, et al. (2005) Lamivudine monotherapy for spontaneous severe acute exacerbation of chronic hepatitis B. J Gastroenterol Hepatol20:426–432.
15. Chen J, Han JH, Liu C, Yu RH, Li FZ, et al. (2009) Short-term entecavir therapy of chronic severe hepatitis B. Hepatobiliary Pancreat Dis Int8:261–266.
16. Chien RN, Lin CH, Liaw YF (2003) The effect of lamivudine therapy in hepatic decompensation during acute exacerbation of chronic hepatitis B. J Hepatol38:322–327.
17. Board of liver diseases, infectious diseases and parasitic diseases of Chinese Medical Association (2000) National viral hepatitis control programme. Chin J Hepatol 6:324–329.
18. Liver failure and artificial liver group, Chinese society of infectious disease, Chinese Medical Association; Severe liver diseases and artificial liver group, Chinese Society of Hepatology, Chinese Medical Association (2006) Diagnostic and treatment guidelines for liver failure. Chin J Hepatol 14:643–646.
19. Jadad AR, Moore RA, Carroll D, Jenkinson C, Reynolds DJ, et al. (1996) Assessing the quality of reports of randomized clinical trials: is blinding necessary? Control Clin Trials 17: 1–12.
20. Deeks JJ, Higgins JPT, Altman DG (2008) Chapter 9: Analyzing data and undertaking meta-analyses. In: Higgins JPT, Green S, editors. Cochrane handbook for systematic reviews of interventions version 5.0.0 (updated February 2008). The Cochrane Collaboration. Available from http://www.cochrane-handbook.org.
21. Higgins JP, Thompson SG, Deeks JJ, Altman DG (2003) Measuring inconsistency in meta-analyses. British Medical Journal 327:557–560.
22. Zhong X, Yuan J, Yang Y,Li W, Chen X (2009) Investigation of the liver failure patients infected with hepatitis B virus treated with entecavir. Chin J Clini Hepatol 25:331–333.
23. Zhao R (2009) Antiviral effect of entecavir in patients with severe chronic hepatitis B.Chin J Public Health 25:758–759.
24. Yang H,Wang Y, Jiang N (2008) Baraclude for treatment of 55 patients with chronic severe hepatitis B.J Practical Medical Technology15:1100–1101.
25. Guo Y (2008) Clinical Observation of entecavir in Treatment of patients with chronic severe hepatitis B.Chin J Prev Contr Chron Non-commun Dis 16:289–290.
26. Han Z, Qin B, Zhang H (2009) Observation on the efficiency and safety of entecavir on chronic hepatitis B.Chin J Clini Hepatol 25:188–190.
27. Xun J, Zhang Y (2004) Observation of short-term therapeutic effect of lamivudine on patients with chronic Severe hepatitis B.J Clini Hepatol 7:214–216.
28. Guo J,Ru R, Ye W (2003) The effect of lamivudine in the treatment of chronic fulminant hepatitis B.China Journal of Modern Applied Pharmacy 20:313–314.
29. Qiu S, Li W, Peng Q (2009) Short-term observation of telbivudine in treatment of chronic severe hepatitis B.Chin J Clini Hepatol 25:190–191.
30. Qin R, Zhu S, Wang G, Den J (2012) Analysis of therapeutic effect of telbivudine on severe chronic hepatitis B.Modern Hospital 12:55–57.
31. Garg H, Sarin SK, Kumar M, Garg V, Sharma BC, et al. (2011) Tenofovir improves the outcome in patients with spontaneous reactivation of hepatitis B presenting as acute-on-chronic liver failure. Hepatology 53(3):774–780.
32. Cui YL, Yan F, Wang YB, Song XQ, Liu L, et al. (2010) Nucleoside analogue can improve the long-term prognosis of patients with hepatitis B virus infection-associated acute on chronic liver failure. Dig Dis Sci 55: 2373–2380.
33. Uemoto S, Inomata Y, Sakurai T, Egawa H, Fujita S, et al. (2000) Living donor liver transplantation for fulminant hepatic failure. Transplantation 70:152–157.
34. Fontana RJ, Hann HW, Perrillo RP, Vierling JM, Wright T, et al. (2002) Determinants of early mortality in patients with decompensated chronic hepatitis B treated with antiviral therapy. Gastroenterology 123:719–727.
35. Hadziyannis SJ, Tassopoulos NC, Heathcote EJ, Chang TT, Kitis G, et al. (2005) Long-term therapy with adefovir dipivoxil for HBeAg-negative chronic hepatitis B.N Engl J Med 352:2673–2681.
36. Sun QF, Lü Y, Xu DZ, Lan XY, Liu JY, et al. (2006) The impact of HBeAg positivity/negativity and HBV-DNA loads on the prognosis of chronic severe hepatitis B.Zhonghua Gan Zang Bing Za Zhi 14:410–413.
37. Vickers C, Neuberger J, Buckels McMaster P, Elias E (1988) Transplantation of liver in adults and children with fulminant liver failure. J Hepatol 7: 143–150.
38. Liaw YF, Raptopoulou-Gigi M, Cheinquer H, Sarin SK, Tanwandee T, et al. (2011) Efficacy and safety of entecavir versus adefovir in chronic hepatitis B patients with hepatic decompensation: a randomized, open-label study. Hepatology 54:91–100.

Author Contributions

Conceived and designed the experiments: FX LY J.Yang. Performed the experiments: FX LY JL TZ. Analyzed the data: FX LY CS RS. Contributed reagents/materials/analysis tools: RS TZ J. Ying. Wrote the paper: FX LY J.Yang.

Anti-HDV IgM as a Marker of Disease Activity in Hepatitis Delta

Anika Wranke[1]*, Benjamin Heidrich[1,15], Stefanie Ernst[2], Beatriz Calle Serrano[1],
Florin Alexandru Caruntu[4], Manuela Gabriela Curescu[5], Kendal Yalcin[6], Selim Gürel[7], Stefan Zeuzem[8],
Andreas Erhardt[9], Stefan Lüth[10], George V. Papatheodoridis[11], Birgit Bremer[1], Judith Stift[12],
Jan Grabowski[1], Janina Kirschner[1], Kerstin Port[1], Markus Cornberg[1], Christine S. Falk[13], Hans-
Peter Dienes[14], Svenja Hardtke[14], Michael P. Manns[1,14,15], Cihan Yurdaydin[3], Heiner Wedemeyer[1,14,15,16]*
and HIDIT-2 Study Group[14]

1 Department of Gastroenterology, Hepatology and Endocrinology, Hannover Medical School, Hannover, Germany, 2 Institute for Biometry, Hannover Medical School, Hannover, Germany, 3 Ankara University Medical Faculty, Ankara, Turkey, 4 Institutul de Boli Infectioase, Bucharest, Romania, 5 Spitalul Clinic de Boli Infectioase, Timisoara, Romania, 6 Dicle University Medical Faculty, Diyarbakir, Turkey, 7 Uludağ University Medical Faculty, Bursa, Turkey, 8 Johann Wolfgang Goethe University Medical Center, Frankfurt/Main, Germany, 9 Heinrich Heine University, Düsseldorf, Germany, 10 University Medical Centre Hamburg-Eppendorf, Hamburg, Germany, 11 Athens University School of Medicine, Athens, Greece, 12 Medical University of Vienna, Vienna, Austria, 13 Institute of Transplant Immunology, IFB-Tx, Hannover Medical School, Hannover, Germany, 14 HepNet Study-House, Hannover, Germany, 15 Integrated Research and Treatment Center Transplantation, Hannover Medical School, Hannover, Germany, 16 German Center for Infection Research (DZIF), Partner Side HepNet Study-House, Hannover, Germany

Abstract

Background: Hepatitis delta frequently leads to liver cirrhosis and hepatic decompensation. As treatment options are limited, there is a need for biomarkers to determine disease activity and to predict the risk of disease progression. We hypothesized that anti-HDV IgM could represent such a marker.

Methods: Samples of 120 HDV-infected patients recruited in an international multicenter treatment trial (HIDIT-2) were studied. Anti-HDV IgM testing was performed using ETI-DELTA-IGMK-2-assay (DiaSorin). In addition, fifty cytokines, chemokines and angiogenetic factors were measured using multiplex technology (Bio-Plex System). A second independent cohort of 78 patients was studied for the development of liver-related clinical endpoints (decompensation, HCC, liver transplantation or death; median follow up of 3.0 years, range 0.6–12).

Results: Anti-HDV IgM serum levels were negative in 18 (15%), low (OD<0.5) in 76 (63%), and high in 26 (22%) patients of the HIDIT-2 cohort. Anti-HDV IgM were significantly associated with histological inflammatory (p<0.01) and biochemical disease activity (ALT, AST p<0.01). HDV replication was independent from anti-HDV IgM, however, low HBV-DNA levels were observed in groups with higher anti-HDV IgM levels (p<0.01). While high IP-10 (CXCL10) levels were seen in greater groups of anti-HDV IgM levels, various other antiviral cytokines were negatively associated with anti-HDV IgM. Associations between anti-HDV IgM and ALT, AST, HBV-DNA were confirmed in the independent cohort. Clinical endpoints occurred in 26 anti-HDV IgM positive patients (39%) but in only one anti-HDV IgM negative individual (9%; p = 0.05).

Conclusions: Serum anti-HDV IgM is a robust, easy-to-apply and relatively cheap marker to determine disease activity in hepatitis delta which has prognostic implications. High anti-HDV IgM levels may indicate an activated interferon system but exhausted antiviral immunity.

Editor: Stephen J. Polyak, University of Washington, United States of America

Funding: The study was funded by the BMBF-funded Integrated Research and Treatment Center Transplantation, Hannover Medical School, Germany (IFB-Tx funding number 01E00802, Project 37 (H. Wedemeyer and B. Heidrich)). Roche and Gilead funded the HIDIT-2 study. The funders had no role in study design, data collection and analysis, decision to publish, or preparation of the manuscript.

* Email: Wedemeyer.Heiner@mh-hannover.de (HW); awranke@freenet.de (AW)

Introduction

Hepatitis delta is caused by infection with the hepatitis D virus (HDV) and represents the most severe form of chronic viral hepatitis [1]. Chronic hepatitis delta is associated with frequent development of liver cirrhosis, hepatic decompensation and hepatocellular carcinoma (HCC) [2]. HDV is a defective satellite virus that requires the help of the hepatitis B surface antigen for viral assembly and propagation [1]. Treatment options for hepatitis delta are limited. As HDV does not encode for a viral enzyme, no specific direct acting antivirals against HDV are available. Pegylated interferon alpha induces HDV-RNA negativity in about one quarter of patients [3], [4]. However, treatment is poorly tolerated with significant side effects in particular in patients with advanced liver disease [4]. In single patients treatment with interferon alpha can be even harmful. Biomarkers are therefore needed to predict the long-term outcome of hepatitis delta and to identify patients at most urgent need for therapy.

There is currently no reliable non-invasive marker associated with disease activity in hepatitis delta. Quantitative HDV-RNA levels do not correlate with grade or stage of liver disease in HDV-infected patients [5]. Quantitative HBsAg levels show some correlation with histological activity but associations are weak [5]. Similarly the HBeAg status is not associated with distinct outcomes in HDV-infected patients [6].

Anti-HDV Immunoglobulin M (IgM) testing was used to diagnose hepatitis delta infection before HDV-RNA assays became available [7]. Anti-HDV IgM can persist in chronic hepatitis delta patients and reappears in patients with relapse after therapy [8], [9], [10]. We previously showed in a smaller cohort of hepatitis delta patients that anti-HDV IgM levels may correlate with histological inflammatory activity [11]. Nevertheless, these findings were not yet reproduced in larger cohorts and the potential role of anti-HDV IgM testing to predict the clinical long-term outcome of hepatitis delta virus infection is unknown. Moreover detailed mechanisms on the immunopathogenesis of HDV infection leading to different anti-HDV IgM activities are largely undefined [12].

Our primary aim was, therefore, to investigate possible associations of anti-HDV IgM with grade and stage of liver disease in hepatitis delta in a cross-sectional approach testing very well characterized samples from a large multicenter study. In a second step, we investigated whether or not anti-HDV IgM activity can predict the clinical long-term outcome in hepatitis delta. Finally, we questioned if specific cytokines, chemokines and angiogentic factors were associated with anti-HDV IgM to understand possible mechanisms regulating humoral immunity against HDV.

Methods

2.1. Patients

Two independent cohorts of patients were studied. First, we analyzed baseline data of the Hep-Net-International-Delta-Hepatitis-Intervention Trial-2 (HIDIT-2) an prospective international, multicentre trial, investigating the efficacy of PEG-IFN alfa-2a plus tenofovir or placebo for 96 weeks in 121 patients chronically infected with HDV (www.clinicaltrials.gov; NCT00932971; EudraCT-No.: 2008-005560-13). Patients with compensated liver disease (Child A) and absence of HIV or HCV coinfection were eligible. Liver biopsies were performed within one year prior baseline.

Central histological pathological reading was performed by two independent and blinded pathologists (H.P.D, J.S.). Grading and staging was performed according to the Ishak score [13]. All biopsies with an Ishak score of F5 or F6 were defined as cirrhosis. Additionally, cirrhosis was also diagnosed when biopsies did not confirm cirrhosis but two of the following criteria coexisted: platelet count below 100000/ml, AST/ALT ratio >1, bilirubin levels at least 1.5 times higher than upper limit of normal (ULN), Albumin <35 g/l or presence of varices.

A total activity index of 0–7 was considered as minimal or mild hepatitis, a score of 8–18 indicated severe hepatitis.

As the HIDIT-2 trial allowed only cross sectional investigation we recruited an additional independent cohort with patients seen at the Hannover medical school from 1995 to 2012 ("MHH cohort"). Of all anti-HDV IgM positive patients a cohort of 78 chronic hepatitis delta patients were screened to correlate liver-related endpoints with the anti-HDV IgM status. Liver-related endpoints were defined as defined as hepatic decompensation (ascites, encephalopathy, variceal bleeding), liver transplantation, HCC or liver-related death. Patients were included in this study if serum samples or anti-HDV IgM testing were available in addition to the following inclusion criteria. Patients were required to have detectable HBsAg and either anti-HDV IgM antibodies or HDV-RNA for at least six months. Only patients with an available follow up of at least 6 months with a minimum of 2 visits and no longer than 2 years between these visits were included. Patients were excluded if they had undergone liver transplantation, or suffered from HCC before the first observation. Virological parameters for hepatitis B and delta were measured as previously described [5,14].

The MHH cohort was recruited from a real world setting and thus patients received various medications during further follow up including nucleoside and nucleotide analogues (n = 16), PEG-IFN alpha (n = 3) and combinations of interferon and HBV polymerase inhibitors (n = 13). 46 patients did not receive any antiviral therapy during follow-up (n = 46).

Ethics Statement. The HIDIT-2 study was obtained by the approving institutional review board of the Hannover Medical School (Ethikkommission der Medizinischen Hochschule Hannover) and the local ethic committees (Landesamt für Gesundheit und Soziales Berlin, Ethikkommission an der Medizinischen Fakultät der Heinrich-Heine-Universität Düsseldorf, Ethikkommission an der Medizinischen Fakultät der Rheinischen Friedrich-Wilhelms-Universität Bonn, Ethikkommission der J.W.-Goethe-Universität Frankfurt, Ethikkommission der Ärztekammer Hamburg, Ethikkommission der Medizinischen Fakultät der Ludwig-Maximillians-Universität, Ethikkommission der Medizinischen Fakultät der Universität Heidelberg, Ethikkommission der Medizinischen Fakultät der Universität Würzburg, Ethikkommission an der Medizinischen Fakultät der Universität Leipzig) (Nr. 5292M, EudraCT-Nr 2008-005560-13). All of the named ethic committees approved this study. For all of the patients informed consent paperwork was written.

For the measurement of cytokines, chemokines and angiogenetic factors the Ethikkommission der Medizinischen Hochschule Hannover had reviewed the experiments and approved this study design (Nr. 5258).

The internal use of data of the MHH cohort was reviewed by the Ethikkommission der Medizinischen Hochschule Hannover and considered that no informed consent was necessary, given the retrospective and noninterventional nature of the study, and that patient's data were analyzed anonymously.

2.2. Anti-HDV IgM

Anti-HDV IgM testing was performed by using ETI-DELTA-IGMK-2 assay (DiaSorin, Saluggia, Italy) according to manufacturer's instructions. In the first step samples were attached to monoclonal IgG directed at human IgM. After one hour of incubation and washing, HDAg was added. Staining was achieved by adding anti-HD horseradish peroxidase and in a last step chromogen to the sample dilution. The optical density (OD) 450/620 values were ascertained by using photometry (Tecan Rainbow Thermo, Tecan, Crailsheim, Germany).

All samples with an anti-HDV IgM OD 450/620 above the mean extinction of the negative control plus 0.1 were considered to be positive. Samples with optical density values of 10% below or above this cut-off were retested.

To investigate to what extent quantitative values of the assay could be used for further analyses we evaluated the performance of the assay with different sera and plasma samples. Sera and plasma samples obtained in parallel from same individuals revealed similar IgM in all individuals tested (data not shown).

We next investigated different incubation periods. While samples with low IgM levels (<0.5 OD) and very high levels (> 2.5) gave similar values irrespective of the incubation period, a high variability was observed for samples with intermediate and high values (0.5–2.5) considering different incubation periods (Figure S1).

We therefore did not further consider evaluation of OD as linear variables for further investigations but rather grouped IgM levels into four categories (negative, <0.5, 0.5–2.5, >2.5).

2.3. Quantification of cytokines, chemokines and growth factors

The concentrations of fifty cytokines, chemokines and angiogenetic factors were measured in sera using the Luminex-base multiplex technology.

Bio-Plex assays (Bio-Rad, Hercules, USA) contain standard concentrations of each analyte and the calculation of respective standard curves allows a precise definition of the concentrations of the protein of interest. The assay was performed according to the manufacturer's protocol. In brief, lyophilized cytokine standard was resuspended in standard diluent. Serial dilution series to generate standard curves for each cytokine, chemokine and growth factor of interest were performed. The bead mixture, specific for cytokines, chemokines or growth factors was incubated for 30 min at RT with 50 µl standard or serum samples that were diluted in sample diluent (1:2 dilution). Several washing steps were performed with 100 µl wash buffer/well, using the automated washer for magnetic beads. After addition of secondary biotinylated antibody mix for 30 min at RT and three more washing steps, Streptavidin-conjugated R-phycoerythrin (SAPE) was added for 10 min at RT (1:100 dilution). After three final washing steps, beads were resuspended with 125 µl assay buffer, acquired and analyzed by the BioPlex Manager 6.0 software.

2.4. Statistics

Statistical analyses were performed by using SPSS software (SPSS Inc., Chicago, Illinois, USA).

All parameters were described as median. P-values <0.05 were considered as significant factors.

Table 1. Baseline characteristics.

	HIDIT-2	MHH cohort
Total	120	78
Sex	male = 79 (66%)	male = 49 (63%)
	female = 41 (34%)	female = 29 (37%)
Age (years) [median (interquartile range)]	39.9 (31.8–49.6) (n = 120)	40 (30.1–48.8) (n = 78)
Country of origin	Eastern Mediterranean = 68 (57%)	Eastern Mediterranean = 27 (35%)
	Eastern Europe = 44 (37%)	Eastern Europe = 31 (40%)
	Italy = 1 (1%)	Italy = 4 (5%)
	Central Europe = 3 (2%)	Central Europe = 6 (8%)
	other = 4 (3%)	other = 10 (12%)
Anti-HCV positive	0	11 (14.1%)
AST (x ULN) [median (interquartile range)]	1.6 (1.1–2.3) (n = 119)	1.9 (1.6–2.6) (n = 75)
ALT (x ULN) [median (interquartile range)]	2.0 (1.3–3.) (n = 119)	1.9 (1.0–3.0) (n = 74)
AP (x ULN) [median (interquartile range)]	0.6 (0.5–0.7) (n = 119)	0.8 (0.6–1.1) (n = 72)
γGT (x ULN) [median (interquartile range)]	0.8 (0.6–1.5) (n = 118)	0.8 (0.6–1.7) (n = 75)
Bilirubin (µmol/L) median (interquartile range)]	11.4 (8.6–17.1) (n = 116)	11.0 (8.0–20.0)(n = 71)
Albumin (g/L) [median (interquartile range)]	42.0 (39.0–45.0) (n = 119)	39 (35.0–42.0) (n = 63)
Platelets (1000/µL) [median (interquartile range)]	172.0 (130.0–208.0) (n = 119)	130.5 (77.3–165.5) (n = 74)
INR [median (interquartile range)]	1.1 (1.0–1.2) (n = 115)	1.1 (1.1–1.2) (n = 70)
APRI-Score [median (interquartile range)]	1.0 (0.9–1.6) (n = 119)	1.7 (1.0–3.1) (n = 74)
AST/ALT-Ratio [median (interquartile range)]	0.7 (0.6–0.8) (n = 119)	0.9 (0.6–1.2) (n = 73)
BEA-Score [median (interquartile range)]	2.0 (1.0–3.0) (n = 109)	2.0 (1.0–3.0) (n = 77)
MELD [median (interquartile range)]	7.5 (6.8–8.2) (n = 112)	8.0 (7.1–9.3) (n = 66)
Child-Pugh classes	A = 112 (93%)	A = 51 (65%)
	B = 0	B = 8 (10%)
	C = 0	C = 1 (1%)
Cirrhosis	51 (43%) (n = 120)	33 (42%) (n = 78)

Parametric values were analysed by T-Test. For non-parametric (distribution-free) parameters Mann-Whitney-U-tests were used. A Fisher exact test was calculated for the comparison of discrete variables.

The association of IgM with liver related clinical endpoints was additionally identified by Cox-regression models and Kaplan-Meier analysis.

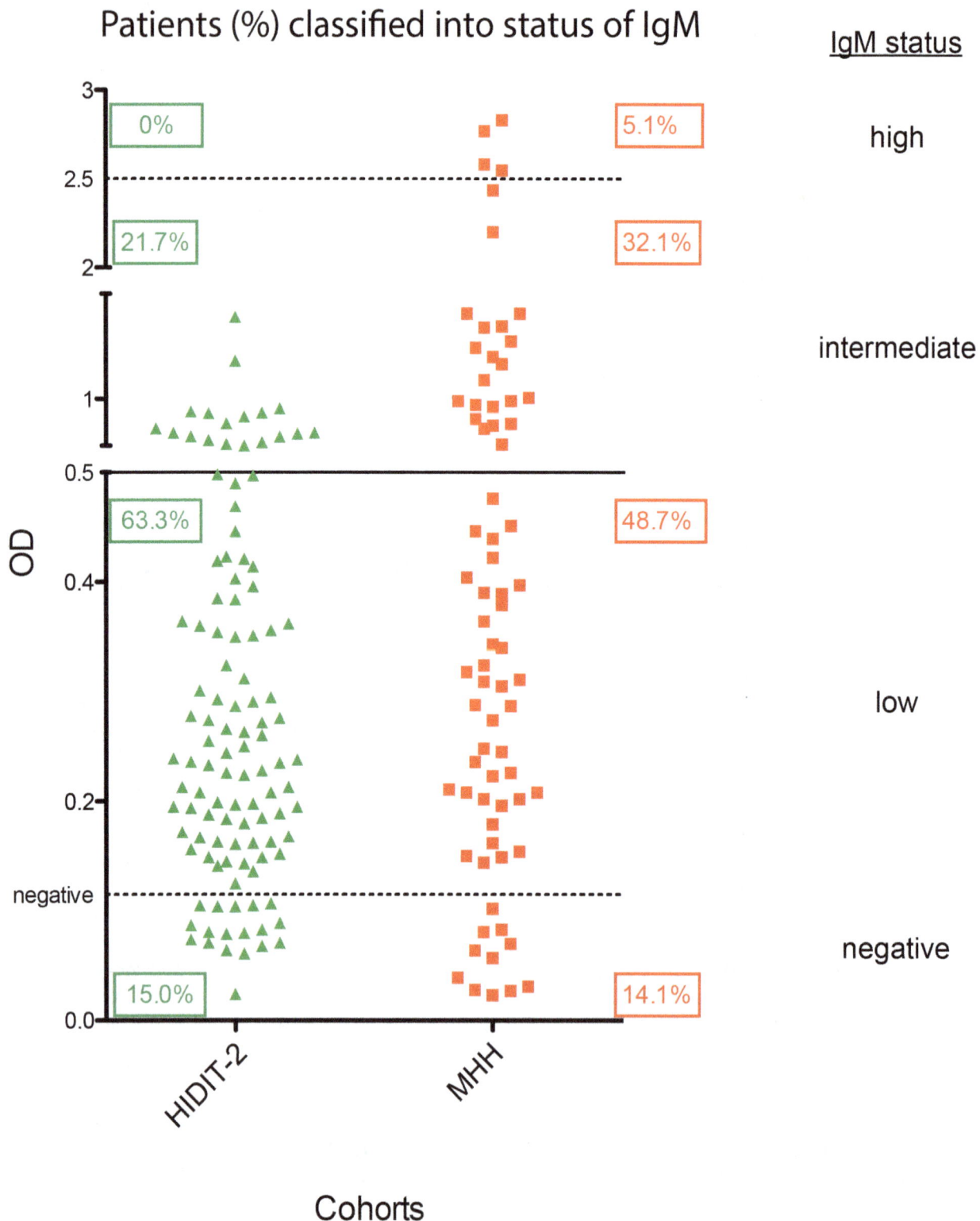

Figure 1. Anti-HDV IgM values in the two cohorts. Grouping into different IgM categories was performed as described in materials and methods.

Results

To investigate the role of anti-HDV IgM testing in hepatitis delta, two independent patient cohorts were studied. Baseline characteristics of patients in both cohorts are shown in Table 1. The HIDIT-2 cohort consisted of individuals fulfilling inclusion criteria for PEG-IFNα-based treatment, thus, individuals with decompensated liver disease were excluded. The second cohort included consecutive patients treated at a tertiary referral center as part of routine clinical follow-up. Both cohorts were similar in terms of gender distribution, mean age, biochemical disease activity and proportion of patients with cirrhosis. Patients in the MHH cohort had slightly more advanced liver fibrosis with a higher mean APRI-Score, higher AST-/ALT- ratios, lower mean albumin levels and lower platelet counts. In the HIDIT-2 cohort most of the patients originated from the Eastern Mediterranean area, whereas in the MHH cohort nearly the same percentage of patients was born in the Eastern Mediterranean area and Eastern Europe regions.

High frequency of anti-HDV IgM in patients with chronic hepatitis delta

Anti-HDV IgM tested positive in 102 patients (85%) of the HIDIT-2 cohort and in 67 patients (85.9%) of the MHH cohort. 63% of patients in the HIDIT-2 cohort and 49% of patients in the MHH cohort presented with low anti-HDV IgM levels. More patients in the MHH cohort showed intermediate IgM values (32%) or even high IgM levels (5%) than in the HIDIT-2 cohort (21% and 0%, respectively) (Figure 1).

Anti-HDV IgM levels are associated with disease activity in hepatitis delta

We next investigated if different categories of anti-HDV IgM levels were associated with clinical, biochemical or virological markers of liver disease in hepatitis delta. As shown in Figures 2

and 3, ALT levels were significantly associated with anti-HDV IgM levels in both cohorts. Similarly, anti-HDV IgM positive individuals had more frequently higher AST levels, higher bilirubin values and lower albumin levels than anti-HDV IgM negative patients in the HIDIT-2 cohort (Table 2). These differences were confirmed for AST and albumin in the MHH cohort (Table 3). Anti-HDV IgM levels were also associated with histological activity when comparing a total histological activity index of 0–7 vs. ≥8 by chi-square analysis (p = 0.02) (Figure 4). In contrast, histological staging was not associated with anti-HDV IgM patients when patients were grouped into cirrhotic and non-cirrhotic individuals (p = 0.4) (Figure 5).

HDV-RNA levels, analyzed both as linear log-transformed values as well as grouped into low, median or high viremia, did not show any association with anti-HDV IgM categories in either of the cohorts (Table 2). Similarly, quantitative HBsAg levels were independent from anti-HDV IgM levels (Table 2). However, HBV-DNA levels were significantly higher in anti-HDV IgM negative patients in the HIDIT-2 cohort (Tables 2 & 3, Figure 6). In the MHH cohort HBV-DNA levels were only available for 35 patients (45%) (anti-HDV IgM negative:4, low:19; intermediate:7; high:1)The differences within the anti-HDV IgM groups were not significant. Nevertheless, the analysis indicated high HBV-DNA levels were more frequently seen in anti-HDV IgM negative patients or in patients with low anti-HDV IgM status (Figure 7).

Thus, high anti-HDV IgM groups were associated with biochemical and histological activity of liver disease and with lower HBV-DNA levels but were independent from HDV replication.

Distinct cytokine and chemokine profiles are associated with anti-HDV IgM levels

To investigate if certain serum inflammatory patterns are associated with anti-HDV IgM levels, a large set of cytokines, chemokines and angiogenic factors was determined in plasma by

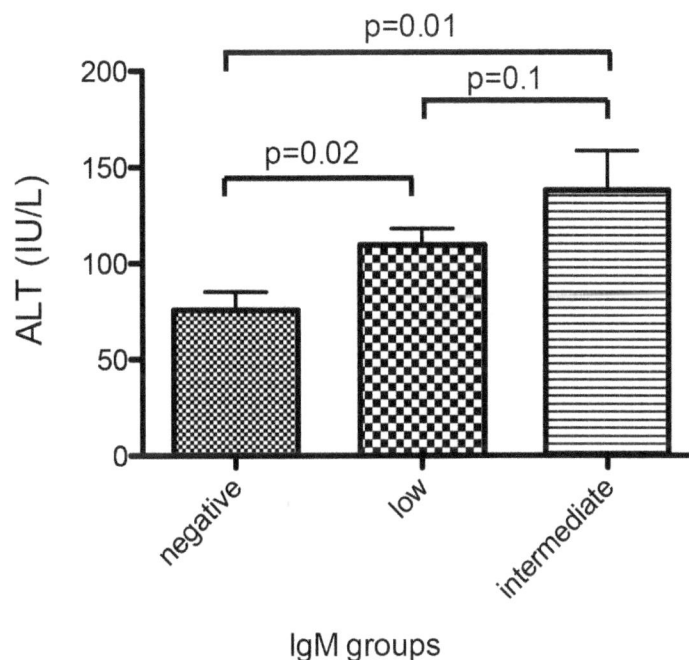

Figure 2. Distribution of ALT values according to Anti-HDV IgM categories in the HIDIT-2 cohort. ALT values were significantly associated with the different anti-HDV IgM groups based on univariate ANOVA (p = 0.04) and univariate T- test in the HIDIT-2 cohort.

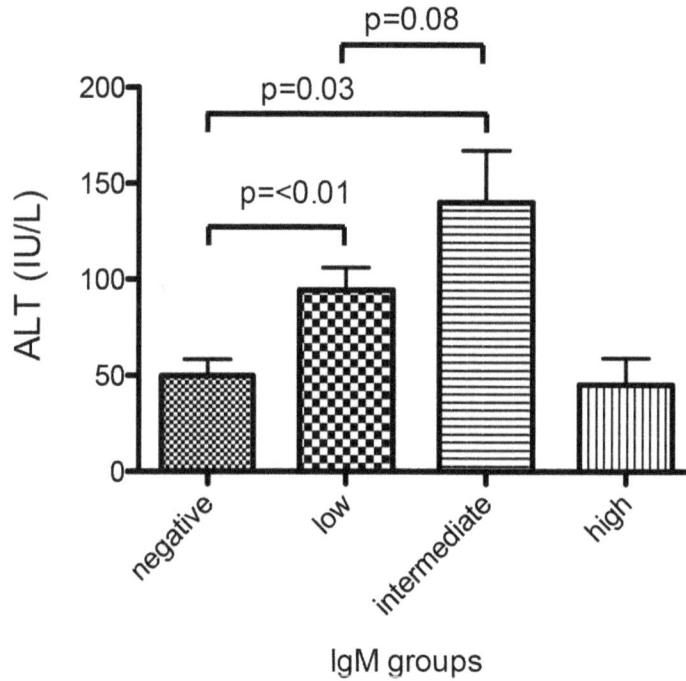

Figure 3. Distribution of ALT values according to Anti-HDV IgM categories in the MHH cohort (only significant p-values). The association of anti-HDV IgM and ALT was confirmed in the MHH cohort with significance over all groups of 0.03.

Grading

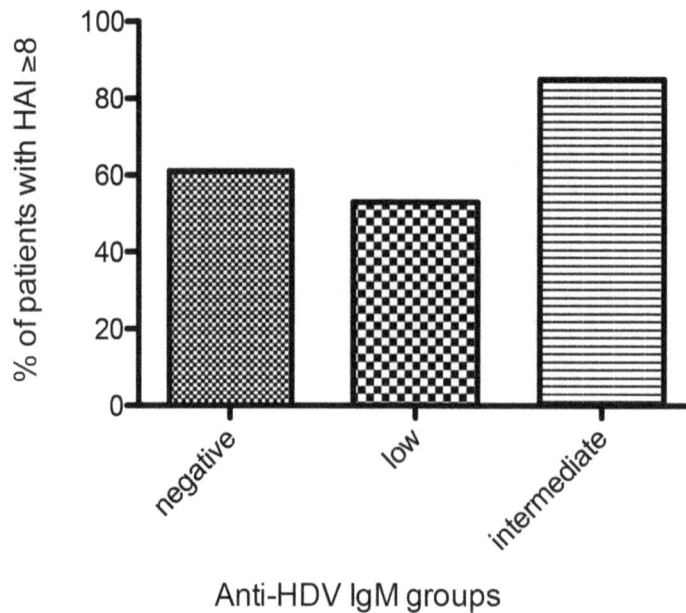

Figure 4. Histological grading of the HIDIT-2 cohort. Diagrammed% of patients with a HAI≥8 within the anti-HDV IgM groups.

Staging

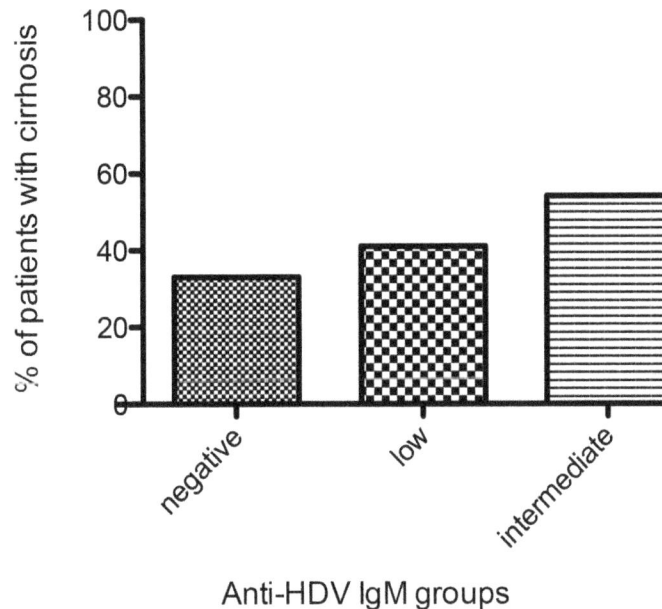

Figure 5. Histological staging of the HIDIT-2 cohort. Diagrammed% of patients with cirrhosis (based on the classification indicated in material and methods) within the anti-HDV IgM groups.

multipex protein arrays (Table S1). Patients with intermediate anti-HDV IgM levels displayed lower serum levels of various pro-inflammatory cytokines including interleukin (IL-) 1, IL- 17, soluble interleukin-2 receptorα (sCD25) and chemokines like IL-8 (CXCL8), SDF-1α (CXCL12) than anti-HDV IgM negative patients (Table 4). The only chemokine that was positively but

not negatively associated with anti-HDV IgM was the interferon gamma-induced protein 10 (IP-10, CXCL10).

To illustrate the univariate ANOVA analysis of all measured parameters we developed a figure indicating which parameters were associated with the three anti-HDV IgM groups in the HIDIT-2 cohort and marked parameters that were high in the intermediate IgM group or low in the low IgM group (Figure 8).

Table 2. Factors associated with anti-HDV IgM positive and negative values according to chi-square analysis in the HIDIT-2 cohort.

HIDIT-2			
	IgM positive	**IgM negative**	p (χ^2-test)
Total	**n = 102**	**n = 18**	
AST (> ULN) [n patients (median AST levels [U/l])]	n = 63 (116.5)	n = 7 (75.7)	0.06
ALT (> ULN) [n patients (median ALT levels [U/l])]	n = 74 (78.3)	n = 11 (55.2)	0.2
γGT (> ULN) [n patients (median γGT levels [U/l])]	n = 41 (73.0)	n = 7 (72.2)	0.6
Bilirubin (> ULN) [n patients (median bilirubin levels [μmol/L])]	n = 29 (13.8)	n = 1 (10.7)	0.03
Albumin (< LLN [n patients (median albumin levels [g/L])]	n = 3 (42.2)	n = 3 (40.1)	0.04
Platelets (< 100000/μL) [n patients (median platelets levels [μL])]	n = 13 (177 727)	n = 0 (174 056)	0.1
HDV-RNA (<20000, 20000–200000, >200000) [n patients (median HDV-RNA levels [IU/m])]	n = 24; 34; 38 (4.9)	n = 5;7; 6 (4.6)	0.9
HBV-DNA (<20000, 20000–200000, >200000) [n patients (median HDV-RNA levels [IU/ml])]	n = 53; 11; 1 (2.4)	n = 6; 5; 3 (3.6)	<0.01
HBsAg (<1000, 1000–10000, >10000) [n patients (median HDV-RNA levels [IU/ml])]	n = 6; 51; 42 (3.9)	n = 1; 7; 10 (4.0)	0.6

Listed bracketed are the median values of the parameters. Virological values are listed in log.
* **LLN**: lower limit of normal. **ULN**: upper limit of normal.

Table 3. Factors associated with anti-HDV IgM positive and negative values according to chi-square analysis in the MHH cohort.

MHH cohort*	IgM positive	IgM negative	p (χ^2-test)
Total	n = 67	n = 11	
AST (> ULN) [n patients (median AST levels [U/l])]	n = 54 (98.8)	n = 5 (44.9)	<0.01
ALT (> ULN) [n patients (median ALT levels [U/l])]	n = 45 (108.0)	n = 4 (50.0)	0.03
γGT (> ULN) [n patients (median γGT levels [U/l])]	n = 29 (82.0)	n = 2 (32.1)	0.09
Bilirubin (> ULN) [n patients (median bilirubin levels [µmol/L])]	n = 20 (18.0)	n = 4 (13.7)	0.5
Albumin (< LLN) [n patients (median albumin levels [g/L])]	n = 21 (37.9)	n = 1 (41.1)	0.09
Platelets (< 100000/µL) [n patients (median platelets levels [µL])]	n = 24 (130 126)	n = 2 (162 363)	0.2
HDV-RNA (<20000, 20000–200000, >200000) [n patients (median HDV-RNA levels [IU/ml])]	n = 48; 6; 12 (4.9)	n = 9; 2; 0 (4.0)	0.2
HBV-DNA (<20000, 20000–200000, >200000) [n patients (median HDV-RNA levels [IU/ml])]	n = 28; 2; 1 (2.7)	n = 3; 1; 0 (3.1)	0.4
Endpoints	n = 26	n = 1	0.05

Listed bracketed are the median values of the parameters. Virological values are listed in log.
* **LLN:** lower limit of normal. **ULN:** upper limit of normal.
*HBsAg levels were available only for a subgroup of patients and could therefore not be analysed.

Anti-HDV IgM negative patients have a more benign clinical course of hepatitis delta

Clinical long-term outcome was investigated in 78 patients who were followed for up to 14 years (median 3 years; range 0.5–14.2). A liver-related clinical decompensation occurred only in one anti-HDV IgM negative patient (9%) but in 26 patients (39%) with positive IgM levels (p = 0.05). In addition to the Fisher exact test (Table 3), endpoints also showed a separation in Kaplan Meier analysis (Figure 9), even though the log-rank (Cox-regression) did not reach a significant value (p = 0.095). Different levels of anti-HDV IgM antibodies (low/high) were not associated with different clinical courses. Of note, the clinical long-term outcome was independent from treatment interventions and response to subsequent antiviral therapies (p = 0.6) or previous exposure to antiviral compounds (p = 0.3) (data not shown).

Thus, anti-HDV IgM testing may identify a subgroup of hepatitis delta patients with a very mild clinical course.

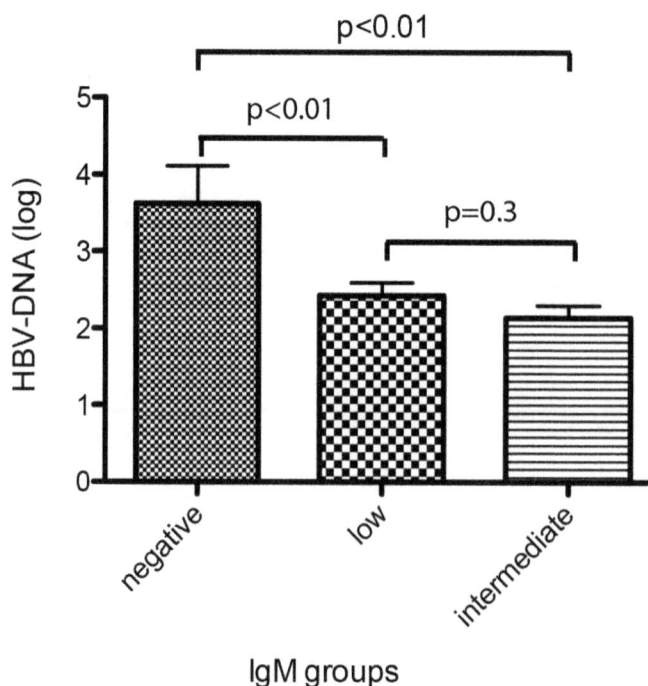

Figure 6. Distribution of HBV values according to Anti-HDV IgM categories in the HIDIT-2 cohort. HBV-DNA (log) is clearly associated with anti-HDV IgM indicated by ANOVA (p<0.01) and by T-test during the different IgM groups.

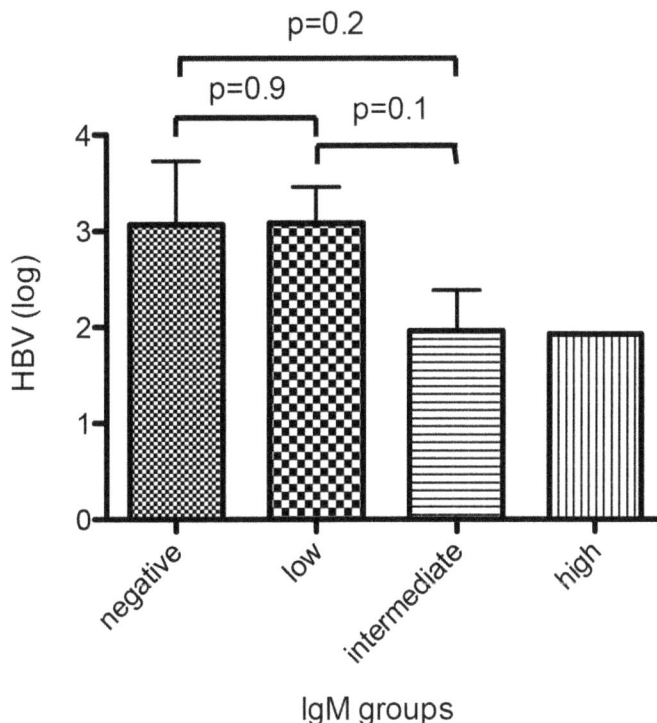

Figure 7. Distribution of HBV values according to Anti-HDV IgM categories in the MHH cohort. HBV-DNA levels were also lower in greater anti-HDV IgM groups in the MHH cohort although no differences could be observed within the anti-HDV IgM groups.

Discussion

Hepatitis delta is the most severe form of chronic viral hepatitis. Considering the limited efficacy and the significant side effect profile of PEG-IFNα therapy, biomarkers are needed to distinguish patients with a more benign natural course of liver disease from individuals who have a higher risk to experience clinical decompensation. We here suggest that anti-HDV IgM may

Table 4. Factors univariatly associated with the groups of anti-HDV IgM based on ANOVA analysis.

	IgM groups			ANOVA
	Negative	**<0.5**	**0.5 - 2.5**	*p-value*
ALT (IU/L) *[median ± standard deviation]*	75.7±40.3	109.5±74.2	137.9±103.5	0.04
AST (IU/L) *[median ± standard deviation]*	55.2±22.6	73.4±42.3	93.0±54.7	0.02
HBV-DNA (log) *[median ± standard deviation]*	3.6±2.1	2.4±1.2	2.4±0.7	<0.01
IL-1β (pg/ml) *[median ± standard deviation]*	5.2±18.6	0.6±1.5	0.1±0.1	0.05
IL-1α (pg/ml) *[median ± standard deviation]*	7.3±25.5	0.7±0.5	0.7±0.4	0.05
IL-8/CXCL8 (pg/ml) *[median ± standard deviation]*	20.01±1.44	8.50±3.50	7.81±3.02	0.04
IL-17 (pg/ml) *[median ± standard deviation]*	115.5±281.2	38.3±18.5	36.7±15.6	0.04
IP-10/CXCL10 (pg/ml) *[median ± standard deviation]*	468.3±202.4	856.5±528.8	1019.0±759.4	0.02
MCP-1/CCL2 (pg/ml) *[median ± standard deviation]*	20.9±23.1	14.0±8.4	11.3±6.4	0.04
M-CSF (pg/ml) *[median ± standard deviation]*	23.1±79.7	2.1±3.0	2.6±2.5	0.05
IL-2Rα/sCD25 (pg/ml) *[median ± standard deviation]*	620.2±1244.3	134.8±63.8	140.2±56.5	<0.01
IL-16 (pg/ml) *[median ± standard deviation]*	221.7±329.1	114.1±50.2	136.6±91.3	0.03
LIF (pg/ml) *[median ± standard deviation]*	63.9±228.1	2.0±3.4	2.1±4.3	0.04
SCF (pg/ml) *[median ± standard deviation]*	116.4±220.9	51.6±26.6	51.7±24.1	0.03
SDF-1α/CXCL12 (pg/ml) *[median ± standard deviation]*	1358.5±4664.1	54.5±31.7	59.4±28.2	0.03
TNF-β (pg/ml) *[median ± standard deviation]*	29.5±107.9	1.1±2.3	1.2±1.5	0.05
b-NGF (pg/ml) *[median ± standard deviation]*	6.9±19.9	1.6±0.8	1.9±0.7	0.05

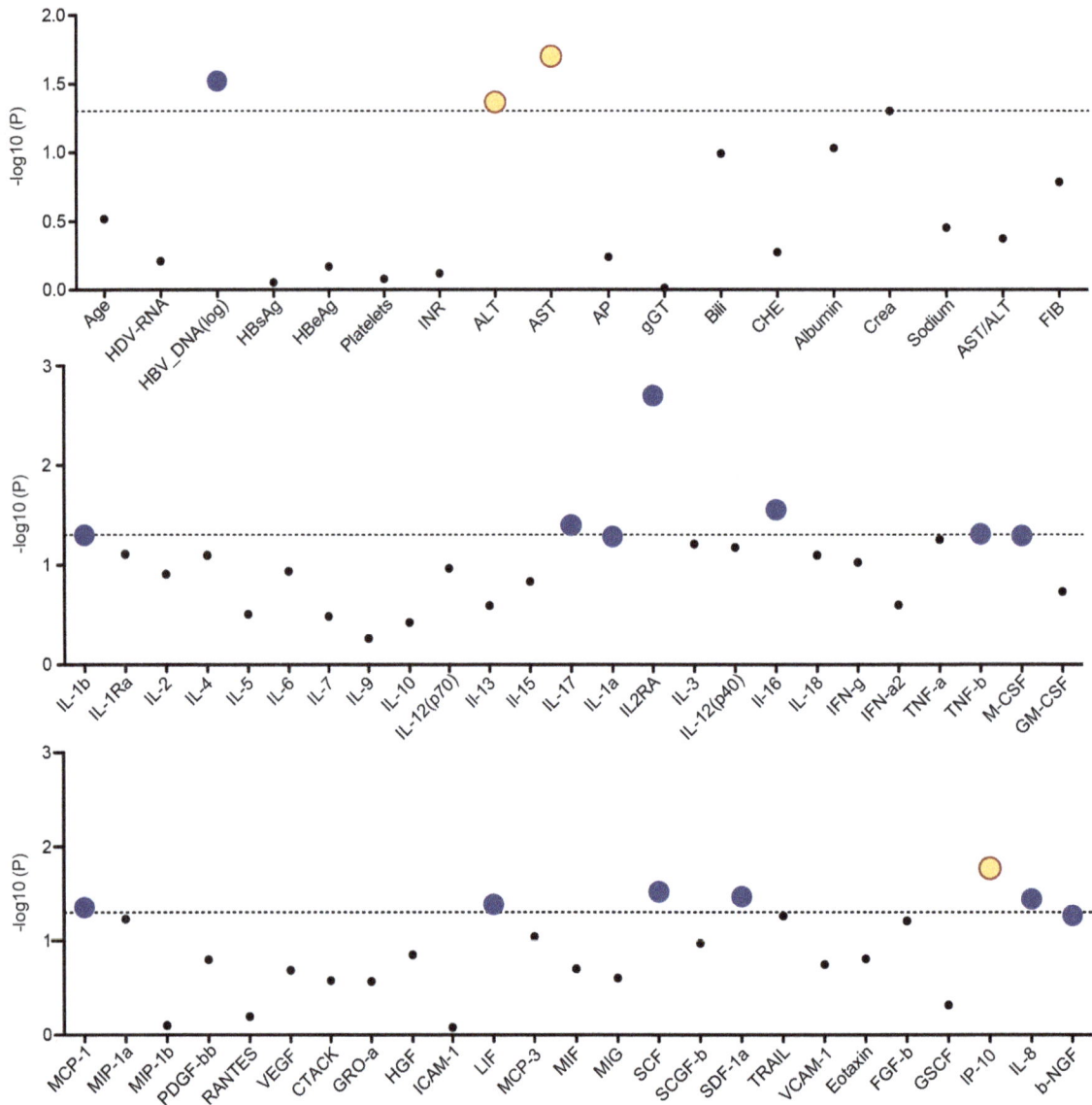

Figure 8. Factors associated with anti-HDV IgM based on univariate ANOVA testing in the HIDIT-2 cohort. The dashed line indicated a p-value of 0.05. All parameters above the line were determined as significantly associated with the four anti-HDV IgM groups. Dots in blue indicate low levels of the value in greater anti-HDV IgM groups while orange dots represent parameters with high levels in a great anti-HDV IgM group shown at x axis.

represent such a marker. IgM levels were associated with histological disease activity and, maybe even more importantly, the absence of anti-HDV IgM identified a subgroup of patients with a very mild course of liver disease that may not require immediate antiviral therapy.

The presence of IgM antibodies against a viral pathogen is usually considered to be associated with early acute infections. However, it is well established for various viral infections including hepatitis B that virus-specific IgM immunogloublins can be detected during all phases of the infection. E.g., anti-HBc IgM antibodies have been observed during flares of chronic hepatitis B [15]. Similarly, increasing levels of anti-HCV IgM have been associated with recurrent hepatitis C after liver transplantation [16]. In chronic hepatitis delta, anti-HDV IgM levels correlated with disease activity and treatment outcome already in earlier studies performed in the 1980ies and early 1990ies [8],[8,10].

However, these study cohorts were rather small and no systematic blinded pathological reading was applied. The present study represents the so far largest cohort of hepatitis delta patients that has been tested for anti-HDV IgM. Another particular strength was that samples were obtained from a very well defined cohort of patients recruited in an international multicenter trial with monitored data and central pathological reading by an experienced pathologist who had no access to other clinical or immunological data. Moreover, a second independent "real-world" cohort of patients collected during routine clinical practice could be studied. With this data set we here demonstrate a rather high frequency of patients testing positive for anti-HDV IgM with more than 80% of patients showing different levels of IgM antibodies in both cohorts. This finding is well in line with our previous sub-analysis of 30 patients treated within the HIDIT-1 study [11].

Cumulative event free survival

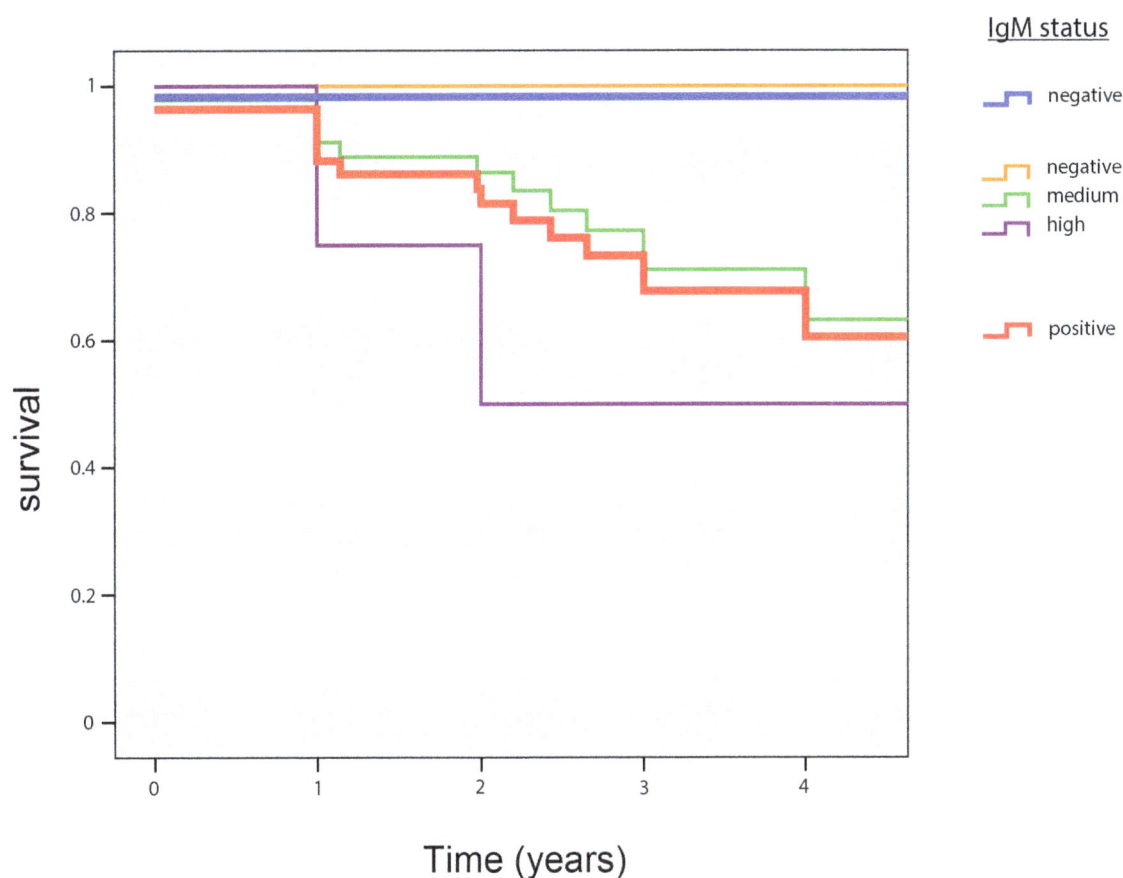

Figure 9. Cumulative event free survival of patients with anti-HDV IgM positive and negative values.

The clinical value of anti-HDV IgM testing in patients with chronic hepatitis delta may be to identify patients with more advanced disease activity. Indeed, ALT and AST levels were significantly higher in patients with intermediate and high anti-HDV IgM levels. More importantly, patients with intermediate anti-HDV IgM levels had more frequently a high inflammatory activity than patients with low levels of or negative anti-HDV IgM. Remarkably, this association with disease activity also translated in differences in the clinical long-term outcome. Only one anti-HDV IgM-negative patient developed a clinical decompensation in the MHH cohort after a follow-up time of up to 12 years. Thus, in clinical practice, the decision to start a potentially toxic treatment based on PEG-IFNα could possibly be delayed in this subgroup of patients which represented around 15% of the cohorts analyzed in the current study. We do not believe that delaying therapy in anti-HDV IgM negative cases would reduce the chance to respond to PEG-IFNα therapy as our preliminary data from another international treatment trial indicated that lower anti-HDV IgM levels maybe associated with weaker but not better treatment responses [11].

Even though the specificity of a negative test to predict a benign clinical course was very high, the sensitivity of anti-HDV IgM testing concerning this particular read-out is still very limited. Grouping patients into low and intermediate anti-HDV IgM levels did not allow to further distinguish different clinical courses of hepatitis delta and thus additional biomarkers would be needed to identify more patients in which treatment may be safely deferred.

Anti-HDV IgM levels were strongly associated with serum CXCL10 (IP-10) levels. CXCL10 has recently been investigated in other hepatitis virus infections and was proposed as a serum marker indicating the activation status of the interferon system. A possible link between serum CXCL10 and anti-HDV IgM could be that IFNα induces CXCL10 and stimulates plasma cells which, thereby, possible leads to an increase anti-HDV IgM levels [17,18]. We previously demonstrated that high levels of CXCL10 can be detected in the serum of hepatitis delta patients and that levels of CXCL10 further increased during PEG-IFNα therapy [19]. High CXCL10 levels have been associated with weaker responses to therapy in hepatitis C virus infection [20], [21], while, in contrast, higher CXCL10 levels correlated with more pronounced declines of HBsAg during polymerase inhibitor therapies in hepatitis B [22] and also PEG-IFNα-based HBV treatment [23]. In line with these findings, we here also describe that patients in a greater anti-HDV IgM group had high levels of CXCL10 levels and lower HBV-DNA values indicating suppressed HBV replication. However, serum HDV-RNA levels were not linked with anti-HDV IgM or serum CXCL10 levels. Thus, these data may suggest that HDV is controlled to a lesser extent by an activated interferon system than HBV. This observation could also partly explain why HDV is usually dominant over HBV as shown by numerous previous studies [5,24,25]. Nevertheless, these findings have to be tested in further experimental studies considering the cellular immunity against HDV.

In contrast to serum CXCL10, all other proinflammatory cytokines investigated in this study showed higher levels when anti-HDV IgM was negative. Thus, controlled HDV infection as indicated by lower disease activity and absence of anti-HDV IgM is associated with a functional broad proinflammatory immune response, indicated by high levels of these cytokines, while more severe disease seems to lead to exhaustion of the antiviral immune defence. Indeed, HDV-specific T cell responses are rather weak in chronic hepatitis delta with active disease [26] but future studies need to investigate this hypothesis in more detail.

Our study has obvious limitations. The clinical course of liver disease in the MHH cohort may have been altered by treatment interventions even though antiviral therapies were not associated with clinical long-term outcome. Moreover, future studies need to investigate anti-HDV IgM dynamics over time, which may even increase the value of IgM testing to predict the clinical outcome. Furthermore, anti-HDV IgM should be investigated in more detail during antiviral therapy. The anti-HDV IgM assay used here allowed reliable determination of semi-quantitative IgM levels; however, improved assays with a broader linear range would be needed to analyse anti-HDV IgM as a continuous linear variable. Finally, although a large cohort of HDV patients was studied, the absolute number of IgM negative patients was still limited. On the other hand, particular strengths of the study are the large sample size, the very well defined cohort of patients recruited in an international multicenter trial, and validation of key findings in an independent cohort.

In summary, our date show that anti-HDV IgM testing is a relatively easy and robust marker which can provide important clinical information as IgM values were associated with disease activity and clinical long-term outcome. We suggest that IgM testing should be introduced in the routine clinical workup of hepatitis delta patients.

Supporting Information

Figure S1 Evaluation of the anti-HDV IgM assay indicated deviations of the optical density values based on variation in time.

Table S1 All measured cytokines, chemokines and angiogenic factors associated with the groups of anti-HDV IgM based on ANOVA analysis.

Acknowledgments

The authors would like to acknowledge the contribution of the HepNet Study-House (a national network sponsored by the German Ministry for Education and Research; BMBF).

Prof. Heiner Wedemeyer is the lead coordinator of its HIDIT-2 Study Group. All lead investigators are listed as authors.

Author Contributions

Conceived and designed the experiments: AW MPM CY HW. Performed the experiments: AW BB JG CSF. Analyzed the data: AW SE. Contributed reagents/materials/analysis tools: AW BH BCS FAC MGC KY SG SZ AE SL GVP JS JK KP MC HPD SH MPM CY HW. Contributed to the writing of the manuscript: AW HW. Suggestions for improvement and proofreading: BH SE BCS FAC MGC KY SG SZ AE SL GVP BB JS JK KP MC CSF HPD SH MPM CY HW.

References

1. Wedemeyer H, Manns MP (2010) Epidemiology, pathogenesis and management of hepatitis D: Update and challenges ahead. Nat Rev Gastroenterol Hepatol 7: 31–40.
2. Hughes SA, Wedemeyer H, Harrison PM (2011) Hepatitis delta virus. Lancet 378: 73–85.
3. Wedemeyer H, Yurdaydin C, Dalekos GN, Erhardt A, Cakaloglu Y, et al. (2011) Peginterferon plus adefovir versus either drug alone for hepatitis delta. N Engl J Med 364: 322–331.
4. Heidrich B, Manns MP, Wedemeyer H (2013) Treatment options for hepatitis delta virus infection. Curr Infect Dis Rep 15: 31–38.
5. Zachou K, Yurdaydin C, Drebber U, Dalekos GN, Erhardt A, et al. (2010) Quantitative HBsAg and HDV-RNA levels in chronic delta hepatitis. Liver Int 30: 430–437.
6. Heidrich B, Serrano BC, Idilman R, Kabacam G, Bremer B, et al. (2012) HBeAg-positive hepatitis delta: Virological patterns and clinical long-term outcome. Liver Int 32: 1415–1425.
7. Rizzetto M (2010) Hepatitis D: Clinical features and therapy. Dig Dis 28: 139–143.
8. Borghesio E, Rosina F, Smedile A, Lagget M, Niro MG, et al. (1998) Serum immunoglobulin M antibody to hepatitis D as a surrogate marker of hepatitis D in interferon-treated patients and in patients who underwent liver transplantation. Hepatology 27: 873–876.
9. Rizzetto M, Shih JW, Gocke DJ, Purcell RH, Verme G, et al. (1979) Incidence and significance of antibodies to delta antigen in hepatitis B virus infection. Lancet 2: 986–990.
10. Farci P, Gerin JL, Aragona M, Lindsey I, Crivelli O, et al. (1986) Diagnostic and prognostic significance of the IgM antibody to the hepatitis delta virus. JAMA 255: 1443–1446.
11. Mederacke I, Yurdaydin C, Dalekos GN, Bremer B, Erhardt A, et al. (2012) Anti-HDV immunoglobulin M testing in hepatitis delta revisited: Correlations with disease activity and response to pegylated interferon-alpha2a treatment. Antivir Ther 17: 305–312.

12. Grabowski J, Wedemeyer H (2010) Hepatitis delta: Immunopathogenesis and clinical challenges. Dig Dis 28: 133–138.
13. Ishak K, Baptista A, Bianchi L, Callea F, De Groote J, et al. (1995) Histological grading and staging of chronic hepatitis. J Hepatol 22: 696–699.
14. Mederacke I, Bremer B, Heidrich B, Kirschner J, Deterding K, et al. (2010) Establishment of a novel quantitative hepatitis D virus (HDV) RNA assay using the cobas TaqMan platform to study HDV RNA kinetics. J Clin Microbiol 48: 2022–2029.
15. Colloredo G, Bellati G, Leandro G, Colombatto P, Rho A, et al. (1996) Quantitative analysis of IgM anti-HBc in chronic hepatitis B patients using a new "gray-zone" for the evaluation of "borderline" values. J Hepatol 25: 644–648.
16. Negro F, Giostra E, Rubbia-Brandt L, Mentha G, Colucci G, et al. (1998) IgM anti-hepatitis C virus core antibodies as marker of recurrent hepatitis C after liver transplantation. J Med Virol 56: 224–229.
17. Jego G, Palucka AK, Blanck JP, Chalouni C, Pascual V, et al. (2003) Plasmacytoid dendritic cells induce plasma cell differentiation through type I interferon and interleukin 6. Immunity 19: 225–234.
18. Liu YJ (2005) IPC: Professional type 1 interferon-producing cells and plasmacytoid dendritic cell precursors. Annu Rev Immunol 23: 275–306.
19. Grabowski J, Yurdaydin C, Zachou K, Buggisch P, Hofmann WP, et al. (2011) Hepatitis D virus-specific cytokine responses in patients with chronic hepatitis delta before and during interferon alfa-treatment. Liver Int 31: 1395–1405.
20. Lagging M, Romero AI, Westin J, Norkrans G, Dhillon AP, et al. (2006) IP-10 predicts viral response and therapeutic outcome in difficult-to-treat patients with HCV genotype 1 infection. Hepatology 44: 1617–1625.
21. Darling JM, Aerssens J, Fanning G, McHutchison JG, Goldstein DB, et al. (2011) Quantitation of pretreatment serum interferon-gamma-inducible protein-10 improves the predictive value of an IL28B gene polymorphism for hepatitis C treatment response. Hepatology 53: 14–22.
22. Jaroszewicz J, Ho H, Markova A, Deterding K, Wursthorn K, et al. (2011) Hepatitis B surface antigen (HBsAg) decrease and serum interferon-inducible

protein-10 levels as predictive markers for HBsAg loss during treatment with nucleoside/nucleotide analogues. Antivir Ther 16: 915–924.

23. Sonneveld MJ, Arends P, Boonstra A, Hansen BE, Janssen HL (2013) Serum levels of interferon-gamma-inducible protein 10 and response to peginterferon therapy in HBeAg-positive chronic hepatitis B. J Hepatol 58: 898–903.

24. Pollicino T, Raffa G, Santantonio T, Gaeta GB, Iannello G, et al. (2011) Replicative and transcriptional activities of hepatitis B virus in patients coinfected with hepatitis B and hepatitis delta viruses. J Virol 85: 432–439.

25. Raimondo G, Brunetto MR, Pontisso P, Smedile A, Maina AM, et al. (2006) Longitudinal evaluation reveals a complex spectrum of virological profiles in hepatitis B virus/hepatitis C virus-coinfected patients. Hepatology 43: 100–107.

26. Nisini R, Paroli M, Accapezzato D, Bonino F, Rosina F, et al. (1997) Human CD4+ T-cell response to hepatitis delta virus: Identification of multiple epitopes and characterization of T-helper cytokine profiles. J Virol 71: 2241–2251.

Genetic Variation in the Interleukin-28B Gene Is Associated with Spontaneous Clearance and Progression of Hepatitis C Virus in Moroccan Patients

Sayeh Ezzikouri[1]*, Rhimou Alaoui[2], Khadija Rebbani[1], Ikram Brahim[1], Fatima-Zohra Fakhir[1], Salwa Nadir[2], Helmut Diepolder[3], Salim I. Khakoo[4], Mark Thursz[5], Soumaya Benjelloun[1]*

1 Virology Unit, Viral Hepatitis Laboratory, Pasteur Institute of Morocco, Casablanca, Morocco, 2 Service de Médecine B, CHU Ibn Rochd, Casablanca, Morocco, 3 Ludwig-Maximilians-Universität München, Marchioninistrasse, München, Germany, 4 University of Southampton, Tremona Road, Southampton, United Kingdom, 5 Department of Hepatology, Division of Medicine, Imperial College, London, United Kingdom

Abstract

Background: Genetic variation in the *IL28B* gene has been strongly associated with treatment outcomes, spontaneous clearance and progression of the hepatitis C virus infection (HCV). The aim of the present study was to investigate the role of polymorphisms at this locus with progression and outcome of HCV infection in a Moroccan population.

Methods: We analyzed a cohort of 438 individuals among them 232 patients with persistent HCV infection, of whom 115 patients had mild chronic hepatitis and 117 had advanced liver disease (cirrhosis and hepatocellular carcinoma), 68 individuals who had naturally cleared HCV and 138 healthy subjects. The *IL28B* SNPs rs12979860 and rs8099917 were genotyped using a TaqMan 5′ allelic discrimination assay.

Results: The protective rs12979860-C and rs8099917-T alleles were more common in subjects with spontaneous clearance (77.9% vs 55.2%; p = 0.00001 and 95.6% vs 83.2%; p = 0.0025, respectively). Individuals with clearance were 4.69 (95% CI, 1.99–11.07) times more likely to have the C/C genotype for rs12979860 polymorphism (p = 0.0017) and 3.55 (95% CI, 0.19–66.89) times more likely to have the T/T genotype at rs8099917. Patients with advanced liver disease carried the rs12979860-T/T genotype more frequently than patients with mild chronic hepatitis C (OR = 1.89; 95% CI, 0.99–3.61; p = 0.0532) and this risk was even more pronounced when we compared them with healthy controls (OR = 4.27; 95% CI, 2.08–8.76; p = 0.0005). The rs8099917-G allele was also associated with advanced liver disease (OR = 2.34; 95% CI, 1.40–3.93; p = 0.0100).

Conclusions: In the Moroccan population, polymorphisms near the *IL28B* gene play a role both in spontaneous clearance and progression of HCV infection.

Editor: Yong-Gang Yao, Kunming Institute of Zoology, Chinese Academy of Sciences, China

Funding: This work was supported by the European Commission under the Health Cooperation Work Programme of the 7th Framework Programme for the Research and Technological Development, HepaCute Project [Grant Agreement n°260844, www.hepacute.eu]. The funders had no role in study design, data collection and analysis, decision to publish, or preparation of the manuscript.

Competing Interests: The authors have declared that no competing interests exist.

* E-mail: sayeh.ezzikouri@pasteur.ma (SE); Soumaya.benjelloun@pasteur.ma (SB)

Introduction

Infection with hepatitis C virus (HCV) is a worldwide health problem, with more than 170 million individuals infected. This infection results in a chronic active hepatitis in more than 80% of the infected patients, of whom 20–30% develop progressive cirrhosis and hepatocellular carcinoma (HCC), conversely only about 10–20% of infected people spontaneously eliminate the virus [1]. In Morocco, the prevalence of anti-HCV antibody in the general population is estimated to be 1.1% [2]. More than 70% of HCV infections in Morocco are genotype 1b, which is the most common genotype in Western North Africa [3]. Therapy with pegintereron-alpha (PegIFN-α) and ribavirin (RVB) is successful in only about 50% of patients infected with genotype 1 [4]. Viral and host factors have been associated with the differences in HCV clearance or persistence, and previous studies have demonstrated

that a strong host immune response against HCV favours viral clearance [5,6]. Ethnic differences in the frequency of virus elimination suggest an involvement of host genetic variation in spontaneous clearance [7]. Four independent genome-wide association studies (GWAS) have recently identified several single nucleotide polymorphisms (SNPs) around the interleukin-28B (*IL28B*) gene, located on chromosome 19q13, coding for IFN-λ3, that are strongly associated with treatment outcome and spontaneous HCV clearance [8,9,10,11]. The two strongest genetic predictors for spontaneous HCV and treatment clearance were SNPs rs12979860 and rs8099917 [8,9,11]. The rs12979860 SNP lies 3 kb upstream of the *IL28B* gene whereas rs8099917 is located 8.9 kb from the IFNλ3-encoding transcript 3′ end in the intergenic region between IFNλ2 and IFNλ3. These polymorphisms exhibit substantial ethnic diversity in their frequency [8,9,11].

Because of its particular geographical location, between the Mediterranean sea, the Atlantic Ocean, and the Sahara desert, Moroccan populations has a dual Berberic and Arabic ethnicity. They show limited genetic diversity as the Arabs and Berbers are closely related [12]. Although the association between *IL28B* polymorphisms and the outcome of HCV infection is well recognised, they have not been studied in Moroccan or in other Maghreb populations. Furthermore there are relatively few studies that have investigated whether this genetic variant also influence the progression of chronic HCV infection [13,14,15,16,17].

In this study, we tested the hypothesis that the SNPs rs12979860 and rs8099917, and their combined effect, are associated with spontaneous clearance and progression of HCV infection in a Moroccan population, in addition to treatment response. To test this hypothesis, we used a prospectively followed up Moroccan cohort that was well characterized in terms of the natural outcome of HCV infection, the stage of disease and treatment response.

Materials and Methods

Patients

To participate in the study, written informed consent for genetic testing including *IL28B* polymorphisms and other potential markers was obtained from all individuals. Each participant was interviewed and completed a structured questionnaire to elicit demographic data and selected risk factors. The study protocol was evaluated and approved by the ethics Committee of the Faculty of Medicine of Casablanca and the study was conducted in accordance with the ethical guidelines of the 1975 Declaration of Helsinki as reflected in a priori approval by the institution's human research committee. Both plasma and peripheral blood mononuclear cells (PBMCs) were stored for all patients. A cohort consisting of 438 Moroccan individuals were enrolled in this study at the Medical Center of Biology at the Pasteur Institute of Morocco and Service of Medicine B CHU Ibn Rochd hospital, Casablanca from January 2010 to October 2012. Two hundred and thirty-two subjects had persistent HCV infection. One hundred and eight were male and 124 female. All were persistently positive for anti-hepatitis C virus (anti-HCV) antibodies and HCV RNA by a quantitative reverse transcriptase-polymerase chain reaction (qRT-PCR) for at least six months. Patients were stratified into two groups according to fibrosis stage as determined by histology. One hundred and fifteen patients had mild chronic hepatitis C (mCHC) (patients with F0 and F1) and 117 patients had advanced liver disease (AdLD) (57 cirrhosis without HCC and 60 cirrhosis with HCC). Sixty-eight individuals (male cases, n = 21 and female cases, n = 47) had spontaneously resolved HCV infection. All were positive for HCV-specific antibodies and negative for HCV RNA in patient's sera by qRT-PCR from at least two measurements more than 6 months apart. Controls consisted of 138 unrelated healthy subjects of mixed Berberic and Arabic ethnicity, who were negative for viral hepatitis markers and had normal serum levels of alanine aminotransferase (ALT) and aspartate aminotransferase (AST). All patients were HBsAg and HIV negative. Serological markers for HBsAg, anti-HCV and anti-HIV were tested with commercially available kits (Axsym, Abbott Diagnostics, Wiesbaden-Delkenheim, Germany and Genscreen Ag/Ab HIV Ultra, Biorad, Marnes La Coquette, France). Plasma HCV-RNA was measured using COBAS AmpliPrep/COBAS TaqMan (Roche Diagnostics, Germany). Hepatitis C virus genotypes were determined by sequencing as described previously [3].

Isolation of Genomic DNA and SNPs Genotyping

Genomic DNA was isolated from PBMC using QIAamp DNA Blood Mini Kit (Qiagen, Valencia, CA) according to the manufacturer's instructions. Genomic DNA concentration was assessed using a NanoVue plus spectrophotometer (GE Healthcare, US). Genotyping for the SNP rs12979860 was performed by means of a TaqMan 5′ allelic discrimination assay. The primers used were forward 5′-TGCCTGTCGTGTACTGAACCA-3′ and reverse 5′-GAGCGCGGAGTGCAATTC-3′. The sequences of the Taqman probes were TGGTTCGCGCCTTC and CTGGTTCACGCCTTC. The probes were labelled with the fluorescent dyes VIC and FAM, respectively. The PCR reaction was carried out in a total volume of 25µl, containing 20 ng of genomic DNA, with the following amplification protocol: pre-incubation at 50°C for 2 min and then 95°C for 10 min, followed by 40 cycles of denaturation at 95°C for 15 s, and annealing/extension at 60°C for 1 min. The genotype of each sample was attributed by the SDS 1.1 software for allelic discrimination (ABI7000, Applied Biosystems, Foster City, CA, USA). Most of the genotypes were confirmed by single base sequencing of PCR products using primers Forward 5′-GCTTATCGCATACGGC-TAGGC-3′ and reverse 5′-TTCCCATACACCCGTTCCTGT-3′, PCR was carried out in a final volume of 25µl, containing 50 ng of genomic DNA, 20 pmol/µl of each primer, 0.5 unit of GoTaq DNA polymerase (Promega, France), 200µM of each dNTP and 1.5 mM $MgCl_2$. The resulting 367-bp PCR product was purified using the Exonuclease I/Shrimp Alkaline Phosphatase (GE Healthcare, US) and sequenced using BigDye Terminator version 3.1 Cycle Sequencing kit (Applied Biosystems, Foster City, CA, USA) and an ABI PRISM 3130 DNA automated sequencer (Applied Biosystems, Foster City, CA, USA). Sequencing data were analyzed using SeqScape v2.5 software (Applied Biosystems, Foster City, CA, USA). The SNP rs8099917 was genotyped using a predesigned TaqMan SNP Genotyping Assay (Applied Biosystems; assay ID C_11710096_10). For 20% of the samples, genotyping was repeated for quality control. The results had 100% concordance.

Statistical Analysis

Continuous variables are presented as mean ± standard deviation or median (range) while categorical variables are expressed as frequencies (%). Differences between continuous variables were analyzed using the Mann-Whitney U test, whilst those between categorical variables were evaluated using the Pearson chi-square test or Fisher's exact test. Departures from Hardy-Weinberg equilibrium were determined by comparing the observed genotype frequencies with expected genotype frequencies in all groups calculated using observed allele frequencies by chi-square G test "Goodness of Fit" with 1 degree of freedom using website http://ihg2.helmholtz-muenchen.de/ihg/snps.html. The existence of differences in allelic and genotypic frequencies between different groups was assessed by means of chi-square test for linear trend when appropriate and calculating the odds ratio (OR) with the 95% confidence intervals (CI). Multiple logistic regression models were used to asses whether *IL28B* rs12979860 C/T and *IL28B* rs8099917 T/G polymorphisms could be considered a predictor of spontaneous resolution and the risk of advanced liver disease. A P value of <0.05 was used as the criterion for statistical significance. All the statistical analyses were performed using Statistical Package for Social Sciences (SPSS) program (version 10.0, SPSS Inc., Chicago, IL, USA).

Results

The demographic data, biochemical features, viral load, viral genotype, and clinical features of our cohort groups are summarized in Table 1. Two hundred and thirty-two patients with HCV persistent infection with a mean age of 63.66±12.26 years [range, 20–90 years], 68 individuals with spontaneous resolution with a mean age of 57.77±15.64 years [range, 17–83 years] and 138 normal controls with a mean age of 56.26±10.57 years [range, 25–85 years] were enrolled in this study. There were no statistically significant differences in the distributions of sex and age between all groups (p>0.05). The mean serum ALT and AST levels was significantly higher in the persistently infected group compared with resolved and control groups (p<0.05). With regard to the viral genotypes, 70% of the patients were infected with viral genotype 1 and 30% of patients with genotype 2 (Table 1). This result is consistent with a recently published report showing the predominance of genotype 1 in Moroccan patients [3].

To estimate the frequencies of the *IL28B* genotypes in Morocco population, the SNPs rs12979860 and rs8099917 were genotyped in healthy controls (Table 2). Overall, the genotype distribution at the rs12979860-C/T locus was as follows: 64 (46%) individuals were C/C homozygous, 59 (43%) were heterozygous and 15 (11%) were T/T homozygotes. At the SNP rs8099917-T/G, the distribution was T/T 80%, T/G 20%, G/G 0%. The allele frequency at the rs12979860 SNP was as follows: 68% for the C allele (95% confidence interval (CI) ±3%) and 90% ±1.69% for the T allele for the rs8099917 SNP. The genotype distributions at both SNPs were in Hardy-Weinberg equilibrium in the healthy control (for the SNP rs12979860, p=0.845 and for the SNP rs8099917, p=0.363).

In order to analyze the impact of polymorphisms of *IL28B* gene in the Moroccan population, we genotyped rs12979860 (C/T) and rs8099917 (T/G) polymorphisms in patients with persistent HCV infection and individuals who had spontaneously cleared the virus (Table 2). Subjects with the rs12979860 C/C genotype cleared HCV infection more often those with the rs12979860-T/T genotype (OR = 4.69; 95% CI, 1.99–11.07; p = 0.0017) or the rs12979860-CT genotype (OR = 2.46 (95% CI, 1.29–4.70;

p = 0.0543) (Table 2). Interestingly, when individuals were stratified according to their rs12979860 genotypes (C/C vs. C/T+T/T), the C/C genotype was overrepresented in the resolved group (66.2%) compared to the persistent HCV infection group (38.4%) (p = 3×10⁻⁵). The rs12979860 C/C genotype was associated with resolution of HCV in both males and females. These results were confirmed by analysis of the linked SNP rs8099917 (Table 2). Genotype distributions were in Hardy-Weinberg equilibrium in both groups (p = 0.345 and 1.00, respectively). 158 of 232 patients (68.1%) with persistent infection were homozygous for T/T, 70 (30.2%) were heterozygous (T/G) and 4 (1.7%) homozygous (G/G), reflecting a T-allele frequency of 83.2%. In individuals with spontaneous clearance the T/T genotype was found in 62 (91.2%) individuals and the G/T genotype in 6 (8.8%). The frequency of the T allele (95.6%) was significantly greater among individuals with HCV clearance as compared to those with persistent infection (83.2%) (p = 0.0025) (Table 2). The *IL28B* T/T genotype was found less frequently in the persistent group compared to spontaneous resolvers (68.1% vs. 91.2%, p = 4×10⁻⁵). Interestingly, when patients with persistent HCV infection were stratified by their viral genotypes, the frequencies of the C/T+T/T genotypes in patients infected with genotype 1 (67.3%) was more prevalent than in patients with genotype 2 (53.5%) (p = 0.0432). Whereas, for the SNP rs8099917, the frequency of G/T+G/G in patients with genotype 1 was 39.8% which was higher than in those infected with genotype 2 (27.9%) (p = 0.0641). This is consistent with a differential effect of the IL-28B polymorphisms on the outcome of genotype 1 versus genotype 2 HCV infection.

To test the association between the SNP rs12979860 and the progression of HCV disease, we genotyped this polymorphism in 117 patients with advanced liver disease (patients with cirrhosis and/or HCC) and compared them with 115 patients with mCHC (Table 3). The frequency of the T/T genotype was significantly overrepresented in advanced liver disease patients compared with mCHC (p = 0.0366) a trend even more pronounced when we compared these frequencies with those of healthy controls (11%, p = 2×10⁻⁵, Table 3). The frequency of the rs12979860-T allele

Table 1. Demographic and clinical characteristics of the study subjects.

	Persistent infection (n = 232)	Spontaneous clearance (n = 68)	Healthy controls (N = 138)
Mean age ± SD, y	63.66±12.26	57.77±15.64	56.26±10.57
Gender (%)			
Male	48	31	48
Female	52	69	52
Alanine aminotransferase (IU/L)	80.38±49.41	31.03±14.90	26.53±9.41
Aspartate aminotransferase (IU/L)	75.59±50.81	29.03±17.08	25.21±9.37
Mean Bilirubin (µmol/L)	26.77±10.20	10.07±2.70	
Mean creatinin (mmol/l)	112.57±105.15	77.28±26.23	
Median Viral Load (IU/ml)	835817 [2030–2.8.10⁸]		
Viral genotypes (%)			
Genotype 1	70		
Genotype 2	30		
mCHC‡	115		
Advanced Liver Disease (AdLD)*	117		

‡Patients with mild chronic hepatitis C.
*including patient with liver cirrhosis and hepatocellular carcinoma.

Table 2. Effect of *IL28B* polymorphisms on the outcomes of HCV infection.

	Healthy controls	Subjects with persistence	Subjects with spontaneous clearance	Subjects with persistence vs. Subjects with spontaneous clearance	OR (95% CI)	P-value[¥]
rs12979860	n = 276	n = 464	n = 136			
C allele	0.680±0.03	0.552±0.026	0.779±0.040	C vs T	2.87 (1.84–4.48)	0.00001
T allele	0.320±0.03	0.448±0.026	0.221±0.040			
	n = 138	n = 232	n = 68			
C/C	64 (46.4%)	89 (38.4%)	45 (66.2%)	C/C vs T/T	4.69 (1.99–11.07)	0.0017
C/T	59 (42.7%)	78 (33.6%)	16 (23.5%)	C/C vs C/T	2.46 (1.29–4.70)	0.0543
T/T	15 (10.9%)	65 (28%)	7 (10.3%)	C/C vs C/T and T/T	3.14 (1.78–5.55)	0.0004
rs8099917	n = 276	n = 464	n = 136			
T allele	0.902±0.017	0.832±0.017	0.956±0.017	T vs G	4.38 (1.86–10.28)	0.0025
G allele	0.098±0.017	0.168±0.017	0.044±0.017			
	n = 138	n = 232	n = 68			
T/T	111 (80.4%)	158 (68.1%)	62 (91.2%)	T/T vs T/G	4.58 (1.89 11.08)	0.0029
T/G	27 (19.6%)	70 (30.2%)	6 (8.8%)	T/T vs G/G	3.55 (0.19–66.89)	0.2110
G/G	0 (0%)	4 (1.7%)	0 (0%)	T/T vs T/G and G/G	4.84 (2.00–11.69)	0.0017

[¥]Bonferroni correction was applied.

in advanced liver disease (50%) was also significantly higher than in patients with mCHC (39.6%) (p = 0.0238). In multivariate logistic regression analysis the association of the rs12979860-T/T genotype with advanced liver disease compared with mCHC revealed an OR of 1.89 (CI, 0.99–3.61; p = 0.0532) after adjustment for age, sex and viral genotype.

We found a similar effect for the SNP rs8099917. In multivariate logistic regression analysis after adjustment for age and sex we found that the genotypes T/G+G/G were higher in those with advanced liver disease as compared to mCHC (42% versus 21%, respectively) (p = 0.0002) (Table 3). Taking the T/T genotype as the reference, the OR and 95% CI for the T/G and

Table 3. Effect of *IL28B* polymorphisms on the progression of HCV infection.

	Healthy controls (N = 138)	mCHC group (n = 115)	HCV-AdLD group (n = 117)	mCHC vs. AdLD OR (95% CI)	P-value[¥]	Healthy controls vs. AdLD OR (95% CI)	P-value[¥]
Mean age ± SD	56.26±10.57	60.58±14.21	66.53±9.26		0.0039		
Male/Female	66/72	44/71	64/53		0.0130		
Genotype 1	-	65%	72%		0.4360		
Genotype 2	-	35%	28%				
rs12979860							
C/C	64 (46.4%)	51 (44.3%)	38 (32.5%)	1.00		1.00	
C/T	59 (42.7%)	37 (32.2%)	41 (35%)	1.49 (0.81–2.74)	0.2025	1.17 (0.66–2.06)	0.5855
T/T	15 (10.9%)	27 (23.5%)	38 (32.5%)	1.89 (0.99–3.61)	0.0532	4.27 (2.08–8.76)	0.0005
C allele	0.680±0.03	0.604±0.037	0.500±0.037	1.00		1.00	
T allele	0.320±0.03	0.396±0.037	0.500±0.037	1.53 (1.06–2.21)	0.0238	2.10 (1.47–3.01)	0.0005
rs8099917							
T/T	111 (80.4%)	91 (79.1%)	68 (58.1%)	1.00		1.00	
T/G	27 (19.6%)	23 (20%)	46 (39.3%)	2.68 (1.48–4.83)	0.0091	2.78 (1.58–4.88)	0.0029
G/G	0 (0%)	1 (0.9%)	3 (2.6%)	4.00 (0.41–39.44)	0.1991	11.94 (0.58–223.97)	0.2898
T allele	0.902±0.017	0.891±0.020	0.778±0.025	1.00		1.00	
G allele	0.098±0.017	0.109±0.020	0.222±0.025	2.34 (1.40–3.93)	0.0100	2.63 (1.59–4.36)	0.0011

*Adjusted for age, gender and viral genotype.
[¥]Bonferroni correction was applied.

G/G genotypes presence in the advanced versus mild groups were 2.68±1.48−4.83 and 4.00±0.41−39.44 respectively (Table 3).

Data for clearance following PegIFN-α plus RVB treatment were available in 41 patients. For the SNP rs12979860, there is a statistical difference (p = 0.035) was observed for the distribution of the genotype C/C [75%, n = 6] and genotypes C/T and T/T [25%, n = 2] between responders and non-responders (genotype C/C [33%, n = 11] and genotypes C/T and T/T [67%, n = 22], Fisher's exact test). Furthermore the rs8099917 polymorphism was associated with SVR. In responders the frequency of patients with T/T genotype (80%) was higher than in non-responders (60%) (OR = 0.46, 95% CI 0.22–1.09; p = 0.019).

The analysis of the combination of SNPs rs12979860 with rs8099917 showed that patients with persistent infection were 8.27 (95% CI, 1.90–36.11; p = 0.0011) times more likely to have the rs12979860-T/T/rs8099917-T/G genotypes (13.80% vs 2.94% in resolved group) and 4.68 (95% CI, 0.25–88.85) fold to have rs12979860-TT/rs8099917-GG genotypes (1.72% vs none in resolved group) but did not reach the significance (p = 0.155) when compared to rs12979860-C/C/rs8099917-T/T carriers.

Therefore, we hypothesized that an increased risk of progression towards advanced liver disease could be detected when unfavourable alleles are combined in a given patient. Consequently, the SNP-SNP combination of rs12979860 with rs8099917 was examined. We found that the rs12979860-T/T/rs8099917-T/G genotype was present in 19.6% of the advanced group versus 6.9% in mCHC (p = 0.0035), conferring an OR of 3.70 (95% CI, 1.49–9.20, p = 0.0035) for advanced liver disease. Additionally, the frequency for patients with rs12979860-T/T/rs8099917-G/G genotypes was 2.6% in the advanced group vs 0.9% in mCHC conferring a 3.87-fold increased risk for advanced liver disease compared to rs12979860-C/C/rs8099917-T/T carriers.

Discussion

The ability of the virus to persist within a host's attributed to its efficient ability to evade the adaptive and innate components of the host's immune system. In addition, a small number of specific host polymorphisms have been correlated with spontaneous HCV clearance [18]. The SNPs near the *IL28B* gene on chromosome 19 coding for type III IFN-λ3 have recently been reported to be associated with clearance and treatment response in HCV [8,19]. First, we analyzed the *IL28B* polymorphisms in the 138 healthy subjects. The rs12979860-C allele frequency observed in the Moroccan population (68%) was similar to that reported in the Egyptian population (67%) [20] and in the Italian population (68%) [13,21] but was significantly higher than those observed within the sub-Saharan African populations (23.1–54.8%) [19]. However, the C allele frequency remains much lower than the highest frequencies found in Eastern Asian (91–100%) and in Oceanian populations (100%) [19]. The frequency of the favourable T allele of the rs8099917 SNPwas 90% amongst Moroccan subjects, which is similar to frequencies reported in African (93%) and European (83%) populations but was higher than those observed in a population with Mexican ancestry (69%) [22]. Thus ethnic differences in the *IL28B* gene polymorphisms may explain, at least in part, the different outcomes rates of HCV infection in different ethnic groups. For this reason, we examined the genetic variation in the *IL28B* gene and the natural clearance of HCV infection in the Moroccan population. Our results demonstrate that the rs12979860- C/C genotype is strongly associated with spontaneous eradication of the virus in the Maghreban populations. Our results are consistent with previous studies of the association of rs12979860-C/C genotype with

spontaneous clearance. We found a relationship with the highest clearance rate among C/C Moroccan subjects (66.2%), an intermediate clearance rate among heterozygous individuals (23.5%), and the lowest rate in the T/T homozygous subjects (10.3%). For spontaneous HCV clearance, Thomas et al. reported that the *IL28B* rs12979860-C/T polymorphism predicted the rate of spontaneous clearance of HCV, with the frequency of spontaneous clearance being 53% in patients with the C/C genotype versus 23% of patients with the T/T genotype [19]. Several larger studies reported that the rs12979860-C/C genotype was associated with spontaneous eradication of the virus [20,23,24,25,26,27] (Table S1). Moreover, Langhans and coworkers demonstrated that high IFN-λ serum levels were prevalent in carriers of the rs12979860-C allele and associated with a favourable outcome of HCV infection confirming the important antiviral properties of type III interferons (IFNs) [28].

The influence of *IL28B* polymorphisms on the severity and progression of liver disease remains unclear with controversial results [13,14,15,16,29,30]. This emphasizes the necessity to replicate these studies in ethnically diverse populations. In our study, the frequency of patients with the rs12979860-T/T genotype differ between mCHC and HCV-AdLD groups (Table 3), suggesting that this polymorphism may play a role in the progression of HCV among Moroccan patients. Actually, in patients with advanced liver disease the frequency of the T allele was 50%, compared to 60.4% of patients with mild liver disease. Carriage of the T allele was found to be an independent predictor of progression to an advanced stage, which is consistent with the reports in other populations [13,16,29,31]. The rs12979860-T/T genotype was previously been associated with a four-fold increase in risk for HCC development in Italian patients, particularly among patients infected with HCV [13]. Recently, Clark and colleagues found that the rs12979860-T/T genotype was associated with fibrosis in patients with chronic hepatitis C [32]. Moreover, several *in vitro* studies and animal models demonstrated that activation of type III IFN induces apoptosis and also that this cytokine possesses anti-tumour activities [33]. Thus, the SNP rs12979860 may serve as an important predictive biomarker of liver disease and offers new insights into the biological pathways involved in liver cirrhosis and carcinogenesis. In addition, it was reported that the rs8099917-T/T genotype was associated with spontaneous clearance of HCV (Table S1) and inflammatory activity and fibrosis in patients with chronic hepatitis C in Japan. Overall our results confirm this positive association between rs8099917 polymorphism and progression of HCV infection [11,34]. Overall, elucidating the mechanism by which the *IL28B* polymorphisms affects the progression to cirrhosis and HCC remains an important future challenge.

In Morocco, HCV genotype 1 is more prevalent than genotype 2. In addition, the SVR rate for individuals infected with genotype 1, is low (40–50%) and requires 12 months of therapy. Results from our small cohort showed that patients who achieved SVR had a higher frequency of the rs12979860-C/C genotype (75%) compared to those carrying the T/T genotype (12.5%).

Finally, the combination of the two polymorphisms is associated with significantly increased persistence and linked to progression towards advanced stages of HCV-associated disease. Individuals with rs12979860-T/T genotype and T/G or G/G of rs8099917 have an 8.27 and 4.68-fold-risk to evolve towards chronicity respectively, and a 3.70 and 3.87 increase in risk to be affected with an advanced liver disease.

We are, however, fully aware that the limitation of the current study is its relatively small size and, further studies warrant the recruitment of a larger cohort with analysis of the above mentioned, and additional polymorphisms and haplotypes of the *IL28B* gene. These will help to clarify their role in HCV clearance and may provide a mechanism for understanding the relationship between IL28B and HCV infection.

In summary, our results are the first providing information about the impact of IL28B polymorphisms on hepatitis C outcomes and progression in the Maghrebian region. We found that rs12979860-C/C and rs8099917-T/T genotypes showed a strong association with resolution of HCV infection. Altogether, our result support that *IL28B* polymorphisms seems to be involved in the progression of HCV infection to cirrhosis and hepatocellular carcinoma. This finding adds evidence to the hypothesis that the host's immunogenetic background modulates the progression of liver disease in chronic hepatitis C in multiple and ethnically diverse populations.

Acknowledgments

We are particularly grateful to Dr Pascal Pineau for reading of Manuscript.

Author Contributions

Conceived and designed the experiments: SE SB SIK. Performed the experiments: SE KR FZF IB. Analyzed the data: SE SB HD SIK. Contributed reagents/materials/analysis tools: RA SN. Wrote the paper: SE SB MT SIK.

References

1. Thomas DL, Seeff LB (2005) Natural history of hepatitis C. Clin Liver Dis 9: 383–398.
2. Benjelloun S, Bahbouhi B, Sekkat S, Bennani A, Hda N, et al. (1996) Anti-HCV seroprevalence and risk factors of hepatitis C virus infection in Moroccan population groups. Res Virol 147. 247–255.
3. Brahim I, Akil A, Mtairag el M, Pouillot R, Malki AE, et al. (2012) Morocco underwent a drift of circulating hepatitis C virus subtypes in recent decades. Arch Virol 157: 515–520.
4. Liver EAftSot (2011) EASL Clinical Practice Guidelines: management of hepatitis C virus infection. J Hepatol 55: 245–264.
5. Cooper S, Erickson AL, Adams EJ, Kansopon J, Weiner AJ, et al. (1999) Analysis of a successful immune response against hepatitis C virus. Immunity 10: 439–449.
6. Rehermann B, Nascimbeni M (2005) Immunology of hepatitis B virus and hepatitis C virus infection. Nat Rev Immunol 5: 215–229.
7. Thomas DL, Astemborski J, Rai RM, Anania FA, Schaeffer M, et al. (2000) The natural history of hepatitis C virus infection: host, viral, and environmental factors. Jama 284: 450–456.
8. Ge D, Fellay J, Thompson AJ, Simon JS, Shianna KV, et al. (2009) Genetic variation in IL28B predicts hepatitis C treatment-induced viral clearance. Nature 461: 399–401.
9. Suppiah V, Moldovan M, Ahlenstiel G, Berg T, Weltman M, et al. (2009) IL28B is associated with response to chronic hepatitis C interferon-alpha and ribavirin therapy. Nat Genet 41: 1100–1104.
10. Tanaka Y, Nishida N, Sugiyama M, Kuroksaki M, Matsuura K, et al. (2009) Genome-wide association of IL28B with response to pegylated interferon-alpha and ribavirin therapy for chronic hepatitis C. Nat Genet 41: 1105–1109.
11. Rauch A, Kutalik Z, Descombes P, Cai T, Di Iulio J, et al. (2010) Genetic variation in IL28B is associated with chronic hepatitis C and treatment failure: a genome-wide association study. Gastroenterology 138: 1338–1345, 1345 e1331–1337.
12. Coudray C, Guitard E, Kandil M, Harich N, Melhaoui M, et al. (2006) Study of GM Immunoglobulin Allotypic System in Berbers and Arabs From Morocco. American Journal Of Human Biology 18: 23–34.
13. Fabris C, Falleti E, Cussigh A, Bitetto D, Fontanini E, et al. (2011) IL-28B rs12979860 C/T allele distribution in patients with liver cirrhosis: role in the course of chronic viral hepatitis and the development of HCC. J Hepatol 54: 716–722.
14. Bochud PY, Bibert S, Kutalik Z, Patin E, Guergnon J, et al. (2012) IL28B alleles associated with poor hepatitis C virus (HCV) clearance protect against inflammation and fibrosis in patients infected with non-1 HCV genotypes. Hepatology 55: 384–394.
15. Joshita S, Umemura T, Katsuyama Y, Ichikawa Y, Kimura T, et al. (2012) Association of IL28B gene polymorphism with development of hepatocellular carcinoma in Japanese patients with chronic hepatitis C virus infection. Hum Immunol 73: 298–300.
16. Eurich D, Boas-Knoop S, Bahra M, Neuhaus R, Somasundaram R, et al. (2012) Role of IL28B polymorphism in the development of hepatitis C virus-induced hepatocellular carcinoma, graft fibrosis, and posttransplant antiviral therapy. Transplantation 93: 644–649.
17. Abe H, Ochi H, Maekawa T, Hayes CN, Tsuge M, et al. (2010) Common variation of IL28 affects gamma-GTP levels and inflammation of the liver in chronically infected hepatitis C virus patients. J Hepatol 53: 439–443.
18. Sklan EH, Charuworn P, Pang PS, Glenn JS (2009) Mechanisms of HCV survival in the host. Nat Rev Gastroenterol Hepatol 6: 217–227.
19. Thomas DL, Thio CL, Martin MP, Qi Y, Ge D, et al. (2009) Genetic variation in IL28B and spontaneous clearance of hepatitis C virus. Nature 461: 798–801.
20. Kurbanov F, Abdel-Hamid M, Latanich R, Astemborski J, Mohamed M, et al. (2011) Genetic polymorphism in IL28B is associated with spontaneous clearance of hepatitis C virus genotype 4 infection in an Egyptian cohort. J Infect Dis 204: 1391–1394.
21. Kobayashi M, Suzuki F, Akuta N, Sezaki H, Suzuki Y, et al. (2012) Association of two polymorphisms of the IL28B gene with viral factors and treatment response in 1,518 patients infected with hepatitis C virus. J Gastroenterol 47: 596–605.
22. Balagopal A, Thomas DL, Thio CL (2010) IL28B and the control of hepatitis C virus infection. Gastroenterology 139: 1865–1876.
23. Shi X, Pan Y, Wang M, Wang D, Li W, et al. (2012) IL28B Genetic Variation Is Associated with Spontaneous Clearance of Hepatitis C Virus, Treatment Response, Serum IL-28B Levels in Chinese Population. PLoS One 7: e37054.
24. Shebl FM, Pfeiffer RM, Buckett D, Muchmore B, Chen S, et al. (2011) IL28B rs12979860 genotype and spontaneous clearance of hepatitis C virus in a multi-ethnic cohort of injection drug users: evidence for a supra-additive association. J Infect Dis 204: 1843–1847.
25. Tillmann HL, Thompson AJ, Patel K, Wiese M, Tenckhoff H, et al. (2010) A polymorphism near IL28B is associated with spontaneous clearance of acute hepatitis C virus and jaundice. Gastroenterology 139: 1586–1592, 1592 e1581.
26. Pedergnana V, Abdel-Hamid M, Guergnon J, Mohsen A, Le Fouler L, et al. (2012) Analysis of IL28B variants in an Egyptian population defines the 20 kilobases minimal region involved in spontaneous clearance of hepatitis C virus. PLoS One 7: e38578.
27. Di Marco V, Bronte F, Calvaruso V, Capra M, Borsellino Z, et al. (2012) IL28B polymorphisms influence stage of fibrosis and spontaneous or interferon-induced viral clearance in thalassemia patients with hepatitis C virus infection. Haematologica 97: 679–686.
28. Langhans B, Kupfer B, Braunschweiger I, Arndt S, Schulte W, et al. (2011) Interferon-lambda serum levels in hepatitis C. J Hepatol 54: 859–865.
29. Rembeck K, Alsio A, Christensen PB, Farkkila M, Langeland N, et al. (2012) Impact of IL28B-related single nucleotide polymorphisms on liver histopathology in chronic hepatitis C genotype 2 and 3. PLoS One 7: e29370.
30. Montes-Cano MA, Garcia-Lozano JR, Abad-Molina C, Romero-Gomez M, Barroso N, et al. (2010) Interleukin-28B genetic variants and hepatitis virus infection by different viral genotypes. Hepatology 52: 33–37.
31. Rivero-Juarez A, Camacho A, Caruz A, Neukam K, Gonzalez R, et al. (2012) LDLr genotype modifies the impact of IL28B on HCV viral kinetics after the first weeks of treatment with PEG-IFN/RBV in HIV/HCV patients. Aids 26: 1009–1015.
32. Clark PJ, Thompson AJ, Zhu Q, Vock DM, Zhu M, et al. (2012) The Association of Genetic Variants with Hepatic Steatosis in Patients with Genotype 1 Chronic Hepatitis C Infection. Dig Dis Sci.
33. Li W, Lewis-Antes A, Huang J, Balan M, Kotenko SV (2008) Regulation of apoptosis by type III interferons. Cell Prolif 41: 960–979.
34. Rao HY, Sun DG, Jiang D, Yang RF, Guo F, et al. (2012) IL28B genetic variants and gender are associated with spontaneous clearance of hepatitis C virus infection. J Viral Hepat 19: 173–181.

Permissions

All chapters in this book were first published in PLOS ONE, by The Public Library of Science; hereby published with permission under the Creative Commons Attribution License or equivalent. Every chapter published in this book has been scrutinized by our experts. Their significance has been extensively debated. The topics covered herein carry significant findings which will fuel the growth of the discipline. They may even be implemented as practical applications or may be referred to as a beginning point for another development.

The contributors of this book come from diverse backgrounds, making this book a truly international effort. This book will bring forth new frontiers with its revolutionizing research information and detailed analysis of the nascent developments around the world.

We would like to thank all the contributing authors for lending their expertise to make the book truly unique. They have played a crucial role in the development of this book. Without their invaluable contributions this book wouldn't have been possible. They have made vital efforts to compile up to date information on the varied aspects of this subject to make this book a valuable addition to the collection of many professionals and students.

This book was conceptualized with the vision of imparting up-to-date information and advanced data in this field. To ensure the same, a matchless editorial board was set up. Every individual on the board went through rigorous rounds of assessment to prove their worth. After which they invested a large part of their time researching and compiling the most relevant data for our readers.

The editorial board has been involved in producing this book since its inception. They have spent rigorous hours researching and exploring the diverse topics which have resulted in the successful publishing of this book. They have passed on their knowledge of decades through this book. To expedite this challenging task, the publisher supported the team at every step. A small team of assistant editors was also appointed to further simplify the editing procedure and attain best results for the readers.

Apart from the editorial board, the designing team has also invested a significant amount of their time in understanding the subject and creating the most relevant covers. They scrutinized every image to scout for the most suitable representation of the subject and create an appropriate cover for the book.

The publishing team has been an ardent support to the editorial, designing and production team. Their endless efforts to recruit the best for this project, has resulted in the accomplishment of this book. They are a veteran in the field of academics and their pool of knowledge is as vast as their experience in printing. Their expertise and guidance has proved useful at every step. Their uncompromising quality standards have made this book an exceptional effort. Their encouragement from time to time has been an inspiration for everyone.

The publisher and the editorial board hope that this book will prove to be a valuable piece of knowledge for researchers, students, practitioners and scholars across the globe.

Contributors

Weixia Ke., Li Liu., Chi Zhang, Xiaohua Ye, Yanhui Gao, Shudong Zhou and Yi Yang
Department of Epidemiology and Biostatistics and Guangdong Key Lab of Molecular Epidemiology, School of Public Health, Guangdong Pharmaceutical University, Guangzhou, Guangdong, China

Jerzy Jaroszewicz, Heiner Wedemeyer and Markus Cornberg
Department of Gastroenterology, Hepatology and Endocrinology, Hannover Medical School, Hannover, Germany

Thomas Reiberger and Markus Peck-Radosavljevic
Division of Gastroenterology and Hepatology,Department of Internal Medicine III, Medical University Vienna, Vienna, Austria

Dirk Meyer-Olson, Matthias Stoll and Reinhold E. Schmidt
Department of Clinical Immunology and Rheumatology, Hannover Medical School, Hannover, Germany.

Stefan Mauss and Stefan Mauss
Center for HIV and Hepatogastro-enterology, Düsseldorf, Germany

Martin Vogel and Jürgen Rockstroh
Department of Internal Medicine I, University of Bonn, Bonn, Germany

Patrick Ingiliz
Medical Center for Infectious Diseases (MIB), Berlin, Germany

Jerzy Jaroszewicz and Robert Flisiak
Department of Infectious Diseases and Hepatology, Medical University of Bialystok, Bialystok, Poland

Jerzy Jaroszewicz, Dirk Meyer-Olson, Martin Vogel, Matthias Stoll, Michael P. Manns, Reinhold E. Schmidt, Heiner WedemeyerJürgen Rockstroh and Markus Cornberg
Department of Gastroenterology, Hepatology and Endocrinology, Hannover Medical School, Hannover, Germany

Thomas Reiberger, Berit Anna Payer and Markus Pcck-Radosavljevic
Division of Gastroenterology and Hepatology,Department of Internal Medicine III, Medical University Vienna, Vienna, Austria

Dirk Meyer-Olson, Matthias Stoll and Reinhold E. Schmidt
Department of Clinical Immunology and Rheumatology, Hannover Medical School, Hannover, Germany

Martin Vogel and Jürgen Rockstroh
Department of Internal Medicine I, University of Bonn, Bonn, Germany

Patrick Ingiliz
Medical Center for Infectious Diseases (MIB), Berlin, Germany

Jerzy Jaroszewicz
Department of Infectious Diseases and Hepatology, Medical University of Bialystok, Bialystok, Poland

Jerzy Jaroszewicz, Dirk Meyer-Olson, Martin Vogel, Matthias Stoll, Michael P. Manns, Reinhold E. Schmidt, Heiner Wedemeyer, Jürgen Rockstroh and Markus Cornberg
German Center for Infectious Disease Research (DZIF)

Renata Leke, Diogo L. de Oliveira, Ben Hur M. Mussulini, Mery S. Pereira, Vanessa Kazlauckas, Guilherme Mazzini and Luis V. Portela
Department of Biochemistry, ICBS, Federal University of Rio Grande do Sul, Porto Alegre, Rio Grande do Sol, Brazil

Carolina R. Hartmann
Department of Pathology, Hospital de Clínicas de Porto Alegre, Porto Alegre, Rio Grande do Sol, Brazil

Themis R. Silveira
Experimental Hepatology and Gastroenterology Laboratory, Research Center of Hospital de Clínicas de Porto Alegre, Post-Graduation in Child and Adolescents Health, Federal University of Rio Grande do Sul, Porto Alegre, Rio Grande do Sol, Brazil

Mette Simonsen and Susanne Keiding
Positron Emission Tomography Centre, Aarhus University Hospital, Aarhus, Denmark

Susanne Keiding
Department of Medicine V, Hepatology and Gastroenterology, Aarhus University Hospital, Aarhus, Denmark

Lasse K. Bak, Helle S. Waagepetersen and Arne Schousboe
Department of Drug Design and Pharmacology, Faculty of Health and Medical Sciences, University of Copenhagen, Copenhagen, Denmark

Abdul Malik and Abdulmajeed Albanyan
Department of Clinical Laboratory Science, College of Applied Medical Sciences, King Saud University, Riyadh, Saudi Arabia

Abdul Malik, Deepak Kumar Singhal and P. Kar
Department of Medicine, Maulana Azad Medical College, University of Delhi, New Delhi, India

Syed Akhtar Husain
Department of Biosciences, Jamia Millia Islamia, New Delhi, India

Christian M. Lange, Philippe Burgisser and Darius Moradpour
Division of Gastroenterology and Hepatology, Centre Hospitalier Universitaire Vaudois, University of Lausanne, Lausanne, Switzerland

Christian M. Lange, Klaus Badenhoop, Jörg Bojunga, Christoph Sarrazin and Stefan Zeuzem
Medizinische Klinik, Klinikum der J. W. Goethe-Universität Frankfurt a.M., Frankfurt a.M., Germany

Stephanie Bibert and Pierre-Yves Bochud
Division of Infectious Diseases, Centre Hospitalier Universitaire Vaudois, University of Lausanne, Lausanne, Switzerland

Zoltan Kutalik
Division of Medical Genetics, Centre Hospitalier Universitaire Vaudois, University of Lausanne, Lausanne, Switzerland

Andreas Cerny
Liver Unit, Ospedale Moncucco, Lugano, Switzerland

Jean-Francois Dufour
University Clinic of Visceral Surgery and Medicine, Inselspital, Bern, Switzerland

Andreas Geier and Stephan Regenass
Division of Gastroenterology and Hepatology,University Hospital Zürich, Zürich, Switzerland

Tilman J. Gerlach
Division of Gastroenterology, Kantonsspital St. Gallen, St. Gallen, Switzerland

Markus H. Heim
Division of Gastroenterology and Hepatology, University Hospital Basel, Basel, Switzerland

Raffaele Malinverni
Hôpital Neuchâtelois, Neuchâtel, Switzerland

Francesco Negro
Division of Gastroenterology and Hepatology, University Hospital Geneva, Geneva, Switzerland

Tobias Müller
Medizinische Klinik mit Schwerpunkt Hepatologie und Gastroenterologie, Charité Campus Virchow Klinikum, Berlin, Germany

Thomas Berg
Klinik für Gastroenterologie und Rheumatologie, Sektion Hepatologie, Universitätsklinikum Leipzig, Leipzig, Germany

Kathleen E. Corey, Jorge Mendez-Navarro, Dienstag and Raymond T. Chung
Gastrointestinal Unit, Massachusetts General Hospital, Boston, Massachusetts, United States of America

Hui Zheng
Massachusetts General Hospital Biostatistics Center, Massachusetts General Hospital, Boston, Massachusetts, United States of America

Aymin Delgado-Borrego
Division of Pediatric Gastroenterology, University of Miami, Miami, Florida, United States of America

Kathleen E. Corey, Jules L.Dienstag and Raymond T. Chung
Department of Medicine, Harvard Medical School, Boston, Massachusetts, United States of America

Erica Villa, Ranka Vukotic,, Stefano Gitto,Elena Turola, Aimilia Karampatou,, Veronica Bernabucci, Nicola De Maria and Elena Bertolini
Department of Gastroenterology, Azienda Ospedaliero-Universitaria and University of Modena and Reggio Emilia, Modena, Italy

Calogero Camma and Salvatore Petta
Sezione di Gastroenterologia, Di.Bi.M.I.S., University of Palermo, Palermo, Italy

Alfredo Di Leo and Maria Rendina
Department of Gastroenterology, University of Bari, Bari, Italy

Luisa Losi
Department of Pathology, Azienda Ospedaliero-Universitaria,Modena, Italy

Annamaria Cenci, Simonetta Tagliavini and Enrica Baraldi
Department of Clinical Pathology, NOCSAE, Modena, Italy

Roberta Gelmini
Department of General Surgery, Azienda Ospedaliero-Universitaria, Modena, Italy

Antonio Francavilla
Istituto di Ricovero e Cura "Saverio de Bellis", Castellana Grotte, Italy

Chen-Shiou Wu, Wei-Chien Huang, Chung-Yi Wu and Yung-Luen Yu
The Ph.D. Program for Cancer Biology and Drug Discovery, China Medical University, Taichung, Taiwan

Ruey-Hwang Chou, Wei-Chien Huang and Yung-Luen Yu
Graduate Institute of Cancer Biology and Center for Molecular Medicine, China Medical University, Taichung, Taiwan

Chia-Jui Yen
Graduate Institute of Clinical Medicine, National Cheng Kung University, Tainan, Taiwan

Chia-Jui Yen
Division of Hematology/Oncology, Department of Internal Medicine, National Cheng Kung University Hospital, Tainan, Taiwan

Chen-Shiou Wu, Shiou-Ting Li, Chien-Tai Ren and Chung-Yi Wu
Genomics Research Center, Academia Sinica, Taipei,Taiwan

Ruey-Hwang Chou and Yung-Luen Yu
Department of Biotechnology, Asia University, Taichung, Taiwan

Juanjuan Zhao and Fu-Sheng Wang
Center for Infection and Immunity, Institute of Biophysics, Chinese Academy of Science, Beijing, China

Yonggang Li
Integrative Medicine Center, Beijing 302 Hospital, Beijing, China

Lei Jin, Shuye Zhang, Rong Fan, Yanling Sun, Chunbao Zhou, Wengang Li, Zheng Zhang and Fu-Sheng Wang
Research Center for Biological Therapy, Institute of Translational Hepatology, Beijing 302 Hospital, Beijing, China, 4 Department of Liver Disease, Tai-An 88 Hospital, Tai-An, Shan Dong Province, China

YuFeng Lou, ManYi Wang and WeiLin Mao
Department of Clinical Laboratory, First Affiliated Hospital, Zhejiang University School of Medicine, Hangzhou, Zhejiang Province, People's Republic of China

Baligh R. Yehia, Craig A. Umscheid and Vincent Lo Re III
Department of Medicine, University of Pennsylvania Perelman School of Medicine, Philadelphia, Pennsylvania, United States of America

Baligh R. Yehia and Craig A. Umscheid
Leonard Davis Institute of Health Economics, University of Pennsylvania, Philadelphia, Pennsylvania, United States of America

Baligh R. Yehia, Craig A. Umscheid and Vincent Lo Re III
Center for Clinical Epidemiology and Biostatistics, Department of Biostatistics and Epidemiology, University of Pennsylvania Perelman School of Medicine, Philadelphia, Pennsylvania, United States of America

Asher J. Schranz
Department of Medicine,New York University School of Medicine, New York, New York, United States of America

Craig A. Umscheid
Center for Evidenced-Based Practice, University of Pennsylvania Health System,Philadelphia, Pennsylvania, United States of America

Calvin Pan
Division of Liver Diseases, Department of Medicine, The Mount Sinai Medical Center, Mount Sinai School of Medicine, New York, New York, United States of America

Yurong Gu, Yubao Zheng, Liang Peng, Hong Deng, Youming Chen,Lubiao Chen, Sui Chen, Min Zhang and Zhiliang Gao
Department of Infectious Disease, The Third Affiliated, Hospital of Sun-Yet-Sen University, Guangzhou, China

Wei Zhang
Department of Infectious Disease, Beijing YouanHospital, Capital Medical University, Beijing, China

Marianne Eisenhardt, Andreas Glässner, Benjamin Krämer, Christian Körner, Bernhard Sibbing,Pavlos Kokordelis, Hans Dieter Nischalke, Tilman Sauerbruch, Ulrich Spengler and Jacob Nattermann
Department of Internal Medicine I, University of Bonn, Bonn, Germany

Seung Up Kim, Ja Kyung Kim and Kwang-Hyub Han
Department of Internal Medicine, Yonsei University College of Medicine, Seoul, Korea

Seung Up Kim, Ja Kyung Kim and Kwang-Hyub Han
Institute of Gastroenterology, Yonsei University College of Medicine, Seoul,Korea

Young Nyun Park
Department of Pathology, Yonsei University College of Medicine, Seoul, Korea

Young Nyun Park
Center for Chronic Metabolic Disease, Yonsei University College of Medicine,Seoul, Korea

Seung Up Kim, Ja Kyung Kim, Young Nyun Park and Kwang-Hyub Han
Liver Cirrhosis Clinical Research Center, Seoul, Korea

Young Nyun Park and Kwang-Hyub Han
Brain Korea 21 Project for Medical Science, Seoul, Korea

Wai-Kay Seto, Danny Ka-Ho Wong, James Fung, John Chi-Hang Yuen, Ivan Fan-Ngai Hung, Ching-Lung Lai and Man-Fung Yuen
Department of Medicine, The University of Hong Kong, Queen Mary Hospital, Hong Kong, Hong Kong

Philip P. C. Ip
Department of Pathology, The University of Hong Kong, Queen Mary Hospital, Hong Kong, Hong Kong

Ching-Lung Lai and Man-Fung Yuen
State Key Laboratory for Liver Research, University of Hong Kong, Queen Mary Hospital, Hong Kong, Hong Kong

Tatsuyuki Tonan, Kiminori Fujimoto and Naofumi Hayabuchi
Department of Radiology, Kurume University School of Medicine, Kurume University Hospital, Kurume, Fukuoka, Japan

Kiminori Fujimoto
Center for Diagnostic Imaging, Kurume University Hospital, Kurume, Fukuoka, Japan

Aliya Qayyum
Department of Radiology and Biomedical Imaging, University of California San Francisco, San Francisco, California, United States of America

Takumi Kawaguchi
Department of Digestive Disease Information and Research and Department of Internal Medicine, Kurume University School of Medicine, Kurume,Fukuoka, Japan

Atsushi Kawaguchi
Biostatics Center, Kurume University School of Medicine, Kurume, Fukuoka, Japan

Osamu Nakashima
Department of Clinical Laboratory Medicine, Kurume University Hospital, Kurume, Fukuoka, Japan

Koji Okuda
Department of Surgery, Department of Medicine, Kurume University School of Medicine, Kurume, Fukuoka, Japan

Michio Sata
Division of Gastroenterology, Department of Medicine, Kurume University School of Medicine, Kurume, Fukuoka, Japan

Satoshi Sekiguchi, Tomoko Chiyo, Takahiro Ohtsuki, Yoshimi Tobita, Yuko Tokunaga, Fumihiko Yasu and Michinori Kohara
Department of Microbiology and Cell Biology, Tokyo Metropolitan Institute of Medical Science, Setagaya-ku, Tokyo, Japan

Kiminori Kimura
Division of Hepatology, Tokyo Metropolitan Komagome Hospital, Bunkyo-ku, Tokyo, Japan

Kyoko Tsukiyama-Kohara
Transboundary Animal Diseases Center, Joint Faculty of Veterinary Medicine, Kagoshima University, Korimoto,Kagoshima, Japan

Takaji Wakita
Department of Virology II, National Institute of Infectious Diseases, Shinjuku-ku, Tokyo, Japan

Toshiyuki Tanaka
Laboratory of Immunobiology, Department of Pharmacy, School of Pharmacy, Hyogo University of Health Sciences, Chuo-ku, Kobe, Japan

Masayuki Miyasaka
Laboratory of Immunodynamics, Department of Microbiology and Immunology, Osaka University Graduate School of Medicine, Suita, Osaka, Japan

Kyosuke Mizuno
Chemo-Sero-Therapeutic Research Institute, Okubo, Kumamoto, Japan

Yukiko Hayashi and Tsunekazu Hishima
Department of Pathology, Tokyo Metropolitan Komagome Hospital, Bunkyo-ku, Tokyo, Japan

Kouji Matsushima
Department of Molecular Preventive Medicine, School of Medicine, University of Tokyo, Bunkyo-ku, Tokyo, Japan

YingLi He and YingRen Zhao
Department of Infectious Diseases, the First Affiliated Teaching Hospital, School of Medicine, Xi'an JiaoTong University, Xi'an, Shaanxi Province, China

Heng Gao
Xi'an Municipal Health College, Xi'an, Shaanxi Province, China

XiaoMei Li
Department of Psychology and Nursing, School of Medicine, Xi'an JiaoTong University, Xi'an, Shaanxi Province, China

YingRen Zhao
Institution of Hepatology, the First Affiliated Hospital of Xi'an JiaoTong University, Xi'an, Shaanxi Province, China

Yu-Ju Lin
Institute of Microbiology and Immunology, School of Life Sciences, National Yang-Ming University, Taipei, Taiwan

Yu-Ju Lin, Mei-Hsuan Lee, Hwai-I Yang, Chin-Lan Jen, San-Lin You, Yu-Ju Lin, Mei-Hsuan Lee, Hwai-I Yang, Chin-Lan Jen and San-Lin You
Genomics Research Center, Academia Sinica, Taipei,Taiwan

Mei-Hsuan Lee
Institute of Clinical Medicine, National Yang-Ming University, Taipei, Taiwan

Hwai-I Yang
Graduate Institute of Clinical Medical Science, College of Medicine, China Medical University, Taichung, Taiwan

Hwai-I Yang
Molecular and Genomic Epidemiology Center, China Medical University Hospital, Taichung, Taiwan

Li-Yu Wang
chool of Medicine, MacKay Medical College, Taipei, Taiwan

Sheng-Nan Lu
Department of Internal Medicine, Kaohsiung Chang-Gung Memorial Hospital, Kaohsiung, Taiwan

Chien-Jen Chen
Graduate Institute of Epidemiology and Preventive Medicine, College of Public Health, National Taiwan University, Taipei, Taiwan

Yuan Li, Jiu-Jun Wang, Shan Gao, Qian Liu, Jia Bai, Xue-Qi Zhao and Xi-Ping Zhao
Department of Infectious Diseases, Tongji Hospital, Tongji Medical College, Huazhong University of Science and Technology, Wuhan, P. R. China

You-Hua Hao, Hong-Hui Ding, Fan Zhu and Dong-Liang Yang
Division of Clinical Immunology, Tongji Hospital, Tongji Medical College, Huazhong University of Science and Technology, Wuhan, P. R. China

Shan-shan Su, Huan He, Ling-bo Kong, Yu-guo Zhang, Su-xian Zhao, Rong-qi Wang and Yue-min Nan
Department of Traditional and Western Medical Hepatology, Third Hospital of Hebei Medical University, Shijiazhuang, China

Huanwei Zheng
Department of Infectious Disease, The Fifth Hospital of Shijiazhuang City, Shijiazhuang, China

Dian-xing Sun
Department of Liver Disease, Bethune International Peace Hospital, Shijiazhuang, China

Jun Yu
Institute of Digestive Disease and Department of Medicine and Therapeutics, State Key Laboratory of Digestive Disease, Li Ka Shing Institute of Health Sciences, The Chinese University of Hong Kong, Hong Kong, China

Hongshan Wei, Renwen Zhang, Xiaohua Hao, Yubo Huang, Yong Qiao, Jun Hou,Xin Li and Xingwang Li
Beijing Ditan Hospital, Capital Medical University, Chaoyang District, Beijing, China

Boan Li
Center of Lab test, 302 Military Hospital, Beijing, China

Benjamin Heidrich, Steffen B. Wiegand, Heiner W. Busch, Benjamin Maasoumy, Undine Baum, Svenja Hardtke, Michael P. Manns,Heiner Wedemeyer and Markus Cornberg
Department of Gastroenterology, Hepatology and Endocrinology, Hannover Medical School, Hannover, Germany

Benjamin Heidrich, Steffen B. Wiegand, Benjamin Maasoumy, Undine Baum, Svenja Hardtke, Michael P. Manns,Heiner Wedemeye and Markus Cornberg
German Liver Foundation, HepNet Study-House,Hannover, Germany, and German Center for Infection Research (DZIF), Partner Site Hannover-Braunschweig, Braunschweig, Germany

Peter Buggisch and Jörg Petersen
IFI Institute for Interdisciplinary Medicine, Asklepios Klinik St Georg, Hamburg, Germany

Holger Hinrichsen
Gastroenterology, Gastroenterologische Schwerpunkt Praxis, Kiel, Germany

Ralph Link
St. Josefs hospital, Offenburg, Germany

Bernd Möller
Medical Practice, Berlin, Germany

Klaus H.W. Böker
Leberpraxis, Hannover, Germany

Gerlinde Teuber
Gastroenterological Practice, Frankfurt, Germany

Hartwig Klinker
Dept. of Internal Medicine II, University of Würzburg, Würzburg, Germany

Elmar Zehnter
Gastroenterological Practice, Dortmund, Germany

Uwe Naumann
Center for Addiction-Medicine, Hepatology and HIV, Praxiszentrum Kaiserdamm, Berlin, Germany

Heiner W. Busch
Medical Practice, Münster, Germany

Raffaella Romeo and Massimo Colombo
AM and A Migliavacca Center for Liver Disease, 1st Division of Gastroenterology, IRCCS Fondazione CàGranda Ospedale Maggiore Policlinico, University of Milan, Milan, Italy

Barbara Foglieni,Marta Spreafico and Daniele Prati
Department of Transfusion Medicine and Hematology, Ospedale A. Manzoni, Lecco, Italy

Giovanni Casazza
Dipartimento di Scienze Biomediche e Cliniche "L. Sacco", University of Milan, Milan, Italy

Lu Zhang
Department of Gynecologic Oncology, Shandong Cancer Hospital and Institute, School of Medicine and life Science, University of Jinan-Shandong Academy of Medical Science, Jinan, Shandong, P.R. China

Jianjun Han
Department of Cancer Interventional Radiology, Shandong Cancer Hospital and Institute, Jinan, Shandong, P.R. China

Huiyong Wu
Department of Cancer Interventional Radiology, Shandong Cancer Hospital and Institute, Jinan, Shandong, P.R. China

Xiaohong Liang
Department of Immunology, Shandong University School of Medicine, Jinan, Shandong, China

Jianxin Zhang
Department of Cancer Interventional Radiology, Shandong Cancer Hospital and Institute, Jinan, Shandong, P.R. China

Jian Li
Department of Cancer Interventional Radiology, Shandong Cancer Hospital and Institute, Jinan, Shandong, P.R. China

Li Xie
Provincial Key Laboratory of Radiation Oncology, Shandong Cancer Hospital and Institute, Jinan, Shandong, P.R. China

Yinfa Xie
Department of Cancer Interventional Radiology, Shandong Cancer Hospital and Institute, Jinan, Shandong, P.R. China

Xiugui Sheng
Department of Gynecologic Oncology, Shandong Cancer Hospital and Institute, Jinan, Shandong, P.R. China

Jinming Yu
Department of Radiation Oncology, Shandong Cancer Hospital and Institute, Jinan, Shandong, P.R. China

Kohei Nagumo, Hiroshi Watanabe, Daisuke Kadowaki, Yu Ishima and Toru Maruyama
Department of Biopharmaceutics, Graduate School of Pharmaceutical Sciences, Kumamoto University, Chuo-ku, Kumamoto, Japan

Motohiko Tanaka,Hiroko Setoyama and Yutaka Sasaki
Department of Gastroenterology and Hepatology, Graduate School of Medical Sciences, Kumamoto University, Chuo-ku, Kumamoto, Japan

Victor Tuan Giam Chuang
School of Pharmacy, Curtin Health Innovation Research Institute, Faculty of Health Sciences, Curtin University, Perth, Western Australia, Australia

Hiroshi Watanabe, Daisuke Kadowaki, Yu Ishima and Toru Maruyama
Center for Clinical Pharmaceutical Science, Kumamoto University, Chuo-ku, Kumamoto, Japan

Naoyuki Yamada And Kazuyuki Kubota
Institute of Innovation, Ajinomoto Co., Inc., Kawasaki-ku, Kawasaki, Japan

Motoko Tanaka and Kazutaka Matsushita
Department of Nephrology, Akebono Clinic, Minami-Ku, Kumamoto,Japan

Akira Yoshida and Hideaki Jinnouchi
Jinnouchi Clinic, Diabetes Care Center, Chuo-ku, Kumamoto, Japan

Makoto Anraku and Masaki Otagiri
Faculty of Pharmaceutical Sciences, Sojo University, Nishi-ku, Kumamoto, Japan

Masaki Otagiri
DDS Research Institute, Sojo University, Nishi-ku, Kumamoto, Japan

Ayesha Ahmed, Dalal M. Al Tamimi and Mohamed A. Shawarby
Department of Pathology, College of Medicine, University of Dammam and King Fahd Hospital of the University, Al-Khobar, Saudi Arabia

Anvarhusein A. Isab
Department of Chemistry, King Fahd University of Petroleum and Minerals, Dhahran, Saudi Arabia

Abdulaziz M. Mansour Alkhawajah
Department of Pharmacology, College of Medicine, University of Dammam, Dammam, Saudi Arabia

Maurizia Rossana Brunetto, Daniela Cavallone, Filippo Oliveri, Francesco Moriconi, Piero Colombatto, Barbara Coco, Pietro Ciccorossi, Carlotta Rastelli, Veronica Romagnoli and Beatrice Cherubini
Laboratory of Molecular Genetics and Pathology of Hepatitis Viruses, Hepatology Unit, Reference Center of the Tuscany Region for Chronic Liver Disease and Cancer, University Hospital of Pisa, Pisa, Italy

Maria Wrang Teilum and Thorarinn Blondal
Division of Dx and Services, Exiqon A/S, Copenhagen, Denmark

Ferruccio Bonino
igestive and Liver Disease, General Medicine II Unit, University Hospital of Pisa, Pisa, Italy

Nawarat Posuwan, Shintaro Ogawa, Shuko Murakami, Sayuki Iijima, Kentaro Matsuura, Noboru Shinkai, Tsunamasa Watanabe and Yasuhito Tanaka
Department of Virology and Liver Unit, Nagoya City University Graduate School of Medical Sciences, Nagoya, Japan

Sunchai Payungporn and Pisit Tangkijvanich
Research Unit of Hepatitis and Liver Cancer,Faculty of Medicine, Chulalongkorn University, Bangkok, Thailand

Nawarat Posuwan, Sunchai Payungporn and Pisit Tangkijvanich
Department of Biochemistry, Faculty of Medicine, Chulalongkorn University, Bangkok, Thailand

Nawarat Posuwan and Yong Poovorawan
Center of Excellence in Clinical Virology, Faculty of Medicine, Chulalongkorn University, Bangkok, Thailand

Feng Xie., Long Yan, Jiongjiong Lu, Tao Zheng, Changying Shi, Jun Ying, Rongxi Shen and Jiamei Yang
Department of Special Treatment and Liver Transplantation, Eastern Hepatobiliary Surgery Hospital, The Second Military Medical University, Shanghai, China

Anika Wranke, Benjamin Heidrich, Beatriz Calle Serrano,Birgit Bremer, Jan Grabowski, Janina Kirschner, Kerstin Port, Markus Cornberg, Michael P. Manns and Heiner Wedemeyer
Department of Gastroenterology, Hepatology and Endocrinology, Hannover Medical School, Hannover, Germany

Stefanie Ernst
Institute for Biometry, Hannover Medical School,Hannover, Germany

Cihan Yurdaydin
Ankara University Medical Faculty, Ankara, Turkey

Florin Alexandru Caruntu
Institutul de Boli Infectioase, Bucharest, Romania

Manuela Gabriela Curescu
Spitalul Clinic de Boli Infectioase, Timisoara,Romania

Kendal Yalcin
Dicle University Medical Faculty, Diyarbakir, Turkey

Selim Gürel
Uludag˘ University Medical Faculty, Bursa, Turkey

Stefan Zeuzem
Johann Wolfgang Goethe University Medical Center,Frankfurt/Main, Germany

Andreas Erhardt
Heinrich Heine University, Düsseldorf, Germany

Stefan Lüth
University Medical Centre Hamburg-Eppendorf, Hamburg, Germany

George V. Papatheodoridis
Athens University School of Medicine, Athens, Greece

Judith Stift
Medical University of Vienna, Vienna, Austria

Christine S. Falk
Institute of Transplant Immunology, IFB-Tx, Hannover Medical School, Hannover,Germany

Peter Dienes, Svenja Hardtke, Michael P. Manns, Heiner Wedemeyer and HIDIT-2 Study Group
HepNet Study-House, Hannover, Germany

Benjamin Heidrich, Michael P. Manns and Heiner Wedemeyer
Integrated Research and Treatment Center Transplantation, Hannover Medical School, Hannover, Germany

Heiner Wedemeyer
German Center for Infection Research (DZIF), Partner Side HepNet Study-House, Hannover, Germany

Sayeh Ezzikouri, Khadija Rebbani, Ikram Brahim,Fatima-Zohra Fakhir and Soumaya Benjelloun
Virology Unit, Viral Hepatitis Laboratory, Pasteur Institute of Morocco, Casablanca, Morocco

Rhimou Alaoui and Salwa Nadir
Service de Me´decine B, CHU Ibn Rochd, Casablanca, Morocco

Helmut Diepolder
Ludwig-Maximilians-Universität München, Marchioninistrasse, München, Germany

Salim I. Khakoo
University of Southampton, Tremona Road, Southampton, United Kingdom

Mark Thursz
Department of Hepatology, Division of Medicine, Imperial College, London, United Kingdom

Index

A

Adefovir, 1, 8, 15, 30, 249-250, 256, 268

Advanced Fibrosis, 40, 97, 105, 110-111, 118

Alanine Aminotransferase, 33-37, 51-52, 58, 65, 73, 78-79, 91, 105, 107, 112-113, 115, 118-119, 126, 129, 140-141, 147-148, 156, 166, 176, 271-272

Anti-disialosyl Galactosyl Globoside, 57

Anti-fibrotic Potential, 96-97, 99

Anti-fucosyl, 57, 60

Antigen Level, 119

Antiretroviral Therapy, 9-10, 15-16, 82

Antiviral Therapy, 1, 8-9, 13, 30, 33, 35, 38, 41, 55, 73, 82-83, 90-91, 103, 137, 152, 156, 165, 171, 180, 184, 232, 237, 241, 249-251, 258, 266, 268, 275

Asterixis, 17, 22

Ataxia, 17, 22

B

Bacterial Translocation, 93

Bile Duct, 17-18, 20, 23

Bradykinesia, 17, 22-23

C

Calcitriol Precursor, 32-33, 37

Carbohydrate Antigen, 58

Cell Size, 76

Chemokines, 67, 71-72, 90, 96, 99-100, 104, 257-259, 261, 263, 268

Chronic Hepatitis, 1, 4-5, 8-10, 16, 25-33, 35-41, 47-48, 65, 69, 78, 84-85, 99, 101, 109, 119, 122, 132, 152, 155-160, 196-201, 207, 219, 238, 250, 274-275

Chronic Liver Disease, 17, 22-23, 31, 40, 42-45, 47, 54, 57-58, 81, 89-90, 93, 122, 156, 166, 175, 197-198, 207, 209-216, 229, 249

Chronic Liver Failure, 17, 22-23, 30, 78, 81, 89, 94-95, 145, 164, 216, 249-250, 256

Cytolytic Activity, 65-66, 68, 71, 73, 100, 159

Cytotoxicity, 65, 75, 104, 134, 136, 138, 140, 157-160, 163-164, 219

E

Echo-planar Imaging, 121, 127

Embryonic Development, 57, 128

Encephalopathy, 17-18, 23-24, 26, 41, 46, 77, 80, 89-90, 106, 195, 249, 258

Entecavir, 1-5, 8, 15-16, 90, 94, 164, 249, 252, 256

F

Fibrotic Tissue, 40, 178

Fulminant Hepatitis, 25, 27-30, 81, 256

G

Gene Encoding, 32

Gene Mutation, 25, 28-29

Genetic Validation, 32, 37-38

Glycan Microarray, 57-60, 63

Glycosylation, 57, 60-61, 64

H

Hepatic Dysfunction, 40

Hepatic Encephalopathy, 17, 23-24, 26, 41, 46, 80, 195, 249

Hepatic Fibrosis, 40-41, 45, 48, 55, 85-86, 100, 104, 112, 156, 175, 182

Hepatic Inflammation, 40, 90, 104, 141

Hepatic Iron Concentration, 121-127

Hepatic Necrosis, 89-90

Hepatic Stellate Cell, 55, 94, 176

Hepatocellular Carcinoma, 1, 16, 25-26, 30-31, 57, 64, 81, 86, 111-113, 120, 131, 138, 140, 147, 149, 151-154, 182, 184, 194, 203, 242, 257, 270, 272, 275

Hepatocellular Damage, 65

Homeostasis, 40, 46, 49, 141, 215-216

Hydroxylase, 32-33, 35, 37, 39

Hydroxyvitamin, 32, 36-37, 46

Hyperammonemia, 18, 23

Hypokinesia, 17, 22

I

Immune System Dysfunction, 18

Immune Tolerance, 114, 117-118, 128, 136, 152, 155, 157, 229

Immunization, 30, 128-129, 132-134, 136-139

Immunodeficiency, 9-10, 13, 16, 49, 73, 75-76, 106, 163-164, 173, 244, 247, 250

Immunomodulatory Drugs, 1-2

Interferon-alfa-based Therapy, 32

L

Lipopolysaccharide, 89, 94

Liver Biopsy, 33, 35-36, 46, 48-50, 73, 83-88, 90, 103, 105-107, 109-114, 119, 121-122, 144, 148, 154, 175-177, 179, 181, 195, 200

Liver Cancer, 57, 64, 87, 106, 156, 194, 203, 207-208, 243

Liver Cirrhosis, 10, 16-17, 21, 23, 26, 28-29, 38, 47, 57, 77, 79, 101, 105-106, 128, 148, 152, 154, 157, 175-178, 184, 188, 209, 211, 243, 257, 272, 274-275

Liver Damage, 17, 30, 65, 68, 75, 90, 96, 104, 152, 158, 160-161, 163-164, 194, 241

Liver Injury, 17, 40, 54, 65-66, 68-69, 72-73, 75, 90, 92-95, 99, 104, 117, 129, 132, 136, 138, 140, 143-144, 146, 148, 164, 217

Locomotor, 17-23

M

Matrix Protein, 205

Monocyte, 248

Multifunctional Cytokine, 40

N

Natural Killer Cells, 65, 75, 99, 104, 157, 164

Necroinflammation, 66, 105-106, 110-111, 113-115, 117-118, 120, 122-125, 152

Nonstructural Protein, 128, 134, 138

Nucleotide Analogue, 250

O

Oncogenesis, 57

P

Pathogenesis, 24, 31, 33, 55, 65-66, 74, 79, 128, 131, 134, 136, 140-141, 144, 152, 157-158, 163-164, 194, 205, 207, 216, 268

Pegylated Interferon, 1, 5, 32, 34, 38, 41-42, 83, 85-86, 119, 165, 183-184, 192-193, 258, 268, 275

Polymerase Inhibitor, 184, 267

Polymorphism, 32-33, 35, 37-39, 146, 191, 268, 270, 272, 274-275

Portal Hypertension, 17-18, 21, 81, 88, 112, 200

Potential Biomarker, 201, 203, 205, 207, 242

Psychological Stress, 140-141, 143, 146

Pulmonary Hypertension, 76, 80

R

Recombinant Vaccinia Virus, 128-129, 136-139

Red Blood Cell, 76, 79-81

Regulatory Phenotype, 165

Ribavirin, 32-38, 41, 46-47, 83, 85-86, 104, 146, 165, 167, 171, 173-174, 183-184, 186, 189, 193, 270, 275

S

Seromarker, 148, 152

Serum A-fetoprotein, 57, 202

Serum Vitamin, 40, 46

Surface Antigen, 9, 16, 26, 28, 30, 78, 113-115, 118-120, 141, 145, 148, 194, 200, 242, 244-245, 257, 268

T

Telbivudine, 1, 16, 249-250, 252, 256

Tenofovir, 1-5, 8-10, 15-16, 90, 92, 94, 249-250, 252, 256, 258

Thioacetamide, 17, 22

Type-2 Cytokine, 140-141, 144-145

V

Vascular Shunting, 17

Viral Hepatitis, 16, 25-26, 28-29, 77, 80-82, 87, 89, 94, 112, 121-122, 126, 139, 156-157, 163-165, 184-185, 256, 258, 265, 270-271, 275

Viral Infection, 48, 76, 182, 243

Viral Protein, 128, 136

www.ingramcontent.com/pod-product-compliance
Lightning Source LLC
Chambersburg PA
CBHW061330190326

41458CB00011B/3948